STRATFORDIANS

Simon Trowbridge was born in Oxford in 1961, and educated at Birmingham University, King's College, London, and University College, London.

By the same author

NECESSITY
THE RETURN
1794

STRATFORDIANS

A Biographical Dictionary of the Royal Shakespeare Company

SIMON TROWBRIDGE

EDITIONS ALBERT CREED

First published in 2008
by Editions Albert Creed
Oxford

ISBN 978-0-9559830-1-6

Some of the content was previously made available, in a different
form, as part of the website *Stratfordians: a Dictionary of the RSC* by
Simon Trowbridge (www.stratfordians.org.uk, 2003-08).
The text has been partly re-written for this book edition.

In memory of my mother
Rita Trowbridge

Contents

Preface

This book surveys the work of the Royal Shakespeare Company from the beginning of Peter Hall's directorship in 1960 to 2008. It includes short essays on many of the most significant members, past and present, of the RSC—actors, directors, designers and others. In choosing to write a dictionary my aim has been to explore the nature and achievement of the RSC through the telling of these individual stories.

Actors and directors who have worked at the RSC over a long period occupy most of these pages; others are included because of their importance or fame. Inevitably, the selection is coloured by my own interests and prejudices. I regret the omissions, and admit that a Stratford dictionary that doesn't include such regular players as Dennis Clinton, Ron Cook, Kevin Doyle, Jimmy Gardner, Peter Geddis, Paul Greenwood, David Killick, Bernard Lloyd, Nicholas Selby, Derek Smith and Graham Turner cannot be considered complete. I hope to be able to increase the coverage in future editions.

I started to write in 1996 at a time when Adrian Noble's first major reforms (particularly the decision to leave the Barbican for six months of the year) were provoking debate and controversy, and I worked to complete the first draft of the manuscript in 2001/02, easily the most turbulent year in the RSC's history. Although the material was written to form the basis of a book, an early version was made available on the Internet (2003-08).

A prelude provides a brief history of the Stratford theatre before 1960. Part One looks at the twenty directors and one actress who have led and guided the RSC: it can be read as a history of the Company. Part Two examines the work of other members of the Company. Finally, a coda explores the nature of today's RSC.

When I first went to Stratford in 1976, the RSC was a repertory company with a core of permanent members. These directors and actors were recognised as being among the leading figures of our theatre, and their identity as members of the RSC was not in doubt. Of England's two national theatres, the one based in Stratford seem pre-eminent most of the time (more radical, more prestigious). The RSC of today is much less influential, and the choice of a courtyard design for the new main house is an indication of a further loss of ambition (the RSC is avoiding the difficult art of visual theatre by deciding to work in a space that favours audience-friendly acting). One positive is that a future director of the RSC will always have the option of reconstituting the RSC as a genuine company.

Toulouse
September 2008

Prelude: the Stratford Theatre, 1879-1959

The creation of the Royal Shakespeare Company in 1960/61 was both a new departure and the continuation of a theatre that had been in operation since 1879. The first Shakespeare Memorial Theatre was destroyed by fire in 1926, although the foyer areas and the shell of the building survived to become, miraculously, the Swan Theatre in 1986. The second Shakespeare Memorial Theatre, dating from 1932, was renamed the Royal Shakespeare Theatre (RST) in 1961. It was closed for re-development in 2007.

The Stratford-upon-Avon theatre was founded by Charles Edward Flower, head of the town's brewery, who in 1875 convened a body called the Council for the Shakespeare Memorial Association to achieve the construction of a theatre, library and art gallery. Registered under the Companies Act, the Council started the process of raising funds from public subscriptions. Charles Flower donated a considerable stretch of land beside the Avon from Clopton Bridge to Holy Trinity Church, the cottages across the road, and most of the funding. Dodgshun and Unsworth's design of a semi-circular redbrick building with medieval and Tudor features—including turrets and a tower—was constructed between 1877 and 1879; the area around it was landscaped into gardens. The horseshoe-shaped interior had a circle and a gallery, and a conventional proscenium stage. The members of the Council for the Shakespeare Memorial Association became the theatre's governors, while the actual work—an annual ten-day festival—was entrusted to visiting companies until 1886, when Frank Benson began thirty-three years as the SMT's director. Charles Flower died in 1892 and was succeeded as chairman by his brother Edgar, who kept the theatre going but who had no enthusiasm for it; he was succeeded in 1903 by his son Archibald, who shared Charles's passion.

The theatre was picturesque and intimate, but its stage and backstage areas were tiny. In 1925 Bernard Shaw, speaking at the birthday luncheon, called for a new building. A year later he responded to the news of its destruction by sending Archibald Flower a congratulatory telegram.

Archibald Flower converted the Stratford Picture House (yet another Flower-owned property) into a temporary theatre, and launched an appeal to raise the £250,000 needed to build a new SMT. He had wanted a new theatre before the fire; the safe option of restoring the original was never considered. The appeal was supported by the party leaders (Stanley Baldwin, Ramsay MacDonald and H.H. Asquith), and by artists of the calibre of Shaw and Thomas Hardy, but there was no possibility of raising such a large sum in the Britain of the 1920s. Flower turned successfully to the financial great of America: John D. Rockefeller alone gave £100,000.

Over seventy architects from Britain and America entered the design competition: the winner, chosen by the Royal Institute, was a modernist design, relatively simple and functional, by the inexperienced Elizabeth Scott, a junior member of a minor London firm. The great niece of Sir George Gilbert Scott, she was the first woman to design a major building in England. Archibald Flower and director William Bridges-Adams sought a world class theatre with the most up-to-date stage machinery and lighting, fine sightlines and a sense of intimacy. They accompanied Elizabeth Scott on a tour of French and German theatres, and took advice from Barry Jackson and Theodore Komisarjevsky, among others. However, costing considerations led to compromises.

The opening on 23 April 1932 (speeches followed by a performance of both parts of *Henry IV*) was a high profile affair that had more to do with civic and national pride than with the contemporary stage (Stratford now had a modern theatre but, with a few exceptions, would fail to attract the finest talent until after the war). The Prince of Wales, having announced that 'Shakespeare was above all an Englishman', made his escape during the first interval. The building was highly controversial. It was considered by many to be an ugly and forbidding structure totally out of keeping with the beautiful riverside setting (it was quickly nicknamed the 'jam factory'). Despite the care taken by Flower and Bridges-Adams, fundamental mistakes were made: the proscenium was too small for the size of the stage, the distance between the proscenium and the front of the stalls was too wide (the forestage could not be used in conjunction with the rolling stages), the circle was too far back, sightlines were inadequate from some sections of the auditorium, and the backstage was rudimentary (too few dressing-rooms; no green room).

Barry Jackson, the first director of the SMT after the war, transformed its fortunes overnight by engaging the emerging young talent (most notably Peter Brook). Anthony Quayle and Glen Byam Shaw, Jackson's successors, continued this policy (discovering Richard Burton, Claire Bloom, Albert Finney and Ian Holm) while persuading the British theatre's greatest stars (John Gielgud, Michael Redgrave, Peggy Ashcroft, Laurence Olivier) to lead the company. This could not have happened without modifications to the theatre (the proscenium was enlarged, the forestage extended) and the building of a green room and new dressing rooms on the river side (1951). Stratford ended the 1950s as a glamorous festival theatre with an international reputation.

Part One: Direction

Peter Hall (b. Bury St Edmunds, Suffolk, 1930) was twenty-nine when he succeeded Glen Byam Shaw as director of the Shakespeare Memorial Theatre. His reputation was already formidable: he was the first all-rounder of the post-war generation, directing Peggy Ashcroft, Laurence Olivier and Charles Laughton at Stratford, Leslie Caron in the West End, running the experimental Arts Theatre Club, and staging the first British production of Samuel Beckett's *Waiting for Godot*. He took charge of the Memorial Theatre with the intention of creating a national company; remarkably, he achieved this bold, unlikely, and controversial *coup de théâtre* within a year. Hall revolutionised Stratford and along with it the whole of English theatre.

Hall's father was a stationmaster who moved along the railway line from Bury St Edmunds to Cambridge and finally to the village of Shelford. Hall attended the Perse, Cambridge's most prestigious school, where he edited the magazine, played Hamlet and rose to become head boy despite his lowly status as a county scholarship pupil. Peter Brook's Stratford production of *Love's Labour's Lost* provoked his interest in directing. At Cambridge, influenced by the English don George Rylands and by John Barton, his older contemporary, he started to formulate the ideas on textual analysis and verse-speaking that would later influence the performance of Shakespeare. Barton and Peter Wood were the star directors. If Hall was in their shadow at Cambridge, he quickly overtook them out in the professional world.

His final student production, Pirandello's *Henry IV*, was reviewed in the London papers (1953). Alec Clunes, director of the Arts Theatre Club, brought it to London for a two-week season.

Within a month Hall found himself directing his first professional production, Somerset Maugham's *The Letter* at the Theatre Royal, Windsor. Alec Clunes had a word with his successor at the Arts Theatre, John Fernald, and Hall returned as a salaried assistant and script-reader while continuing to work as a guest director elsewhere (for six months in 1954 he ran the Oxford Playhouse).

The radical Arts was the right theatre for a young director. For years it had mounted daring work, obscure classics and plays that could not be staged by 'legitimate' theatres because of the censor. Hall made his name directing bold productions of García Lorca's *Blood Wedding* (1954), an adaptation of André Gide's *The Immoralist* (1954), Ionesco's *The Lesson* (1955) and Julien Green's *South* (1955), and succeeded Fernald as director later that year. If Hall enjoyed the patronage of influential people, he mostly made his own luck through the originality of his choices. His next production, *Waiting for Godot*, became the talking point of the theatrical year. It started Hall's rapid rise to celebrity status (consolidated by his marriage to Leslie Caron). It also brought him to the attention of Tennessee Williams (Hall staged *Camino Real* at the Phoenix in 1957) and of Stratford's Anthony Quayle and Glen Byam Shaw.

Ten years after seeing Brook's *Love's Labour's Lost* Hall began his Stratford career with the same play (1956). *Cymbeline* with Peggy Ashcroft in 1957 and *Twelfth Night* in 1958, both designed with pictorial elegance by Lila De Nobili, were greatly admired. He became Glen Byam Shaw's chosen successor. Hall had wanted the Stratford job since his schooldays. He wanted a company, and the Arts, with its limited finances and short runs, could not offer this. A close relationship developed between the young director and Fordham Flower, the SMT's remarkable chairman and head. By selecting Hall as director (the succession was settled informally by an exchange of letters), Flower gave the go-ahead to a revolution that would end the conservative, self-financing Stratford of limited seasons. It was perhaps not a difficult decision to make since his theatre was in danger of becoming a glamorous but fusty corner of heritage England. The imminent birth of a state-funded national theatre under Laurence Olivier made this most likely. The details were discussed during the Company's historic winter 1958 tour of Russia, in Leningrad's Hotel Astoria: three-year contracts to create a genuine company, not just of actors but of directors and designers, the introduction of contemporary and experimental work, and—to make it all possible—a London base funded by the state. A national theatre in all but name, pre-empting Olivier's official troupe (the strategic and tactical ingenuity of this aspect of the scheme must have appealed to an old soldier like Flower). A new name, the Royal Shakespeare Company, would underline the Stratford theatre's modernisation, and its considerable reserves of £175,000 would be spent to achieve it. By dawn Flower had agreed to gamble everything on the talent of Peter Hall and the expectation of an Arts Council grant.

The time was right for the RSC. The strength of Hall's ideas, provoking thousands of words in the newspapers, caught the imagination of the public and made the Aldwych adventure seem less of a gamble than it actually was. The passionate involvement of Peggy Ashcroft was of paramount importance. Other senior actors followed, but some were wary of the three-year contracts. Paul Scofield at first said yes, then changed his mind. Hall brought in a young actor called Peter O'Toole, who became a star during the first RSC season, but who broke his contract at its end to make *Lawrence of Arabia*. Those who remained had to cope with an arrangement that divided their lives between Stratford and London. But it was an adventure that vitalised nearly everyone involved.

Initially the RSC struggled to find a voice. Hall programmed Shakespeare's comedies and contemporary French plays that failed to gel. However, his own production of *Troilus and Cressida* and John Whiting's *The Devils*, the RSC's first commission, pointed to the future. Ian Holm, Eric Porter, Ian Richardson, Vanessa Redgrave and Judi Dench were among the talented actors brought to prominence by the Company's first wave of work.

Hall's innovative decision to share the directorship, to make the Company an ensemble of directors and designers, was crucial. In 1962 Peter Brook, the acknowledged genius of post-war theatre, and the oracle-like Michel Saint-Denis, one of the century's most influential theatre artists (teacher, theorist and director), joined Hall as co-directors. Brook formed an experimental group; Saint-Denis established a workshop studio. John Barton and Clifford Williams were associate directors; John Bury, from Joan Littlewood's Theatre Workshop, became head of design, supported by the Algerian designer Farrah, a protégé of Saint-Denis's. Harold Pinter became the Company's second house dramatist. Later, the young directors David Jones, Trevor Nunn and Terry Hands joined the team. Jones initially worked as an administrator at the Aldwych, and Hands headed the Company's touring wing, Theatregoround (1966). Hall and his colleagues challenged the traditions of the previous era, replacing painted cloths with solid sets, pictorial fantasy with realism, stilted verse-speaking with a modern conversational style that, paradoxically, observed the iambic pentameter to the letter. Most importantly, they sought contemporary relevance in Shakespeare and mounted a repertory consisting of both classical and new work.

The RSC's future was secured by the quality of its work between 1962 and 1966: Saint-Denis's *Cherry Orchard* (1962); the experimental season at the Arts (1962); Brook's *King Lear* (1962) and 'Theatre of Cruelty' seasons (1963/64); Vanessa Redgrave in *As You Like It* (1962); Clifford Williams's *Comedy of Errors* (1962); Hall's *Wars of the Roses* (1963); the history cycle of 1964; Pinter's *The Homecoming* (1965); David Warner in Hall's *Hamlet* (1965); and Brook's *Marat/Sade* (1966). Success at the box-office meant that the RSC was able to sustain its operation at the Aldwych until October 1962, when the Arts Council, under public pressure (a letter of support from the leading theatre critics was published in *The Telegraph*) but still reeling from Hall and

Flower's refusal after months of negotiations to take Stratford into the National Theatre, awarded the Company its first small subsidy. (The principle had been won, but the first grant of £47,000 was barely a fifth of the sum earmarked for the NT; resentment over Hall's *fait accompli* lingered for years within the Arts Council.) The RSC was leasing the Aldwych from the commercial sector. Consequently, Hall committed the Company's future to the City of London's Barbican Arts Centre, then being built.

Hall's risk-taking was apparent in all aspects of his management of the RSC and greatly contributed to the Company's success. It was there in his casting of young actors like Peter O'Toole and David Warner in leading roles, in his support of Peter Brook's experimental work, in his decision to devote an entire season to the history plays (epic cycles of this kind were new in Britain), and in his very public taking-on of the censor, the Arts Council and the National Theatre.

Hall and Brook's campaign against censorship was part of the RSC's radical agenda. In the 1960s the Lord Chamberlain was still enforcing the Theatre Act of 1843, which gave his office the power to ban the production of plays on grounds of 'good manners', 'decorum' and 'public peace'. The rules forbade profanity, indecency, sedition and the representation of living persons. All new works had to be submitted before their presentation; the Lord Chamberlain could refuse a licence without consultation, but in practice was more likely to ask for specific changes. Theatre clubs could operate more freely.

Playwrights were unable to use four letter words, or to explore, overtly, themes of sexuality; theatres were unable to satirise politicians or to criticise Britain's allies or to question organised religion. The RSC under Peter Hall, by taking things to the limit and beyond, was instrumental in ending a system of censorship that allowed a Court official, at that time a former governor of the Bank of England, to remove the word 'piss' from a contemporary play.

Hall initially staged work likely to offend the censor in theatre clubs—the season at the Arts in 1962 and Brook's 'Theatre of Cruelty' project at LAMDA and the Donmar in 1963-64 (the Lord Chamberlain's letter objecting to Jean Genet's *The Screens*, one of the plays performed, was mockingly read out to the audience); but this changed in 1964 when he staged a challenging programme at the Aldwych, including David Rudkin's *Afore Night Come*, Roger Vitrac's *Victor* and Peter Weiss's *Marat/Sade*. Hall told the Lord Chamberlain that every cut would be printed in the programmes. The cumulative effect of the 1964 season outraged the Establishment and Hall's enemies (including Emile Littler, an RSC governor, who complained to the *London Evening News* that the RSC was staging 'dirty plays'), and, as intended, initiated a high-profile debate on the anachronistic absurdity of theatre censorship.

Hall's workload was damaging to his personal life. His marriage to Leslie Caron ended in divorce and he suffered a breakdown while rehearsing *The Wars of the Roses*. His doctor prescribed months of rest, but Peter Brook told him to keep working—Hall believes that this saved his career (see *Making an Exhibition of Myself*, Sinclair-Stevenson, 1993).

1966 was a decisive year. The Arts Council would not increase the RSC's grant and Hall responded with uncharacteristic negativity, mounting a cost-cutting season of revivals. For the first time he worked outside of the RSC, directing *The Magic Flute* at Covent Garden. Most significantly, that summer Fordham Flower died. Within a year Hall had decided to step down as artistic director. It seems remarkable that he walked away so suddenly, after only eight years. Looking back Hall is surprised himself, confessing in this autobiography that he has felt homeless since leaving the RSC. He made a final inspired decision: the recommendation that Trevor Nunn should succeed him.

Hall did not impose a rigid house style, but his own productions were influential enough to make it appear otherwise. His early Shakespeare work was light-footed and romantic—the 1957 *Cymbeline* was conceived as a dark fairytale—but also full of youthful energy and playful sexuality, as in the acting of Dorothy Tutin and Geraldine McEwan (*Twelfth Night*, 1958). The setting for *A Midsummer Night's Dream* (1959) was a Tudor banquet hall into which the forest ingeniously intruded. Titania was a young woman (Mary Ure); Puck, perhaps for the first time, was streetwise and sardonic (Ian Holm). *Coriolanus* (1959) featured Laurence Olivier at his most dynamic, but despite Hall's ability to get the best out of star actors his love of big performances played third fiddle to language and unity of tone. In the early 1960s he started to view the plays politically, projecting them through a lens of modernity. He developed a production style based on plain but emblematic imagery that complemented the psychological realism of the acting. The 1960 *Troilus and Cressida* featured a sandpit and a rust-red cyclorama: the set made an appropriate visual statement while offering a bare arena for the actors. His productions of the *Henry VI* plays and *Richard III* (*The Wars of the Roses*) won acclaim for their narrative clarity and thematic cohesion (the central theme being the self-perpetuating brutality of power-politics). A dark, metallic environment was used to create the clamour of battle. The RSC came into its own as an ensemble in these productions. Hall's *Hamlet* (1965) was a notable cultural event of the 1960s, the theatrical equivalent of a new LP by the Beatles. Young audiences identified with David Warner's unconventional Hamlet and with the production's central theme—the plight of the non-conformist in the face of an oppressive state (John Bury's black set consisted of two anterooms for spying).

After 1968 Hall remained a co-director of the RSC, staging (at the Aldwych) new plays by Edward Albee (*A Delicate Balance*, 1969; *All Over*, 1972), Simon Gray (*Dutch Uncle*, 1969), and Harold Pinter (*Landscape* and *Silence*, 1969; *Old Times*, 1971). Nunn and others half-expected Hall to return to lead the RSC again; they were shocked by his decision to succeed Olivier as director of the National (1973). For some time Hall and Nunn tried to find a means of merging the two companies.

Hall oversaw the National's move to the South Bank, and made the building popular with audiences despite an often hostile press and a strike-happy workforce (his *Diaries*, published in 1983, give the definitive account of these years). His decision to divide the work between separate ensembles, each led by a director or actor, was particularly successful. Since leaving the National in 1988 he has found commercial backing for the Peter Hall Company, in the West End and elsewhere. In 1997 he took charge of the Old Vic and produced a season of work— including *King Lear* with Alan Howard, *Waiting for Godot* with Howard and Ben Kingsley and *The Seagull* with Victoria Hamilton and Michael Pennington—that was the envy of the RSC and the National. Regrettably, the backers withdrew, the Old Vic was put up for sale, and, true to form, the Arts Council showed no interest in subsidising Hall's work there. In 2003 he ran another fine repertory season at the Theatre Royal, Bath, directing the same trio of actors in Coward's *Design For Living* and Pinter's *Betrayal*, and his daughter, Rebecca Hall, in a wise and beautiful production of *As You Like It*.

In 1992 he returned to the RSC after an absence of twenty years to direct *All's Well That Ends Well* in the Swan. This was followed Peter Shaffer's *The Gift of the Gorgon* (Pit, 1992), *Julius Caesar* in the main house (1995), and John Barton's *Tantalus*, which he co-directed with his son Edward Hall (2000).

It is often said of Peter Hall that he is an 'empire builder'. Perhaps the label is inevitable for a man who ran and irrevocably changed both the RSC and the National. Looking back at his record the evidence reveals that at every stage he has supported his younger associates. Of all the leading European directors of the contemporary theatre, Hall is arguably the least concerned with his own status as an artist. Like a general he is a master of strategy and tactics, ruthless in the pursuit of victory—for the RSC, the NT, the playwright, and, indeed, for every single production he has directed. To save a production, Hall is prepared to replace an actor or even, in the case of *Tantalus*, to damage a life-long friendship.

The RSC was, and is, far removed from the clichés pertaining to the theatre. Actors have often compared Stratford to a university campus, describing an experience that is an exhausting but rewarding combination of performance and learning. Despite the changes of recent years, the RSC still bears the stamp of Peter Hall.

John Barton (b. London, 1928). The origins of the Stratford revolution of the 1960s can be traced back to Peter Hall's student days at Cambridge. Cambridge theatre of the late 1940s and early 1950s owed much to John Barton, then a student at King's but already an all-round theatre man who combined scholarship with stagecraft (this most analytical examiner of texts was also a fight director). Barton has remained a don-like figure, while his eccentricities have provided anecdotes for generations of actors. Despite his training as a Shakespeare scholar, Barton has always been a fearless interpreter, prepared to adapt, cut and even write new dialogue: *The Wars of the Roses* (1963) and *King John* (1974) are the most obvious examples. For Barton, the practical requirements of actors and the theatre are paramount.

The son of a senior civil servant, Barton went to Eton. At Cambridge he was an academic high-flyer as well as a one-man theatre company. He remained at King's (as fellow and Lay Dean) until 1960, when Peter Hall asked him to join the RSC as his number two. Hall wanted his friend's depth of knowledge as a textual scholar and was a little reckless in giving him the season's most difficult assignment, Peggy Ashcroft and Peter O'Toole in *The Taming of the Shrew*. Used to undergraduate actors, Barton needed time to learn that directing Ashcroft and O'Toole required a higher level of tact: O'Toole led a rebellion and Hall took over the production. For the next four years Barton's RSC work consisted of teaching, adaptations and co-direction (he was now an associate rather than Hall's deputy or a member of the directorate). His influence was felt, however, in his adaptation of the *Henry VI* plays (*The Wars of the Roses*) and his work on the history cycle of 1964. His anthology *The Hollow Crown* became an RSC favourite.

He returned to solo directing in 1965. Consistency of tone gave his productions an un-Shakespearean sense of pure logic. *Twelfth Night* (1969-72) is remembered with affection as a sublime romantic comedy imbued with Chekhovian melancholy. It is a mistake to view Barton as solely a text man: he employed considerable stagecraft—sounds of the sea, candlelight, painterly compositions—to achieve the beguiling atmosphere of his *Twelfth Night*. *Richard II* (1973-74) is the best example of Barton's method of interpreting a play, of taking an intellectual view and changing the text to make it work. Ian Richardson and Richard Pasco alternated the roles of Richard and Bolingbroke to emphasise their interchangeability as tragic figures. To this end Barton's Bolingbroke spoke the great speech on sleeplessness and the strain of kingship from *Henry IV* ('uneasy lies the head that wears the crown'). Barton also used stylised staging devices (the actors started the play in their rehearsal clothes; they frequently spoke directly to the audience) and a few symbolic objects, including a mirror, to make implicit the correlation between the king, forced to assume a role, and the actor playing him. His 'adaptation' of the problematic *King John* (1974) was more justified.

In the mid-1970s Barton returned to the comedies. *Much Ado About Nothing* (1976) was ingeniously set in India at the height of the British Raj. The social rules of military and colonial life fitted the play perfectly. Even more evocative was his melancholy version (set on bare boards beneath autumnal trees) of the early comedy *Love's Labour's Lost* (1978). In Barton's interpretation, the King of Navarre and his friends began the play as immature undergraduates; by its end each had been transformed by a much more knowing young woman. *Hamlet* (1980) used theatre as a metaphor (the platform stage was surrounded by all the props needed for the performance), but it was the least self-advertising of Barton's major productions, as rich, complex and thrilling as the text.

Also in 1980 Barton fulfilled a long-standing ambition by staging at the Aldwych a cycle of Greek plays. He adapted the work of Euripides, Sophocles, Aeschylus and Homer into a single narrative telling the story of the Trojan War. Ten plays were performed over three evenings. As co-author he added his own scenes and freely changed the meaning of the texts to achieve a continuous narrative. After *The Greeks* Barton started to write an original play based on the myth of Tantalus, and during the twenty years he worked on the project he gradually became less active as a director. To stage *Tantalus* the RSC formed a partnership with the Denver Center for the Performing Arts. Peter Hall's production opened in 2000, but without its author who objected to Hall's changes and cuts. Given Barton's history as an adaptor and editor of playwrights' texts, his indignation provokes a certain irony. The rift was a reminder that the Hall/Barton axis has always been prone to volatility, with flare-ups occurring in 1960 (Hall demotes Barton at the RSC), 1974 (Hall moves to the National and 'poaches' the RSC actress Susan Fleetwood) and 1978 (Barton's decision to stage *The Greeks* steals the thunder on Hall's planned production of *The Oresteia*).

Perhaps Barton's achievement and influence as a director of Shakespeare is closely aligned to his skill as a teacher, and therefore usefully summed up by the series of workshops he conducted with RSC actors for Channel Four in 1984 (*Playing Shakespeare*). They formed the basis of a book that is used by actors throughout the English-speaking world as a manual on the acting of Shakespeare. Barton's special ability to inspire actors through a process of enquiry and interpretation (often of a single phrase or word), as revealed in *Playing Shakespeare*, is the reason why his productions are remembered for the quality of the ensemble playing: Judi Dench, Donald Sinden, Lisa Harrow and Emrys James in *Twelfth Night*; Pasco and Richardson in *Richard II*; Dench and Sinden in *Much Ado About Nothing*; Michael Pennington, Jane Lapotaire and Richard Griffiths in *Love's Labour's Lost*.

Under Adrian Noble Barton remained influential. During a question and answer session in 2002, Dominic Cooke, director of the RSC's production of John Marston's *The Malcontent*, was asked about the difficulty of interpreting this rarely performed 17th century text: he replied that John Barton had dropped by to tell the company the meaning of the words. This anecdote, however slight and amusing, seems to sum up the contribution of a director who has, perhaps uniquely, devoted his entire career to one theatre company.

Peggy Ashcroft (1907-1991, b. Croydon). In England, Peggy Ashcroft was the first modern classical actress. In her twenties and thirties she occupied a unique position of exclusivity, the only girl in a men's club. More than that, she had a quality of simplicity and grace that eluded the greatest of her male colleagues. While John Gielgud was in love with the grand poetic statement and Laurence Olivier with dressing-up, the artifice of performance, Peggy Ashcroft was spontaneous, intuitive and transparently herself. She was also perennially youthful and forward-looking. At the age of fifty-three she embraced the radicalism of Peter Hall's RSC, eventually joining the artistic directorate and leading the Company for three decades.

Peggy Ashcroft's mother was an amateur actress and former pupil of Elsie Fogerty, founder of the Central School of Speech and Drama. Ashcroft enrolled at Central (then based in the Albert Hall) in 1924, the same year as Laurence Olivier, and made her professional debut before the end of the course, aged nineteen, at the Birmingham Rep: she took over the role of Margaret in J.M. Barrie's *Dear Brutus* (W.G. Fay, 1926), and then worked with Olivier in John Drinkwater's *Bird in Hand* (1927). In London, her early opportunities included Betty in Congreve's *The Way of the World* (Nigel Playfair, Wyndham's, 1927), Anastasia in Shaw's *The Fascinating Foundling* (Henry Oscar, Arts Theatre,

1928), and Kristina in Strindberg's *Easter* (Allan Wade, Arts, 1928).

Her first Shakespearean role was Desdemona to Paul Robeson's *Othello* (Ellen van Volkenburg, Savoy, 1930), followed by Juliet in an Oxford University Dramatic Society production of *Romeo and Juliet* directed by Gielgud (New Theatre, 1932). In 1932-33 she was a member of Lilian Baylis's drama factory at the Old Vic, playing Cleopatra in Shaw's *Caesar and Cleopatra*, Imogen in *Cymbeline*, Rosalind in *As You Like It*, Portia in *The Merchant of Venice*, Perdita in *The Winter's Tale*, Kate in *She Stoops to Conquer*, the title role in John Drinkwater's *Mary Stuart*, Juliet in *Romeo and Juliet*, Lady Teazle in *The School for Scandal*, and Miranda in *The Tempest*. Gielgud directed *The Merchant*; Harcourt Williams the rest. She repeated her Juliet for the famous revival at the New in 1935 (Gielgud and Olivier alternated the roles of Romeo and Mercutio).

Ashcroft appeared in three films during these years, *The Wandering Jew* (Maurice Elvey, 1933), Hitchcock's *The Thirty-Nine Steps* (1935), and *Rhodes of Africa* (Berthold Viertel, 1936). She is irresistible in the Hitchcock; those five or so minutes of film give us an indication of her Juliet. In 1936 she played Nina alongside Gielgud and Edith Evans in *The Seagull* (Theodore Komisarjevsky, her former husband, New). In 1937-38, as a member of Gielgud's remarkable company at the Queen's, she was Irina in Michel Saint-Denis's production of *Three Sisters*, Lady Teazle in *The School for Scandal* (Tyrone Guthrie), and Portia in *The Merchant of Venice* (Gielgud and Glen Byam Shaw). After the Blitz she played Catherine in Rodney Ackland's *The Dark River* (Whitehall, 1943); Ophelia opposite Gielgud in *Hamlet* (George Rylands, Haymarket, 1944); Titania in *A Midsummer Night's Dream* (Nevill Coghill, Haymarket, 1945); and the title role in *The Duchess of Malfi* (Rylands, Haymarket, 1945). Her films during the war years were *Channel Incident* (Anthony Asquith, 1940) and *New Lot* (Carol Reed, 1942).

The Stratford theatre had been dismissed as a backwater before the war, but with the appointment of Barry Jackson as director in 1946 the focus of classical theatre shifted from London to Warwickshire. When Anthony Quayle took over in 1949 the key players of the 1930s, Ashcroft among them, came together with a new generation led by Peter Brook and Peter Hall. Suddenly Stratford was both glamorous and innovative. Ashcroft played Beatrice opposite Gielgud in *Much Ado About Nothing* (Gielgud, 1950); Cordelia in *King Lear* (Gielgud, 1950); Portia in *The Merchant of Venice* (Denis Carey, 1953); a triumphant Cleopatra opposite Michael Redgrave in *Antony and Cleopatra* (Glen Byam Shaw, 1953); Beatrice in a revival of Gielgud's *Much Ado* and Cordelia in a new production of *King Lear* by George Devine which featured controversial, modernist designs (European Tour, 1955); Rosalind opposite Richard Johnson in *As You Like It* (Glen Byam Shaw, 1957); and Imogen, regarded as one of her finest performances (she was fifty, but words such as 'beauty', 'rapture' and 'grace' have been used to describe it), in *Cymbeline* (Hall, 1957).

This last was a landmark production, the beginning of Ashcroft and Hall's friendship. When Hall set about transforming the Summer Festival into a semi-permanent, year-round, national company, with radical plans for a London base requiring state subsidy, he knew that conflict with the National Theatre movement and West End managers was inevitable. Ashcroft was the first actor he approached and her involvement gave the project instant legitimacy. She had long dreamed of a permanent company. Her RSC roles, not only Shakespeare but also Pinter and Duras, showed the extent of her ambition for the Company: Kate opposite Peter O'Toole in *The Taming of the Shrew* (John Barton, RST, 1960); Paulina in *The Winter's Tale* (Peter Wood, RST, 1960); the title role in *The Duchess of Malfi* (Donald McWhinnie, RST, 1960); *The Hollow Crown* (Barton, Aldwych, 1961); Emilia in Franco Zeffirelli's disastrous production of *Othello* (RST, 1961); Madame Ranevsky alongside Gielgud, Dorothy Tutin, Ian Holm and Judi Dench in *The Cherry Orchard* (Michel Saint-Denis, RST, 1961); Queen Margaret, regarded as her masterpiece, in *The Wars of the Roses* (Hall, RST,

1963); Mother in Marguerite Duras's *Days in the Trees* (John Schlesinger, Aldwych, 1966); Mrs Alving in *Ghosts* (Alan Bridges, Aldwych, 1967); Agnes in Edward Albee's *A Delicate Balance* (Hall, Aldwych, 1969); Beth in Harold Pinter's *Landscape* (Hall, Aldwych, 1969); Katherine in *Henry VIII* (Nunn, RST, 1969); Volumnia in Günter Grass's *The Plebeians Rehearse the Uprising* (Jones, Aldwych, 1970); the Wife in Albee's *All Over* (Hall, Aldwych, 1972); Flora in Pinter's *A Slight Ache* (Hall, Aldwych, 1973); Lidya in Aleksei Arbuzov's *Old World* (Terry Hands, Aldwych, 1976); and the Countess of Rossillion, a wonderful swansong of warmth and compassion, in *All's Well That Ends Well* (Trevor Nunn, RST, 1981). Her last RSC appearance was for a performance of *The Hollow Crown* in the Swan (1986).

During the SMT/RSC years she occasionally moonlighted elsewhere. In 1951 she played the title role in *Electra* (Saint-Denis) and Mistress Page in *The Merry Wives of Windsor* (Hugh Hunt) at the Old Vic; in 1952, Hester in Rattigan's *The Deep Blue Sea* (Frith Banbury) at the Duchess; and in 1954, the title role in *Hedda Gabler* (Peter Ashmore) at the Lyric Hammersmith. She was also the first established star to join George Devine's radical Royal Court, playing Shen Te/Shui Ta in Brecht's *The Good Woman of Setzuan* (Devine, 1956), and Rebecca West in Ibsen's *Rosmersholm* (Devine, 1959). She had been against Peter Hall's decision to move to the National, feeling it to be a betrayal of the RSC, but out of friendship she joined him there for three productions: *John Gabriel Borkman* (Old Vic, 1975), in which she played Ella opposite Ralph Richardson and Wendy Hiller; Beckett's *Happy Days* (Old Vic, 1975); and Lilian Hellman's *Watch on the Rhine* (Mike Ockrent, Lyttelton, 1980), in which she played Fanny. She also enjoyed her most prolonged and creative period as a screen actress. She won an Oscar for her performance as Mrs Moore in David Lean's *A Passage to India* (1984) and was unforgettable as Aunt Hanna in Joseph Losey's *Secret Ceremony* (1968), Frau Messner in Stephen Poliakoff's *Caught on a Train* (BBC, 1980), and Barbie Batchelor in *The Jewel in the Crown* (Christopher Morahan and Jim O'Brien, ITV, 1984).

Michel Saint-Denis (1897-1971, b. Beauvais, France). It is hard to think of an important English classical actor of the 20th century who was not influenced, either directly or indirectly, by the great French director and teacher Michel Saint-Denis.

A native of Burgundy, Saint-Denis survived the Great War and spent the formative years of his career with his uncle Jacques Copeau's company at the Théâtre du Vieux Colombier in Paris. Initially Copeau's secretary, he acted, directed and wrote plays in collaboration with Jean Villard. In 1930 he formed his own troupe, La Compagnie des Quinze.

La Compagnie des Quinze caused a sensation when they visited London in 1931. Saint-Denis's highly stylised direction and the physicality of the acting—utilising masks, mime and music—inspired many young actors and directors, including Michael Redgrave, Peggy Ashcroft and John Gielgud. Working in England from 1935, the year he founded the London Theatre Studio, Islington, Saint-Denis advocated permanent companies and in-house training and taught a method of creating theatre that was essentially new on this side of the Channel. Insisting upon long rehearsal periods, the autocratic Saint-Denis looked for truth and meaning in improvisation; he believed that reality on the stage depended upon the discovery of a collective style, and expected his actors to bring to the work everything in their experience of life. Between 1935 and 1937 he directed John Gielgud in *Noah* (New Theatre), Edith Evans in *The Witch of Edmonton* (Old Vic), and Laurence Olivier in *Macbeth* (Old Vic), but it was not until 1938, at the Queen's Theatre and then the Phoenix Theatre, that the benefits of his approach became clear. John Gielgud, Peggy Ashcroft, Michael Redgrave, Alec Guinness and George Devine were asked to work together on each play for seven weeks and to consider the smallest of details. The result was Saint-Denis's *Three Sisters*, a production universally acclaimed as an ensemble masterpiece. Although the outbreak of the war cut short this important episode, there can be little doubt that it inspired Gielgud to base his theatre work of the 1940s and 50s around repertory seasons, and left Ashcroft looking for the theatrical home she would eventually find at the RSC.

Saint-Denis joined the Infanterie Coloniale, and from 1940 ran the BBC's French Section. After the war he started again. He was general director of the Old Vic Theatre School from 1946 to 1952, and co-director of the Old Vic from 1950 to 1952. In this capacity, he oversaw the reconstruction of the stage and auditorium and directed Olivier in *Oedipus Rex* and Ashcroft in *Electra*. Between 1952 and 57 he was back in France, the first director of the Centre National Dramatique de l'Est in Strasbourg.

Peter Hall's conversations with Saint-Denis during the 1950s crystallized his own thoughts about theatre companies. In 1962 he invited Saint-Denis and Peter Brook to join the RSC as his co-directors. By asking Saint-Denis to direct Ashcroft and Gielgud in *The Cherry Orchard* (1961) Hall was making a particular statement about the significance and role of his new company, and it is appropriate to view the RSC of Hall, Brook, Ashcroft and Saint-Denis as the final destination of 20th century English theatre. Saint-Denis's particular RSC task was to set up and run a centre for experimentation and training (The Studio), but he also acted as Hall's confidant. In his autobiography Hall depicts Saint-Denis as a figure of wisdom who provided both 'ballast' and 'direction'. The Studio had a brief but significant history. It was initially a marquee in the garden of Avonside (the artistic director's house); later, a temporary building was erected on waste ground in Southern Lane. Many of the most important young RSC actors of the early to mid-1960s were taught by Saint-Denis. The Studio was abandoned on Saint-Denis's retirement in 1966, but the tin hut would be reborn as The Other Place theatre in 1974.

Peter Brook (b. London, 1925) was a fully-formed artist by the age of twenty. The son of scientists, both of Russian origin, both distinguished, he was brought up in Chiswick, west London. He went to prestigious schools (Westminster, Gresham's and Magdalen College, Oxford) without having much liking or use for them, and was just too young to fight in the war. And yet, for whatever reason, he was a young man in a hurry who possessed from the off those technical and managerial skills of the theatre normally only acquired through experience.

If the young Brook was a theatre man waiting in the wings—he writes in *Threads of Time* (Methuen, 1998) that when he first went to the theatre his interest was held not by the play but by a curiosity in the unseen backstage activity that made it happen—what he wanted most was to direct films. He left school at sixteen to take up an apprenticeship at Merton Park Studios in south London, but quickly found the work boring and unglamorous. He learned that becoming a film director meant many years of hard graft climbing the industry ladder, whereas play directing could be achieved through personal enterprise and guile. Going up to Oxford in 1942 he directed—in a hired theatre near Hyde Park Corner in London (the university theatre society was a closed shop)—a student production of Marlowe's *Doctor Faustus*. However, he found that he could not give up his ambition to make films. With a group of fellow enthusiasts he shot a movie of Laurence Sterne's *A Sentimental Journey*. This was the first example of Brook's extraordinary ingenuity and drive. He circumvented the wartime ban on the selling of film by purchasing rejected stock from the RAF, and the ban on commercial developing by employing a Soho pornographer. It was Brook's impudence, as much as the illegality of the project, that led his college, Magdalen, to threaten to send him down unless he abandoned directing for good (amusingly, the dons made him sign such a declaration). Within months of graduating he achieved fame in the theatre. He would return to movie making, directing Laurence Olivier in *The Beggar's Opera* (1953), Jeanne Moreau and Jean-Paul Belmondo in *Moderato Cantabile* (1960) and, most notably, an adaptation of William Golding's *Lord of the Flies* (1963), but it would never become his metier.

Brook made his name in a small theatre in an unassuming street behind a station in Birmingham (perhaps he had a sense of coming full circle when, decades later, he entered another theatre behind a station—the Bouffes du Nord). Without Barry Jackson, director of the Birmingham Rep, who took a risk on the young director, and Paul Scofield, the actor who starred in those first remarkable productions, his career might have taken longer to ignite. *Man and Superman*, *King John* and *The Lady from the Sea* (1945) signalled a generational change. Brook directed without reference to tradition, concentrating on interpretation and visual inventiveness and curbing the actors' long-established propensity for melodrama and bombast, and it was perhaps surprising that he took so many with him (one of the actors remarked to Jackson, 'That young man knows what he wants, and he is going to get it'). The following year Jackson took charge of the Stratford Memorial Theatre and engaged Brook to direct *Love's Labour's Lost*. Few critics had seen the Birmingham work, so it was Brook's fresh take on *Love's Labour's*—the charm, mystery and melancholy of a Watteau painting, but with provocative anachronisms (a Dull in bobby's helmet carrying a truncheon; a water-pistol; a telescope)—that established his reputation as the wunderkind of the English stage.

Throughout the 1950s Brook was something of a jack-of-all-trades, always on the move, a mountebank carrying in his suitcase a box of tricks that delighted audiences at Covent Garden, in the West End and at Stratford (he would exhaust his interest in theatrical devices by the end of the decade). His originality was most apparent in his productions of Shakespeare, particularly of the then little known *Measure for Measure* and *Titus Andronicus* at Stratford in 1950 and 1955. The theatre of the immediate post-war years understandably sought to offer escape and fantasy. Brook, though, brought the contemporary Europe of police states, paranoia and fear into his versions of *Measure for Measure*—interpreted as a play about government and society rather than as a problem comedy—and *Hamlet* (1956). The latter formed the central part of a season of plays with Scofield at the Phoenix Theatre that seemed connected by these themes (an adaptation of Graham Greene's *The Power and the Glory* and T.S. Eliot's *The Family Reunion* completed the repertory). The 1955 rediscovery of *Titus Andronicus*, starring Laurence Olivier, was Brook's most flamboyant classical production.

In 1962 Peter Hall invited Brook to join him in the running of the RSC. Brook accepted on condition that he could form a group that would operate outside of the formal structures and deadlines of the Company. Brook wanted theatre-making to be a collective endeavour and an evolving process. In rehearsals and on the stage he introduced disorder, surprise and rough edges in an attempt to make dramatic performance truer to life. His collaborator on the project, Charles Marowitz, selected twelve young actors, all new to the RSC, and devised the exercises and improvisations that evolved into the *Theatre of Cruelty* performances at LAMDA in 1964. By the end of the year Brook had expanded the group to perform Jean Genet's *The Screens* at the Donmar Rehearsal Studios and taken the workshop aesthetics of the *Theatre of Cruelty* project into the creation of his great production of Peter Weiss's *Marat/Sade* at the Aldwych. The anti-establishment and agitprop aspects of Brook's radical RSC came to the fore when he developed the theatre piece *US*, a condemnation of American policy in Vietnam (Aldwych, 1966). Similarly, in staging Shakespeare's *King Lear* (1962) and *A Midsummer Night's Dream* (1970) Brook dismissed romantic notions and pretty pictures to discover plays obsessively concerned with psychology, metaphors and the absurdity of the human condition.

After the opening of *A Midsummer Night's Dream* Brook settled permanently in Paris. In Paris Brook is financially supported by the French state and therefore able to run his own group and theatre in the way he wants, non-commercially. But it would be wrong to assume that Brook settled in Paris for financial reasons. His interest in French culture goes back a long way. He began his professional career with a production of Jean Cocteau's *La machine infernale* (*The Infernal Machine*, Chanticleer

Theatre Club, London, 1945), and went on to direct the London premieres of Jean-Paul Sartre's *Huis clos* (*Vicious Circle*, Arts, 1946, starring Alec Guinness) and *Morts sans sépulture/La putain respectueuse* (*Men Without Shadows/The Respectable Prostitute*, Lyric Hammersmith, 1947); and Jean Anouilh's *L'invitation au château* (*Ring Round the Moon*, Globe, 1950, starring Scofield and Claire Bloom), *Colombe* (New, 1951) and *L'aouette* (*The Lark*, Lyric Hammersmith, 1955, starring Dorothy Tutin). His Stratford productions of *Titus Andronicus* and *King Lear* visited Paris (Théâtre Sarah Bernhardt, today's Théâtre de la Ville) in 1957 and 1963 respectively. He first worked in Paris at the Théâtre Antoine, a private theatre run by a grande dame who asked the uncomplaining young actresses to lift their skirts at the audition. Here theatre culture and practices seemed stuck in the 19th century: there were few fat cat commercial producers and the director was both artist and master. Brook staged Tennessee Williams's *A Cat on a Hot Tin Roof* (*La chatte sur un toit brûlant*), starring Jeanne Moreau, in 1957, followed by Arthur Miller's *A View from the Bridge* (*Vu du Pont*) in 1958. His Parisian career continued with the French premiere of Jean Genet's *Le balcon* at the Théâtre de Gymnase (1960); and John Arden's *La danse de Sergent Musgrave* and Rolf Hochhuth's *Le vicaire* at the Théâtre de l'Athénée (1963). In May 1968 he was in the city working on a production of *The Tempest* for Jean-Louis Barrault's 'Théâtre de nations' festival at the Odéon; when the government closed the theatres after the student revolt Brook took his group to the Roundhouse in London. Their very physical presentation of *The Tempest* (spectators were forced to move as the actors rushed mobile scaffolding into new positions) astounded some and alienated others.

On moving to Paris Brook established the Centre International de Recherche Théâtrale (CIRT). The name makes one think of Pierre Boulez's intimidating avant-garde institute at the Pompidou, but Brook's centre had nothing to do with modern technology. Research for Brook meant going in the opposite direction—a quest to see what could be learned from the perceived simplicity, truth and wonder of primitive forms that would take him and his actors on journeys to Africa and the Middle East (1971-73). Rejecting the conventions of the contemporary stage, Brook used only the most basic elements of performance—a space (which could be anywhere), a troupe of actors, a devised text (derived by the troupe from non-theatre source material—the poetry of Ted Hughes and the Persian epic *Conference of the Birds*) and a few simple props. And when Brook stopped travelling and opened his own theatre in Paris, returning, therefore, to the conventional, a style of unadorned simplicity, of rough magic, of storytelling, was retained. Brook's base, the Bouffes du Nord, is in the 10th arrondissement, a quarter where west meets east, where shopkeepers display little red and yellow heaps of aromatic spices and trays of fresh fish on the pavements beneath the six-storey apartment blocks of Haussmann's Paris; and where the metro clatters on metal stilts above the Boulevard de la Chapelle—the district of the outer boulevards described in Émile Zola's *L'Assommoir*. The theatre itself is situated behind the Gare du Nord, the end of a terrace rising above the cutting through which trains travel to and from London (spectators in the auditorium can hear the rumble of the trains). This, then, is a quarter far removed from the tourist heart of the city and its ornate palace theatres. The Bouffes, a 19th century boulevard theatre, had been dark for twenty years, used only by the homeless. If from the outside the building is disappointingly nondescript, its interior, similar in shape and size to that of an Elizabethan playhouse, both courtyard and room, is perfect for Brook's needs. He repaired the fabric but as far as possible left the theatre as he had found it—dilapidation gives the Bouffes the quality of an improvised space.

Brook's productions of Shakespeare's *Timon d'Athènes* (1974) and *Mesure pour mesure* (1978) and Chekhov's *La cerisaie* (*The Cherry Orchard*, 1981) established the Bouffes as one of the leading Paris theatres. The *Mahabharata* (1985), an epic dramatisation of an ancient Indian story, was the culmination of his later style. Brook and Jean-Claude Carrière spent ten years developing the text, knowing it to be the perfect vehicle for an international troupe. In another sense, it was the product of the dubious European idea of the 1960s that less technologically advanced parts of the world contain in their civilisations levels of spiritual meaning lost to people in the capitalist West. There is, in Brook, an unexplained turning away from the Western tradition.

During the last twenty-five years Brook has staged only one play by Shakespeare in English, *Hamlet*, and then in an abridged chamber form (2000), and only one in French, *La tempête* (1990). There have been no other productions of a classic play from any period. If a director of Brook's stature does not interpret great plays is there not a sense that he is in semi-retirement? There are plenty of lesser talents delivering chamber-sized deconstructions and distillations, adapting playwrights' work in an attempt to achieve the prestige of authorship. Such pieces, even when notable, are merely flotsam.

For Brook, what has come to matter most is the journey, not the destination, as if after a single performance the work, inevitably, becomes stale, moribund, a part of the 'Deadly Theatre' of convention and repetition. But theatre is only performance. If rehearsals function as a way of living, a secular religion, who (outside of the group) needs to care? Brook's RSC Shakespeares were created in less than seven weeks by professional actors who went home at night. Few would argue that his later productions, created without deadlines by dedicated disciples of the cause (using experimental techniques in an attempt to make, as Brook has said, the invisible visible), were of greater significance.

Clifford Williams (1926-2005, b. Cardiff) initially worked as an actor. He had no formal training (from school he went into the army). His five years as a bit player in the provinces started at the end of the war and included the 1948 Stratford season— Prince Henry in *King John* (Michael Benthall); Servant/Player in the Robert Helpmann/Paul Scofield *Hamlet* (Michael Benthall);

Shepherd in *The Winter's Tale* (Anthony Quayle); Alexander in *Troilus and Cressida* (Anthony Quayle); and Soldier in *Othello* (Godfrey Tearle).

At the age of twenty-four he re-thought his career. He established the Mime Theatre Company, the first troupe of its kind in Britain (1950); wrote his first play, *The Disguises of Arlecchino* (1951); and travelled to South Africa to work as a director (National Theatre of South Africa, mid-1950s). Following staff appointments at the Marlowe Theatre, Canterbury, and the Queen's Theatre, Hornchuch, he directed noteworthy work at the Arts Theatre in London: García Lorca's *Yerma* (1957); Friedrich Dürrenmatt's *The Marriage of Mr Mississippi* (1959); Eugene O'Neill's *A Moon for the Misbegotten* (1960); and Ionesco's *Victims of Duty* (1960).

In 1962 Williams joined the RSC as a staff producer. Peter Hall quickly offered him one of the plays in the Company's experimental season at the Arts. David Rudkin's *Afore Night Comes* was an exceptional first play, its strong language and depiction of violence controversial for the time, and Williams's production did the text full justice. Later that year he was given his first Stratford production. Peter Hall needed to fill the gap created by the postponement of the Peter Brook/Paul Scofield *King Lear* and asked his most junior director to produce *The Comedy of Errors* in three weeks. Williams found a style for the play that was fast and inventive, and encouraged his fine cast (led by Ian Richardson, Alec McCowen and Diana Rigg) to perform with an uncomplicated and infectious enjoyment. The actors began the play in grey costumes on a bare wooden stage. As the play progressed they acquired coloured items of clothing. A severe Brechtian prologue gave way to a carnival. Williams's *Comedy of Errors* was a brilliantly plotted farce with an undertone of disquiet and distress.

After *The Comedy of Errors* Hall made Williams an associate director. He worked with Peter Brook on a production of *The Tempest* (RST, 1963), and staged Rolf Hochhüth's controversial play *The Representative* (Aldwych, 1963) as historical fact, projecting newsreel images on the walls of the set. The production was applauded for its powerful spectacle and fine acting, but caused debate as to the legitimacy of the play's central theme—the Catholic Church's failure to condemn the persecution of the Jews. He next worked on the 1964 histories, and staged a fascinating double of Marlowe's *The Jew of Malta* and Shakespeare's *The Merchant of Venice* with the same actor, Eric Porter, playing Barabas and Shylock (RST, 1965).

He directed Judi Dench in *Major Barbara* (Aldwych, 1970) and *The Duchess of Malfi* (RST, 1971). *Wild Oats* with Alan Howard was a huge popular hit, remaining in the repertoire for four years (1976-79). The most interesting of his later RSC productions was Alexander Solzhenitsyn's *The Love-Girl and the Innocent* (Aldwych, 1981).

Based at the RSC until the 1980s, Williams maintained a parallel career as a versatile freelance director. Among his credits were such diverse pieces as the National's all male *As You Like It* (Old Vic, 1967); the sex revue *Oh! Calcutta!* (Round House, 1970); Anthony Shaffer's thriller *Sleuth* (St Martin's, 1970); Alan Bennett's *The Old Country* (Queen's, 1977); and Hugh Whitemore's *Breaking the Code* (Theatre Royal Haymarket, 1986).

David Jones (1934-2008, b. Poole) studied at Christ's College, Cambridge, and made is name at the BBC, one of the talented young directors produced by Huw Wheldon's *Monitor* arts programme (1958-64). As well as directing and editing editions of the show, he made classic short films on the Berliner Ensemble, Joan Littlewood's Theatre Workshop, William Golding and E.M. Forster. In 1961 at the Mermaid Theatre he staged T.S. Eliot's *Sweeney Agnostes*, W.B. Yeats's *Purgatory* and Samuel Beckett's *Krapp's Last Tape*. He directed his first RSC production—Boris Vian's *The Empire Builders*—at the Arts in 1962, and accepted the largely administrative position of Artistic Controller two years later. Only rarely directing Shakespeare at Stratford, he helped to plan the varied programme of new plays and European classics at the Aldwych (he was responsible for the day-to-day running of the Aldwych from 1969 to 72, and again in 1976/77). In particular, he championed the plays of David Mercer and revived the theatre of Maxim Gorky—his productions of *Enemies*, *The Lower Depths*, *Summerfolk* and *The Zykovs* were highlights of the Aldwych seasons of the early 1970s.

From 1977 to 78 he produced the BBC's *Play of the Month*, commissioning television productions of Shaw, Harley Granville-Barker, Chekhov, Jean-Paul Sartre, David Mercer (*Flint*), and Edward Bond (*The Sea*), and directing *The Beaux Stratagem*, Tankred Dorst's *Ice Age* and Harold Pinter's *Langrishe, Go Down*. The exceptional *Langrishe* starred Jeremy Irons and Judi Dench. In 1979, at Stratford, he directed Judi Dench in *Cymbeline* and Ben Kingsley in Brecht's *Baal*. Later that year he left the RSC to take up the position of Artistic Director of the Brooklyn Academy of Music in New York. *Betrayal*, his first feature film, based on Harold Pinter's play, was released in 1983. A journeyman director in Hollywood, his work included *84 Charing Cross Road* (1987); *Jacknife* (1989); Pinter's version of Kafka's *The Trial* (1992); and *The Confession* (1999).

Trevor Nunn (b. Ipswich, 1940) followed in Peter Hall's footsteps before making his own way as an innovative producer—the master logistician of the world's largest theatre company (he took his mentor's model and expanded it in all directions)—and one of the founders of the modern musical theatre.

His task at the beginning was daunting. Although Nunn had been chosen by Hall he was only twenty-eight and his appointment was met with considerable scepticism. He had come to the RSC with a brilliant CV from Cambridge (he had taken student productions to the Edinburgh Festival) and the Belgrade Theatre, Coventry (1962-65), but his first solo RSC shows—*The Thwarting of Baron Bolligrew* and *Tango*—were failures. It was said that he lacked authority in the rehearsal room. He turned things round with his next project, the Jacobean rarity *The Re-*

venger's Tragedy (RST, 1966), partly by working with young actors and a designer from the Belgrade, Christopher Morley. Stylised and overtly theatrical, a *dance macabre* in black and silver, it challenged the prevailing house style. In the next year Nunn confirmed his new status with assured productions of *The Taming of the Shrew*, starring Janet Suzman (whom he later married) and Michael Williams, and *The Relapse*.

His elevation divided the RSC along generational lines (although Peggy Ashcroft took to Nunn as she had taken to Hall a decade before). From the outside it initially looked like a caretaker appointment. Nunn turned out to be so capable an artistic director in difficult circumstances (Hall had resigned suddenly) that the doubters were silenced. First, he organised the RSC's work around a two-year cycle with more transfers of Stratford productions to London: this allowed a smaller company of actors to stay together longer. Second, his first full season (1969) felt like a departure: a new stage configuration was designed by Christopher Morley (a white box that placed emphasis on space, colour and light) and the choice of plays—*Pericles*, *The Winter's Tale*, *Women Beware Women*, *Twelfth Night* and *Henry VIII*—was the most challenging in years. The season was a critical and popular success (the RSC's audience grew during Nunn's first years). Third, he introduced more international touring: this filled the gap between Stratford and London (the Stratford season ended in November until 1974, when Nunn extended it into the New Year); it was also financially profitable. All of Nunn's early changes were made in the context of the RSC's precarious financial state—his choices were both creative and fiscally cunning.

The integrated approach and box set style of 1969 remained influential, not least on two of the RSC's greatest productions—Peter Brook's *A Midsummer Night's Dream* (1970) and Buzz Goodbody's *Hamlet* (1975). Nunn believed in continuity but was restlessly creative. In the early 1970s he began the process that led to the opening of a studio theatre in Stratford. Small-scale and experimental work had always been important to the RSC, but, with the exception of Peter Brook's 'Theatre of Cruelty' seasons (1963-64) and Michel Saint-Denis's workshop studio in Stratford (influential internally in terms of the training and development of actors), it had been peripheral to the Company's main operation. Because of limited funds—the Arts Council would not permit any portion of the RSC's subsidy to be spent on extracurricular activities—seasons of small-scale work at the Arts Theatre in 1962 (Hall had wanted to acquire the Mercury Theatre in Notting Hill) and at The Place in 1971, 1973 and 1974 had not been sustainable. The RSC's small-scale touring outfit, Theatregoround, was viewed as a 'second eleven' until the early 1970s when Nunn included its productions in the Stratford programme. As Theatregoround's operation grew it became too costly.

This small-scale work had been centred on new plays and rarely performed classics. In 1970 the RSC mounted a Theatregoround Festival at the Roundhouse in London. Peter Brook's *A Midsummer Night's Dream*, Trevor Nunn's *Hamlet* and Terry Hands's *Richard III* were performed without their décor or costumes. The RSC saw the potential of producing Shakespeare in a small space, where the actors could speak directly and intimately to spectators and where the poetic power of the words would be undiminished. Nunn decided to convert Michel Saint-Denis's former studio in Southern Lane, a prefabricated tin hut erected without any intention of permanence back in 1964 and at that time used as the headquarters of Theatregoround, into a performance space.

In 1973 the RSC tried out the Studio, as it was still called, by mounting a limited season of four plays. Sensing the remarkable quality of this inauspicious venue, Nunn invited Buzz Goodbody to formulate a policy and a programme for the theatre she named The Other Place. Except for two dressing rooms there was no backstage; there was no stage door; no bar. The Other Place offered a very austere and uncomfortable environment, but the close proximity of actors and spectators heightened the excitement of both performing and watching theatre. From the

41

start The Other Place was looked upon as the Stratford company's second theatre rather than as a fringe venue, although Goodbody ensured that it had a particular role by forming new links with the local community and schools, and by offering an experience that was affordable, unstuffy and excitingly unpredictable. The Other Place would become the RSC's main theatre for new plays and rare classics, but its initial importance was in giving new life to the Company's performance of Shakespeare. Goodbody's *Hamlet*, with Ben Kingsley, and Nunn's *Macbeth*, with Ian McKellen, were among the most influential productions of the 1970s, leading to the view, still widely held in England, that Shakespeare's plays are most powerfully presented as studies in character psychology rather than as narratives of action and spectacle. After Goodbody's tragic death in 1975 Nunn entrusted The Other Place to Ron Daniels.

The case for a second theatre had been won, and Nunn looked for a sister venue in London, eventually selecting the Donmar Warehouse in Covent Garden and entrusting its operation (as a space for radical new work as well as TOP transfers) to Howard Davies (1977).

Nunn further re-invigorated the RSC by establishing the Newcastle residency (1977) and small-scale tour (1978). Perhaps most importantly he brought on a new generation of artists—actors, directors and designers who gave the Company its identity, momentum and strength in depth for nearly two decades. By the beginning of the 1980s, creative and administrative duties were shared out among a team of associate directors (the aforementioned Daniels and Davies, plus Barry Kyle, John Caird, Bill Alexander and Adrian Noble). Because Nunn asked his associates to begin as assistant directors, and to make a lasting commitment, he gave the RSC a new cohesion.

Most of Nunn's changes did not begin until 1974; 1972 and 1973 were his years of crisis. In April 1972 Peter Hall told his RSC colleagues that he was leaving to run the National. The break was hard for Hall, Nunn, David Brierley and Peggy Ashcroft and led to a shared fantasy that the National and the

RSC could merge. Nunn took the merger seriously because he feared that the more heavily subsidised National, moving into the new building on the South Bank, would monopolise the best actors. Laurence Olivier viewed the plan as an attempt by Stratford to take over the National. The merger idea was abandoned. Nunn had to deal with the consequences of Hall's departure just as the demands of running the RSC were beginning to catch up on him. He was exhausted from staging the four plays of *The Romans*; then his comment in a letter to *The Times* that the RSC was 'basically a left-wing organisation' caused a furore. In contrast to Hall in 1967, however, Nunn came through his moment of crisis. His fears proved unfounded, for the RSC of 1975 to 1982 eclipsed Hall's troubled NT.

As a director Nunn is versatile and eclectic, a master of both structure and interpretation. The white spaces and clean lines of his acclaimed production of *The Winter's Tale* in 1969, gave way to the spectacular visuals of *The Romans* in 1972. His Other Place *Macbeth* grew out of a frustration with the requirements of the main house. The performance had the directness of a folk tale, with the actors sitting around a bare circle of wooden planks. Its dark, ritualistic atmosphere emanated from the actors' vivid presentation of the text. In the same year Nunn also directed main house productions of *Romeo and Juliet, King Lear* and *The Comedy of Errors*, the latter brilliantly re-interpreted as a musical. One scene of *The Comedy of Errors* was staged in and around an outdoor movie show, a clever but seemingly organic sequence and the perfect example of Nunn's ability to act as a 'co-author' without advertising the fact.

An intimate *Three Sisters* in The Other Place (1979) was more memorable than a wintry *As You Like It* (1977) and naturalistic *Merry Wives of Windsor* (1979) in the main house. Nunn's concentration on social worlds had given many of his productions a novelistic sweep. In 1980 he went the next step and staged, with John Caird, a two-part adaptation of Dickens's *Nicholas Nickleby* (Aldwych). For years he had used wooden, balconied sets and large casts to orchestrate scenes, and *Nickleby* was the climax of this style. With *Juno and the Paycock* (1980) and *All's Well That Ends Well* (1981) he took the intimate style of his studio work into the Aldwych and the RST with spellbinding results. *All's Well* was set at the outbreak of the Great War, an elegant Edwardian world of chambermaids and cafés, but also of soldiers disembarking through locomotive steam. The callous snobbery of Mike Gwilym's Bertram made sense in a society of public schoolboy soldiers; Helena's assertion of her rights made sense in the age of the suffragettes. The production also looked to Chekhov, not least in the beautiful scenes between Peggy Ashcroft's Countess and Harriet Walter's Helena. Nunn was at the height of his powers as a director of classical texts but he had already made the move into musicals that would end his tenure at the RSC. Lloyd Webber's *Cats* (1981) started a new phase of his career, and although he remained in joint charge of the RSC until 1986 he was for part of that time away.

The beginning of his break from the RSC coincided with the move to the Barbican (1982) and the end of a golden period in the Company's history. Nunn directed *Henry IV*, the Barbican's inaugural production, in his *Nickleby* style. In 1985 he struck a deal with Cameron Mackintosh and staged *Les Misérables* as an RSC production, thereby providing the Company with a valuable source of income. His final act as chief executive was to oversee the opening of the Swan Theatre (1986). Years earlier he had planned the construction of a new theatre within the shell of the original Shakespeare Memorial Theatre, and the Swan was the glorious result of his vision and perseverance.

The 1926 fire had destroyed the roof and gutted the auditorium but left the shell of the building, including the foyer and gallery rooms, intact. After the construction of the new SMT, the original became a storeroom and eventually the RSC's main rehearsal room (called the Conference Hall). The shape and size of the space led Nunn and associate designer John Napier to the exciting conclusion that the Conference Hall could be reborn as a Jacobean-style galleried playhouse, dedicated to the works of Shakespeare's contemporaries (the persuasive artistic justification for a third Stratford theatre). The local architect Michael Reardon delivered an exceptional design (late 1970s), but despite an exhaustive campaign at home and in America the RSC failed to raise even a fraction of the cost. For years Nunn's dream was placed on hold, waiting for the day when an American called Frederick Koch would see the model of the Swan in Stratford and say, 'I'd like to pay for that'.

The Swan and its attic rehearsal room cost two million pounds. The combination of the Swan's horseshoe shape, height, bare bricks and wooden galleries provokes a good feeling the moment you enter the auditorium. The four hundred or so spectators line the walls, and surround the platform stage. Those closest sit with their knees against it. It is a public space in the truest sense—spectators look across at each other, and the actors, surrounded, have to include them, subtly, in the performance.

The Swan is primarily an actors' space. They can work the spectators like comedians, excite them with action, or still them into a rapt silence. I imagine the close and very visible scrutiny of the audience can be nerve-wracking for inexperienced performers, but many RSC members of the 1980s and 90s were so exhilarated by the experience that they came to dislike working in the main house (an unfortunate consequence of the Swan's success). Directors and designers are less in thrall of an auditorium that is impossible to disguise or re-configure: the Swan is the design.

Nunn directed an exuberant production of Thomas Heywood's *The Fair Maid of the West* during the opening season and then left the Company. His departure came at a time of trouble—a growing deficit, an unsuccessful Barbican, and the beginning of a hostile press—but he left the RSC in the good hands of Terry Hands, John Barton, David Brierley and Adrian Noble. If there was a noticeable change it was due to the fact that many of the major actors of the Nunn years—Helen Mirren, Ben Kingsley, Patrick Stewart, David Suchet, Bob Peck, Judi Dench, Roger Rees, Mike Gwilym—also departed.

After ten years as a gun-for-hire Nunn succeeded Richard Eyre as Director of the National (1998-03). It was interesting to watch as he attempted to turn the National of the 1990s into the RSC of the 1970s and 80s. He worked alongside his old RSC colleagues John Caird, Howard Davies and Genista McIntosh and even repeated the repertoire—*Peter Pan* (RSC 1982; NT 1997), *Antony and Cleopatra* with Helen Mirren (RSC 1982; NT 1998), *The Forest* (RSC 1980; NT 1999), *Money* (RSC 1981; NT 1999), and *Summerfolk* (RSC 1974; NT 1999). More to the point, after the rather bland, middlebrow programming of his predecessor, he was typically ambitious and enterprising, creating a National Theatre company and staging a rare play by Tennessee Williams rather than the latest David Hare.

Nunn has remained connected to the RSC, directing McKellen and Willard White in a fine *Othello* (the costumes alluded to the period of reconstruction after the American Civil War) to close the original Other Place in 1989; *Measure for Measure* to open its replacement in 1991; and McKellen in *King Lear* and *The Seagull* at the Courtyard in 2007.

Terry Hands (b. Aldershot, Hampshire, 1941) came to epitomise the idea of the theatre director in the 1970s: enigmatic, European-minded, habitually dressed in black. His productions of that time, dynamically staged, utilising cavernous darkness and intense white light, showed a mastery of the main stage. As Artistic Director he successfully steered the Company through the financial crisis of 1986-90.

Hands, from an army family, studied English literature at Birmingham University before training at RADA. While still in his early twenties he founded the Liverpool Everyman (1964)—productions included *Richard III*, *Look Back in Anger* and Arnold Wesker's *The Four Seasons*. He joined the RSC in 1966 to run the Company's touring group, Theatregoround, and established his reputation with a main stage version of *The Merry Wives of Windsor* (1968) lovingly set in period. Its popularity led to revivals in

1969 and 1975, but Hands was seldom this traditional. Frontal attack and spot-lighting made his work highly distinctive, as did the presence of the RSC's most attractive and talented young performers: *The Man of Mode* (Aldwych, 1971), *The Balcony* (Aldwych, 1971) and *Henry VI* (RST, 1977) featured Helen Mirren; *Romeo and Juliet* (RST, 1973), Timothy Dalton and Estelle Kohler; *Henry IV, Henry V* (RST, 1975), *Henry VI, Coriolanus* (RST, 1977), *Richard II, Richard III* (RST, 1980), Alan Howard. The Hands/Howard history play cycle dominated Stratford in the mid-1970s; in particular, their unabridged production of the three parts of *Henry VI*, performed in a single day with visceral intensity, was a landmark. Sexually charged productions of *As You Like It* (RST, 1980)—rarely has this play's rush from winter to spring, from repression to feeling, been so ecstatically realised—and *Troilus and Cressida* (Aldwych, 1981) followed.

From 1972 to 78 Hands was a Consultant Director at the Comédie-Française in Paris, where he directed *Richard III, Pericles, Twelfth Night, Le Cid* and *Murder in the Cathedral*, and married the great actress Ludmila Mikaël (their daughter, Marina Hands, would emerge as a star of French stage and screen in the early 2000s—she joined the Comédie-Française in 2006). On the continent Hands's linguistic skill and production style made him (after Peter Brook) the best placed and most admired British director—he also worked in Vienna at the Burgtheater (*Troilus and Cressida, As You Like It*) and in Italy at the Teatro Stabile di Genova (*Women Beware Women*). He dominated Paris theatre during one memorable month in 1976 with *Twelfth Night* at the Comédie-Française, *Otello* at the Opera, and his RSC *Henry V* at the Odéon.

Hands's appointment in 1978 as joint Artistic Director of the RSC came just in time to prevent his defection to the National— see Peter Hall's *Diaries* (Hamilton, 1983). Nunn and Hands were a formidable team. By sharing the leadership of the Company Nunn was able to spend time away. Hands oversaw the move to the Barbican (1982), and became sole Artistic Director in 1987. During these years he mounted stylish productions of *Much Ado*

About Nothing (RST, 1982), featuring reflective surfaces and a lone female cellist, and *Cyrano de Bergerac* (Barbican, 1983), but *Othello* (RST, 1985), with Ben Kingsley and David Suchet, *The Winter's Tale* (RST, 1986), *Julius Caesar* (RST, 1987) and *Coriolanus* (RST, 1989), with Charles Dance, failed to have the impact of his earlier Shakespeare work.

The RSC grew in size during the 1980s. The opening of the Swan and its London equivalent, the Mermaid, in 1987, meant that Hands was running six theatres at a time when the RSC's grant was frozen. A government inquiry into the RSC had concluded, in 1984, that the Company was well-managed and under-funded, but ministers and officials were soon ignoring this inconvenient truth. The RSC withdrew from the Mermaid in 1988 (expansion only made economic sense in the short term), and by 1989 the financial situation was so bad that Hands closed the Barbican Theatre over the winter. This was a direct challenge to the Arts Council and the government, a risky policy of brinkmanship that succeeded because the government couldn't allow a flagship arts organisation to go under. The RSC's grant was increased and the Barbican Theatre re-opened in the spring.

Hands took the brunt of media hostility. Prompted in part by the need to find a new source of finance for the RSC, he directed a musical of Stephen King's *Carrie* (RST and New York, 1988): the unsavoury result—the production was critically panned on both sides of the Atlantic—may have hastened his departure. His last few years in charge were exceptional: he brought in important new talent (Nicholas Hytner, Deborah Warner, Sam Mendes), gave Adrian Noble control of the 1988-89 programme, brought to the fore a new generation of actors (including Ralph Fiennes, Amanda Root, Simon Russell Beale, Amanda Harris, Linus Roache, Imogen Stubbs, Mark Rylance, Richard McCabe), and directed excellent revivals of *Romeo and Juliet* (Swan) with Rylance, Peter Flannery's *Singer* (Swan) with Sher, and *Love's Labour's Lost* (RST) with Fiennes, Beale, Amanda Root and John Wood. *The Seagull*, his swansong as Artistic Director, was a triumph of ensemble acting. *Love's Labour's Lost* ended with a coup derived from character (see: Richard Ridings).

As a freelance director Hands staged *Arden in Faversham* in Zurich (1991) and *Hamlet* in Paris (Marigny Theatre, 1994). He returned to the RSC in 1992 to direct Marlowe's *Tamburlaine the Great* (Swan and Barbican). In 1997 he was appointed Artistic Director of Clwyd Theatr Cymru, and began his regime with *Equus*, Peter Barnes's *A Christmas Carol* and Siân Evans's Jack the Ripper play *The Journey of Mary Kelly* (1998). *Mary Kelly's* grave and disturbing atmosphere was established, in typical Hands style, from very little—a grey stage and red lighting. Subsequent work at Clwyd: *Twelfth Night* (1999); Owen Teale in a studio *Macbeth* (1999); *Under Milk Wood* (2000); Nicol Williamson in *King Lear* (2001); Tom Stoppard's *Rosencrantz and Guildenstern Are Dead* (2002); *Romeo and Juliet* (2002); Arnold Wesker's *The Four Seasons* (2002); Noël Coward's *Blithe Spirit* (2003); Malcolm Storry in Arthur Miller's *The Crucible* (2003); *One Flew Over the Cuckoo's Nest* (2004); Gerard Murphy in *Troilus and Cressida* (2005); Alan Ayckbourn's *A Chorus of Disapproval* (2006); Jonathan Lichtenstein's *Memory* (2006); and Stoppard's *Arcadia* (2007). In October 2001, unable to support Adrian Noble's restructuring of the RSC, he resigned as an advisory director.

Buzz Goodbody (1946-1975, b. London) was the discovery of the 1966 National Student Drama Festival (Cardiff). Her Sussex production of *Notes from the Underground*, which subsequently played for a short season at the Garrick in London, so impressed John Barton that he brought her into the RSC, aged twenty-one.

She only worked for a short time as Barton's personal assistant (a feminist, she did not take kindly to running errands). She was the assistant director on Terry Hands's *The Merry Wives of Windsor* (RST, 1968), *Pericles* (RST, 1969) and *Women Beware Women* (RST, 1969); Trevor Nunn's *The Winter's Tale* (RST, 1969) and *Henry VIII* (RST, 1969); and Barton's *Twelfth Night* (RST, 1969).

For Theatregoround she devised and directed the anthologies *To Be or Not to Be* and *Eve and After* followed by her first major production, *King John* (1970), with Patrick Stewart and Norman Rodway. For several months she collaborated with Terry Hands, David Benedictus and Guy Woolfenden on a documentary drama with songs about the 1926 General Strike, called *Strike*; when this project fell through she directed *Arden of Faversham* at short notice, but withdrew before the first performance because of a dispute with Dorothy Tutin (Theatregoround Festival at the Roundhouse, 1970). *Strike* reflected her political views (she was a member of the Communist Party), as did Trevor Griffiths's *Occupations* and *The Oz Trial*, the plays she directed for the RSC's studio season at The Place (1971). By this time she was working regularly with a strong group of young RSC actors, led by Patrick Stewart, Ben Kingsley and Estelle Kohler, and, as the RSC's only female director, had provoked the passing interest of tabloid journalists. Also in 1971 she co-founded the Women's Street Theatre Group.

In 1972 she worked on Trevor Nunn's Roman season as co-director—*Coriolanus, Julius Caesar, Antony and Cleopatra* and *Titus Andronicus. As You Like It* (1973), her first solo main house production, featuring Eileen Atkins, David Suchet and Richard Pasco, combined in its ideas and design (a 'forest' of metal tubes, a hammock, modern dress for some characters, Edwardian for others) disparate influences—Chekhov, music hall, and contemporary sexual politics.

In 1973 Trevor Nunn placed her in charge of the RSC's new studio theatre in Stratford, a corrugated tin hut previously used as a rehearsal room. Goodbody was an inspired choice because she brought a new dimension to the Company: she was the most promising young director, the only woman, and she had connections with the radical fringe. She began to formulate a policy for The Other Place that would link it to the local community and to younger audiences. During her first season in charge (1974) she directed *King Lear*, with Tony Church, Mike Gwilym and David Suchet, and *The World Turned Upside Down*. *King Lear* toured America in February 1975. The season, an instant success, also included productions by Howard Davies, Ron Daniels (*Afore Night Come*) and Nicol Williamson (*Uncle Vanya*). She planned a second season of *Hamlet*, Ben Jonson's *Epicene* and Brecht's *Man is Man*. *Hamlet*, which opened the season in April 1975, was a landmark. Staged with economy on a white set, it was performed in modern dress with conversational intensity by Ben Kingsley, George Baker, Mikel Lambert, Yvonne Nicholson, Bob Peck, Stuart Wilson and Griffith Jones.

Four days after the first performance, Buzz Goodbody committed suicide. Trevor Nunn took over The Other Place season, and transferred *Hamlet* to London.

Barry Kyle (b. 1947), like Terry Hands, studied at the RSC's local university, Birmingham, and started his career in Liverpool (he was an associate director at the Liverpool Playhouse, 1970-72). He joined the RSC as an assistant director in 1973 and staged his own piece *Sylvia Plath* alongside Plath's *Three Women*, The Other Place's first productions. For the next few years he directed in the main house in conjunction with John Barton and Trevor Nunn (more than an assistant but not the dominant voice) while continuing to mount his own productions in the studio, including *Richard III* (1975) with Ian Richardson. He became an associate director in 1978.

Kyle is an adaptable director, particularly good at ensemble pieces. His productions in The Other Place of Howard Brenton's *The Churchill Play* (1978) and the rarely performed classics *The Maid's Tragedy* (1980) and *The Witch of Edmonton* (1981) were raw, vivid and powerful. His main house work was, overall, less successful, although the 1984 *Love's Labour's Lost*, featuring an elegant semi-abstract setting (tall Chinese parasols rising like trees; a headless Cupid), was very fine—witty, melancholy and dreamily seductive. He excelled in the Swan with imaginative and probing productions of James Shirley's *Hyde Park* (1987), Marlowe's *The Jew of Malta* (1987) and *Doctor Faustus* (1989), and, particularly, Shakespeare and Fletcher's *The Two Noble Kinsmen* (1986), which revealed an enviable sleight of hand—a suspended cage, tall poles and a ribbon of green lace became a prison, a forest and a garden. John Fletcher wrote *The Two Noble Kinsmen*'s strong subplot, the story of a young girl's unrequited love. This, in Imogen Stubbs's affecting performance, was the revelation of Kyle's production. Like Helena in *A Midsummer Night's Dream* she leaves home and sleeps rough in pursuit of the man who has rejected her; like Ophelia in *Hamlet* she loses her reason to the distress of those who love her—the scenes are by turns humorous, tender and heartbreaking, and Fletcher was both canny and affectionate in offering his mentor these acts of homage in the midst of their play. Kyle's staging was an erotically charged exploration of longing and betrayal.

Among Kyle's finest RSC productions was *The Dillen* (1983), the story of a Stratford working-class family from 1897 to after the Great War. The production began in The Other Place but mostly played in promenade throughout Stratford. The past was brought to haunting life in the streets of the Old Town and in the fields beside the Avon as day turned into night. Kyle conjured simple but unforgettable images—pea-pickers working in a meadow; a torch-lit procession through the streets—while the actors performed with vigour and feeling.

When the Nunn/Hands era came to an end Barry Kyle moved to the United States, surprisingly taking up a position at Louisiana State University in Baton Rouge. As head of the directing course in the Department of Drama he founded and ran the University's resident professional theatre company, Swine Palace Productions (1992-01). Louisiana may be as provincial as you can get in the States without moving to Alaska, but Kyle created something there while occasionally directing in New York (*Henry V*, 1992) and Washington (*Romeo and Juliet* at the Shakespeare Theater).

Since returning to England, Kyle has worked at Shakespeare's Globe directing Julian Glover in *King Lear* (2001) and an all-female *Richard III* (2003).

Ron Daniels (b. Niteroi, Brazil, 1942). Born in Brazil to British parents, Ron Daniels came to England in 1963 on a drama scholarship and worked initially as an actor (his professional career had started as a teenager; following an abortive spell at drama school he co-founded the Teatro Oficina in São Paulo). He joined the RSC in 1968 to play the small role of Metellus Cimber in *Julius Caesar* (John Barton, RST) and John Grass in *Indians* (Jack Gelber, Aldwych). His reputation as a director was established at the Victoria Theatre, Stoke-on-Trent, where he worked on both classical and modern texts.

Trevor Nunn brought Daniels back into the RSC in 1974 to direct new plays, and the occasional classic, at The Other Place. He became Artistic Director of TOP in 1977 and along with Howard Davies (Director of the Warehouse) spearheaded the RSC's new writing work for the next decade. There was no obvious division in quality between the new plays and the classics that played side by side. Daniels's productions of David Edgar's *Destiny* (1976), David Rudkin's *The Sons of Light* (1977), Ford's *'Tis Pity She's a Whore* (1977) and Shakespeare's *Pericles* (1979) were lucid and gripping—new plays staged as classics, classics staged as new plays.

The success of *Pericles* and *Timon of Athens* (1980) led to his first main house production, a fine *Romeo and Juliet* (1980) with Anton Lesser and Judy Buxton. *A Midsummer Night's Dream* (1981), starring Mike Gwilym and Juliet Stevenson, used the mechanics of Victorian theatre as a metaphor. *The Tempest* (1982) was designed with extravagance, but Daniels returned to the leaner style of *Romeo* for his remarkable productions of *Hamlet* (1988) and *Richard II* (1990). In *Hamlet* he took imaginative risks (Mark Rylance's Hamlet wore pyjamas for much of the play) to emphasise dislocation and mental disturbance: the set's slanting walls were plain white, like those of an institution, and the outdoor scenes were played before a vast, turbulent seascape. In *Richard II* he contrasted an elegant court with the urban landscape of a modern civil war.

Daniels left the RSC at the end of the Terry Hands era and moved to America. As Associate Artistic Director of the American Repertory Theatre (Cambridge, Massachusetts) from 1992 to 96, he directed *Hamlet*, with Mark Rylance; *The Seagull*, with Rylance; *Henry IV*; *The Cherry Orchard*, with Claire Bloom; *Henry V*; *The Threepenny Opera* (1995); *The Tempest* (1995), with Paul Freeman as Prospero; *Long Day's Journey into Night* (1996), with Claire Bloom; and Naomi Wallace's *Slaughter City* (1996). During this time he was also the Director of the A.R.T.'s Institute for Advanced Theatre Training.

Since 1996 he has worked as a freelance director. In late 1996 he returned to the RSC to direct the world premiere of *Slaughter City* in the Pit (his A.R.T. production opened a few months later). In 1997 he staged a main house *Henry V* (RST) with Michael Sheen in the title role: played in modern dress before black walls etched with the names of the dead, it was an unremittingly sombre, often angry, production.

Howard Davies (b. 1940) worked as a stage manager at the Bristol Old Vic before the company's head, Val May, gave him a production to direct—Edward Bond's *Narrow Road to the Deep South*. He was subsequently made an associate director with responsibility for the Old Vic Studio. He directed Stephen Moore in *Who's Afraid of Virginia Woolf?*, Paul Eddington in *Long Day's Journey into Night*, and Anna Calder-Marshall in *Troilus and Cressida*. The plays of English political writers like Edward Bond and the modern classics of American theatre have remained at the centre of his work.

One of Davies's late night shows at the Old Vic Studio was a drama-documentary by David Illingworth based on the Oz trial. The RSC's Buzz Goodbody saw the show and acquired the work for the Company's season at The Place in London (1971). Through this connection Davies eventually joined the RSC as an assistant director, working on productions by John Barton (*King John*) and David Jones, and staging Snoo Wilson's *The Beast* at The Place (1974). He worked with Goodbody to open The Other Place in Stratford (Brecht's *Man is Man*, 1975), and after her untimely death Trevor Nunn placed him in charge of the RSC's new play policy: it was in this role, as director of the Warehouse, that he made his most important contribution. From 1977 to 1982 the RSC ran the Warehouse as a theatre dedicated to innovative and challenging new work. Plays by Edward Bond, Howard Barker and Howard Brenton shared the stage with revivals of Brecht, Shakespeare and the occasional rarity. Davies supported the writer, served the text and never self-advertised.

As well as remaining doggedly faithful to those difficult masters Bond and Barker by directing revivals of *Bingo* (1976) and *The Fool* (1980) and the premieres of *The Bundle* (1977) and *The Loud Boy's Life* (1980), Davies fashioned hits from three quality middlebrow entertainments: Pam Gems's *Piaf* (1978), C.P. Taylor's *Good* (1981) and Christopher Hampton's *Les liaisons dangereuses* (1985) all transferred to the West End and eventually to Broadway. As a director more interested in contemporary plays than in the classics, Davies was almost unique within the RSC. During his twelve years with the Company he only directed three of Shakespeare's plays in the main house, *Macbeth* with Bob Peck and Sara Kestelman (1982), *Henry VIII* with Richard Griffiths and John Thaw (1983), and *Troilus and Cressida* with Anton Lesser and Juliet Stevenson. Of the three, *Troilus* was the most unusual and revealing. If Davies's instincts are for literal readings, on this occasion he took an imaginative leap and transposed Shakespeare's bitterly cynical account of the Trojan War to the conflict between England and Russia in the Crimea (1850s). The emblematic décor, suggesting a dilapidated mansion, was striking in itself but eventually limiting since it had to serve for both camps and all scenes. The decision to depict Cressida (Juliet Stevenson) as unambiguously virtuous ran counter to the text, but Davies's final image of Pandarus playing plangent notes on a piano as the battle raged outside was unforgettable.

One senses that Davies was never entirely happy at the RSC after the closure of the Warehouse and the move to the Barbican. One also senses that his interests shifted during the 1980s. He stopped directing Brecht, Bond and other playwrights of the political left and sought a theatre of lightness, feeling, poetry and pure entertainment. After directing Brian Cox in John Whiting's *A Penny for a Song* on the Barbican's main stage (1986) he left the RSC for the National, where he began with a crowd-pleasing revival of Dion Boucicault's expert piece of blarney, *The Shaughraun* (1988). Inspired by the Olivier's revolving stage, Davies's designer, Bill Dudley, created a picturesque Irish cliff top and cottage that rose like a telescope and span like a spinning wheel. Davies directed the play as a sophisticated pantomime. Continuing at the National he was suddenly eclectic, directing Ibsen's *Hedda Gabler* (1989), David Hare's *The Secret Rapture* (1989), Shaw's *Pygmalion* (1992), Schiller's *Mary Stuart* (1996), and Wesker's *Chips With Everything* (1997), as well as two modern American classics—Tennessee Williams's *Cat on a Hot Tin Roof* (1988) and Arthur Miller's *The Crucible* (1990). American theatre has become his specialty in the sense that it has inspired his finest recent work—Edward Albee's *Who's Afraid of Virginia Woolf?* (1996) and Eugene O'Neill's *The Iceman Cometh* (1998) at the Almeida; O'Neill's *Mourning Becomes Electra* at the National (2003-04). As one of Nicholas Hytner's associates at the NT, he has also directed Rostand's *Cyrano de Bergerac* (2004), García Lorca's *The House of Bernarda Alba* (2005), Brecht's *Galileo* (2006), Gorky's *Philistines* (2007), and David Hare's *Gethsemane* (2008). In 1996 he returned to the RSC to direct Richard Nelson's *The General from America* in the Swan.

John Caird (b. Canada, 1948). John Caird's early childhood was spent in Montreal, where his father, a congregational minister and scholar, was teaching at McGill University. The family returned to England and to Oxford in 1959. Caird went to Magdalen College School and trained to be an actor in Bristol.

From 1974 to 76 he was an associate director at the Contact Theatre, Manchester, responsible for productions of *Look Back in Anger*, *Downright Hooligan* and *Twelfth Night*. He joined the RSC in 1977 to assist Ron Daniels (*'Tis Pity She's a Whore*; *The Lorenzaccio Story*) and Trevor Nunn. His contribution to Nunn's *As You Like It* (1977-79) was such that Nunn made him his co-director. During the next few years he became best known as Nunn's junior partner, co-directing *The Merry Wives of Windsor* (RST, 1979), *Nicholas Nickleby* (Aldwych, 1980), *Peter Pan* (Barbican, 1982) and *Les Misérables* (Barbican, 1985).

At the same time, in the studios, he directed Emrys James in Strindberg's *The Dance of Death* (1978), the young David Threlfall and Leslie Manville in Peter Flannery's *Savage Amusement* (1978), Alun Armstrong in *The Caucasian Chalk Circle* (1979), Mike Gwilym and Harriet Walter in Farquhar's *The Twin Rivals* (1981), and Flannery's *Our Friends in the North* (1982). In the main house he was responsible for an autumnal production of *Twelfth Night* (1983), beautifully acted by Emrys James, John Thaw, Daniel Massey, Miles Anderson, Zoë Wanamaker, Sarah Berger and Gemma Jones, and an exuberant, deliciously satirical production of *A Midsummer Night's Dream* (1989) — the forest was a junk yard, the fairies wore doc martins, tutus and pretend wings, and Mendelssohn's famous score was parodied by a rock band. In the Swan he led the Ben Jonson revival with robust productions of *Every Man in His Humour* (1986) and *The New Inn* (1987), and staged Gay's *The Beggar's Opera* (1992) as though it was *Les Misérables*.

Since the early 1990s he has worked most prominently at the National (from 1997 to 2000 he was Nunn's deputy in all but name): *Trelawny of the Wells* (Olivier, 1993); *The Seagull* (Olivier, 1994); *Stanley* (Cottesloe, 1996); *Peter Pan* (Olivier, 1997); *Candide* (Olivier, 1999); *Money* (Olivier, 1999); the Simon Russell Beale

Hamlet (Lyttelton, 2000); and Charlotte Jones's *Humble Boy* (Cottesloe, 2001).

Elsewhere, he has directed *Siegfried and Roy at the Mirage* (Las Vegas, 1989); *Children of Eden* (West End, 1991); Mozart's *Zaïdé* (Battignano, 1991); *Life Sentences* (New York, 1993); Shaw's *The Millionairess* (UK Tour, 1995); *Jane Eyre* (Toronto, 1996); Michael Weller's *What the Night is For* (Comedy, 2002); Anouilh's *Becket* (Theatre Royal Haymarket, 2004); and the Simon Russell Beale *Macbeth* (Almeida, 2005).

Bill Alexander (b. 1948) acted with The Other Company in London before winning a Thames Television Trainee Director bursary that took him to the Bristol Old Vic in 1973. Bristol was a good training ground for the RSC in the 1970s: Howard Davies was already there and Adrian Noble, also on a Thames bursary, was to succeed Alexander. Among the productions Alexander directed at Bristol were Simon Gray's *Butley* (starring Peter Postlethwaite and John Nettles), Noël Coward's *Blithe Spirit*, and Alan Ayckbourn's *How the Other Half Loves*. From Bristol he went briefly to the Royal Court, and then worked as a freelance director. In 1977 he joined the RSC. As Resident Director he concentrated on new plays in the studio theatres. Three productions with Antony Sher enhanced his reputation: *Molière* (TOP, 1982), *Tartuffe* (Pit, 1983), and *Richard III* (RST, 1984).

Alexander followed *Richard III*, a solid reading enlivened by Sher's *tour de force*, with two further successes, *The Merry Wives of Windsor* (RST, 1985) and *The Merchant of Venice* (RST, 1987). The first was ingeniously set in the 1950s; the second targeted the racism of the Christian characters. *A Midsummer Night's Dream* (RST, 1986) initially featured a pretty forest out of Arthur Rackham; in London Alexander abandoned this entirely and set much of the play on a black stage with the actors picked out by spot lighting. *Twelfth Night* (RST, 1987) and *Much Ado About Nothing* (RST, 1990) featured exceptional casts but were hampered by permanent sets and pictorial predictability.

Alexander was responsible for the 1988 London season, and he was a strong contender for the top position when Terry Hands announced his resignation. From 1992 to 2000 he was Artistic Director of the Birmingham Rep. A skilled administrator, he rejuvenated the Rep by casting RSC actors, programming successes such as Janet Suzman's *The Cherry Orchard* (1997) and Lucy Bailey's *Baby Doll* (1999), establishing a new writing policy for the reconfigured studio (The Door, 1998), winning lottery funding to improve the building (1999), holding free events and open days, and staging impressive productions of *Othello* (with Jeffery Kissoon) and *Hamlet* (with Richard McCabe and Gerard Murphy). His other productions at the Rep were *Volpone* (1993), *Old Times* (1993), *The Snowman* (1993), *The Tempest* (1994), *Macbeth* (1995), *The Way of the World* (1995), *The Alchemist* (1996), *The Nativity* (1999), and *Twelfth Night* (2000).

Since leaving the Rep Alexander has directed Shelagh Stephenson's *Mappa Mundi* at the National (Cottesloe, 2002), and *Titus Andronicus* and *King Lear* at the RSC (RST, 2003, 2004).

Adrian Noble (b. Chichester, 1950). Adrian Noble's original, visually compelling productions of the classics dominated the RSC's main stage from 1982 to 2002. At a time when most directors, confronted by the size of the RST, sought refuge in permanent sets, Noble kept the stage bare and open to the back wall. Stark but striking scenography, the metaphorical use of objects and colour, and the fluent elision of scenes, made his work highly distinctive.

The son of an undertaker, Noble studied at Bristol University and the Drama Centre, London, and began his career working in community theatre in Birmingham. He came to the RSC from the Bristol Old Vic, where he had directed Brecht's *Man is Man* (1976) and *Ubu Rex* (1977); Shakespeare's *Titus Andronicus* (1978) and *Timon of Athens* (1979); Arthur Miller's *A View From the Bridge* (1978); Middleton and Rowley's *The Changeling* (1978); Congreve's *Love for Love* (1979); and Farquhar's *The Recruiting*

Officer (1979). At the RSC he started as an assistant director but was quickly brought into the directorial team after the success of his Manchester Royal Exchange productions of *The Duchess of Malfi* (1980), with Helen Mirren and Bob Hoskins, and *Doctor Faustus* (1981), with Ben Kingsley. He directed two acclaimed productions in The Other Place, Ostrovsky's *The Forest* and Ibsen's *A Doll's House* (both 1981), then his first main house production, the Michael Gambon/Antony Sher *King Lear* (1982). Noble created a unique theatrical world for the play through the imaginative use of images (such as Lear's discarded workman's boots, which remained on stage). The expression of ideas in visual terms is a common factor in his work. *Measure for Measure* (RST, 1983) featured 18th century clothes and a beautiful cyclorama, but also a prison wall, modern lamps and an electric chair; *Henry V* (RST, 1984) magnificent tableaux of banners and light juxtaposed with images showing the realism of war (soldiers huddled together beneath tarpaulin in driving rain); and *Macbeth* (RST, 1986), starring Jonathan Pryce and Sinéad Cusack, the recurring motif of small children, a black mass for the witches and a black set which gradually contracted until long spears pierced the walls. *Macbeth* and *As You Like It* (RST, 1985)—modern-dress, parachute silk, an Arden that in all respects but colour mirrored the court—showed Noble's preoccupation with metaphors and dreams.

The Plantagenets (RST, 1988), a trilogy drawn from the *Henry VI* plays and *Richard III*, was more traditionally conceived, but the visual storytelling was unmistakably the work of the Adrian Noble/Bob Crowley partnership. Towards the end of the second play the white floor cloth, by now smeared with blood like a butcher's apron, was lifted to hang as a backcloth against which the shadow of Anton Lesser's Richard edged towards Ralph Fiennes's Henry, imprisoned in a cage that rose up to the flies. The second play closed with a blackout following Richard's triumphant cry of 'Now', the first word of the third, which opened with a sudden lights-up. From the top of a table Richard began 'Now is the winter...' as a public speech, only to jump down to address the audience, the other characters frozen in time. If there was a feeling that *The Plantagenets* repeated an earlier RSC triumph (*The Wars of the Roses*), Noble's production of *The Master Builder* (Barbican, 1989) with John Wood and Joanne Pearce was inimitable—lucid, poetic and erotic.

In his first three years as Artistic Director Noble directed *Henry IV, The Thebans, The Winter's Tale, Hamlet,* and *King Lear*. In the *Henries* (RST, 1991) the décor was colour-coded, grey for the court, red for the tavern. Gads Hill was represented by misty blue light and a corpse tied to a post. One example of the production's cinematic style: as Henry's corpse was carried from his death chamber the scene 'dissolved' into Shallow's orchard (beekeepers like ghosts). *The Winter's Tale* (RST, 1992) featured a gauze cube of travelling clouds, in which figures were conjured, and the recurrent use of coloured balloons. The play's contrasts were achieved with rapid transitions, and the overall theme of redemption was movingly realised. *Hamlet* (Barbican, 1992), set in the early 20th century with references to Ibsen and Munch, found visual equivalents for the themes of decay and death. The ash-grey set of the last act—a grey sheet covered the stage until Ophelia (Joanne Pearce) pulled it away to reveal decayed funeral wreaths and the upright piano she had played in Act One—provided an atmosphere of loss and sterility. Hamlet (Branagh, never better) met the players at a railway station—a reference to RSC history, since every spring from 1886 to 1919 Stratford people met Frank Benson's company at the station. The early performances ended with Hamlet and the other victims of the play forming a group at the rear of the stage, a tableau that suggested a sepia photograph of long dead figures, but this idea was abandoned by the time of the press night. Noble's second version of *King Lear* (RST, 1993) was more direct, less radical, than the 1982 production. A sense of humankind's insignificance in the cosmos was conveyed by the massive planetary symbol that dominated the play, spectacularly fracturing to pour sand after Gloucester's blinding. Real rain during the storm, graphic acts of violence throughout. The interpretation complimented the haunted and haunting performance, his last, of Robert Stephens.

A Midsummer Night's Dream (RST, 1994) featured inappropriate objects (a 'forest' of swaying light bulbs, umbrellas, doors without rooms) and electric colours. It was dazzling but the fine cast of young actors found it difficult to flesh out their characters. *Romeo and Juliet* (RST, 1995) was dark and original, but the 19th century setting was a mixed blessing. *Cymbeline* (RST, 1997) was staged as both a fable and a dream: a billowing white cloth rose and fell within a wide sky-blue box. *Twelfth Night* (RST, 1997) lacked the cinematic flow usually associated with Noble. Its originality lay in its rejection of autumnal melancholy for a brightly-coloured setting in which cruelty and pain were not hidden beneath nostalgia. The garish costumes fixed the actors within predictable archetypes. In the Swan Noble delivered intimate, beautifully choreographed productions of Chekhov, Ibsen and T.S. Eliot.

Adrian Noble succeeded Terry Hands as Artistic Director in 1991 (he had been the clear favourite for some time, and had successfully directed the 1988-89 season). His period in charge was one of innovation and controversy, culminating in the RSC's first fundamental change of direction since 1960/61: the redevelopment of Stratford (creating new theatres and a training academy for young actors), the withdrawal from the Barbican (leaving the RSC without a London home, but with more flexibility to open new productions in appropriate performing spaces), and the introduction of a structure based around short contracts and one-off productions (to suit the working lives of actors, particularly the Company's senior alumni).

His appointment continued the Stratford tradition of promoting from within. Terry Hands advocated joint artistic directors, but Noble rejected this option, preferring to work with an Executive Producer, effectively a deputy (Michael Attenborough, an outsider, was appointed), and a General Manager (David Brierley). Two producers, Lynda Farran and Nicky Pallot, were brought in to oversee productions and to form new links between acting companies and management. Noble disbanded the team of associate directors (some had left anyway, and all remained connected to the RSC as honorary associates), and worked on his first season (1991) with newcomers, although Trevor Nunn returned to open the new Other Place.

Noble initially focused on the classical repertory. Some commentators misread this as a rejection of new work. Like Trevor Nunn in 1969, Noble was concentrating on first principles and needed time to find and commission work of sufficient merit and originality. He was not interested in perpetuating the outdated view that serious theatre should first and foremost be political, a left-wing monitor of the state of the nation. So much of post-war British drama and theatre had been parochial, polemical, earnest, worthy and theatrically dull. At the RSC, beginning in the 1980s, one could detect a more sophisticated European attitude, a belief in a theatre of ideas, style and sensuality. His first major innovation came in 1995 with the decision to withdraw from the Barbican for six months of the year and to set up a second provincial residency (Plymouth). The objectives of the change, which came into operation in 1997, were to increase access to a national company, to address the problem of the Barbican's unpopularity, and to focus attention on Stratford. Noble had tried to make the Barbican a success with the public by scheduling prestigious revivals (including the Branagh *Hamlet*) and by organising a festival called *Everyone's Shakespeare*, but attitudes remained stubbornly negative. It had become increasingly difficult to risk anything other than Stratford transfers.

Noble's decision to run the Stratford season from autumn to autumn (1996) was not successful. From 1999 the Stratford year was divided between winter and summer seasons. Over time, like Trevor Nunn and Terry Hands before him, he established a new team of associate directors (Michael Attenborough, Katie Mitchell, Steven Pimlott, Michael Boyd and Gregory Doran). This was a clear achievement, allowing the creative management of the RSC to be shared (by 2000 the structures were strong enough for Noble to spend part of the year in Aix-en-Provence, directing Monteverdi's *Le retour d'Ulysse dans sa patrie*). In 1997 he announced plans to develop the old Collins Music Hall in Islington as a new London home for the RSC. The lottery commission turned down the bid, but agreed to part-finance the re-building of the RST.

Dissatisfaction with the main house had increased in the 1990s. Too few directors could master the space, and actors compared it unfavourably with the Swan. The theatre was forbidding from the balcony. By 2000 it was clear that the RSC had a preference for the most radical solution: a new RST, a new TOP, and a centre for training, to be designed by the Dutch architect Erick van Egeraat. The Arts Council turned down an initial application for funding, but agreed to contribute £755,140 towards the cost of a feasibility study in May 2000. Donations from individuals, from Advantage West Midlands (£304,000), Stratford District Council (£50,000), and Warwickshire County Council (£50,000), completed the £3.3 million total. The Arts Council agreed to earmark £50 million to the cost of the development, which left the RSC needing to raise the same amount (nearly £30 million had been promised by 2000). The feasibility study, carried out in 2001, produced a business plan and a scheme for the surrounding roads and public places. The RSC consulted its staff, audience and the local community.

In the meantime new attempts were made to improve the actor-audience relationship. In 1999 the stage was re-designed to become a semi-circular disk stretching into the stalls. It worked, but was cautious, a denial of the full depth of the stage and that great back wall. In 2001 the forestage was brought forward by seventeen feet and extended across the whole width of the auditorium (fifty feet) to create a wide and long acting area in front of the proscenium. At the same time the full depth of the stage behind the proscenium was utilised. Both the stage and auditorium (designed by Alison Chitty) were painted the same shade of grey. 2002 saw the return of the standard configuration.

During the 1990s Noble's RSC was gradually becoming smaller, less a play factory, than the Company he had inherited. Peter Hall returned in 1992 and 1995 (his first main stage production since 1967), and directed John Barton's *Tantalus* in 2000. Barton himself directed a fine *Peer Gynt* in 1994, and his verse workshops (based on Shakespeare's sonnets) once more became an integral part of RSC life in Stratford. In this way the RSC was moving forward while acknowledging the past. Major classical actors—Robert Stephens, Antony Sher, Kenneth Branagh, David Troughton, David Calder, Philip Voss, Joanne Pearce, Samantha Bond, Harriet Walter—were doing their best work; exciting younger players—Toby Stephens, Jeremy Northam, Joseph Fiennes, Ray Fearon, William Houston, Emma Fielding, Alexandra Gilbreath, Emily Watson, Olivia Williams, Zoë Waites—were emerging; important playwrights—David Edgar, Peter Whelan, Richard Nelson, Ann Devlin, Martin McDonagh, David Greig, Robert Holman—were under commission. The complete history play cycle (2000/01) and The Other Place season of new plays by Peter Whelan, Martin McDonagh and David Edgar (2001) received particular acclaim.

Then, in May 2001, came the announcement of radical change. The replacement of the RST proved the controversial tenet of 'Project Fleet', in that it received most of the publicity and provoked letters of protest from Judi Dench and Donald Sinden. Noble's plan to modernise the Stratford theatre and its environs to the highest European standards fell victim to a conservative alliance of Stratford pensioners (who formed a protest group called HOOT or 'Hands Off Our Theatre'), theatre critics, and a few veteran star actors. However, it was Noble's decision to make the RSC homeless in London and to divide the ensemble into temporary units that caused the real concern. To what extent would the RSC remain a genuine company? And would the artistic results be worth the cost (redundancies and the destruction of the Stratford theatre's century-old sense of community)?

Despite the turmoil within the RSC, the work produced by the changes was of a high quality. The productions at the Roundhouse were fascinatingly diverse, and Gregory Doran's Jacobean season was unforgettable. However, poor attendances in London exposed the recklessness of a policy that depended upon box office hits. More importantly, Noble's loss of support within the Company was compounded by his decision to direct *Chitty Chitty Bang Bang* in the West End. Criticism, much of it personal and vitriolic, snowballed, and in March 2002 Noble announced that he would step down at the end of his contract in March 2003. With hindsight the resignation looks inevitable, but the feeling persists that Michael Boyd will benefit from Noble's decision to break the mould at the RSC. The conveyor belt transfer of productions from Stratford to the Barbican had become a deadening routine, predictable and inflexible.

Noble closed his RSC career with Ibsen's *Brand* (Swan, 2003). He has since directed Oscar Wilde's *A Woman of No Importance* (Theatre Royal Haymarket, 2003); Mozart's *Die Zauberflöte* (Glyndebourne, 2004); Brian Friel's *The Home Place* (Gate, Dublin, 2005); Verdi's *Falstaff* (Göteborg Opera, 2005); a Mozart-Da Ponte cycle conducted by William Christie at the Opéra national de Lyon (*Cosi fan tutte*, 2006; *Le nozze di Figaro*, 2007); Tennessee Williams's *Summer and Smoke* (Nottingham Playhouse, 2006); Sartre's *Kean* (West End, 2007); Verdi's *Macbeth* (Met, New York, 2007-08); and *Hamlet* (Stratford Shakespeare Festival, Ontario, Canada, 2008).

Michael Attenborough (b. 1950) was president of the drama society at Sussex University and began his career at the Mercury Theatre, Colchester. As an associate director at the Leeds Playhouse (1974-79) he directed Shakespeare, Shaw, Chekhov and new plays by Willy Russell and Alan Bleasdale. He worked for a year at the Young Vic under Michael Bogdanov, directing *The Merchant of Venice* and *What the Butler Saw*, before taking up the position of Artistic Director at the Palace Theatre, Watford

(1980-84). Productions at Watford included *The Girl in Melanie Klein*, *The Big Knife*, *Romantic Comedy*, and *Terra Nova*. From 1984 to 1989 he ran the Hampstead Theatre to constant acclaim, revealing a knack for selecting important new plays. Most notably he directed Frank McGuinness's *Observe the Sons of Ulster Marching Towards the Somme* (1986) with John Bowe and Ciaran Hinds, and Tom Kempinski's *Separation* (1986) with David Suchet and Saskia Reeves. He was briefly Artistic Director of the Turnstyle Group before joining the RSC as Adrian Noble's deputy (1991).

His brief covered casting, publicity, the commissioning of new writing, and producing. In 1996 he stepped back from administration to concentrate on directing. His work was initially confined to the smaller spaces. *Amphibians* (Pit, 1992), *The Changeling* (Swan, 1992), *After Easter* (TOP, 1994) and David Edgar's *Pentecost*, (TOP, 1994) were followed by two impressive hits, Peter Whelan's *The Herbal Bed* (TOP, 1996) and *Romeo and Juliet* (Pit, 1997). Both featured strong performances from young actors (Teresa Banham, Joseph Fiennes; Zoë Waites, Ray Fearon). Attenborough's concept for *Romeo and Juliet* (rural Italy in the first decades of the 20th century) refashioned an overexposed play.

Attenborough reunited Ray Fearon and Zoë Waites for *Othello*, his first main house production (1999). Impressive use was made of the season's stage configuration, a white disk jutting out into the stalls. The stage was divided by a row of tall flagpoles; canvas screens were lowered for the interior scenes. The production was set in the early years of the 20th century and had the feel of a garrison town in a desert region of the British Empire (one could detect the influence of the films of his father, Sir Richard Attenborough). The handsome uncluttered design made evocative use of desert yellows and night blues. Othello and Desdemona strolled beneath fireworks. The gulling of Cassius was brilliantly staged as a regimental party. It was gripping, well-spoken and only lacked a sense of visceral horror. The mutually enthralled young leads, frozen in the sights of Richard McCabe's Iago, gave the play an unusual poignancy.

In 2002 Attenborough succeeded Jonathan Kent and Ian McDiarmid as Artistic Director of the Almeida.

Steven Pimlott (1953-2007, b. Manchester). In a profession of artistic schizophrenics Steven Pimlott had more personalities than most: a skilled organiser of big shows at the trashier end of the music theatre industry (*Carmen* at Earl's Court; *Doctor Dolittle* at the Hammersmith Apollo), he also championed the work of Phyllis Nagy, and directed thought-provoking productions of Shakespeare, T.S. Eliot and Tennessee Williams.

Pimlott was educated at Manchester Grammar School and Sidney Sussex College, Cambridge. His career began in opera. He was a staff producer at ENO (1976-78) before making his name at Opera North (1978-80)—Puccini's *La bohème* and *Tosca*, Verdi's *Nabucco*, and Massenet's *Werther*. It wasn't until the late 1980s that he achieved notice as an interpreter of plays. In particular, as an associate director at the Sheffield Crucible, he directed delightfully strange, visually poetic productions of Shakespeare's *Twelfth Night* and *The Winter's Tale*, and Botho Strauss's *The Park* (1987-88).

The quality of this work took him to the National in 1989/90—*Sunday in the Park with George* (Lyttelton), *The Miser* (Olivier)—and to the RSC in 1990. For the next twelve years he worked alongside Adrian Noble. The Germanic monumentalism of *Julius Caesar*, his first RSC production (1990), was quickly abandoned. T.S. Eliot's *Murder in the Cathedral* (Swan, 1993) and Shakespeare's *Measure for Measure* (RST, 1994), both set in the 1930s, were theatre *noirs*, sombre in tone but thrilling as dramatic stories. *Richard II* (TOP, 2000) and *Hamlet* (RST, 2001) were performed on plain, laboratory-like sets. The style was iconoclastic and contemporary.

Pimlott was co-artistic director of the Chichester Festival Theatre from 2003 to 05.

Katie Mitchell (b. Reading, 1964). For a time, during the 1990s, it looked as if the future of the RSC would rest on the shoulders of Katie Mitchell. She went from one heavyweight text to another, surveying each with the precise, fearless eye of a surgeon. Shakespeare, Ibsen, Strindberg, Greek tragedy, the Mysteries, Samuel Beckett. Katie Mitchell is unlikely to direct a light comedy.

She likes sombre colours (particularly grey and brown), half-light, religious imagery, East European folk music and dance. She can create powerful images but she is most interested in the way people think and interact. She prefers studio theatres, intimate spaces, the theatrical equivalents of X-ray machines.

Katie Mitchell was educated at Magdalen College, Oxford. She joined the RSC in 1988 as an assistant director. She assisted Adrian Noble on *The Master Builder* (1989), and became an associate director in 1996. At The Other Place and Pit she directed Thomas Heywood's *A Woman Killed With Kindness* (1991), Ibsen's *Ghosts* (1992), Strindberg's *Easter* (1995), and *The Mysteries* (1997), bringing to each her clinical eye but also, paradoxically, passion. Jane Lapotaire, Simon Russell Beale, Joanne Pearce and Lucy Whybrow are among the actors who have given intense performances under her guidance.

Since the late 1990s Katie Mitchell has worked most prominently at the National: *Rutherford and Son* (Cottesloe, 1994); *The Machine Wreckers* (Cottesloe, 1995); Ted Hughes's version of *The Oresteia* (Cottesloe, 1999); Chekhov's *Ivanov* (Cottesloe, 2002), *Three Sisters* (Lyttelton, 2003) and *The Seagull* (Lyttelton, 2006); Euripides's *Iphigenia at Aulis* (Lyttelton, 2004) and *Women of Troy* (Lyttelton, 2007); Caryl Churchill's version of Strindberg's *A Dream Play* (Cottesloe, 2005); and an adaptation of Virginia Woolf's *Waves* (Cottesloe, 2006-07).

Gregory Doran (b. Huddersfield, 1958). Following his student years at Bristol University and the Bristol Old Vic Theatre

School, Gregory Doran acted on stages in Nottingham, York, Harrogate and Leeds (roles included Marchbanks in *Candida*, Cosway in *Scenes from a Voyage to the Indies*, and Albert in *Albert's Bridge*). His early directing assignments gave a better indication of his ambition. As an associate director at the Nottingham Playhouse (1980-86) he directed *Long Day's Journey into Night*, *Waiting for Godot* and Alan Ayckbourn's *The Norman Conquests*; while productions elsewhere included *A Midsummer Night's Dream* (State University of New York), *The Booke of Sir Thomas Moore* (Young Vic), *Romeo and Juliet* (Mayfair Theatre), and *The Atheist's Tragedy* (Bristol). In 1987 he joined the RSC to play Solanio in *The Merchant of Venice* (Bill Alexander, RST); Octavius in *Julius Caesar* (Terry Hands, RST); Don Mathias/Bashaw in Marlowe's *The Jew of Malta* (Barry Kyle, Swan); and Beaufort in Jonson's *The New Inn* (John Caird, Swan). He continued at the RSC as an assistant director, working on Bill Alexander's *Cymbeline* in the RST, Terry Hands's *Romeo and Juliet* and Barry Kyle's *Dr Faustus* in the Swan, and Janice Honeyman's *Have* in the Pit (all 1989). He worked as a freelance director for a few years, before directing his first RSC production in 1992. He joined the team of associate directors in 1997.

Doran's productions are compellingly direct. *The Odyssey* (TOP, 1992) started as a workshop on Homer (1991) and ended as a play by Derek Walcott. *Titus Andronicus* (Market Theatre, Johannesburg/NT Studio, 1995), a multi-racial, modern-dress production featuring Antony Sher, was influenced by the recent history of South Africa (the concept became strained). *Henry VIII* (Swan, 1996) re-established an underrated play. *The Winter's Tale* (RST, 1998), with Sher as a Leontes, was set mostly in a receding tunnel below a billowing canopy of grey silk. Sombre and oppressive, the first half of the play was beautifully realised. Because there was little sense of unity between the two halves (curiously and fatally, Autolycus was erased from the final act) the ending lacked impact. The same actress played the boy Mamillius (in a wheelchair) and Perdita, an original stroke. *Macbeth* (Swan, 1999) was a basic reading, fast, ferocious and set predictably in perpetual night. Its bare boards, expressionistic lighting and all-round dynamism owed much to Terry Hands. It began with an unforgettable coup—a sudden and total blackout of the stage *and* auditorium (the witches were heard but not seen).

As part of the reforms of 2002, Adrian Noble asked Doran to take charge of a season of neglected plays in the Swan. A dedicated ensemble of twenty-eight actors was formed to perform five works—Shakespeare's *Edward III*, Jonson's *Eastward Ho!*, Massinger's *The Roman Actor*, Fletcher's *The Island Princess*, and Marston's *The Malcontent*. In an attempt to replicate the fluent working methods of the Jacobean stage (and to get the full repertoire on the stage quickly), Doran asked his actors and fellow directors to create a production after only three weeks of rehearsal. Born under the vitriolic criticism of the reforms and threatened in its first weeks of rehearsal by the illness of one director and the resignation of another, Doran's brilliant project defied all expectations.

For a few years Doran seemed the most articulate director of Shakespeare of his generation. The illuminating pairing of Shakespeare's *Shrew* and Fletcher's *The Tamer Tamed* (Swan, 2003) was typical of an artist who is passionate about the language and history of English classical theatre. *All's Well That Ends Well* (2003), with Judi Dench as the Countess, was handsome, lyrical and alive to the haunting peculiarity of 'problem' Shakespeare. But the theatre is a merciless art form. Doran's musical *Merry Wives of Windsor* (RST, 2006) was a rare unqualified failure, and *A Midsummer Night's Dream*, although excellent in the RST (2005), came across as forced, over-acted and visually uninspired when revived in the Courtyard (admittedly a minority view—most spectators, being so visible in this theatre, seem to feel obliged to have a good time). *Hamlet*, built around the popularity of David Tennant, likewise suffered from the party atmosphere in the galleries (2008).

Michael Boyd (b. Belfast, 1955). Michael Boyd was born in Northern Ireland, the son of a doctor who moved his family to London and then to Scotland. He directed student productions at Edinburgh University and, funded by the British Council, studied under Anatoly Efros at the Malaya Bronnaya Theatre in Moscow (1979).

His early work included Ron Hutchinson's *Risky City* and *The Mystery Plays* at the Belgrade, Coventry (1980-82), and Marcella Evaristi's *Hard to Get* at the Traverse, Edinburgh (1980). As an associate director at the Sheffield Crucible he directed *A Midsummer Night's Dream* and Howard Barker's *A Passion in Six Days* (1983).

His directorship of Glasgow's Tron from 1985 to 1996 established a major new theatre and provided a showcase for contemporary Scottish writing. In a theatrical style influenced by performance art, dance and music, he directed Chris Hannan's *The Baby*; Iain Heggie's *Clyde Nouveau*; Peter Arnott's *Losing Alec*; Alasdair Gray's *McGrotty and Ludmilla*; Michel Tremblay's *The Guid Sisters* and *The Real Wurld*; an adaptation of Ted Hughes's *Crow*; C.P. Taylor's *Good*; and *The Trick is to Keep Breathing*, his own adaptation of Janice Galloway's novel. His most famous production at the Tron was the Iain Glen *Macbeth* (1993).

In 1994 he directed his first RSC production, John Ford's tragedy *The Broken Heart* (Swan). Performed in period costumes, the production's formal dances were juxtaposed against modern music by his regular collaborator Craig Armstrong (sustained notes on the strings, creating a mood of menace)—a brilliant stroke. Ford's suffering people were movingly brought to life by a fine cast (Iain Glen, Emma Fielding, Olivia Williams). *Much Ado About Nothing* (RST, 1996), his inaugural production as an RSC associate, was notable for its darkness of tone. *Measure for Measure* (RST, 1998) concentrated on paranoia and danger, on personal and public breakdown. The play was set in an enclosed space until the final moments, when the full depth of the stage was revealed—the Duke and Isabella walked slowly away into this previously hidden world. In *A Midsummer Night's Dream* (RST, 1999) the forest was a laboratory of desire, sensuality and transformation. Roses bloomed from the floorboards; fairies—mostly aroused girls in modern dress—burst through trap doors. Boyd began the play in monochrome and ended it with the abandonment of an intimate dance. *Romeo and Juliet* (RST, 2000) was set, less successfully, in a similar off-white space bounded by two curved walls: there were telling ideas—sombre music (solo cello) accompanied the Mercutio/Tybalt fight—but the Romeo and Juliet of David Tennant and Alexandra Gilbreath were too mature.

He is fascinated by the macabre. The murdered heroine of *The Broken Heart* sat beside a table of decaying food as the buzz of flies filled the auditorium. The murdered of *The Spanish Tragedy* (Swan, 1997), doomed, one by one, in purgatory, to re-live the terrible events, waited silently behind a blood-red curtain. Similarly, the ghosts of Mercutio and Tybalt witnessed the final scenes of *Romeo and Juliet*. In 2000/01 he staged the three parts of *Henry VI* and *Richard III* (Swan and Young Vic).

In April 2003 Michael Boyd succeeded Adrian Noble as artistic director. He may have been chosen over the other leading candidate, Gregory Doran, because his production style seems, on the surface, to be more original. The fact that Doran stayed on meant that Boyd was able to spend the first year of his directorship reviewing all aspects of the RSC's operation. He kept Noble's summer and winter seasons, and the shorter contracts, but abandoned the scheme to build a new RST in favour of the conversion of the existing building. For reasons that remain unclear, he split the company into RST and Swan Theatre ensembles. The former was designated the 'core' company. He devoted his first main house summer season (2004) to the tragedies, and his second (2005) to the comedies. Then, for 2006/07, he organised a Shakespeare complete works festival in Stratford. Visiting companies joined the RSC in the performing of all of Shakespeare's plays. This grand project generated good publicity, but its artistic value was weakened by the inclusion of too few major productions from abroad and by the decision to fragment the RSC into many separate ensembles. One of those ensembles revived Boyd's 2000/01 productions of the three parts *Henry VI* and *Richard III*. Boyd kept the group together and staged *Richard II*, the two parts of *Henry IV* and *Henry V* in Stratford during 2007. Then, early in 2008, all eight history plays were performed in sequence at the Roundhouse in London.

The rebuilding and opening of the RST will occupy Boyd during the next few years. He chose a 'courtyard' configuration for the new theatre. His tenure will be judged on the consequences of that decision.

Part Two: Dictionary

A

Joss Ackland (b. London, 1928). As a character actor in British and American films, Joss Ackland has brought weight to a string of insubstantial roles. He is physically imposing, expert at accents, and can seem authentic even when playing a caricature: his Mafia chief in *The Sicilian* (Michael Cimino, 1987) and South African in *Lethal Weapon 2* (Richard Donner, 1989) are the prime examples. He was seen at his best as the betrayed husband— emotion kept in check behind a polite smile and a rigid dress code—in the colonial Kenya of *White Mischief* (Michael Radford, 1987).

Perhaps an unlikely actor, his early years in the English theatre were interrupted by a spell in Africa: he worked as a tea planter in Malawi (1954) and as a disc jockey in South Africa (1955-57). On his return he joined the Oxford Playhouse Company and then the Old Vic (1958-61), where his roles included Falstaff, Sir Toby Belch, Caliban and Pistol. He was an associate director and a leading actor at the Mermaid Theatre from 1961 to 1963. His commitment to the stage has diminished over the years. In middle age he showed an appetite for musicals: Frederick in *A Little Night Music* (1975-76), Perón in *Evita* (1978), and Romain Gary in *Jean Seberg* (Peter Hall, NT Olivier, 1983).

His two periods of work with the RSC were separated by thirty-five years. At the beginning of his career he was a member of the 1947 Stratford company—he played Beelzebub in a production of *Doctor Faustus* (Walter Hudd) which also featured Paul Scofield and Donald Sinden—and he returned to the RSC thirty-five years later to play a formidable Falstaff in the two parts of *Henry IV* (Trevor Nunn, 1982), the Barbican's opening production. Later in the season he played Captain Cook and Mr Darling in *Peter Pan* (Nunn and John Caird).

Jenny Agutter (b. Taunton, 1952). A movie actress from an early age, Jenny Agutter came to notice playing the eldest daughter in *The Railway Children* (Lionel Jeffries, 1970). In Nicholas Roeg's *Walkabout* (1971) she was leggy, sunburnt and innocently provocative as the schoolgirl abandoned in the Outback. Among her later films were *The Eagle Has Landed* (1976), *Logan's Run* (1976), *Equus* (Sidney Lumet, 1977), *The Riddle of the Sands* (1979), and *An American Werewolf in London* (John Landis, 1981).

From 1972 to 75, when she was in most demand as a film actress, she concentrated on the stage, appearing in productions of *The School for Scandal*, *Rooted*, *Arms and the Man* and *The Ride Across Lake Constance* before joining the National Theatre at the Old Vic for Peter Hall's first season as director (1974): Miranda to John Gielgud's Prospero in *The Tempest* (Hall), and *Spring Awakening* (Bill Bryden). This was the beginning of an occasional stage career. She has appeared in *Hedda Gabler* at the Roundhouse (Charles Marowitz, 1980), *Breaking the Code* on Broadway (1987), *Peter Pan* on the South Bank (John Caird, Olivier, 1997-98), and *Equus* at the Gielgud Theatre (Thea Sharrock, 2007). Her longest commitment was made to the RSC, where in 1982/83 she gave memorable performances as Regan in *King Lear* (Adrian Noble, RST); Alice, an Elizabethan *femme fatale*, in *Arden of Faversham* (Terry Hands, TOP); Fontanelle in Edward Bond's *Lear* (Barry Kyle, TOP); and Grace in Nick Darke's *The Body* (Nick Hamm, Pit). In 1985 she played Polya in Stephen Poliakoff's *Breaking the Silence* (Ron Daniels, Mermaid); in 1995, the Princess of France in *Love's Labour's Lost* (Ian Judge, Barbican).

Bruce Alexander is one of those invisible craftsmen of the stage who belong to no obvious type, and who appear to follow no method or technique—in other words, he is an actor whose great skill is simply to put on the character with the costume. During seven years with the RSC, the best and most sustained theatre work of his career, he conjured characters who were funny, loathsome, pitiable and dangerous (sometimes all at once): McCarthy in *The Time of Your Life* (Howard Davies, TOP, 1983); Norfolk in *Henry VIII* (Davies, RST, 1983); Canon Melville/Black George in *The Dillen* (Barry Kyle, TOP, 1983); Sir Politic Would-Be in *Volpone* (Bill Alexander, TOP, 1983); Tupik/Stanislas in Charles Wood's *Red Star* (John Caird, Pit, 1984); Swiss Cheese in *Mother Courage* (Davies, Barbican, 1984); Justin O'Connell in *Waste* (John Barton, Pit, 1985); Sir Hugh Evans in *The Merry Wives of Windsor* (Alexander, RST, 1985); Oliver in *As You Like It* (Adrian Noble, RST, 1985); Diomedes in *Troilus and Cressida* (Davies, RST, 1985); Bonifacio in *Il Candelaio* (Clifford Williams, Pit, 1986); Hank opposite Frances Barber in Nick Darke's two-hander *The Dead Monkey* (Roger Michell, Pit, 1986); Feste in *Twelfth Night* (Alexander, RST, 1987); Tranio in *The Taming of the Shrew* (Jonathan Miller, RST, 1987); Cloten in *Cymbeline* (Alexander, TOP, 1987); Prozorov in *Three Sisters* (Barton, Barbican, 1988); Parolles in *All's Well that End's Well* (Kyle, RST, 1989); and Ferdinand in the Harriet Walter *Duchess of Malfi* (Alexander, Swan, 1989).

Alexander's earlier theatre appearances included Joint Stock's productions of David Hare's *Fanshen* (1975) and Stephen Lowe's *The Ragged Trousered Philanthropists* (William Gaskill, 1978); and Gaskill's *A Fair Quarrel* at the National (Olivier, 1979).

In the 1990s his career was dominated by the long-running series *Frost* (ITV), in which he played Superintendent Mullett. Since 2000 he has been back on the stage: Cauchon in *Saint Joan* (Anthony Clark, Birmingham Rep, 2000); Alonso in *The Tempest* (Jonathan Kent, Almeida, 2001); Kent in *King Lear* (Barry Kyle,

Globe, 2001); Lockit in Vaclav Havel's version of *The Beggar's Opera* (Geoffrey Beevers, Orange Tree, Richmond, 2003); Huxley in Crispin Whittel's *Darwin in Malibu* (Birmingham Rep, 2003); and Cleon/Bawd in *Pericles* (Neil Bartlett, Lyric Hammersmith, 2003).

Roger Allam (b. London, 1953). One of the leading Shakespeareans of his generation, with few equals as a verse-speaker, Roger Allam is also a versatile exponent of character types—his range extends from musicals to television comedy.

He studied drama at Manchester University and gained his early experience at the Contact Theatre, the Birmingham Rep and the Glasgow Citizens' (roles included Macbeth, Angelo in *Measure for Measure*, Macheath in *The Threepenny Opera*, and the Sheriff of Nottingham in *Babes in the Wood*). In 1975 he co-founded the feminist company Monstrous Regiment. His work on the fringe included Marcel in *Scum*, Mr Packer in *Vinegar Tom*, Carl in *Kiss and Kill*, Wilby in *Sus* (Soho Poly), and Angelo in *Oona Pooka* (Tricycle).

Allam joined the RSC in 1981 and became an associate artist in 1989. He has given distinctive and expressive accounts of Mercutio in *Romeo and Juliet* (John Caird, Small-scale Tour, 1983); Clarence in the Antony Sher *Richard III* (Bill Alexander, RST, 1984); Brutus in *Julius Caesar* (Hands, RST, 1987); Sir Toby Belch in *Twelfth Night* (Alexander, RST, 1987); the Duke to Josette Simon's Isabella in *Measure for Measure* (Nicholas Hytner, RST, 1987); Benedick to Susan Fleetwood's Beatrice in *Much Ado About Nothing* (Alexander, RST, 1990); Trigorin in *The Seagull* (Hands, Swan, 1990); Trissotin in Molière's *The Learned Ladies* (Steven Pimlott, TOP, 1996); and Macbeth (Tim Albery, RST, 1996). Alongside this classical work, Allam starred as Javert in *Les Misérables* (Nunn/Caird, Barbican, 1985) and took parts in a number of contemporary plays: Conrad/Browne/Kruger in Peter Flannery's *Our Friends in the North* (John Caird, TOP, 1982); Lin Tse-Tsii in Peter Nichols's *Poppy* (Terry Hands, Barbican, 1982);

Ford in Trevor Griffiths's *The Party* (Howard Davies, TOP, 1984); Victor Ellison in Robert Holman's *Today* (Alexander, TOP, 1984); Adrian in Arthur Miller's *The Archbishop's Ceiling* (Nick Hamm, Pit, 1986); and Pimm in Deborah Levy's *Heresies* (Susan Todd, Pit, 1986);

Since 1992 Allam has mostly worked away from the RSC: Oberon in *The Fairy Queen* (Adrian Noble, Peter Hall Company, Aix-en-Provence Festival, 1989); Madras in Harley Granville-Barker's *The Madras House* (Lyric Hammersmith, 1992); Stone in the musical *City of Angels* (Michael Blakemore, Prince of Wales, 1993); Bernard Nightingale in *Arcadia* (Nunn, Theatre Royal Haymarket, 1994); John Worthing in *The Importance of Being Earnest* (Hands, Birmingham Rep, 1995); Mirabell in *The Way of the World* (Phyllida Lloyd, NT Lyttelton, 1995); Serge in *Art* (Matthew Warchus, Wyndham's, 1997); and Marc in *Art* (Warchus, Wyndham's, 1998). In 1999 he joined Trevor Nunn's first repertory ensemble at the National to play a dangerous, superior Ulysses in *Troilus and Cressida* (Olivier), Graves in Edward Bulwer-Lytton's *Money* (John Caird, Olivier), and Bassov in Maxim Gorky's *Summerfolk* (Nunn, Olivier). He continued on the South Bank as Hitler in David Edgar's *Albert Speer* (Nunn, Lyttelton, 2000); Lopakhin in *The Cherry Orchard* (Nunn, Cottesloe, 2000); and Willy Brandt in Michael Frayn's *Democracy* (Michael Blakemore, Cottesloe, 2003). Then: Ray in David Harrower's *Blackbird* (Peter Stein, Edinburgh Festival, 2005); Lambert le Roux in *Pravda* (Jonathan Church, Chichester, 2006); and Bernard in Marc Camoletti's *Boeing-Boeing* (Matthew Warchus, Comedy, 2007).

Miles Anderson (b. Zimbabwe, 1947) trained at RADA and started his RSC career in 1970 at the Aldwych playing James in Dion Boucicault's *London Assurance* (Ronald Eyre); Snobby Price in Shaw's *Major Barbara* (Clifford Williams); and Sir Henry Guildford in *Henry VIII* (Trevor Nunn). In the following year's Stratford season he was restricted to the minor roles of Salarino in *The Merchant of Venice* (Terry Hands); Valentine in *Twelfth Night* (John Barton); Officer in *Much Ado About Nothing* (Eyre); Soldier in *Othello* (Barton); and Harold Rabbit in *Toad of Toad Hall* (Euan Smith).

His profile was raised by Peter Ustinov's *The Unknown Soldier and His Wife* (New London Theatre, 1973). For much of the rest of the 1970s he was a leading member of Richard Cottrell and Adrian Noble's Bristol Old Vic company: Leruska in *Once Upon a Time*; James Joyce in *Travesties*; Antonio in *The Duchess of Malfi*; Norman in *The Norman Conquests*; Schweyk in *Schweyk in the Second World War*; Algernon in *The Importance of Being Earnest*; Turner in *Destiny*; Tattle in *Love for Love* (Noble); Captain Plume in *The Recruiting Officer* (Noble); Aeneas in *Troilus and Cressida* (Richard Cottrell); and Buckler in *Donkey's Years*. He also worked at the Oxford Playhouse and the Manchester Royal Exchange—Philby in *Philby Going Home*, Peter Mortensgaard in *Romersholm* (Caspar Wrede, 1981).

From 1981 to 1989, back at the RSC, Anderson created a compellingly unorthodox body of work: Hermes Wouldbe, bespectacled and punctilious, in *The Twin Rivals* (John Caird, TOP, 1981); Dog, naked and sinister, in *The Witch of Edmonton* (Barry Kyle, TOP, 1981); Sir Frederick Blount, unable to pronounce the letter 'r', in *Money* (Bill Alexander, TOP, 1981); Poins in *Henry IV* (Nunn, Barbican, 1982); the title role in *Peter Pan* (Nunn/Caird, Barbican, 1982); Dudley in *The Time of Your Life* (Howard Davies, TOP, 1983); Orsino in *Twelfth Night* (Caird, RST, 1983); Welborne in *A New Way to Pay Old Debts* (Noble, TOP, 1983); Mosca in *Volpone* (Alexander, TOP, 1983); Sigismund in Calderón's *Life's a Dream* (John Barton, TOP, 1983); Antipholus of Ephesus, succeeding Peter McEnery, in *The Comedy of Errors* (Noble, Barbican, 1984); Eilif in *Mother Courage* (Howard Davies, Barbican, 1984); Lefranc in *Deathwatch* and Claire in *The Maids* (Gerard Murphy/Ultz, Pit, 1987); the title role opposite Amanda Root in *Macbeth* (Noble, RST, 1988); and Dorimant in *The Man of Mode* (Garry Hynes, Swan, 1988).

Essentially a television actor in the 1990s and 2000s, appearing in such popular pieces as Anthony Minghela's *What If It's Raining?* (Channel Four, 1986), *House of Cards* (BBC, 1990), *Soldier Soldier* (ITV, 1990), *Oliver's Travels* (Giles Foster, BBC, 1995), *The Scold's Bridle* (David Thacker, BBC, 1998) and *The Ruby in the Smoke* (BBC, 2006), Anderson returned to the stage to play a menacing Bill Sikes in Sam Mendes's production of *Oliver!* (London Palladium, 1994-95), Charles in Joe Penhall's *The Bullet* (Dominic Cooke, Donmar Warehouse, 1998), and Finbar in Conor McPherson's *The Weir* (Ian Rickson, Duke of York's, 1999-00).

Francesca Annis (b. London, 1944) trained to be a dancer. She appeared in films from an early age, starting with the minor British features *The Cat Gang* (1959) and *No Kidding* (1960). She played Eiras in Hollywood's *Cleopatra* (1963). Her other early films were *The Eyes of Annie Jones* (1963), *Flipper and the Pirates* (1964), *Saturday Night Out* (1964), *The Pleasure Girls* (1965), *The Walking Stick* (1970), and Polanski's *Macbeth* (1971), in which she gave her most striking screen performance. In the 1970s she appeared on television as Emma in *Madame Bovary* (Rodney Bennett, 1975) and Lillie Langtry in *Lillie* (1978).

Francesca Annis is an acclaimed classical actress who has never settled to being a stage performer. Her theatre appearances have included Ophelia opposite Nicol Williamson in *Hamlet* (Roundhouse, 1969); Natalya in Turgenev's *A Month in the Country* (Peter Gill, NT Olivier, 1981); Lady Windermere in *Lady Windermere's Fan* (Philip Prowse, Birmingham Rep, 1994); Gertrude opposite Ralph Fiennes in *Hamlet* (Jonathan Kent, Almeida Company, Hackney Empire, 1995); the title role in *Hedda Gabler* (Annie Castledine, Richmond Theatre, 1999); Mrs Alving in *Ghosts* (Robin Phillips, Comedy, 2001); Florence Lancaster in Noël Coward's *The Vortex* (Michael Grandage, Donmar Warehouse, 2002-03); Rosa in Lars Noren's *Blood* (James Macdonald, Royal Court, 2003); Matilda in Pirandello's *Henry IV*

(Grandage, Donmar Warehouse, 2004); and Ruth in John Osborne's *Epitaph for George Dillon* (Peter Gill, Comedy, 2005).

Her one prolonged stage commitment was made to the RSC, where over a four year period she played Isabella in *Measure for Measure* (Keith Hack, RST, 1974); Juliet opposite Ian McKellen in Trevor Nunn's Elizabethan *Romeo and Juliet* (RST, 1976); Cressida opposite Mike Gwilym in *Troilus and Cressida* (John Barton/Barry Kyle, RST, 1976); and Luciana (blonde wig and spectacles) in Nunn's musical version of *The Comedy of Errors* (RST, 1976). She was in her early thirties, but used her slender physique and thin voice to maximum effect, creating a convincingly young, impassioned Juliet.

Alun Armstrong (b. Anfield Plain, Durham, 1946). The versatile and distinctive Alun Armstrong worked as a gravedigger before securing his first acting job, at the Cambridge Arts Theatre. Soon afterwards he won an important supporting role in the Michael Caine thriller *Get Carter* (1971). At the Royal Court he created roles in David Storey's *The Changing Room* (Lindsay Anderson, 1971), *Cromwell* (Anthony Page, 1973) and *Mother's Day* (Robert Kidd, 1976). He was in Bill Bryden's *The Passion* at the National (Cottesloe, 1977).

His work at the RSC included dazzlingly Dickensian performances as the sadistic Squeers in *Nicholas Nickleby* (Trevor Nunn, Aldwych, 1981); Thersites in *Troilus and Cressida* (Howard Davies, RST, 1985); Thénadier—bringing the house down—in *Les Misérables* (Nunn/John Caird, Barbican, 1985); and Barabas in *The Jew of Malta* (Barry Kyle, Swan, 1987). He was a biting Petruchio to Sinéad Cusack's Kate in *The Taming of the Shrew* (Kyle, RST, 1982). Also: Dogberry in *Much Ado About Nothing* (Davies) and Azdak in *The Caucasian Chalk Circle* (Caird, Small-scale Tour, 1979); Alun in Barrie Keeffe's *Bastard Angel* (Bill Alexander, Warehouse, 1980); Leathers/Frontage/Baker in Howard Barker's *The Loud Boy's Life* (Davies, Warehouse, 1980); Trinculo in *The Tempest* (Ron Daniels, RST, 1982); Ralph Trap-door in *The Roaring Girl* (Kyle, Barbican, 1983); Leontes in *The Winter's Tale* (Adrian Noble) and John Proctor in *The Crucible* (Kyle/Nick Hamm, Small-scale Tour, 1984); and Stuart Clarke in Doug Lucie's *Fashion* (Hamm, TOP, 1987).

Since leaving the RSC Armstrong has appeared in 20th century classics, new plays and the occasional musical: Adolf in Strindberg's *The Father* (David Leveaux, NT Cottesloe, 1988); Aimable in *The Baker's Wife* (Nunn, Phoenix, 1989); the title role—Dickensian once more—in Stephen Sondheim's *Sweeney Todd* (Declan Donnellan, NT Cottesloe, 1993); Einstein in Terry Johnson's *Insignificance* (Donmar Warehouse, 1995); Hamm in *Endgame* (Katie Mitchell, Donmar Warehouse, 1996); Willy Loman in *Death of a Salesman* (David Thacker, NT Lyttelton, 1996); the scheming editor—giving Walter Matthau a run for his money and blowing Griff Rhys Jones off the stage—in *The Front Page* (Sam Mendes, Donmar Warehouse, 1998); replacing Ian Holm in Shelagh Stephenson's *Mappa Mundi* (Alexander, NT Cottesloe, 2002); Pizarro in Peter Shaffer's *The Royal Hunt of the Sun* (Nunn, NT Olivier, 2006).

Armstrong has appeared regularly in character roles on the big screen, from Britain's *A Bridge Too Far* (Richard Attenborough, 1977), *The Duellists* (Ridley Scott, 1977), and *The French Lieutenant's Woman* (Karel Reisz, 1981), to Hollywood's *White Hunter, Black Heart* (Clint Eastwood, 1990), *The Saint* (Philip Noyce, 1997) and *The Mummy Returns* (2001). His work on television has included leading parts in *Our Friends in the North* (BBC, 1996); *Witness Against Hitler* (1996); *Breaking the Code* (Herbert Wise, BBC, 1996); *Aristocrats* (BBC, 1999); *Adrian Mole: the Cappuccino Years* (BBC, 2001); *Sparkhouse* (BBC, 2002); *Bedtime* (BBC, 2002); *Messiah 2* (BBC, 2003); *New Tricks* (BBC, 2003-06); *Between the Sheets* (ITV, 2003); *Carrie's War* (BBC, 2003); and *Bleak House* (BBC, 2005).

Eileen Atkins was born in a Salvation Army women's hostel in Clapton, north London (1934). Her mother, a seamstress, was forty-six years old. Her father worked for the Gas Board. Eileen was their third child and her arrival qualified the family for a council house in Tottenham.

She was a child dancer, performing in working men's clubs. Mrs Atkins had mapped out her future as a showgirl, and was seemingly unaware of the sordid subtext. It was not something the daughter wanted for herself, and she broke free when she was fifteen. By this time she had won a scholarship to Latymer School in Edmonton. She excelled in school plays and, encouraged by a teacher, decided to become an actress. There was no money to send her to drama school, so she trained to be a drama teacher at the Guildhall School, supported by a council grant.

Robert Atkins, director of the Outdoor Theatre, Regent's Park, was the important influence at the beginning of her career. Impressed by her at twelve (she had written to him after seeing a performance of *King John* in the park), he brought her into the company at nineteen (1953). She was cast as the country girl Jacquenetta in *Love's Labour's Lost*, and would have played Titania in *A Midsummer Night's Dream* if rain had not washed away the season. She made little professional headway until her late twenties. In the 1950s a leading actress had to be conventionally pretty; even tortured characters like Ophelia were played by English roses. Eileen Atkins was tall and gangling, and her face, wonderful at registering hurt and longing, intelligence and irony, had yet to come into fashion. She moved to Stratford as the wife of an actor—Julian Glover. She worked as an usherette and a shop assistant before finally walking on stage as a lady or citizen (1957-59).

She emerged gradually. She played for a season at the Old Vic—Lady Anne in *Richard III* (Colin George), Viola in *Twelfth Night* (Colin Graham), and Miranda in *The Tempest* (Oliver Neville, 1961-62)—and appeared opposite Laurence Olivier in David Turner's *Semi-Detached* in the West End (1962). Frank Marcus's controversial play about a lesbian relationship, *The Killing of Sister George* (Bristol Old Vic, 1965), brought her to wide notice. She was Celia in T.S. Eliot's *The Cocktail Party*

(Wyndham's, 1968) and Elizabeth I in Robert Bolt's *Vivat! Vivat Regina!* (Piccadilly, 1970). At the Royal Court she created roles in David Storey's *The Restoration of Arnold Middleton* (Robert Kidd, 1967) and Peter Gill's *The Sleepers' Den* (Gill, Theatre Upstairs, 1969).

She returned to the RSC as a leading actress, but her work for the Company has been disappointingly sporadic. In 1973 she played the title role in Marguerite Duras's *Suzanna Andler* (Howard Sackler, Aldwych), and Rosaland in Buzz Goodbody's production of *As You Like It* (RST)—she clashed with Goodbody over the production's concept (Rosalind wore blue jeans), but her performance was admired. Eight years later she created the role of Nell in Peter Nichols's *Passion Play* (Mike Ockrent, Aldwych, 1981). In 1998 she played a sublime duet with Michael Gambon in Yasmina Reza's *The Unexpected Man* (Matthew Warchus, Pit).

Elsewhere, since the 1970s: the title role in *Saint Joan* (Prospect, Old Vic, 1977); Viola in *Twelfth Night* (Prospect, 1978); the title role in *Medea* (Young Vic, 1986); Agnes in Edward Albee's *A Delicate Balance* (Anthony Page, Theatre Royal Haymarket, 1997); Meg in Harold Pinter's *The Birthday Party* (Lindsay Posner, Duchess, 2005); Bridget in Frank McGuinness's *There Came a Gypsy Riding* (Michael Attenborough, Almeida, 2007); and, at the National, Hesione in *Heartbreak House* (Old Vic, 1975), Paulina in *The Winter's Tale* and the Queen in *Cymbeline* (Peter Hall, Cottesloe, 1988), the Old Woman in Harold Pinter's *Mountain Language* (Pinter, Lyttelton, 1988), Hannah in Tennessee Williams's *The Night of the Iguana* (Richard Eyre, Lyttelton, 1992), Gunhild alongside Vanessa Redgrave and Paul Scofield in *John Gabriel Borkman* (Eyre, Lyttelton, 1996), and Honor in Joanna Murray-Smith's *Honour* (Roger Michell, Cottesloe, 2003).

Virginia Woolf has dominated her recent career. She portrayed the writer on television; in a one-woman show, *A Room of One's Own* (Patrick Garland, Hampstead Theatre, 1989); and in her own play, based on letters, *Vita and Virginia* (Ambassadors, 1993). In 1997 she adapted *Mrs Dalloway* for the screen. Also behind the cameras, she created, with Jean Marsh, the drama serials *Upstairs Downstairs* (ITV) and *The House of Elliott* (BBC).

As a screen character actress she has given many incisive and tender performances, including Lilian Bentley in *Let Him Have It* (Peter Medak, 1991), Jack Nicholson's secretary in *Wolf* (Mike Nichols, 1994), Richard E. Grant's quietly grieving mother-in-law in *Jack and Sarah* (Tim Sullivan, 1995), and the cook in *Gosford Park* (Robert Altman, 2001).

Hayley Atwell (b. London, 1982) travelled in Europe and worked for a casting director before entering the Guildhall School. She started her career at the highest level playing Io in *Prometheus Bound* (James Kerr, Sound Theatre, 2005), Catherine in the BBC's adaptation of Alan Hollinghurst's *The Line of Beauty* (Saul Dibb, 2006) and Bianca in the RSC's *Women Beware Women* (Laurence Boswell, Swan, 2006).

While poignantly beautiful and self-destructive in the Hollinghurst, she presented the corrupted Bianca as a petulant party girl (the violent ending — Bianca clambered over the other actors to straddle the dying duke (Tim Pigott-Smith), her face and breasts becoming smeared with his blood — was the best authentically Jacobean moment of recent years).

The following months saw her progress from the BBC's *Fear of Fanny* and *Ruby in the Smoke* to leading roles in the films *How About You, Cassandra's Dream* (Woody Allen) and *Brideshead Revisited* (Julian Jarrold). At the National, for Nicholas Hytner, she played Belinda in George Etherege's *The Man of Mode* (2007) and the title role in Shaw's *Major Barbara* (2008).

B

George Baker (b. Varna, Bulgaria, 1931). George Baker's father was a businessman in the cotton trade who became the British honorary vice-consul in Varna. At the beginning of the Second

World War, his Irish mother, a nurse, took the children home to Britain, a treacherous journey that almost saw them stranded in Paris. His father was posted to Egypt, where he died in 1943. Tall and mature for his age (the circumstances of his early life had left him caring for his mother and younger siblings), Baker was only fifteen when he conned his way into a job in the regional theatre. He made his West End debut in Frederick Lonsdale's *Aren't We All?* at the Theatre Royal Haymarket in 1953, and soon afterwards was placed under contract by Associated British Pictures.

British cinema of the 1950s consisted largely of war films and romantic comedies about doctors and nurses, and Baker was restricted to such standard product as *The Dam Busters* (1954); *The Ship That Died of Shame* (1955); *The Woman For Joe* (1955); *The Feminine Touch* (1956); *A Hill in Korea* (1956); *No Time for Tears* (1957); and *The Moonraker* (1958).

He continued to work in the theatre, travelling to New York as Phillipe in Noël Coward's *Look After Lulu* (1957), and establishing his reputation as a classical actor at the Old Vic (supporting roles, 1959-61). At the RSC his key roles were the Son, opposite Peggy Ashcroft, in Marguerite Duras's *Days in the Trees* (John Schlesinger, Aldwych, 1966) and Claudius in the Ben Kingsley *Hamlet* (Buzz Goodbody, TOP, 1975). His other work for the Company consisted of the Theatregoround shows *Room for Company* (Gareth Morgan, Aldwych, 1968) and *The Trial and Execution of Charles I* (1969)—he performed in the former and devised the latter; Worcester in *Henry IV Part One* (Terry Hands, TOP, 1975); Clarence/Mayor of London in *Richard III* (Barry Kyle, TOP, 1975); and Austin Proctor in David Mercer's *Cousin Vladimir* (Jane Howell, Aldwych, 1978).

For five years from 1968 he ran his own company, Candida Plays. In 1978 he directed *The Lady's Not For Burning* at the Old Vic. In 1979, at the Riverside Studios, he played the Duke opposite Helen Mirren in *Measure for Measure* (Peter Gill).

Baker's television appearances were as ephemeral as they were numerous. Two roles stood out: Tiberius in *I, Claudius*

(BBC, 1976), and Detective Chief Inspector Reg Wexford in the *Ruth Rendell Mysteries* (ITV, 1987-98).

Sean Baker. Sean Baker's early theatre work included the National's 1980/81 season: Ballad Singer in *The Life of Galileo* (John Dexter, Olivier); Apprentice in Thomas Dekker's *The Shoemakers' Holiday* (Dexter, Olivier); and Chorus in *The Oresteia* (Peter Hall, Olivier).

An often chillingly puritanical figure (on the stage), he was at the RSC from 1985 to 89: Pyotr Vasilyevich in Gorky's *Philistines* (John Caird, TOP, 1985); Paris in *Troilus and Cressida* (Howard Davies, RST, 1985); Chevalier Danceny in Christopher Hampton's *Les liaisons dangereuses* (Davies, TOP, 1985); Sebastian Brückner in *Mephisto* (Adrian Noble, Barbican, 1986); Rainer Werner Fassbinder's *Blood on the Neck of the Cat* (Alan Rickman, fringe festival production, Almeida, 1986); Ernesto Pico in Richard Nelson's *Principia Scriptoriae* (David Jones, Pit, 1986); Cassius in *Julius Caesar* (Terry Hands, RST, 1987); Giles Pearson in Heidi Thomas's *Indigo* (Sarah Pia Anderson, TOP, 1987); Hippolito in *The Revenger's Tragedy* (Di Trevis, Swan, 1987); Angelo in *Measure for Measure* (Nicholas Hytner, RST, 1987); Shade in Howard Barker's *The Bite of the Night* (Danny Boyle, Pit, 1988); Lawrence/Ted in Stephen Lowe's *Divine Gossip* (Barry Kyle, Pit, 1988); Peter Reese/A Black Dog in Howard Brenton's *The Churchill Play* (Kyle, Barbican, 1988); and Cassio in *Othello* (Trevor Nunn, TOP, 1989).

Appearances since 1990: Leontes in *The Winter's Tale* (Phyllida Lloyd, Manchester Royal Exchange, 1991); Ball in Howard Barker's *Victory* (Greenwich Theatre, 1991); Stefano in *The Tempest* (Michael Bogdanov, English Shakespeare Company, 1992); Krogstad in Ibsen's *A Doll's House* (Stephen Unwin, English Touring Theatre, 2004); Arnholm in Ibsen's *The Lady from the Sea* (Lindsay Posner, West Yorkshire Playhouse, 1994); Frans Hals in John Constable's *Tulip Futures* (Abigail Morris, Cockpit, 1994); Krak in Howard Barker's *The Castle* (Kenny Ireland, The

Wrestling School, Riverside Studios, 1995); Timberlake Werten-baker's *Our Country's Good* (Caroline Hall), Brecht's *The Caucasian Chalk Circle* (Gerard Murphy), and Claudius in *Hamlet* (Ireland, Royal Lyceum, Edinburgh, 1995); the Duke in *Measure for Measure* (Stéphane Braunschweig, Nottingham Playhouse, 1997); Freud in Terry Johnson's *Hysteria* (Joanna Read, Octagon Theatre, Bolton, 1998); Pastor Manders in Ibsen's *Ghosts* (David Hunt, Theatre Royal, Plymouth, 1999); Ash in Patrick Marber's *Dealer's Choice* (Angus Jackson, Clwyd Theatr Cymru, 2002); the Cardinal Inquisitor in Brecht's *The Life of Galileo* (David Salter, Battersea Arts Centre, 2002); Andrew Marvell in Oliver Ford Davies's *King Cromwell* (Sam Walters, Orange Tree, 2003); John Steinbeck's *Of Mice and Men* (Jonathan Church, Birmingham Rep company, Old Vic, 2004); and Jean Anouilh's *Becket* (John Caird, Theatre Royal Haymarket, 2004).

Teresa Banham (b. Surrey, 1964) first appeared at the RSC playing a townsperson in Adrian Noble's production of *The Master Builder* (Barbican, 1989). She was then cast as Frau Pflug in *The Blue Angel* and Julia in *Measure for Measure*, the Trevor Nunn double-bill that opened the new Other Place in 1991. Because of the indisposition of Claire Skinner she stood in as Isabella during the previews of *Measure for Measure*, and on the transfer to the Young Vic she played Mariana.

A sometime singer with a band, she gained her early experi-ence on regional stages in roles as diverse as Linda in *Blood Brothers*, Judy in *The Adventures of Paddington Bear*, Fran in *Mod-ern Languages*, Sophie in *Tom Jones*, Petra in *A Little Night Music*, Lucy in Ayckbourn's *Woman in Mind*, and Agnes in *School for Wives*. Her first significant television play was Leslie Megahey's *Cariani and the Courtesans* (BBC, 1987).

She made her name as a leading actress playing the title role in *Anna Karenina* (Shared Experience, 1992), Cath opposite Iain Glen in Michael Frayn's *Here* (Michael Blakemore, Donmar Warehouse, 1993), and Dinah Morris in *Adam Bede* (Orange

Tree). On television she co-starred in *The Healer* (Mike Hodges, 1992), the powerful oilrig drama serial *Roughnecks* (1994-95), and *Six Sides of Cougan* (1995). Returning to Stratford, she created the role of Susanna, Shakespeare's daughter, in Peter Whelan's *The Herbal Bed* (Michael Attenborough, TOP, 1996)—an exceptional performance, full of ordinary feeling. She was also Isabella in *The White Devil* (Gale Edwards, Swan).

For an actress of quality she has worked infrequently on the stage: a revival of *Anna Karenina* (Lyric Hammersmith, 1998); Em in Tamsin Oglesby's *My Best Friend* (Anthony Clark, Hampstead Theatre, 2000); Miss A alongside Michael Pennington and Jamie Glover in David Mamet's *The Shawl* (Angus Jackson, Sheffield Crucible, 2001); the mother in Simon Stephens's *One Minute* (Sheffield Crucible, 2003); and a movingly neglected Emilia in Rupert Goold's Second World War *Othello* (Royal Theatre, Northampton, 2003)—she provocatively lifted her skirt and placed the handkerchief in her stocking, but Finbar Lynch's Iago coldly ignored this attempt at seduction. In 2005/06, back at the RSC ('Gunpowder' season, Swan), she played Lady More in *Thomas Moore* (Robert Delamere), Cornelia in *Believe What You Will* (Josie Rourke), and Queen Anne in *Speaking Like Magpies* (Goold).

Frances Barber (b. Wolverhampton, 1958). The fourth of six children born to a dog track bookmaker and a school cook, Frances Barber was educated at Wolverhampton Grammar School and Bangor University, where she read English and Drama and deliberately erased her Black Country accent. In the first phase of her career she appeared on the London fringe in new plays by emerging writers—Snoo Wilson's *Spaceache* (Tricycle, 1980), Mike Bradwell's *Ooh La La!* (Hull Truck, Bush, 1980), Doug Lucie's *Hard Feelings* (Bradwell, Bush, 1983), and Brian Thompson's *Turning Over* (Bush, 1983).

It was at the RSC, 1984-86, that she emerged as a promising classical actress: the tragic courtesan—bruised eyes in a pale oval face—in Pam Gems's *Camille* (Ron Daniels, TOP); Ophelia to Kenneth Branagh's Laertes in the Roger Rees *Hamlet* (Daniels, RST); Jacquenetta in *Love's Labour's Lost* (Barry Kyle, RST); and Dolores opposite Bruce Alexander in Nick Darke's *The Dead Monkey* (Roger Michell, Pit). During the following year, perhaps the best of her career, she played a striking Viola in Branagh's production of *Twelfth Night* at the Riverside Studios and starred in the film *Sammy and Rosie Get Laid* (Stephen Frears).

She has created a succession of strong-minded women in television drama serials and films, but the theatre has stretched her more. Key performances have included Maxine opposite Alfred Molina in Tennessee Williams's *The Night of the Iguana* (Richard Eyre, NT Lyttelton, 1992); Eliza Doolittle opposite Alan Howard in *Pygmalion* (Howard Davies, NT Olivier, 1992); 'Marilyn Monroe' in Terry Johnson's *Insignificance* (Donmar Warehouse, 1995); Sonya in *Uncle Vanya* (Bill Bryden, Chichester, 1996); and Anna, succeeding Sally Dexter, in Patrick Marber's *Closer* (NT Lyric, 1998). She returned to the RSC in 2007 to play Goneril in the Ian McKellen *King Lear* and Arkadina in *The Seagull* (Trevor Nunn, Courtyard). Sadly a knee injury forced her to miss the early performances (the excellent Melanie Jessop took over).

In the cinema, Barber has worked for Richard Loncraine (*The Missionary*, 1983), Peter Greenaway (*A Zed and Two Noughts*, 1985), Frears (*Prick Up Your Ears*, 1987), Nicholas Roeg (*Castaway*, 1987) and Dennis Potter (*Secret Friends*, 1992), and for the French directors Jacques Doillon (*Du fond du coeur*, 1994), Arnaud Desplechin (*Esther Kahn*, 2000), Michel Blanc (*The Escort*, 2000) and Laurent Bouhnik (*24 heures de la vie d'une femme*, 2002).

Desmond Barrit (b. Wales, 1940) worked as an accountant before breaking into professional acting at the age of thirty-five. He appeared with a children's theatre company, and then in repertory at Lincoln, Swansea, York, Cardiff and East Grinstead. He was 'discovered' by Nicholas Hytner, who cast him as Brogard in *The Scarlet Pimpernel* (Chichester, 1985). He next joined the National to play the Chauffeur in *Jacobowsky and the Colonel* (Jonathan Lynn, Olivier, 1986), Achille Blond in *The Magistrate* (Michael Rudman, Lyttelton, 1986), and Charlie in *Three Men on a Horse* (Lynn, Cottesloe, 1987).

Hytner was partly responsible for his entry into the RSC (1988-89 cycle). As well as his remarkable Trinculo—a massive, mournful clown with a collapsed pudding of a face—in Hytner's *The Tempest* (RST), he was Tom Errand in *The Constant Couple* (Roger Michell, Swan); Ross/Porter in *Macbeth* (Adrian Noble, RST); Banjo in *The Man Who Came to Dinner* (Gene Saks, Barbican); Gloucester in *King Lear* (Cicely Berry, Almeida); and Feste in *Twelfth Night* (Stephen Rayne, RSC College Tour).

He went with his RSC colleague Alex Jennings to the Old Vic for Corneille's *The Liar* (Jonathan Miller, 1989), then returned to the National to play Toad in Hytner's production of Alan Bennett's *The Wind in the Willows* (Olivier, 1991). Over the next few years he starred as Brazen in *The Recruiting Officer* (Hytner, NT Olivier, 1992), Billy in David Ashton's *The Chinese Wolf* (Dominic Dromgoole, Bush, 1993), and Cotrone in Pirandello's *The Mountain Giants* (William Gaskill, NT Cottesloe, 1993).

For much of the 1990s Barrit was at the RSC. He was in masterful comic form as Antipholus of Ephesus *and* Antipholus of Syracuse in *The Comedy of Errors* (Ian Judge, RST, 1990); Malvolio—majestically ugly, vain and self-bloated—in *Twelfth Night* (Judge, RST, 1994); and Bottom in *A Midsummer Night's Dream* (Noble, RST, 1994). Barrit's Bottom was a self-centred but talented amateur ham transformed into incredulity ('methought I was, and methought I had ...' was spoken with a downwards glance inside his trousers). He returned to play Falstaff in the two parts *Henry IV* (Michael Attenborough, Swan, 2000). Injury forced his withdrawal from Gregory Doran's musical version of *The Merry Wives of Windsor* (2006).

Barrit's other theatre work: the sadistic Tropatchov in Turgenev's *Fortune's Fool* (Gale Edwards, Chichester, 1996); Dame Trott in *Jack and the Beanstalk* (Norwich, 1996); the revue *Then*

Again (Lyric Hammersmith, 1997); Caryl Churchill's *This is a Chair* (Stephen Daldry, Royal Court at the Duke of York's, 1997); Birdboot/Harold in *The Real Inspector Hound/Black Comedy* (Gregory Doran, Comedy Theatre, 1998); Widow Twankey in his own production of *Aladdin* (Norwich, 1998-99); Monsieur Henri, death in a fedora, in Anouilh's *Euridice* (Simon Godwin, BAC, 1999); Zangler in Tom Stoppard's *On the Razzle* (Peter Wood, Chichester, 2001); leading Steven Pimlott's first season at Chichester (2003) as Shylock in *The Merchant of Venice* (Gale Edwards) and Sorin in *The Seagull* (Pimlott); and Pseudolus in *A Funny Thing Happened on the Way to the Forum* (Edward Hall, NT Olivier, 2004).

Alan Bates (1934-2003, b. Allestree, Derbyshire) was one of the discoveries of George Devine's English Stage Company at the Royal Court, the first Cliff in John Osborne's *Look Back in Anger* (1956). Before breaking into films in the early 1960s he played Mick in the premiere production of Harold Pinter's *The Caretaker*. Throughout his career he remained committed to the stage, working regularly with such writers as David Storey and Simon Gray. His profile as a film star obscured the importance of his place in the contemporary theatre.

He trained at RADA and, after national service in the RAF, began his career with the Midland Theatre Company — Denis Cannan's *You and Your Wife*, Molière's *School for Wives* and Shakespeare's *The Comedy of Errors* (Coventry, 1955). The following year he joined the new English Stage Company. As well as Cliff in *Look Back in Anger* (Tony Richardson), he played Simon in Angus Wilson's *The Mulberry Bush* (George Devine, 1956); Hopkins in *The Crucible* (Devine, 1956); Stapleton in Nigel Dennis's *Cards of Identity* (Richardson, 1956); Harcourt in *The Country Wife* (Devine, 1956-57); Le Crachton in Jean Giraudoux's *The Apollo de Bellac* (Richardson, 1957); and Dr Brock in Michael Hastings's *Yes — and After* (John Dexter, 1957). He went with *Look Back* to New York in 1958, and then left the Royal Court to play the forlorn younger son in O'Neill's *Long Day's Journey into Night* (British premiere, Jose Quintero, Edinburgh Festival and Globe). His performance as the arrogant young landlord to Donald Pleasance's tramp in *The Caretaker* (Donald McWhinnie, Arts, 1960) climaxed the first phase of his career.

His good looks, unaffected charm and intuitive style of playing allowed for a smooth transition into features (he was better at understatement and more adaptable than most of his Royal Court contemporaries). The resulting body of work was impressively diverse and compelling: Frank Rice in *The Entertainer* (Richardson, 1960); The Man in *Whistle Down the Wind* (Bryan Forbes, 1961); *A Kind of Loving* (John Schlesinger, 1962); *The Running Man* (Carol Reed, 1963); Mick in *The Caretaker* (Clive Donner, 1964); the English writer opposite Anthony Quinn in *Zorba the Greek* (Michael Cacoyannis, 1964); *Nothing But the Best* (Donner, 1964); *Georgy Girl* (Silvio Narizzano, 1966); *King of Hearts* (Philippe de Broca, 1966); Gabriel Oak in *Far from the Madding Crowd* (Schlesinger, 1967); *The Fixer* (John Frankenheimer, 1968); Birkin in *Women in Love* (Ken Russell, 1969); Vershinin in *Three Sisters* (Laurence Olivier, 1970, based on the National Theatre production); *A Day in the Death of Joe Egg* (Peter Medak, 1971); *The Go-Between* (Joseph Losey, 1971); the writer opposite Dominique Sanda in *Story of a Love Story* (Frankenheimer, 1973); *Butley* (Harold Pinter, 1974); *In Celebration* (Lindsay Anderson, 1975); *Royal Flash* (1975); *An Unmarried Woman* (Paul Mazursky, 1977); *The Shout* (Jerzy Skolimowsky, 1978); *The Rose* (1979); Diaghilev in *Nijinsky* (1981); *Quartet* (James Ivory, 1982); *The Return of the Soldier* (1983); *The Wicked Lady* (1984); *Duet for One* (1986); *Prayer for the Dying* (1987); *We Think the World of You* (1989); *Mr Frost* (1990); *Dr M* (Claude Chabrol, 1990); Claudius in *Hamlet* (Franco Zeffirelli, 1991); *Losing Track* (1992); *Secret Friends* (Dennis Potter, 1992); *Shuttlecock* (1994); *Silent Tongue* (1994); *The Grotesque* (1996); Gayev in *Varya* (Michael Cacoyannis, 1999); the butler in *Gosford Park* (2001); *The Mothman Prophecies* (2002); *Evelyn* (Bruce Beresford, 2002); *The Sum of All Fears* (2002); *The Statement* (Norman Jewison, 2003).

On the stage, his work for Simon Gray amounted to a set of variations on themes of failure and regret, blackly comic, the characters becoming increasingly dishevelled and melancholic: the title role in *Butley* (Harold Pinter, Criterion, 1971); Simon Hench in *Otherwise Engaged* (Pinter, Queen's, 1975); *Stage Struck* (Stephen Hollis, Vaudeville, 1979); the title role in *Melon* (Christopher Morahan, Theatre Royal Haymarket, 1987); Simon Hench in *Simply Disconnected* (Richard Wilson, Minerva, Chichester, 1996); and J.G. in *Life Support* (Aldwych, 1997). He also created roles for David Storey in productions directed by Lindsay Anderson—*In Celebration* (Royal Court, 1969), *Life Class* (Royal Court, 1974), *Stages* (NT Cottesloe, 1992); Harold Pinter—the sadistic interrogator in *One for the Road* (Lyric Studio, 1984); Arnold Wesker—*The Four Seasons* (Saville, 1965); and Peter Shaffer—the title role in *Yonadab* (Peter Hall, NT Olivier, 1985).

Alan Bates selected his classical roles carefully, at intervals. In 1967 he appeared at Stratford, Ontario, as Richard III and Ford in *The Merry Wives of Windsor*; in 1970 at the Nottingham Playhouse as Hamlet; in 1976 at the Derby Playhouse as Trigorin in *The Seagull*; in 1985 at the Riverside Studios as Edgar in Strindberg's *The Dance of Death* (Keith Hack); in 1989 at the Strand as Chekhov's Ivanov and Benedick to Felicity Kendall's Beatrice in *Much Ado About Nothing* (Morahan); in 1995 at the Haymarket as Solness in *The Master Builder* (Peter Hall); and in 1996 at Chichester as Kuzovkin in Turgenev's *Fortune's Fool* (Gale Edwards).

His work at the RSC was separated by a gap of over twenty-five years. He joined the Company in 1973 to play Petruchio opposite Susan Fleetwood in *The Taming of the Shrew* (Clifford Williams, RST). He returned in 1999 to play Antony opposite Frances de la Tour in *Antony and Cleopatra* (Steven Pimlott, RST) and the title role in *Timon of Athens* (Gregory Doran, RST). Hidden behind an unkempt beard, his Antony looked like a man lost in the wilderness—it was a big, emotionally-charged performance. Sadly, illness prevented him from playing Timon.

Major writers and directors lured him onto the small screen at intervals: Simon Gray's *Plaintiffs and Defendants* and *Two Sundays* (BBC, 1975); Dennis Potter's version of *The Mayor of Casterbridge* (BBC, 1978); John Mortimer's *A Voyage Round My Father* (ITV, 1982); Alan Bennett's *An Englishman Abroad* (Schlesinger, BBC, 1983); Graham Greene's *Doctor Fisher of Geneva* (BBC, 1984); Tom Stoppard's *The Dog It Was That Died* (ITV, 1988); Proust in Bennett's *102 Boulevard Haussmann* (BBC, 1991); Gray's *Unnatural Pursuits* (BBC, 1992); Bounderby in Peter Barnes's version of *Hard Times* (BBC, 1994); and Alan Plater's *Oliver's Travels* (BBC, 1995).

Simon Russell Beale (b. Penang, Malaysia, 1961) joined the RSC in 1986 having previously worked at the Traverse Theatre, Edinburgh, and the Royal Exchange, Manchester. During eight continuous years with the RSC he progressed from clowns and fops to Richard III, Konstantin in *The Seagull* and Edgar in *King Lear*.

His RSC career began with the Young Shepherd in *The Winter's Tale* (Terry Hands, RST, 1986). In that first season he also played a dissolute aristocrat in Nick Dear's *Art of Success* (Adrian Noble, TOP); Ed Know'ell in *Every Man in His Humour* (John Caird, Swan); Fawcett in *The Fair Maid of the West* (Trevor Nunn, Swan); Kulygin in *The Storm* (Nick Hamm, Pit); and Nick in Tony Marchant's play about City dealers, *Speculators* (Barry Kyle, Pit). In 1988/89 he delivered three fops in the Swan, Clincher Senior in *The Constant Couple* (Roger Michell), Sir Fopling Flutter in *The Man of Mode* (Garry Hynes) and Lord Acre in Edward Bond's *Restoration* (Michell). His achievement was to suggest loneliness and pain. In direct contrast he ended the season in three new plays in the Pit: Henry in Richard Nelson's *Some Americans Abroad* (Michell), Engels in Frank McGuinness's *Mary and Lizzie* (Sarah Pia Anderson) and Danny in Stephen Poliakoff's *Playing With Trains* (Ron Daniels).

The next few years revealed the range of his talent: his seedy Thersites in tramp's coat and balaclava was the most memorable character in a production of *Troilus and Cressida* by Sam Mendes that also featured Ralph Fiennes, Amanda Root, Ciaran Hinds and David Troughton (Swan, 1990); his Richard III (Mendes, TOP and Small-scale Tour, 1992), a shaven head jutting out from a leather greatcoat, was gleefully psychotic; his Konstantin in *The Seagull* (Terry Hands, Swan, 1990) and Oswald in *Ghosts* (Katie Mitchell, TOP, 1993) had a despair that went beyond act-ing; for Edgar in *King Lear* (Noble, RST, 1993) he drew on all four. In Noble's production Beale's Edgar was given many memorable moments: seen in tableaux against a vast moon as he took on the persona of Poor Tom for the first time; sharing snatches of song with the Fool during the storm ('I smell the blood of an Englishman'); beating Oswald to death with a club. He also played Navarre in *Love's Labour's Lost* (Hands, RST, 1990); the title role in Marlowe's *Edward II* (Gerard Murphy, Swan, 1990); Mr Hyde in *The Strange Case of Dr Jekyll and Mr Hyde* (Peter Wood, Barbican, 1991); and a revisionist Ariel, stiff-backed and humourless, to Alec McCowan's Prospero in *The Tempest* (Mendes, RST, 1993).

Since 1995 Simon Russell Beale has been based at the Na-tional: Mosca in *Volpone* (Matthew Warchus, Olivier, 1995); Rosencrantz in *Rosencrantz and Guildenstern Are Dead* (Matthew Francis, Lyttelton, 1996); Iago in *Othello* (Sam Mendes, Cottesloe, 1997); Voltaire/Dr Pangloss in *Candide* (John Caird, Olivier, 1999); Alfred Evelyn in Edward Bulwer-Lytton's *Money* (Caird, Olivier, 1999); Dudakov in *Summerfolk* (Trevor Nunn, Olivier, 1999); George IV in Nick Stafford's *Battle Royal* (Howard Davies, Lyttelton, 2000); the title role in *Hamlet* (Caird, Lyttelton, 2000); Charlotte Jones's *Humble Boy* (Caird, Cottesloe, 2001); George in Tom Stoppard's *Jumpers* (David Leveaux, Lyttelton, 2003); the title role in Brecht's *The Life of Galileo* (Davies, Olivier, 2006); Face to Alex Jennings's Subtle in *The Alchemist* (Hytner, Olivier, 2006); Benedick opposite Zoë Wanamaker in *Much Ado About*

Nothing (Hytner, Olivier, 2007-08); Undershaft in Shaw's *Major Barbara* (Hytner, Olivier, 2008).

Elsewhere: the title role in *Uncle Vanya* and Malvolio in *Twelfth Night* (Mendes, Donmar, 2002); the title role, opposite Emma Fielding, in *Macbeth* (Caird, Almeida, 2005); Philip in Christopher Hampton's *The Philanthropist* (David Grindley, Donmar, 2005); and the King in *Spamalot* (Palace Theatre, 2007).

Sean Bean (b. Sheffield, 1959) appears on the stage so rarely that it has been generally forgotten that he was once a member of the RSC. A former welder from Sheffield, he has become one of Britain's best film stars. And yet the star of *Sharpe* (ITV, 1993-97, 2006) stayed with the RSC for two years (1986-87), playing Romeo in *Romeo and Juliet* (Michael Bogdanov, RST), Robin Starveling in *A Midsummer Night's Dream* (Bill Alexander, RST), and Spencer in *The Fair Maid of the West* (Trevor Nunn, Swan). Speaking the verse in his Yorkshire accent, he was refreshingly low-key as Romeo in Michael Bogdanov's chic modern-dress production.

He had already acted in his first feature, Derek Jarman's *Caravaggio* (1986), and his first television drama, *Winter Flight*, while his early theatre work included *Cabaret* (Rotherham); Tybalt in *Romeo and Juliet* (Watermill Theatre, Newbury); Journalist in *The Last Days of Mankind* and Animal Seller in *Rosenkavalier* (Glasgow Citizens', 1983); Lederer in *Deathwatch* (Foco Novo, Young Vic, 1985); and, for the Young Writers' Festival at the Royal Court (Theatre Upstairs, 1985), Art in *Gone*, Estate Agent in *Stalemate* and Terry in *Who Knew Mackenzie*. On leaving the RSC he landed the lead in Mike Figgis's first feature, *Stormy Monday* (1988), and his film career took off immediately. Most notably, he has played Tadgh McCabe in *The Field* (Jim Sheridan, 1990); a libertine in *Clarrisa* (BBC, 1991); an Irish terrorist pursuing Harrison Ford in *Patriot Games* (Philip Noyce, 1992); Mellors in *Lady Chatterley's Lover*, opposite his RSC contemporary Joely Richardson (Ken Russell, BBC, 1992); the villain, cleverly ironic, in the Bond film *Goldeneye* (1995); and Boromir in *Lord of the Rings* (Peter Jackson, 2001).

Bean's rare post-RSC stage appearances have included Danny in *Killing the Cat* at the Royal Court (Soho Theatre Company, Theatre Upstairs, 1990), and an underrated *Macbeth*, opposite Samantha Bond, in the West End (Edward Hall, Albery, 2002).

Maureen Beattie (b. Bundoran, Ireland, 1953). The daughter of the Scottish music hall comedian and actor Johnny Beattie, Maureen Beattie was raised in Glasgow (she was born during a summer season in Bundoran, County Donegal). She trained for the stage at the Royal Scottish Academy of Music and Drama, and gained her early experience in variety at Perth and repertory at Dundee. It was only at the end of her twenties that she started to achieve recognition. Two roles for Michael Boyd were particularly significant—Emilia in *Othello* at the Lyric Hammersmith (1984), and Lady Macbeth in *Macbeth* at the Tron, Glasgow (1985). Maureen Beattie compelled attention, and not simply because her eyes, for a brunette, were so nakedly blue: her appealing Scottish voice was at ease with Shakespeare's verse.

She was first at the RSC in 1988-89, playing, with typical élan, Lady Lurewell in *The Constant Couple* (Roger Michell, Swan); Lady Macduff in *Macbeth* (Adrian Noble, RST); Pert in *The Man of Mode* (Garry Hynes, Swan); Cordelia in *King Lear* (Cicely Berry, TOP); Maggie Cutler in *The Man Who Came to Dinner* (Gene Saks, Barbican); and Mary Burns in Frank McGuinness's *Mary and Lizzie* (Sarah Pia Anderson, Pit). She was a sinister White Witch in the 2001 Sadler's Wells revival of *The Lion, the Witch and the Wardrobe* (Noble). She returned to Stratford in 2003—Queen Elizabeth in *Richard III* (Sean Holmes, RST) and a ferocious Tamora in *Titus Andronicus* (Bill Alexander, RST)—and in 2006/07 to appear in the Histories—Eleanor in *Henry VI*, the Duchess of York in *Richard III* and *Richard II*, Mistress Quickly in *Henry IV* and *Henry V* (Boyd, Courtyard).

Elsewhere, since 1990: Kate in *The Taming of the Shrew* (Mark Brickman, Sheffield Crucible, 1990); Elmire in *Tartuffe* (Lou Stein, Palace Theatre, Watford, 1990); the title role in John Clifford's *Ines de Castro* (Ian Brown, Riverside Studios, 1991); Ruby in David Ashton's *The Chinese Wolf* (Dominic Dromgoole, Bush, 1993); Klaus Pohl's *Waiting Room Germany* (Mary Peate, Royal Court, 1995); Mistress Page in Terry Hands's *The Merry Wives of Windsor* (NT Olivier, 1995); Damon in *Damon and Pythias* (Globe, 1996); Emilia in Sam Mendes's *Othello* (NT Cottesloe, 1997); Hester in *The Deep Blue Sea* (Dana Fainaru, Nottingham Playhouse, 2000); magnificent as *Medea* (Graham McLaren, Theatre Babel, Edinburgh Festival, 2000); Peter Gill's *Small Change* (Rufus Norris, Sheffield Crucible, 2002); and Ma opposite David Troughton in Thornton Wilder's *The Skin of Our Teeth* (David Lan, Young Vic, 2004).

On television, she has played regular leading roles in *Casualty* (BBC, 1992-93), *Bramwell* (ITV, 1997-98), and *The Bill* (ITV, 2003).

Katy Behean (1961-1996, b. Sutton Coldfield, West Midlands) trained at the National Youth Theatre and RADA. She made an impression during her first RSC season, 1982/83, playing a Weird Sister alongside Christine Kavanagh and Josette Simon—three crazed young girls in modern dress—in the Bob Peck *Macbeth* (Howard Davies, RST); Ursula in *Much Ado About Nothing* (Terry Hands, RST); a tender Solveig to Derek Jacobi's *Peer Gynt* (Ron Daniels, TOP); Mariette Rivalle in *Molière* (Bill Alexander, TOP); Mary in *The Roaring Girl* (Barry Kyle, Barbican); Marianne in *Tartuffe* (Alexander, Pit); Wendy in *Peter Pan* (Trevor Nunn/John Caird, Barbican); and Gravedigger's Boy's Wife, succeeding Alice Krige, in Edward Bond's *Lear* (Kyle, Pit, 1984). On her return in 1988 she was a shameless Belinda, grappling with her undone dress following her seduction by Miles Anderson's Dorimant, in *The Man of Mode* (Garry Hynes, Swan), and she was remarkable as Philomele in *The Love of the Nightingale* (Hynes, TOP). In London she added Jenny Marx in Frank McGuinness's *Mary and Lizzie* (Sarah Pia Anderson, Pit). A member of Terry Hands's last company, 1990/91, she played a sinister Queen Isabella in *Edward II* (Gerard Murphy, Swan), a desperately sad Masha in *The Seagull* (Hands, Swan), and Jessie in Peter Whelan's *The Bright and Bold Design* (Alexander, Pit).

Katy Behean's screen work included the RSC's *Tartuffe* (Alexander, BBC, 1983); Maria in *Love's Labour's Lost* (BBC, 1985); Beatrice in Alan Bennett's *The Insurance Man* (Richard Eyre, BBC, 1985); Young Marcia in *Wetherby* (David Hare, 1986); *Tai-Pan* (Daryl Duke, 1986); Sarah Loveless in *Comrades* (Bill Douglas, 1987); *Hidden City* (Stephen Poliakoff, 1988); Fyolka in *Chekhov in Yalta* (ITV, 1988); and Young Sophia in the drama series *Sophia and Constance* (BBC, 1988).

Christopher Benjamin (b. Trowbridge, Wiltshire, 1934). A distinguished character actor, Christopher Benjamin initially joined the RSC to play Vincent Crummles and Walter Bray in *Nicholas Nickleby* (Trevor Nunn/John Caird, Aldwych, 1980). He has since performed an impressive range of characters: Stephano in *The Tempest* (Ron Daniels, RST, 1982); Dogberry in *Much Ado About Nothing* (Terry Hands, Barbican, 1983); Archie in Nick Darke's *The Body* (Nick Hamm, Pit, 1983); Arden in *Arden of Faversham* (Hands, Pit, 1983); Montfleury in *Cyrano de Bergerac* (Hands, Barbican, 1983); Polonius in *Hamlet* (Daniels, Barbican, 1985); Pope Clement VI in Peter Barnes's *Red Noses* (Hands, Barbican, 1985); Holofernes in *Love's Labour's Lost* (Barry Kyle, Barbican, 1985); Sir Nicholas in *The Virtuoso* (Phyllida Lloyd, Pit, 1992); the Prince in Ostrovsky's *Artists and Admirers* (Lloyd, Pit, 1992); Martin Alonzo Pinzon in Richard Nelson's *Columbus and the Discovery of Japan* (Caird, Barbican, 1992); Capulet in *Romeo and Juliet* (Adrian Noble, RST, 1995); Sir Tunbelly in *The Relapse* (Ian Judge, Swan, 1995); the title role in

Julius Caesar (Peter Hall, RST, 1995); Bottom in the 1996 revival of Adrian Noble's *A Midsummer Night's Dream* (Barbican); Kent in the Nigel Hawthorne *King Lear* (Yukio Ninagawa, Barbican, 1999); and Dogberry in *Much Ado About Nothing* (Gregory Doran, RST, 2002).

Elsewhere, Benjamin's work has included Alan Ayckbourn's *How the Other Half Loves* (Ian Strachan, Greenwich Theatre, 1988); Orgon in *Tartuffe* (Lou Stein, Palace Theatre, Watford, 1990); General Bridgenorth in Shaw's *Getting Married* (Chichester, 1993); Sterling in *The Clandestine Marriage* (Nigel Hawthorne, Queen's Theatre, 1994); the mayor in *The Front Page* (Sam Mendes, Donmar Warehouse, 1997); and Mangan in *Heartbreak House* (Christopher Morahan, Chichester, 2000). On television, he was in *The Forsyte Saga* (BBC, 1967), *The Avengers* (ITV, 1967), *The Prisoner* (ITV, 1967-68), *Poldark* (BBC, 1975), *Inspector Morse* (ITV, 1992), *Pride and Prejudice* (BBC, 1995), and many other productions.

Paul Bentall (b. London) trained at the Drama Centre, London, and made his name at the Glasgow Citizens'—Trigorin in *The Seagull*, Owen Marshall in Noël Coward's *Semi-Monde*, and Fedya in Robert David MacDonald's *Chinchilla* (all Philip Prowse, 1977). He was a regular player at the National from 1980 to 86, playing Sexton in *Much Ado About Nothing* (Peter Gill, Olivier, 1981); Horatio in *The Spanish Tragedy* (Michael Bogdanov, Cottesloe, 1982); Strozzi in John Fowles's version of Alfred de Musset's *Lorenzaccio* (Bogdanov, Olivier, 1983); and Ian Hubbard in Alan Ayckbourn's *A Chorus of Disapproval* (Olivier, 1985).

Bentall's first RSC roles were Pete Gavin in *Showboat* (Ian Judge, RST, 1990) and Larry Banks in Alan Ayckbourn's *Wildest Dreams* (Ayckbourn, Pit, 1993). He then concentrated on the classics: Artemidorus in *Julius Caesar* (Peter Hall, RST, 1995); Lord Hastings in *Richard III* (Steven Pimlott, RST, 1995); Poet in Howard Brenton's version of Goethe's *Faust* (Bogdanov, Pit,

1996); Gardiner in *Henry VIII* (Gregory Doran, Swan, 1996-97); Pisanio in *Cymbeline* (Adrian Noble, RST, 1997); Don Cyprian in *The Spanish Tragedy* (Michael Boyd, Swan, 1997); Pantaloon in Goldoni's *A Servant to Two Masters* (Tim Supple, TOP, 1999-00); Gripe in *Love in a Wood* (Supple, Swan, 2001); Shakespeare in Peter Barnes's *Jubilee* (Doran, Swan, 2001); and Doran's season of rarities (Swan, 2002)—Copland/Douglas/Villiers in *Edward III* (Anthony Clark), Security in *Eastward Ho!* (Lucy Pitman-Wallace), Equato in *The Malcontent* (Dominic Cooke). In 2005 he returned to the National to appear alongside Jim Broadbent in Lee Simpson and Phelim McDermott's *Theatre of Blood* (Lyttelton).

Cicely Berry (b. 1926) is the RSC's influential voice coach and teacher but also something of an unsung director since, in the area of text, many RSC directors of the last thirty-five years have benefited from her expertise.

Her work goes way beyond the basic technical considerations of vocal strength, diction and projection. She begins with the premise that an actor, like a classical singer, needs to find his or her own voice. Put simply, she helps actors to speak heightened language naturally. Her method is based on physical exercises that the actor performs while speaking the text. The aim is to prevent self-consciousness in verse-speaking, making it as spontaneous as physical movement.

Despite the close correlation between her work and direction, she has only once created her own RSC production, a studio *King Lear* in 1989 (TOP and Almeida). It was a vividly immediate staging, the knots of difficulty in the language untied and the words ringing out with utter clarity. It is surprising that she has never been asked (or persuaded) to direct again.

Cicely Berry taught at the Central School of Speech and Drama before joining the RSC in 1969. Her publications include *Voice and the Actor* (Harrap, 1973), *The Actor and the Text* (Harrap, 1987), and *Text in Action* (Virgin, 2001).

Many RSC actors have cited Berry as a defining influence on their ability to perform Shakespeare's plays.

Paul Bettany (b. London, 1971). One of the leaders of a new generation of British film stars, Paul Bettany came to prominence playing a sadistic London gangster in *Gangster No. 1* (Paul McGuigan, 2000). It was a part that released him from the British heritage cinema and TV of his most prominent previous work—*Sharpe's Waterloo* (1997), *Coming Home* (1998), *The Land Girls* (David Leland, 1998), *David Copperfield* (2000). He has since been cast in mainstream American movies—*A Knight's Tale* (2001); *A Beautiful Mind* (Ron Howard, 2001) alongside Russell Crowe and Jennifer Connelly, his future wife; again with Crowe in *Master and Commander* (Peter Weir, 2003); *Wimbledon* (Richard Loncraine, 2004); *The Da Vinci Code* (Howard, 2006); and *Firewall* (Loncraine, 2006). European films have included *The Heart of Me* (Thaddeus O'Sullivan, 2003); Lars von Trier's idiosyncratic *Dogville* (2003) opposite Nicole Kidman; and *The Reckoning* (McGuigan, 2004).

Bettany's early work in the theatre included Stephen Daldry's *An Inspector Calls*, his debut, at the Aldwych (1993); the 1995/96 season at the RSC—Paris in *Romeo and Juliet* (Adrian Noble), Decius Brutus/Strato in *Julius Caesar* (Peter Hall, Ian Charleson nomination), Richmond in *Richard III* (Steven Pimlott, all RST), and the Drum Major in *Woyzeck* (Sean Holmes, TOP)—he followed in the footsteps of his father, Thane Bettany, an alumni of the 1956 to 58 Stratford seasons; Richie in Joe Penhall's *Love and Understanding* at the Bush (Mike Bradwell, 1997); and Christophe Pellet's *One More Wasted Year* at the Royal Court (Mary Peate, 1997).

Colin Blakely (1930-1987, b. Bangor, Northern Ireland). Colin Blakely was a late starter who looked as if he'd walked into the theatre by mistake from a rugby pitch or a building site. His talent, though, in a wide range of work, was artful and subtle.

He managed his family's retail business in Belfast before making the transition from the amateur to the professional stage. Following work in Belfast and Wales, he moved to London and made his name at the Royal Court in Sean O'Casey's *Cock-a-Doodle Dandy* (George Devine, 1959); John Arden's *Serjeant Musgrave's Dance* (Lindsay Anderson, 1959); Max Frisch's *The Fire Raisers* (Anderson, 1961); and as Bottom in *A Midsummer Night's Dream* (Tony Richardson, 1962).

Between Royal Court engagements Blakely joined the RSC's 1961 Stratford company to play Touchstone in the Vanessa Redgrave *As You Like It* (Michael Elliott), Hastings in *Richard III* (William Gaskill), and the Duke of Venice in *Othello* (Franco Zeffirelli). From 1963 he was a core member of Laurence Olivier's new National Theatre at the Old Vic: Kite in *The Recruiting Officer* (Gaskill, 1964); Hobson in *Hobson's Choice* (John Dexter, 1964); Pizarro to Robert Stephens's Atahuallpa in Peter Shaffer's *The Royal Hunt of the Sun* (Dexter, 1964)—both actors were at their most formidable; Proctor in Arthur Miller's *The Crucible* (Laurence Olivier, 1965); Boyle in O'Casey's *Juno and the Paycock* (Olivier, 1966); the title role in *Volpone* (Tyrone Guthrie, 1968); and Creon in *Oedipus* (Peter Brook, 1968). (Stephens and Blakely shared a dressing room, and took turns to buy in bottles of Guinness during performances; they would later star as Holmes and Watson in Billy Wilder's *The Private Life of Sherlock Holmes*.)

In 1970 Blakely played Astrov in a Royal Court revival of *Uncle Vanya* (Anthony Page), and the following year, at the RSC, he created the role of Deeley—caught between Vivien Merchant and Dorothy Tutin—in Harold Pinter's *Old Times* (Peter Hall, Aldwych). Blakely remained with the RSC for the next two years, playing the title role in *Titus Andronicus* (Trevor Nunn, RST, 1972), Roger Casement, alongside his wife Margaret Whiting, in David Rudkin's *Cries from the Casement* (Terry Hands, The Place, 1973), and General Muster in Philip Magdalany's *Section Nine* (Charles Marowitz, The Place, 1973). Blakely, a bear-like man, made Titus as wounded, vulnerable and culpable as Lear.

The beginning of Blakely's film career coincided with the new wave of realist filmmaking: he was cast in Karel Reisz's *Saturday Night and Sunday Morning* (1960) and Lindsay Anderson's *This Sporting Life* (1963). *This Sporting Life*, Fred Zinnemann's *A Man for All Seasons* (1966), Albert Finney's *Charlie Bubbles* (1967), *The Private Lives of Sherlock Holmes* (1970), Joseph Losey's *Galileo* (1975) and Peter Brook's *Meetings with Remarkable Men* (1979) contain Blakely's most significant work in film.

If primarily a film actor during the 1970s and 80s, he returned to the stage to star in *Heartbreak House* (John Schlesinger, NT Old Vic, 1975); Peter Shaffer's *Equus* (Dexter, NT Albery, 1976); Alan Ayckbourn's *Just Between Ourselves* (Queen's, 1977); Alan Bennett's *Enjoy* (Vaudeville, 1980); Arthur Miller's *All Our Sons* (Wyndham's, 1981); and Pinter's *Other Places* (consisting of *Victoria Station*, *One for the Road* and *A Kind of Alaska*, Kenneth Ives, Duchess Theatre, 1985).

Michael Bogdanov (b. London, 1938). Michael Bogdanov's approach to Shakespeare is both irreverent and doctrinal. Irreverent because he freely edits the texts to make his own points. Doctrinal, because he follows, every time, the same basic concept—modern dress. Some of his ideas have been inspired—Jonathan Pryce's realistic tramp invading the RST at the beginning of the 1978 RSC *Taming of the Shrew* for instance—but often he has appeared to be thinking like a bright six-former or student director: this is the inevitable result of pitching the work at the young, and Bogdanov may say that it is a price he is willing to pay to achieve accessibility.

He studied at Trinity College, Dublin, and at the Sorbonne. After an early career in television (he co-wrote the ITV series *Broad and Narrow*, 1965, and worked as a producer/director at Telefis Eireann in Dublin from 1966 to 68), he surfaced at the Royal Court (*A Comedy of the Changing Years*) and the Oxford Playhouse (his own version of Molière's *Le bourgeois gentil-*

homme, 1969). He next joined the RSC to work as Peter Brook's assistant director on *A Midsummer Night's Dream* (1970-72).

While working for Brook he also assisted Jean-Louis Barrault in Paris (*Rabelais,* 1971). During the 1970s he ran the Phoenix Theatre in Leicester (1973-77) and the Young Vic (1978-80). By the end of the decade he had developed a signature style from the iconic objects of contemporary life. If the use of flak jackets and machine guns, designer suits and sports cars, was often clever and amusing, the productions never caught the zeitgeist in any considerable way. His growing reputation as a *provocateur* was confirmed by his RSC debut, the aforementioned irreverent, chauvinistic *Shrew* with Jonathan Pryce at his most charismatic, and by Howard Brenton's *Romans in Britain* at the National (1980), a production that included a scene of male rape (Mary Whitehouse, the media's favourite champion of censorship and prudery, took Bogdanov to court on grounds of obscenity).

Bogdanov worked at the National from 1977 and was an associate director there until 1988, directing such shows as *Sir Gawain and the Green Knight* (Lyttelton, 1977); *The Hunchback of Notre Dame* (Cottesloe, 1977); Calderón's *The Mayor of Zalamea* (Cottesloe, 1981); Molière's *The Hypochondriac* (Olivier, 1981); *Uncle Vanya* (Lyttelton, 1982); *The Spanish Tragedy* (Cottesloe, 1982); John Fowles's translation of Alfred de Musset's *Lorenzaccio* (Olivier, 1983); and Mark Rozovsky's dramatisation of Tolstoy's *Strider, the Story of a Horse* (Cottesloe, 1984).

In 1986, with Michael Pennington, he formed the English Shakespeare Company to tour his own large-scale, deliberately populist productions of Shakespeare: *Henry IV* and *Henry V* (1986-87, also Old Vic); *The Wars of the Roses* (1987-89); *Coriolanus* and *The Winter's Tale* (1990-91); *Macbeth* and *The Tempest* (1992); *Beowulf* (1997); *As You Like It* and *Antony and Cleopatra* (1998). From 1989 to 92 he ran the Deutsche Schauspielhaus in Hamburg.

At the RSC he has continued to work, intermittently, as a guest director: Sean O'Casey's *The Shadow of a Gunman* (TOP,

1980); an exuberant production of Beaumont's *The Knight of the Burning Pestle* on the *Nicholas Nickleby* set (Aldwych, 1981); a stylish *Romeo and Juliet*, interpreted to make points about the destructiveness of capitalism, starring Sean Bean and Niamh Cusack as the lovers, Hugh Quarshie as Tybalt (driving a red Alfa Romeo sports car) and Michael Kitchen as Mercutio (RST, 1986); Carlo Goldoni's *The Venetian Twins* with David Troughton (Swan, 1993); Brendan Behan's *The Hostage* (Barbican, 1994); and Howard Brenton's adaptation of the two parts of Goethe's *Faust* (Swan, 1995).

Samantha Bond (b. 1961) is among the brightest and most elegant of contemporary theatre actresses. Her similarity in appearance to the young Judi Dench was formerly recognised when the two were cast by the National as mother and daughter in David Hare's *Amy's View* (Richard Eyre, Lyttelton, 1997). However, her ability has not been fully revealed on television where she has tended to play dull, worthy heroines—Mary in *The Ginger Tree* (BBC, 1989), Bridget in *The Black Candle* (1991)—or harassed wives—Sarah in *Tears Before Bedtime* (BBC, 1995), Isabel in *Family Money* (Renny Rye, Channel Four, 1997). Her early opportunity in a series of *Rumpole of the Bailey*, and her cameos as Helga in *Erik the Viking* (Terry Jones, 1989) and Miss Moneypenny in the Pierce Brosnan Bonds—*Goldeneye* (1995), *Tomorrow Never Dies* (1997), *The World is Not Enough* (1999), *Die Another Day* (2002)—give a better indication of her appeal.

In the theatre her breakthrough came when she joined the Renaissance Theatre Company. She was outstanding as Juliet in *Romeo and Juliet* (Kenneth Branagh, Lyric Hammersmith Studio, 1986) and Beatrice in *Much Ado About Nothing* (Judi Dench, Birmingham Rep Studio, 1987), both in partnership with Branagh. Also in 1987 she joined the RSC to play La Présidente de Tourvel in *Les liaisons dangereuses* (Howard Davies, Ambassadors). Returning in 1992/93, she was a delightful Rosalind in *As You Like It* (David Thacker, RST) and a heartbreaking Hermione ('the Emperor of Russia was my father...') in *The Winter's Tale* (Adrian Noble, RST). In London (on her return from maternity leave) she played Celia in *As You Like It* while her replacement, Kate Buffery, continued as Rosalind.

For other theatres, she has played The Wife in *Never in My Lifetime* (Soho Poly); Jill Rillington in Alan Ayckbourn's *Man of the Moment* (Globe, 1990); the Infanta in Corneille's *Le Cid* (Jonathan Kent, NT Cottesloe, 1994); Mary in Shelagh Stephenson's *The Memory of Water* (Terry Johnson, Vaudeville, 1998-99); Karen in Donald Margulies's *Dinner With Friends* (Simon Curtis, Hampstead Theatre, 2001); Lady Macbeth opposite Sean Bean in *Macbeth* (Edward Hall, Albery, 2002); Mrs Arbuthnot in *A Woman of No Importance* (Noble, Theatre Royal Haymarket, 2003-04); Esther in James Phillips's *The Rubenstein Kiss* (Hampstead Theatre, 2005); and Lady Driver in Michael Frayn's *Donkeys' Years* (Jeremy Sams, Comedy, 2006).

Ken Bones (b. Kent) worked as a civil servant before training for the stage at RADA. He appeared extensively in provincial repertory during the first decade of his career. An actor of all round ability, he possesses one of the great contemporary voices.

Bones first worked at the RSC in 1982/83, cast as Borachio and then Don Pedro in *Much Ado About Nothing* (Terry Hands), Burgundy in *King Lear* (Adrian Noble), Sir Beauteous Ganymede in *The Roaring Girl* (Barry Kyle), Miklos Poloczi in David Edgar's *Maydays* (Ron Daniels) and Castel Jaloux in *Cyrano de Bergerac* (Hands) in the main house; and Dick Reede in *Arden of Faversham* (Hands) and Thidias/Alexas in *Antony and Cleopatra* (Noble) in the studio. He was Edward IV in *The Plantagenets* (Noble, RST) in 1988/89, and during Noble's directorship starred powerfully in Schiller's *Wallenstein* (Tim Albery, Pit, 1993) and brought considerable presence to the supporting roles of Theridamas in Marlowe's *Tamburlaine the Great* (Hands, Swan, 1992); De Guiche in *Cyrano de Bergerac* (Gregory Doran, Swan,

1997-98); Polixenes in *The Winter's Tale* (Doran, RST, 1998); Banquo in *Macbeth* (Doran, Swan, 1999); and the Cardinal in *The Duchess of Malfi* (Gale Edwards, Barbican, 2000). For Michael Boyd he has played Brabantio in *Othello* (Doran, Swan, 2004); Enobarbus in *Antony and Cleopatra* (Doran, Swan, 2006); and Antonio in *The Tempest* (Rupert Gould, RST, 2006).

Elsewhere, Bones's theatre appearances have included the title role in the first modern performance of *Sir Thomas More* (Shaw Theatre, London, 1990); the King of France in the Derek Jacobi/Robert Lindsay *Becket* (Elijah Moshinsky, Theatre Royal Haymarket, 1991); the Earl of Warwick to Imogen Stubbs's Joan in Shaw's *Saint Joan* (Gale Edwards, Strand, 1993); Julian in Alan Ayckbourn's *Communicating Doors* (Ayckbourn, Gielgud Theatre, 1995); the butler in Noël Coward's *Relative Values* (Joe Harmston, Tour, 2002); Ernest in Coward's *Design For Living* (Marianne Elliott, Manchester Royal Exchange, 2002); Pope Urban VIII to David Troughton's Galileo in Richard N. Goodwin's *The Hinge of the World* (Edward Hall, Yvonne Arnaud Theatre, Guildford, 2003); and the Duke in *The Revenger's Tragedy* (Melly Still, NT Olivier, 2008).

Hugh Bonneville (b. London, 1963) read theology at Corpus Christi College, Cambridge, and trained for the stage at Webber Douglas. His real name is Hugh Richard Bonneville Williams; he used the stage name Richard Bonneville until the mid-1990s.

At Cambridge, where his contemporaries included Sam Mendes, Christopher Luscombe, Steve Punt and Nick Hancock, he played Romeo and co-wrote the Footlights show *Tropical Heatwave* (1985). His professional career began at the Open Air Theatre, Regent's Park. Within a year he was working at the National: *School for Wives* (Di Trevis, Lyttelton, 1987); *Yerma* (Trevis, Cottesloe, 1987); David Edgar's *Entertaining Strangers* (Peter Hall, Cottesloe, 1987); *Juno and the Paycock* (Peter Gill, Lyttelton, 1989); *The School for Scandal* (Peter Wood, Olivier, 1990); and Peter Pears in Paul Godfrey's *Once in a While the Odd Thing*

Happens (Godfrey, Cottesloe, 1990). At the Leicester Haymarket in 1988 he appeared in Terence Rattigan's *French Without Tears* (Simon Usher).

He joined the RSC in 1991, a tall, physically commanding actor with a boyish face. His work ranged from the gleefully dim, riotously funny, Sir Samuel Hearty in *The Virtuoso* (Phyllida Lloyd, Swan, 1991) to Laertes in the Kenneth Branagh *Hamlet* (Adrian Noble, Barbican, 1992). Memorably, he played Laertes as a dignified, grief-stricken everyman in a brown suit. In-between he was cast as Valentine in *The Two Gentlemen of Verona* (David Thacker, Swan), Bergetto in *'Tis Pity She's a Whore* (David Leveaux, Swan), Kastril in *The Alchemist* (Sam Mendes, Swan), Brian Taylor in Billy Roche's *Amphibians* (Michael Attenborough, Pit) and Surly in *The Alchemist* (Mendes, Barbican).

Since leaving the RSC he has played Tony in Jonathan Harvey's *Beautiful Thing* (Hettie MacDonald, Donmar Warehouse, 1994); Dick Dudgeon in *The Devil's Disciple* (Christopher Morahan, NT Olivier, 1994); Throbbing in Alan Bennett's *Habeas Corpus* (Sam Mendes, Donmar Warehouse, 1996); Martin in Tamsin Oglesby's *Us and Them* (Jennie Darnell, Hampstead Theatre, 2003); and Jan in Maria Goos's *Cloaca* (Kevin Spacey, Old Vic, 2004). He has concentrated on screen work, progressing from bit parts in Branagh's *Frankenstein* (1994) and the Bond film *Tomorrow Never Dies* (1997) to highly accomplished, distinctive and varied character work in major television dramas— *Mosley* (1998); the hapless husband in *Madame Bovary* (Tim Fywell, BBC, 2000); Julian Ormerod in *Take a Girl Like You* (BBC, 2000); finding complexity in the Victorian villain of *Daniel Deronda* (BBC, 2002); Philip Larkin in *Love Again* (BBC, 2003); the Prince Regent in *Beau Brummell* (BBC, 2006); the compassionate detective in *Five Days* (BBC, 2007); the majestically dull Pooter in *Diary of a Nobody* (BBC, 2007); Hugh Greene in *Filth: the Mary Whitehouse Story* (BBC, 2008)—and films of varying quality— *Notting Hill* (Roger Michell, 1999); *Blow Dry* (2001); John Bayley opposite Kate Winslet in *Iris* (Richard Eyre, 2001); Samuel Pepys in *Stage Beauty* (Eyre, 2004); *Asylum* (David Mackenzie, 2005);

Man to Man (Régis Wargnier, 2005); *Scenes of a Sexual Nature* (Ed Blum, 2006).

In 1994, as Hugh Williams, he produced the West End transfer of *Beautiful Thing* (Duke of York's) and co-wrote and directed Christopher Luscombe's one-man show *Half-Time* (Donmar, previously seen during the 1992 RSC fringe festival in Stratford, and originally conceived for the Footlights).

Laurence Boswell (b. Coventry, 1959) was an assistant director at the RSC in 1983, working on productions by Adrian Noble (*Measure for Measure*), John Caird (*Twelfth Night*) and Howard Davies (*Henry VIII*). This was his first job in the theatre on leaving Manchester University with a drama degree and an impressive portfolio of student productions, including two National Student Drama Festival award winners, Ben Jonson's *The Silent Woman* (1981) and Lope de Vega's *The Dog in the Manger* (1982).

He first came to notice at the Gate Theatre in Notting Hill, where he was Stephen Daldry's associate director (1990-92) before succeeding him as artistic director. A champion of neglected classics, Boswell directed Lope de Vega's *Punishment Without Revenge* and Tirso de Molina's *Don Gil of the Green Britches* during his first year at the Gate, and instigated the acclaimed Spanish Golden Age season of 1991-92, staging the opening and closing plays—Lope de Vega's *The Gentleman from Olmedo* and *The Great Pretenders*—and providing the translation for Daldry's landmark production of Tirso de Molina's *Damned for Despair*. As artistic director he staged Euripides's *Hecuba* (1992); Lope de Vega's *Madness in Valencia* (1992-93); Ramon Maria del Valle-Inclan's *Bohemian Lights* (1993); Marivaux's *The Cheating Hearts* (1994); Marie Laberge's *Aurelie, My Sister* (1994); and *Agamemnon's Children*, a trilogy consisting of Euripides's *Electra*, *Orestes* and *Iphigenia* (1995). He adapted Goldoni's *The Lovers* (1995).

In 1995 he left the Gate to work as a freelance director. Adrian Noble invited him back to the RSC to adapt and direct a Gate-style production of Calderón's neglected *The Painter of Dishonour* at The Other Place. All the ingredients were there but, mysteriously, the final result failed to generate the excitement of Boswell's Gate equivalents. His second RSC production was a vibrant and colourful modern-dress version of Jonson's *Bartholomew Fair* (Swan, 1997).

Increasingly, the pioneering spirit of his early work has given way to Ben Elton adaptations and mainstream classics. Since 1995 he has directed *A Voyage Round My Father* (Nuffield Theatre, Southampton, 1995); Ben Elton's *Popcorn* (Nottingham Playhouse, 1996) and *Inconceivable* (West Yorkshire Playhouse, 2001); Penelope Wilton and Richard Johnson in Eugene O'Neill's *Long Day's Journey into Night* (Young Vic, 1996); a breathtaking *Beauty and the Beast* (Young Vic, 1996-97); Kelly McGillis in *As You Like It* (Shakespeare Theatre, Washington, 1997); *The Country Wife* (Tour, 1997); Paul Rhys in a fine *Hamlet* (Young Vic, 1999); Steven Froelich's *Weekend in Rio* (Pleasance Dome, Edinburgh Festival, 2001); Clive Owen and Victoria Hamilton in *A Day in the Death of Joe Egg* (New Ambassadors, 2001); Kenneth Lonergan's *This Is Our Youth* (Garrick, 2002); and Madonna in David Williamson's *Up For Grabs* (Wyndham's, 2002).

In 2003 Boswell joined Michael Boyd's new directorial team at the RSC. His first projects were repeats of previous work— *Beauty and the Beast* (RST) and a Spanish Golden Age season (Swan, 2004). *Women Beware Women* (Swan, 2006) was dynamically performed by Penelope Wilton, Tim Pigott-Smith, Peter Guinness, Julian Curry, Susan Engel and the outstanding newcomer Hayley Atwell.

John Bott (1923-1994, b. Douglas, Isle of Man). A late starter, John Bott was forty-one when a BBC radio job initiated his career as a professional actor (1964). His subsequent early stage work included Pierre Lannes in *The Lovers of Viorne* (Royal Court, 1971), the Duke of Venice in *Othello* (Mermaid, 1971), Cotton in *Cato Street* (Young Vic, 1971), and Pradah Singh in *Conduct Unbecoming* (Queen's, 1970-71).

The rest of his career was dominated by two periods of work at the RSC (1972-77 and 1988-94): Titus Lartius in *Coriolanus* (Trevor Nunn/Buzz Goodbody, RST, 1972); Balthazar in *The Comedy of Errors* (Clifford Williams, RST, 1972); Soothsayer in *Julius Caesar* (Trevor Nunn/Buzz Goodbody, Aldwych, 1973); Bennett in Tom Stoppard's *Travesties* (Peter Wood, Aldwych, 1974); Count Von Stalberg in *Sherlock Holmes* (Frank Dunlop, US Tour, 1974); Banks in *Wild Oats* (Williams, Aldwych, 1976); Old Man/Scottish Doctor in *Macbeth* (Adrian Noble, RST, 1988); Handy in *The Man of Mode* (Garry Hynes, Swan, 1988); Gaoler in Edward Bond's *Restoration* (Roger Michell, Swan, 1988); Baldwin in Richard Nelson's *Some Americans Abroad* (Michell, Pit, 1989); Dr Herdal in *The Master Builder* (Noble, Barbican, 1989); Balthasar in *The Comedy of Errors* (Ian Judge, RST, 1990); Warwick in *Edward II* (Gerard Murphy, Swan, 1990); John Sefton/Washington Irving in Nelson's *Two Shakespearean Actors* (Michell, Swan, 1990); Bishop of Carlisle in *Richard II* (Ron Daniels, RST, 1990); Archdeacon Daubeny in *A Woman of No Importance* (Philip Prowse, Barbican, 1991); Poole in *Dr Jekyll and Mr Hyde* (Peter Wood, Barbican, 1991); Corin in *As You Like It* (David Thacker, RST, 1992); Archidamus/Paulina's Steward in *The Winter's Tale* (Noble, RST, 1992); and Bardolph in *The Merry Wives of Windsor* (Thacker, RST, 1992). In 1974 he published *The Figure of the House: the Remarkable Story of the Building of Stratford's Royal Shakespeare Theatre*. He died in America during the RSC's 1994 tour of *The Winter's Tale*.

John Bowe (b. Greasby, Merseyside, 1950) trained at the Bristol Old Vic Theatre School and gained his early theatre experience with Prospect and the New Shakespeare Company. At the RSC, 1978-87, he was both a long-haired leading player and a versatile character actor: Gratiano in *The Merchant of Venice* (John Barton, TOP, 1978); Jack Slipper in Peter Whelan's *Captain Swing* (Bill Alexander, TOP, 1978); Corporal Taylor in Howard Brenton's *The Churchill Play* (Barry Kyle, TOP, 1978); Philo/Scarus in *Antony and Cleopatra* (Peter Brook, RST, 1978); Alexander Studzinsky in Bulgakov's *The White Guard* (Kyle, Aldwych, 1979); Orlando to Susan Fleetwood's Rosalind in *As You Like It* (Terry Hands, RST, 1980); Diphilus/Neptune in *The Maid's Tragedy* (Kyle, TOP, 1980); Laertes in the Michael Pennington *Hamlet* (Barton, RST, 1980); Mowbray in *Richard II* (Hands, RST, 1980); Sir Richard Ratcliffe in *Richard III* (Hands, RST, 1980); Feast in Howard Brenton's *Thirteenth Night* (Kyle, Warehouse, 1981); Knull in *The Swan Down Gloves* (Hands, Aldwych, 1981); Black Will in *Arden of Faversham* (Hands, TOP, 1982); King of France in *King Lear* (Adrian Noble, RST, 1982); First Workman in Edward Bond's *Lear* (Kyle, TOP, 1982); Tranio in *The Taming of the Shrew* (Kyle, RST, 1982); Lieutenant in Nick Darke's *The Body* (Nick Hamm, Pit, 1983); Le Bret in *Cyrano de Bergerac* (Hands, Barbican, 1983); Bouton, succeeding David Troughton, in *Molière* (Bill Alexander, Pit, 1983); and Tinman/Hickory in *The Wizard of Oz* (Ian Judge, Barbican, 1987).

Since 1990 Bowe has worked most prominently on television. He is unlikely to better the performance he gave as the chillingly smooth, spaniel-eyed killer in *Prime Suspect I* (ITV, 1991).

Raymond Bowers is a veteran of pantomimes, revues, television comedy, and the classical stage. From 1982 to 1997 he was a senior supporting player at the RSC, where his varied classical work included Justice Clement in Ben Jonson's *Every Man in His Humour* (John Caird, Swan, 1986); Antigonus in *The Winter's Tale* (Terry Hands, RST, 1986); Bedford and other roles in *The Plantagenets* (Noble, RST, 1988); Angelo in *The Comedy of Errors* (Ian Judge, RST, 1990); Gaseno in Tirso de Molina's *The Last Days of Don Juan* (Danny Boyle, Swan, 1990); Lord Mortimer in Marlowe's *Edward II* (Gerard Murphy, Swan, 1990); Physician in the

115

Robert Stephens *King Lear* (Noble, RST, 1993); Old Gobbo in *The Merchant of Venice* (David Thacker, RST, 1993); Sir Nathaniel in *Love's Labour's Lost* (Judge, RST, 1993); and Calchas in *Troilus and Cressida* (Judge, RST, 1996). He created roles in David Edgar's *Maydays* (Ron Daniels, Barbican, 1983); Peter Barnes's *Red Noses* (Hands, Barbican, 1985); Nicholas Wright's *The Desert Air* (Noble, Pit, 1985); Howard Barker's *The Castle* (Nick Hamm, Pit, 1985); Tony Marchant's *Speculators* (Barry Kyle, Pit, 1987); and Peter Whelan's *The Herbal Bed* (Michael Attenborough, TOP, 1996).

Robert Bowman (b. Washington State, USA) came to England to study acting at the Guildhall School. His career began in Dublin, where he worked for a year at the Abbey Theatre. Returning to London he joined Stephen Daldry's company at the Gate Theatre. Two years later he played the son in Daldry's landmark production of *An Inspector Calls* at the National (Lyttelton, 1992). He dropped out of Tim Supple's production of *Omma* at the Young Vic, but has since worked frequently with the director: *Grimm's Tales* (1994), *More Grimm Tales* (1997), Malvolio in *Twelfth Night* (1998), and *As I Lay Dying* (1998) at the Young Vic; *Haroun and the Sea of Stories* at the National (1998); and Antipholus of Syracuse in *The Comedy of Errors* (Small-scale Tour, 1996-97), and Ranger in Wycherley's *Love in a Wood* (Swan, 2001) at the RSC. Other RSC appearances: 1994-95—Sebastian in *Twelfth Night* (Ian Judge, RST), Mr Friendall in *The Wives' Excuse* (Max Stafford-Clark, Swan), and Ithocles in *The Broken Heart* (Michael Boyd, Swan); 2001-02—outstanding as Roman in David Edgar's *The Prisoner's Dilemma* (Michael Attenborough, TOP); and 2006—the Reverend Hale in *The Crucible* (Dominic Cooke, RST).

Elsewhere: Leonard in *Maria Magdalena* (Malcolm Edwards, Gate, 1990); Edgar in *King Lear* (Jude Kelly, West Yorkshire Playhouse, 1995); *The Oresteia* (Katie Mitchell, NT Cottesloe, 2000); Rebecca Gilman's *Spinning into Butter* (Royal Court, 2001); Kurt opposite Elizabeth Hurran in Franz Xaver Kroetz's *The*

Nest (Elen Bowman, Arcola Theatre, London, 2003); and the title role in *Cyrano de Bergerac* (Simon Reade, Bristol Old Vic, 2007).

Stephen Boxer (b. Sidcup, 1948) trained at Rose Bruford and worked in provincial repertory (Lancaster, Leicester, Southampton, Edinburgh and Sheffield) before beginning a London career that has been consistently acclaimed: Alyosha in *The Brothers Karamazov* (Fortune, 1981); *Faith, Hope and Charity* and Sartre's *The Devil and the Good Lord* (John Dexter, Lyric Hammersmith, 1984); Peter Quilpe in *The Cocktail Party* (Dexter, Phoenix, 1986); Sturman in *The Clearing* (Bush, 1993); the Duke in *Measure for Measure* (Declan Donnellan, Cheek By Jowl, International Tour, 1994); and, at the National, Auden in Peter Godfrey's play about Benjamin Britten, *Once in a While the Odd Thing Happens* (Paul Godfrey, Cottesloe, 1990), David Edgar's *The Shape of the Table* (Jenny Killick, Cottesloe, 1990), Christopher Hampton's *White Chameleon* (Richard Eyre, Cottesloe, 1991), Daniel Mornin's *At Our Table* (Killick, Cottesloe, 1991), and Voltore in the Michael Gambon/Simon Russell Beale *Volpone* (Matthew Warchus, Olivier, 1995).

At the RSC, from 1989 to 98, he played Bosola in *The Duchess of Malfi* (Bill Alexander, Swan, 1989); Monakhov in Gorky's *Barbarians* (David Jones, Barbican, 1990); Buckingham in *Richard III* (Sam Mendes, TOP and Small-scale Tour, 1992); Francisco de Medici in *The White Devil* (Gale Edwards, Swan, 1996); the cold-as-steel Goche—judges and clerics fit this actor like a glove—in Peter Whelan's *The Herbal Bed* (Michael Attenborough, TOP, 1996); Kemble in Richard Nelson's *The General from America* (Howard Davies, Swan, 1996); a surprisingly callous Feste in *Twelfth Night* (Adrian Noble, RST, 1997); Littlewit in *Bartholomew Fair* (Lawrence Boswell, Swan, 1997); and Angelo in *Measure for Measure* (Michael Boyd, RST, 1998). He returned in 2008 to star as Petruchio in *The Taming of the Shrew* (Conall Morrison, Courtyard).

Boxer's other recent work has included Stephen Hawking in Robin Hawdon's *God and Stephen Hawking* at the Theatre Royal, Bath (Jonathan Church, 2000); the father in Pirandello's *Six Characters Looking for an Author* at the Young Vic (Richard Jones, 2001); Colbert in Nick Dear's *Power* at the National (Lindsay Posner, Cottesloe, 2003); Argan's brother in Molière's *The Hypochondriac* at the Almeida (Posner, 2005); and the Hunter in Strindberg's *The Great Highway* at the Gate (Wally Sutcliffe, 2006).

Danny Boyle (b. Radcliffe, Lancashire, 1956). From a working-class Catholic family, brought up near Bolton (his parents, a power station worker and a hairdresser, were originally from Galway), Danny Boyle went to a Salesian school and discovered theatre on a school trip to Stratford to see *Richard II* (John Barton's production). He started to direct as an English and Drama student at Bangor University.

He came to prominence at the Royal Court, where he ran the Theatre Upstairs (1982-85) before becoming the Court's Deputy Director (1985-87). Boyle brought flare to a typical collection of Royal Court plays, including Hanif Kureishi's adaptation of Janusz Glowacki's *Cinders* (1981); Louise Page's *Salonika* (1982); Howard Brenton's *Victory* (1983) and *The Genius* (1983); Edward Bond's *The Pope's Wedding* (1984) and *Saved* (1984); and Timberlake Wertenbaker's *The Grace of Mary Traverse* (1985). At the RSC, 1988-91, he directed visually striking productions of rare classics and radical premieres, a fascinating body of work: Howard Barker's *The Bite of the Night* (Pit, 1988); Ben Jonson's *The Silent Woman* (Swan, 1989); Howard Brenton's *Hess is Dead* (Almeida, 1989); a sensual, vibrant staging of Nick Dear's adaptation of Tirso de Molina's *The Last Days of Don Juan* (Swan, 1990); and Ibsen's *The Pretenders* (Pit, 1991).

After the success of *Don Juan* one might have expected Boyle to direct a main house Shakespeare, but his ambitions lay elsewhere. He had already worked in television, producing Alan

Clarke's chilling depiction of sectarian murders *Elephant* (BBC, 1989), and directing *The Hen House* (BBC, 1989) and the *Inspector Morse* drama 'Masonic Mysteries' (ITV, 1990). He now made *Mr Wroe's Virgins* (BBC, 1993), four interlocking films starring Jonathan Pryce, Lia Williams, Kerry Fox, Kathy Burke and Winnie Driver, followed by his first feature films, *Shallow Grave* (1994), a stylish suspense thriller about yuppie greed set in Edinburgh, and *Trainspotting* (1995), an unlikely but dynamic black comedy involving heroin addiction and violence. The success of the latter provoked Boyle to direct films financed by and aimed at America: *A Life Less Ordinary* (1997) and *The Beach* (1999). He has since made *28 Days Later* (2002); *Millions* (2004); *Sunshine* (2007).

David Bradley (b. York, 1942) worked as an engineer before winning a place at RADA, aged twenty-four. He made his debut playing Dr Pinch in *The Comedy of Errors* at the Sheffield Crucible, and his early progress included the NT's 1971 season (Old Vic) and *The Mystery Plays* at York.

In his first ten years at the RSC he played supporting roles, gradually gaining in prominence: Antonio in *The Merchant of Venice* (John Barton, TOP, 1978); Hardeness in Peter Whelan's *Captain Swing* (Bill Alexander, TOP, 1978); Peter Reese in *The Churchill Play* (Barry Kyle, TOP, 1978); Soothsayer in Peter Brook's production of *Antony and Cleopatra* (RST, 1978); Second Shepherd in *The Shepherd's Play* (Barton, TOP, 1978); Andy in Tom McGrath's *The Innocent* (Davies, Warehouse, 1979); Oliver Fulton/Policeman in *Once in a Lifetime* (Trevor Nunn, Aldwych, 1979); Shakebag in *Arden of Faversham* (Terry Hands, TOP, 1982); Albany in *King Lear* (Adrian Noble, RST, 1982); the Prison Doctor in Edward Bond's *Lear* (Kyle, TOP, 1982); Charron in *Molière* (Alexander, TOP, 1982); Openwork in *The Roaring Girl* (Kyle, Barbican, 1983); Cleante in *Tartuffe* (Alexander, Pit, 1983); Dr Jameson in Nicholas Wright's *The Custom of the Country* (David Jones, Pit, 1983); Camillo in *The Winter's Tale* (Noble, Small-scale Tour, 1984); Dr Caius in *The Merry Wives of Windsor* (Alexander,

RST, 1985); Bartolomeo in *Il Candelaio* (Clifford Williams, Pit, 1986); Humpage in John Whiting's *A Penny for a Song* (Howard Davies, Barbican, 1986); Fistula in Václav Havel's *Temptation* (Roger Michell, TOP, 1987); Sir Andrew Aguecheek in *Twelfth Night* (Alexander, RST, 1987); the title role in *Cymbeline* (Alexander, TOP, 1987); Kulygin in *Three Sisters* (Barton, Barbican, 1988); Morose in *The Silent Woman* (Danny Boyle, Swan, 1989); and Mephistopheles in *Dr Faustus* (Kyle, Swan, 1989).

He was a leading member of Adrian Noble's first ensemble, 1991-93, playing Shallow in *Henry IV Part Two* (Noble, RST); Polonius in the Branagh *Hamlet* (Noble, Barbican); and Subtle in *The Alchemist* (Sam Mendes, Swan). He made Shallow vain and manipulative, while delivering the comedy, and looked for good motives in Polonius, a highly original reading. In 1993/94 his skill was showcased by the improbable double of Trinculo in *The Tempest* (Mendes) and Gloucester in the Robert Stephens *King Lear* (Noble, RST).

At the National in 1997 he gave a performance of menace and bile as Max in Harold Pinter's *The Homecoming* (Roger Michell, Lyttelton). In 1998 he played Thèramène in *Phèdre* and Burrus in *Britannicus* (Jonathan Kent, Almeida at Malvern and the Albery); in 1999, God in *The Mysteries* (Bill Bryden, NT Cottesloe). Following several years of concentrated screen work—including Filch in the *Harry Potter* films—he returned to the stage: the title role in *Titus Andronicus* at the RSC (Alexander, RST, 2003); the title role in both parts of *Henry IV* at the National (Nicholas Hytner, Olivier, 2005); Davies in Pinter's *The Caretaker* at the Sheffield Crucible (Jamie Lloyd, 2006); and Spooner in Pinter's *No Man's Land* at the Gate, Dublin (Rupert Goold, 2008).

Kenneth Branagh (b. Belfast, 1960). The son of a Belfast builder who moved his family to England at the beginning of the Troubles, Kenneth Branagh lived in Reading from the age of ten and attended Meadway Comprehensive School. From the moment of his first experience of acting in a school play (*Oh!*

What a Lovely War) he worked towards a career in the theatre. Trips to Oxford to see Derek Jacobi's *Hamlet* (1977) and to Stratford (1978) initiated his enthusiasm for Shakespeare. At RADA, where he played Hamlet in a production directed by Malcolm McKay, he was singled out as an actor of exceptional promise.

Three performances brought him to prominence: Judd in Adrian Mitchell's *Another Country* (Stuart Burge, Queen's, 1982), Billy in Graham Reid's Belfast television play *Too Late to Talk to Billy* (Paul Seed, 1982), and the title role in Adrian Noble's RSC production of *Henry V* (1984). The twenty-four year old was suddenly the 'new Olivier'. He could command a big stage, but other similarities were merely superficial. Branagh was no matinee idol, he looked like a regular person and sought to internalise Henry (a meeting with Prince Charles inspired the quality of troubled introspection that made the performance so memorable). Henry was his first RSC role; later in the 1984-85 season, at Stratford and the Barbican, he played Laertes in *Hamlet* (Ron Daniels), Navarre in *Love's Labour's Lost* (Barry Kyle) and Mike in Louise Page's *Golden Girls* (Barry Kyle). For the acting company's fringe festival (Newcastle, Almeida and Donmar Warehouse, 1985) he wrote and directed a play called *Tell Me Honestly*, a satire on the end of year interviews each actor had with Terry Hands. By this time he was feeling constrained by the actor's role in a large repertory company.

With the wages from his cameos in Clare Peploe's *High Season* and Pat O'Connor's *A Month in the Country*, Branagh directed *Romeo and Juliet* at the Lyric Hammersmith Studio (1986). The production had directness and energy and featured a fine Juliet from Samantha Bond; its emphasis on performance over interpretation was to become the presiding idea of Renaissance, the company Branagh formed in 1987. Renaissance began with a season of diverse shows at the Riverside Studios: Branagh's play *Public Enemy* (directed by Malcolm McKay), John Sessions's one-man show *Napoleon*, and a wintry *Twelfth Night*. In early 1988 he moved the company to the Birmingham Rep Studio for the launch of three Shakespeare productions directed by famous actors. Branagh played Benedick opposite Samantha Bond's Beatrice in Judi Dench's production of *Much Ado About Nothing*, the title role in Derek Jacobi's *Hamlet*, and Touchstone in Geraldine McEwan's *As You Like It*. The productions were vehicles for good performances: Branagh and Bond duelled expertly in *Much Ado*, and Branagh's fiery Hamlet was admired. The subsequent tour lasted for nine months and ended in London at the Phoenix Theatre.

The media pack that followed Branagh during the next few years was fed by his marriage to Emma Thompson and the success of his film version of *Henry V*, but had very little to do with his finest work, which was understated and perceptive in its response to character—Osvald in Ibsen's *Ghosts* (Elijah Moshinsky, BBC, 1985), and Guy Pringle in *Fortunes of War* (James Cellan-Jones, BBC, 1987). *Henry V* (1989), the first large-scale Shakespeare movie since Polanski's *Macbeth* in 1971, was both a stirring epic and a further exploration of the dark themes highlighted by Adrian Noble in the 1984 production. As a result of his Oscar nomination Branagh went to Hollywood to make an entertaining but unconvincing thriller, *Dead Again* (1991). Back home he filmed his own script *Peter's Friends* (1992), a kind of English *Big Chill*, utterly contrived, and a too-sunny *Much Ado About Nothing* (1993) featuring American stars. During this period Renaissance toured America with productions of *King Lear* (Richard Briers played Lear, Branagh Edgar and Emma Thompson The Fool) and *A Midsummer Night's Dream*.

By the early 1990s Renaissance had run its course. Branagh accepted Adrian Noble's invitation to return to the RSC to play the title role in *Hamlet* (Barbican, 1992). It was his best work, a subtle, multifaceted, beautifully spoken account of the role. The character's grief and stoicism remained poignantly alive throughout.

After this highpoint he worked for eight years exclusively in films. *Frankenstein* (1994), a Hollywood epic starring Robert De Niro as the monster, had some impressive sequences and good performances throughout, but it was critically savaged. He found refuge in the shooting of a small film from his own script about a group of 'resting' actors mounting a production of *Hamlet, In the Bleak Mid Winter* (1995), and as a fine Iago in Oliver Parker's film of *Othello* (1996). He then filmed an unabridged *Hamlet* with an international cast, in 70mm. Released in the US on Christmas Day 1996, the film was masterly for two-thirds of its length, but lacked the subtlety and depth of his 1992 stage *Hamlet*. As an actor for hire, he played a lawyer in Robert Altman's *The Gingerbread Man* (1998); the Woody Allen role in Allen's *Celebrity* (1998); a pantomime villain in *Wild Wild West* (1999); Heydrich in *Conspiracy* (TV, 2001); the title role in *Shackleton* (Charles Sturridge, TV, 2002); Lockhart in *Harry Potter and the Chamber of Secrets* (Chris Columbus, 2002); Neville in *Rabbit-Proof Fence* (Phillip Noyce, 2002); Uncle Albert in *Five Children and It* (2004); Franklin Roosevelt in *Warm Springs* (TV, 2005); and Henning Von Tresckow in *Valkyrie* (Bryan Singer, 2008). As a filmmaker he remains obsessed with the theatre: *Love's Labour's Lost* (2000); *As You Like It* (2006); and *The Magic Flute* (2006). These movies struggled to find an audience despite their overtly populist intentions. Branagh's next project, Michael Caine and Jude Law in Harold Pinter's adaptation of *Sleuth* (2007), was at least a departure.

Branagh returned to the stage in 2001, director of the hit comedy *A Play What I Wrote* (Liverpool Playhouse Studio and Wyndham's). He played Richard III at the Sheffield Crucible (Michael Grandage, 2002), and the title role in David Mamet's *Edmond* at the National (Edward Hall, Olivier, 2003). For the Donmar Warehouse's 2008/09 season at the Wyndham's, he starred as Chekhov's Ivanov (Grandage).

David Brierley (b. 1936). While studying at Clare College, Cambridge, David Brierley worked for John Barton on student productions, and it was because of Barton that he joined the RSC as an assistant stage manager in January 1961 (he had spent the previous two years teaching English at the Perse School in

Cambridge and the King Edward VI School in Macclesfield). Brierley stage managed the Vanessa Redgrave *As You Like It* and the John Gielgud *Othello*, among other shows, and was quickly promoted to oversee the department (he writes about these early years in *Summerfolk: Essays Celebrating Shakespeare and the Stratford Theatres*, Long Barn Books, 1997). He worked as Peter Hall's assistant from 1966 and became General Manager (the RSC's top administrator) in 1968. The Company benefited from Brierley's outstanding qualities as a manager for the next eighteen years.

Stephen Brimson Lewis (b. London) studied under John Gunter at the Central School and began his career working for Peter Wood, first as an assistant at the National and then as the designer of a Plácido Domingo *Otello* at the Wiener Staatsoper (1987). He consolidated his growing reputation designing for Sean Mathias at the National—*Uncle Vanya* (Cottesloe, 1992); *Les parents terribles* (Lyttelton, 1994); and *A Little Night Music* (Olivier, 1995).

At the RSC he has been Gregory Doran's designer of choice since 1999: *Timon of Athens* (RST, 1999); *Macbeth* (Swan, 1999); *King John* (Swan, 2001); *Much Ado About Nothing* (RST, 2002); *The Taming of the Shrew* (RST, 2003); *The Tamer Tamed* (Swan, 2003); *All's Well That Ends Well* (Swan, 2003); *Othello* (Swan, 2004); *A Midsummer Night's Dream* (RST, 2005); *Antony and Cleopatra* (Swan, 2006); and *The Merry Wives of Windsor* (RST, 2006).

Jasper Britton (b. London, 1962) grew up around actors (his father is Tony Britton) and knew from an early age that he wanted to act himself. His initial progress was unorthodox. Instead of training at drama school, he worked as an assistant stage manager and later as a sound operator, and had to wait six years before securing his first acting job.

As if compensating for his late start, during his first RSC season (1992-93) he played supporting parts with attention-seeking originality: Ben Budge in *The Beggar's Opera* (John Caird, Swan); Masterless Man in *A Jovial Crew* (Max Stafford-Clark, Swan); Calyphas/Meander in *Tamburlaine the Great* (Terry Hands, Swan); an ever-present soothsayer, a chorus of death, in *Antony and Cleopatra* (Caird, RST); and the enigmatic under-footman in Michael Hastings's *Unfinished Business* (Steven Pimlott, Pit). From the outset he was a performer who liked to create a strong visual image, and was particularly adept at projecting traits that are often mistaken for charisma—moodiness and distain.

He steadily built a reputation as a leading actor of style and range, at the National, the Globe and elsewhere: the Dauphin in the Imogen Stubbs *Saint Joan* (Gale Edwards, Theatr Clwyd, 1993); Chief Weasel in Alan Bennett's *Wind in the Willows* (Nicholas Hytner, NT Olivier, 1994-95); the title role in *Richard III* (Brian Cox, Open Air Theatre, Regent's Park, 1995); Leonardo opposite Alexandra Gilbreath in García Lorca's *Blood Wedding* (Tim Supple, Young Vic, 1996); Rupert in *Rope* (Gareth Armstrong, Salisbury Playhouse, 1997); Bendrix opposite Caroline Faber in Graham Greene's *The End of the Affair* (Rupert Goold, Bridewell, 1997); Romeo opposite Jayne Ashbourne in *Romeo and Juliet* (Jonathan Church, Salisbury Playhouse, 1998); Solyony in *Three Sisters* (Bill Bryden, Birmingham Rep, 1998); Trevor Nunn's 1999 NT Ensemble—Thersites in *Troilus and Cressida* (Olivier), Ryumin in *Summerfolk* (Lyttelton), and Cat in *Honk!* (Julia McKenzie, Olivier); the Globe's 2000 season—Caliban in the Vanessa Redgrave *Tempest*, and Palamon in *The Two Noble Kinsmen* (Tim Carroll); outstanding, and less the showman, as the brother betrayed by Toby Stephens and Clare Swinburne in Simon Gray's *Japes* (Peter Hall, Theatre Royal Haymarket, 2001); the Globe's 2001 season—the title role opposite Eve Best in *Macbeth* (Carroll); Malcolm in Alan Ayckbourn's *Bedroom Farce* (Loveday Ingram, Aldwych, 2002); Henry II in Jean Anouilh's *Becket* (John Caird, Theatre Royal Haymarket, 2004); Judge Brack in *Hedda Gabler* (Matthew Lloyd, West Yorkshire Playhouse, 2006); Satan in *Paradise Lost* (Rupert Goold, Oxford Stage Company, Tour, 2006); Adolf opposite Teresa Banham in

Strindberg's *The Father* (Angus Jackson, Minerva, Chichester, 2006); and the dentist in *Little Shop of Horrors* (Matthew White, Menier Chocolate Factory, 2006-07).

Britton returned to the RSC in 2003 to play Petruchio in both Shakespeare's *The Taming of the Shrew* (RST) and John Fletcher's repost, *The Tamer Tamed* (Swan, both Doran). His dishevelled Petruchio in *The Shrew* was more hard-drinking vagabond than romantic lead, as emotionally wary as Alexandra Gilbreath's Kate: they were beautifully matched.

Jim Broadbent (b. Lincoln, 1949). The son of a furniture maker who established a Lincolnshire commune for conscientious objectors during the war, Jim Broadbent trained at the London Academy of Music and Dramatic Art and first came to wide notice working for Mike Leigh—*Ecstasy* (Hampstead Theatre, 1979); *Goose-pimples* (Hampstead Theatre, 1981)—and as one-half of the National Theatre of Brent. With a face that Phiz could have drawn, he is arguably the most distinctive character actor of his generation. The quintessential Mike Leigh actor, he flirts constantly with caricature: it is a style that allows humour and pain to co-exist.

Broadbent's early screen work included small parts in the films *Time Bandits* (Terry Gilliam, 1981), *The Hit* (Stephen Frears, 1984), and *Brazil* (Gilliam, 1985), and Del Boy's nemesis, DCI Roy 'The Slag' Slater, in *Only Fools and Horses* (BBC, from 1983—he was originally offered the role of Del Boy). Acclaimed performances in Leigh's *Life is Sweet* (1990), *The Crying Game* (Neil Jordan, 1992), *Bullets Over Broadway* (Woody Allen, 1994), *Little Voice* (Mark Herman, 1998), and, especially, Leigh's *Topsy-Turvy* (1999), established his reputation internationally, and he has since been in high demand: *Bridget Jones's Diary* (2001); Baz Luhrmann's *Moulin Rouge!* (2001); *Iris* (Richard Eyre, 2001, Oscar for Best Supporting Actor); Martin Scorsese's *Gangs of New York* (2002); *Nicholas Nickleby* (2002); *Bright Young Things* (Stephen Fry, 2003); *Around the World in 80 Days* (2004); *Vanity*

Fair (Mira Nair, 2004); *Vera Drake* (Leigh, 2004); *Bridget Jones: the Edge of Reason* (2004); *The Chronicles of Narnia* (2005); *Art School Confidential* (2006); *The Street* (BBC, 2006); *Longford* (Channel Four, 2006); *Hot Fuzz* (Edgar Wright, 2007); *And When Did You Last See Your Father?* (Anand Tucker, 2007).

On the English stage Broadbent has slowly (and regrettably) become an endangered species: the title role in *The Government Inspector* (Richard Eyre, NT Olivier, 1985); Pekala in Ronald Harwood's *The Deliberate Death of a Polish Priest* (Kevin Billington, Almeida, 1985); Kafka's father in Alan Bennett's *Kafka's Dick* (Eyre, Royal Court, 1986); Leontes in *The Winter's Tale* (Steven Pimlott, Sheffield Crucible, 1987); Sergeant Kite in Farquhar's *The Recruiting Officer* and Harry/Arscott in Timberlake Wertenbaker's *Our Country's Good* (Max Stafford-Clark, Royal Court, 1988); Chandebise/Poche in Feydeau's *A Flea in Her Ear* (Richard Jones, Old Vic, 1989); Wicksteed in Alan Bennett's *Habeas Corpus* (Sam Mendes, Donmar Warehouse, 1996); and Tupolski in Martin McDonagh's *The Pillowman* (John Crowley, NT Cottesloe, 2003).

He was at the RSC for one season (1982/83): Austin Donohue/Weir in Peter Flannery's *Our Friends in the North* (John Caird, Pit); the Colonel in Tom Stoppard's *Every Good Boy Deserves Favour* (Trevor Nunn, Barbican); and Pat in Peter Whelan's *Clay* (Bill Alexander, Pit).

Bille Brown (b. Biloela, Queensland, Australia, 1952) studied at Queensland University and began his career with the Queensland Theatre Company. As well as playing leading roles, he wrote a trilogy of plays for the company's education department: *Springle* (1975), *Tufff* (1976), and *Prunes* (1977).

Based in England from 1976 to 95, Brown worked most prominently at the RSC as a supporting player: First Ruffian in *Wild Oats* (Clifford Williams, Aldwych, 1976); Thomas Gargrave in *Henry VI* (Terry Hands, RST, 1977); Jaques de Boys in *As You Like It* (Trevor Nunn, RST, 1977); Second Volscian Citizen in

Coriolanus (Hands, RST, 1977); Soldier in *The Women-Pirates Ann Bonney and Mary Read* (Ron Daniels, Aldwych, 1978); Carter in *Saratoga, or, Pistols for Seven* (Ronald Eyre, Aldwych, 1978); Le Beau in *As You Like It* (Hands, RST, 1980); Barnardo in *Hamlet* (John Barton, RST, 1980-81); Sir Henry Green in *Richard II* (Hands, RST, 1980); Lord Lovel in *Richard III* (Hands, RST, 1980); Griselda in his own pantomime *The Swan Down Gloves* (Ian Judge/Hands, RST, 1981); Paris in *Troilus and Cressida* (Hands, Aldwych, 1981); Wicked Witch in *The Wizard of Oz* (Judge, Barbican, 1987-88); Sir Andrew Aguecheek in *Twelfth Night* (Judge, RST, 1994); and Elbow in *Measure for Measure* (Steven Pimlott, RST, 1994).

As classical actor, playwright (*Bill and Mary*, QTC, 2002) and teacher (Queensland University), Brown is one of the Australian theatre's most distinguished figures. His version of *Aladdin*, starring Ian McKellen, was a hit for Kevin Spacey's Old Vic in 2004/05. Films (all Australian): *Oscar and Lucinda* (Gillian Armstrong, 1997); *The Dish* (2000); *The Man Who Sued God* (2001); *Black and White* (2002); *Dirty Deeds* (2002).

Susan Brown (b. Bristol, 1946) trained at the Rose Bruford College of Speech and Drama. It was in the 1980s that she began to find recognition for her vivid but subtle characterisations. For Bill Pryde's Cambridge Theatre Company she appeared in mainstream classics — Mrs Sullen in *The Beaux' Stratagem*, Helen in *The Vortex*, multiple roles in Shaw's *Back to Methuselah*, and Millamant in *The Way of the World* (1984-89). Things could hardly have been more different at the Royal Court, where she was cast in Andrea Dunbar's *Shirley* (Carole Hayman, 1986), Gregory Motton's *Downfall* (1988), Hugh Stoddart's *Gibraltar Strait* (Simon Curtis, 1990), and, most importantly, Jim Cartwright's *Road* (Curtis, 1986-87).

She has since played La Poncia in *The House of Bernarda Alba* (Katie Mitchell, Gate, 1992); Jenny Ross in Phyllis Nagy's *Butterfly Kiss* (Steven Pimlott, Almeida, 1994); Stella in Simon Smith's

You Be Ted and I'll Be Sylvia (Jonathan Church, Hampstead Theatre, 1999); the mother in Peter Gill's *Small Change* (Rufus Norris, Sheffield Crucible, 2002); Clytemnestra in Edna O'Brien's version of Euripides's *Iphigenia* (Anna Mackmin, Sheffield Crucible, 2002-03); Hetty in Imogen Stubbs's *We Happy Few* (Stephen Rayne, Malvern Festival Theatre, 2003); Old Woman opposite Nicholas Woodeson in Ionesco's *The Chairs* (Thea Sharrock, Gate, 2006); and the washerwoman in Nikolai Erdman's *The Suicide*, renamed *Dying For It* (Mackmin, Almeida, 2007).

She joined the RSC in early 1995 to play Mrs Heyst in Katie Mitchell's production of Strindberg's *Easter* (Pit). Moving on to Stratford she was an unusually young and melancholy nurse to Lucy Whybrow's Juliet in *Romeo and Juliet* (Adrian Noble, RST), and a powerful Queen Elizabeth in the David Troughton *Richard III* (Steven Pimlott, RST). She returned in 1998 to create the role of Kay in Robert Holman's *Bad Weather* (Pimlott, TOP).

Brenda Bruce (1918-1996, b. Manchester). The fascinating, versatile and sorely-missed Brenda Bruce enjoyed a career that was delightfully unorthodox. She started as a teenage chorus girl in *1066 and All That* at the Strand Theatre in the 1930s and ended as an acclaimed interpreter of Shakespeare. In-between she trained under Barry Jackson at the Birmingham Rep (1936-39), presented a television show with her husband Roy Rich called *Rich and Rich* (1950s), and ran a hotel near Stratford (1970s). On the stage, her successes included the iconic roles of Eliza (opposite Alec Clunes) in Bernard Shaw's *Pygmalion* (Lyric Hammersmith, 1947) and Winnie in the British premiere of Samuel Beckett's *Happy Days* (George Devine, Royal Court, 1962).

Brenda Bruce joined the RSC in 1964. She was the ideal vessel for Shakespeare's humanism, the RSC's resident Mistress Page in *The Merry Wives of Windsor* (performing the role for John Blatchley in 1964 and for Terry Hands in 1968 and 1975); Dionyza and the Bawd in *Pericles* (Hands, RST, 1969); Paulina in *The Winter's Tale* (Trevor Nunn, RST, 1969); Maria in *Twelfth Night*

(John Barton, RST, 1969); Queen Elizabeth in *Richard III* (Hands, RST, 1970); Gertrude in *Hamlet* (Nunn, RST, 1970); Lady Capulet in *Romeo and Juliet* (Hands, RST, 1973); Queen Margaret in *Richard III* (Barry Kyle, TOP, 1975); Mistress Quickly in *Henry V* (Hands, International Tour, 1976); and the Nurse in *Romeo and Juliet* (Ron Daniels, RST, 1980).

In London, at the Aldwych, she created roles in the British premieres of Henry Livings's *Eh?* (1964), Jules Feiffer's *Little Murders* (1967) and José Triana's *The Criminals* (1967). More appreciably, she embraced the eclecticism of the programming, delivering during one memorable season (1971) the sparkling international hat trick of Paulina in Maxim Gorky's *Enemies* (David Jones), Lady Townley in George Etherege's *The Man of Mode* (Hands) and Irma in Jean Genet's *The Balcony* (Hands). An early participant in the RSC's development of small-scale work, she was a member of the first ensemble at The Other Place (1973) and played Mrs Hall in Strindberg's *Comrades* (Kyle) and Mrs Crowley in Snoo Wilson's *The Beast* (Howard Davies) at the Place, London (1974).

Throughout her career Brenda Bruce worked as a character actress in British films: *Millions Like Us* (Frank Launder/Sidney Gilliat, 1943); J.B. Priestley's *They Came to a City* (Basil Dearden, 1944); *Night Boat to Dublin* (Lawrence Huntington, 1945); *Piccadilly Incident* (Herbert Wilcox, 1946); *Carnival* (Stanley Haynes, 1946); Terence Rattigan's wartime comedy *While the Sun Shines* (Anthony Asquith, 1947); *When the Bough Breaks* (Lawrence Huntington, 1947); *My Brother's Keeper* (Alfred Roome, 1948); *Marry Me* (Terence Fisher, 1949); *Don't Ever Leave Me* (Arthur Crabtree, 1949); Terence Rattigan's *The Final Test* (Anthony Asquith, 1953); *Law and Disorder* (Charles Crichton, 1958); *Behind the Mask* (Brian Desmond Hurst, 1958); Dora in Michael Powell's *Peeping Tom* (1960); *Nightmare* (Freddie Francis, 1964); *Steaming* (Joseph Losey, 1985); *Little Dorrit* (Christine Edzard, 1988); *December Bride* (Thaddeus O'Sullivan, 1990); and *Splitting Heirs* (1993).

Alfred Burke (b. 1918) was in his late sixties when he first joined the RSC. During the next fourteen years he played a succession of incisive cameos with the gravity and grace of a master: Duncan in the Jonathan Pryce *Macbeth* (Adrian Noble, RST, 1986); Savel Dikoy in *The Storm* (Nick Hamm, Pit, 1987); Jolyon in Robert Holman's *Across Oka* (Sarah Pia Anderson, TOP, 1988); Gonzalo in *The Tempest* (Nicholas Hytner, RST, 1988); Gabriel Hedges in *Restoration* (Roger Michell, Swan, 1988); Knut Brovik in *The Master Builder* (Noble, Barbican, 1989); Nestor in *Troilus and Cressida* (Sam Mendes, Swan, 1990); Wemyss in Richard Nelson's *Two Shakespearean Actors* (Michell, Swan, 1990); Sorin in *The Seagull* (Terry Hands, Swan, 1990); Adam in *As You Like It* (David Thacker, RST, 1992); Lord Lafew in *All's Well That Ends Well* (Peter Hall, Swan, 1992); Lepidus in *Antony and Cleopatra* (John Caird, RST, 1992); the Button-Moulder in *Peer Gynt* (John Barton, Swan, 1994); Egeus in *A Midsummer Night's Dream* (Noble, RST, 1994); Old Gentleman in *Roberto Zucco* (James Macdonald, TOP, 1997); Gonzalo in *The Tempest* (Noble, RST, 1998); John of Gaunt in *Richard II* (Steven Pimlott, TOP, 2000); and Escalus in *Romeo and Juliet* (Michael Boyd, RST, 2000). The latter found him physically frail — his legs like two bent walking sticks — but as alert as ever.

In the 1960s and 70s he had been a television actor, the star of the popular series *Public Eye* (ITV).

Alan Burrett (b. London) first worked at the RSC in 1989/90, lighting John Caird's productions of *A Midsummer Night's Dream* and *As You Like It* (RST), and Barry Kyle's *Moscow Gold* (Barbican). The next few years saw him collaborating with Adrian Noble and the designers Bob Crowley, Ultz and Anthony Ward to achieve the striking images of *Henry IV Parts 1 and 2* (RST, 1991), *The Thebans* (Swan, 1991), *Hamlet* (Barbican, 1992), and *King Lear* (RST, 1993).

Other RSC work: Noble's *Macbeth* (Barbican, 1993); Michael Attenborough's *The Changeling* (Swan, 1992) and *The Herbal Bed*

(TOP, 1996); David Leveaux's *Romeo and Juliet* (Barbican, 1992); David Thacker's *Julius Caesar* (TOP, 1993), *The Two Gentlemen of Verona* (Barbican, 1993), *Coriolanus* (Swan, 1994), *Bingo* (Swan, 1995) and *The Tempest* (Swan, 1995); Ian Judge's *Love's Labour's Lost* (RST, 1993); and Matthew Warchus's *Henry V* (Barbican, 1995). Burrett has been based in the United States since the late 1990s.

John Bury (1925-2000, b. Aberystwyth). From 1946 to 1963 John Bury worked for Joan Littlewood's Theatre Workshop, initially as an actor but then as Stratford East's resident designer. He designed some of the Theatre Workshop's most notable productions, including Shelagh Delaney's *A Taste of Honey* (1958), *Fings Ain't Wot They Used to Be* (1958) and *Oh! What a Lovely War* (1963). He developed a method, based on the 'building' of sets, which can be inadequately described as Brechtian. If the production required a brick wall, then Bury would build a brick wall. This was the opposite of the style of pictorial simulation (painted cloths, etc.) that dominated Stratford-upon-Avon in the 1950s.

Bury took his method to the RSC in 1962. Peter Hall wanted an unadorned, unsentimental theatre, and Bury was the right designer. Their work, austere and deliberately plain (they avoided colour), gave the early RSC its house style. Within the confines of this aesthetic Bury created sets that had imagistic power—the all-metal environment of *The Wars of the Roses* (RST, 1963), or the grey house of *The Homecoming* (Aldwych, 1965). As head of design, he introduced a basic grey box set and a standard rake—to achieve unity, all directors and designers were expected to use this configuration, and it remained prevalent until 1968. He played a key part in the design of the Barbican Theatre.

For Hall, Bury also designed *The Collection* (Aldwych, 1962); *Richard II* (RST, 1964); *Henry IV* (RST, 1964); *Henry V* (RST, 1964); *Eh?* (Aldwych, 1964); *Hamlet* (RST, 1965); *The Government Inspec-*

tor (Aldwych, 1966); *Macbeth* (RST, 1967); *A Delicate Balance* (Aldwych, 1969); *Dutch Uncle* (Aldwych, 1969); *Landscape* and *Silence* (Aldwych, 1969); *Old Times* (Aldwych, 1971); *All Over* (Hall, 1972); and *A Slight Ache* (Aldwych, 1973). His other RSC productions included *Afore Night Come* (Williams, Arts Theatre, 1962); *The Physicists* (Brook, Aldwych, 1963); *Coriolanus* (Barton, RST, 1967); *The Criminals* (Hands, Aldwych, 1967); *The Silver Tassie* (Jones, Aldwych, 1969); *Henry VIII* (Nunn, RST, 1969); and *Exiles* (Harold Pinter, Aldwych, 1971).

Bury's tenure as head of design came to an end when Hall stepped down as artistic director. When Hall moved to the National Theatre Bury went with him; he was head of design there until 1985.

Judy Buxton trained at the Rose Bruford College of Speech and Drama. During two and a half years with the RSC, she was a memorable Juliet, dark, supple and sensuous, in *Romeo and Juliet* (Ron Daniels, RST, 1980); Iphigenia in John Barton's *The Greeks* (Aldwych, 1980); Phrynia in *Timon of Athens* (Daniels, TOP, 1980); Jessica in *The Merchant of Venice* (Barton, Aldwych, 1981); Kit in *The Swan Down Gloves* (Hands, Aldwych, 1981); and Sweet Girl in *La Ronde* (Barton, Aldwych, 1982). Curiously, this hugely promising classical work was both preceded and followed by a sporadic screen career of sitcoms, drama serials and B-movies.

Before joining the RSC she was best known for her role as a nurse in the long-running medical soap *General Hospital* (1972-79), but also appeared in *The Likely Lads* (BBC, 1976), *Rising Damp* (1977), *Blake's Seven* (BBC, 1979) and the films *The Devil Within Her* (Peter Sasdy, 1975), *The Bawdy Adventures of Tom Jones* (Cliff Owen, 1976) and *Aces High* (Jack Gold, 1976).

C

David Calder (b. Portsmouth, 1946). The redoubtable David Calder was an indispensable senior player at the RSC during the Adrian Noble era. His qualities include fine verse-speaking, an authoritative presence and adaptability.

Like so many leading actors who came of age in the 1960s Calder was a member of the National Youth Theatre. Following his training at the Bristol Old Vic School he appeared with the Old Vic company, and went on to make his name as Shylock, Macbeth and Eddie in Arthur Miller's *A View from the Bridge* on regional stages. As a member of the Prospect Theatre Company in 1969 he played Lord Ross in *Richard II* and Young Spencer in *Edward II* (Tour).

Calder was first a member of the RSC during the early 1970s, playing Lorenzo in *The Merchant of Venice* (Terry Hands, RST, 1971); Chorus in the Michael Williams *Henry V* (John Barton, Theatregoround, 1971); Cassio in *Othello* (Barton, RST, 1971); Chief Ferret in *Toad of Toad Hall* (Euan Smith, RST, 1972); Krivoy Zob in Gorky's *The Lower Depths* (David Jones, Aldwych, 1972); and Balin in John Arden's *Island of the Mighty* (Jones, Aldwych, 1972). Since his return in 1988 he has created a formidable York in Adrian Noble's *The Plantagenets* (RST, 1988); Manly in *The Plain Dealer* (Ron Daniels, Swan, 1988); Larry Palmer in Howard Brenton's *H.I.D.* (Danny Boyle, Almeida, 1989); Gorbachev, an uncanny resemblance, in Brenton's *Moscow Gold* (Barry Kyle, Barbican, 1990); Skule in Ibsen's *The Pretenders* (Boyle, Pit, 1991); a charismatic, deeply-felt Kent in the Robert Stephens *King Lear* (Noble, RST, 1993); a contemporary Shylock in *The Merchant of Venice* (David Thacker, RST, 1993); Sir Toby Belch in *Twelfth Night* (Noble, RST, 1997-98); and a powerful Prospero in *The Tempest* (Noble, RST, 1998).

Elsewhere, since 1980, his work has been equally engrossing: Sarah Daniel's *Ripen Our Darkness* (Royal Court Upstairs, 1981); Creon in *Medea* (Traverse, Edinburgh, 1983); Iago in *Othello*

(David Thacker, Young Vic, 1984); Gorky to Daniel Day-Lewis's Mayakovsky in *Futurists* (Richard Eyre, NT Cottesloe, 1986); de Sade in *Marat/Sade* (Jeremy Sams, NT Olivier, 1997); Yasmina Reza's *Conversations After a Burial* (Howard Davies, Almeida, 2000); Lillian Hellman's *The Little Foxes* (Marianne Elliott, Donmar Warehouse, 2001); Joanna Laurens's *Five Gold Rings* (Michael Attenborough, Almeida, 2003); Harry in David Storey's *Home* (Sean Holmes, Oxford Stage Company, Tour, 2004); and Max in Tom Stoppard's *Rock 'n' Roll* (Trevor Nunn, Duke of York's, 2006-07).

On television, Calder co-starred in the popular drama serials *Widows* (ITV, 1983); *Bramwell* (ITV, 1995-96); *Drovers' Gold* (BBC, 1997); and *Holding On* (BBC, 1997). He played John Lawrence in Richard Eyre's *Tumbledown* (BBC, 1989); Krogstad opposite Juliet Stevenson in *A Doll's House* (David Thacker, BBC, 1991); Chubb in Alan Bennett's drama about Anthony Blunt, *A Question of Attribution* (John Schlesinger, BBC, 1992); Sir Paul Condon in *The Murder of Stephen Lawrence* (Paul Greengrass, ITV, 1999); and Churchill in *Wallis and Edward* (ITV, 2005). He can claim a broad collection of movies: *Superman* (1978); *American Friends* (Tristram Powell, 1991); *Hollow Reed* (Angela Pope, 1996); *The World is Not Enough* (Michael Apted, 1999); *The King is Alive* (2000); *Perfume* (Tom Tykwer, 2006); *Goya's Ghosts* (Milos Forman, 2006).

Cheryl Campbell (b. St Albans, 1949). The daughter of a pilot, Cheryl Campbell trained at the London Academy of Music and Dramatic Art and worked at the Watford Palace Theatre, the Birmingham Rep and the Glasgow Citizens' before coming to notice in 1975 at the National (Old Vic) as Freda in the Ralph Richardson/Peggy Ashcroft/Wendy Hiller *John Gabriel Borkman* (Peter Hall) and Maggie in W.S. Gilbert's *Engaged* (Michael Blakemore).

Blonde, pallid and emotionally wrecked, she played the rural schoolmistress in Dennis Potter's *Pennies from Heaven* (Piers

Haggard, BBC, 1978), followed by Sarah Bernhardt in *Lillie* (ITV, 1978) and Vera Brittain in *Testament of Youth* (Moira Armstrong, BBC, 1979). In 1981 she joined the RSC and was a startlingly provocative Nora in *A Doll's House* (Adrian Noble, TOP) and a coquettish Diana to Harriet Walter's Helena in *All's Well That Ends Well* (Trevor Nunn, RST). On the big screen, she played Sheila McVicar in *McVicar* (Tom Clegg, 1980), Sister Monica in *Hawk the Slayer* (Terry Marcel, 1980), Jenny Liddell opposite Ian Charleson in *Chariots of Fire* (Hugh Hudson, 1981), Lady Aline Hartlip in *The Shooting Party* (Alan Bridges, 1984), and the shipwrecked Lady Alice Clayton in *Greystoke* (Hudson, 1984).

She has worked less prominently since, mostly on the stage: Asta in *Little Eyolf* (Lyric Hammersmith, 1985); the title role in *The Daughter-in-Law* (Hampstead Theatre, 1985); Margery Pinchwife to Gary Oldman's Horner in *The Country Wife* (Nicholas Hytner, Manchester Royal Exchange, 1986-87); Michael Frayn's Chekhov selection *The Sneeze* (Ronald Eyre, Aldwych, 1988); Constance in Somerset Maugham's *The Constant Wife* (Lucy Parker, Theatr Clwyd, 1990); Blanche in *A Streetcar Named Desire* (Leicester Haymarket, 1990); Emma in Harold Pinter's *Betrayal* (David Leveaux, Almeida, 1991); Phyllis Nagy's *The Strip* (Royal Court, 1995); Lady Wouldbe in *Volpone* (Matthew Warchus, NT Olivier, 1995); Arthur Miller's *The Last Yankee* (Michael Grandage, Mercury Theatre, Colchester, 1996); Arkadina in *The Seagull* (Stephen Unwin, English Touring Theatre, Donmar Warehouse, 1997); Peter Nichols's *Passion Play* (Michael Grandage, Donmar Warehouse, 2000); Hannie Rayson's *Life After George* (Michael Blakemore, Duchess Theatre, 2002); and Michael Frayn's *Noises Off* (Jeremy Sams, NT Piccadilly, 2003).

She returned to the RSC for the 1992-94 cycle and played Mistress Ford in *The Merry Wives of Windsor* (David Thacker, RST); Beatrice-Joanna in *The Changeling* (Michael Attenborough, Swan); Natasha in *Misha's Party* (David Jones, Pit); and Lady Macbeth opposite Derek Jacobi in *Macbeth* (Noble, Barbican).

John Carlisle. John Carlisle has created an RSC gallery of cold but urbane manipulators—among them a hawk-like Ulysses in *Troilus and Cressida* (Terry Hands, Aldwych, 1981); Don John in *Much Ado About Nothing* (Hands, RST, 1982); Ralph Nickleby in *Nicholas Nickleby* (Trevor Nunn/John Caird, RST, 1986); a racist Antonio in *The Merchant of Venice* (Bill Alexander, RST, 1987); Machevil in *The Jew of Malta* (Barry Kyle, Swan, 1987); Oberon in *A Midsummer Night's Dream* (Caird, RST, 1989); and Iachimo in *Cymbeline* (Alexander, RST, 1989). During fifteen continuous years with the Company, he was also a forceful figure in Jacobean rarities—the King in Beaumont and Fletcher's *The Maid's Tragedy* (Kyle, TOP, 1980), Lovel in Ben Jonson's *The New Inn* (Caird, Swan, 1987); in Ibsen and Chekhov—Pastor Manders in *Ghosts* (Katie Mitchell, TOP, 1993), Dorn in *The Seagull* (Hands, Swan, 1990); and in contemporary plays—the Parson in Edward Bond's *The Fool* (Howard Davies, TOP, 1980), the Rector in Nick Darke's *The Body* (Nick Hamm, Pit, 1983), the Minister in Caryl Churchill's *Softcops* (Davies, Pit, 1984), Serioja's Voice in John Berger's *A Question of Geography* (Caird, TOP, 1987), Schliemann in Howard Barker's *The Bite of the Night* (Danny Boyle, Pit, 1988), William Macready in Richard Nelson's *Two Shakespearean Actors* (Roger Michell, Swan, 1990), and Jaeger in David Pownall's *Elgar's Rondo* (Di Trevis, Swan, 1993).

Carlisle returned to the RSC to play Gloucester in the Nigel Hawthorne *King Lear* (Yukio Ninagawa, Barbican 1999), but left the cast of John Barton's *Tantalus* when Peter Hall decided the actors should wear masks (2000). He has worked most prominently elsewhere in recent years: Dr Rank in the Janet McTeer/Owen Teale *A Doll's House* (Anthony Page, Playhouse, 1996); Jowett and Stead in Tom Stoppard's *The Invention of Love* (Richard Eyre, NT Cottesloe, 1997); Old Bakunin in Stoppard's *The Coast of Utopia* (Trevor Nunn, NT Olivier, 2002); Lord Boreal in *His Dark Materials* (Nicholas Hytner, NT Olivier, 2003); and the uncle in Pirandello's *As You Desire Me* (Jonathan Kent, Playhouse, 2005).

Nancy Carroll (b. London, 1974) was a member of the vibrant drama society at Leeds University, playing leading roles in Alan Ayckbourn's *Season's Greetings*, the musical *Cabaret*, and Molière's *Tartuffe*. *Tartuffe* visited the 1996 Edinburgh Festival, and Nancy Carroll went on to train at the London Academy of Music and Dramatic Art, graduating in 1998. Her professional career started at the RSC, where as a member of the winter 1998/99 company in Stratford and London she played small roles in *The Lion, the Witch and the Wardrobe* (Adrian Noble) and *The Winter's Tale* (Gregory Doran). Following her breakthrough as Ophelia in *Hamlet* (Gemma Bodinetz) at the Bristol Old Vic she returned to the RSC to play a stylish Celia in *As You Like It* (Doran, RST), and a tender Lady Percy in *Henry IV* ('This England: the Histories', Michael Attenborough, Swan, 2000).

She is both a leading and a character actress: Cordelia in *King Lear* (Jonathan Kent, Almeida at King's Cross, 2002); Jennet in Christopher Fry's *The Lady's Not for Burning* (Samuel West, Minerva, Chichester, 2002); Frau Jung opposite Ralph Fiennes in Christopher Hampton's *The Talking Cure* (Howard Davies, NT Cottesloe, 2002-03); the female leads opposite Jo Stone-Fewings in the Noël Coward double-bill *Astonished Heart/Still Life* (Philip Wilson, Liverpool Playhouse, 2004); the Chevalier to Charlotte Rampling's Countess in Marivaux's *The False Servant* (Kent, NT Cottesloe, 2004); Lorna in Amelia Bullmore's *Mammals* (Anna Mackmin, Bush, 2005); Gloria in Bernard Shaw's *You Never Can Tell* (Peter Hall, Theatre Royal, Bath, 2005); Alice in Harley Granville-Barker's *The Voysey Inheritance* (Peter Gill, NT Lyttelton, 2006); Penelope in Philip King's farce *See How They Run* (Douglas Hodge, Duchess, 2006); Mrs Loveit in *The Man of Mode* (Nicholas Hytner, NT Olivier, 2007); and Louise Strandberg in Victoria Benedictsson's *The Enchantment* (Paul Miller, NT Cottesloe, 2007).

Elaine Cassidy (b. Dublin, 1979) was still at school in Kilcoole, County Wicklow, when Atom Egoyan cast her as Felicia in *Felicia's Journey* (1999). It was a remarkable beginning. Her serious brown eyes and bare legs were the outward signs of a performance that captured perfectly the character's sweet determination, naivety and vulnerability.

She has since fulfilled the promise of *Felicia* in an impressive range of work: the mute maid in *The Others* (Alejandro Amenábar, 2001); Runt in *Disco Pigs* (Kirsten Sheridan, 2001); Agnes in *The Lost World* (Stuart Orme, BBC, 2001); Carrie in *The Bay of Love and Sorrows* (Tim Southam, 2002); Martin McDonagh's terrifying child-woman in *The Lieutenant of Inishmore* at the RSC (Wilson Milam, Garrick, 2002); Anna in *Watermelon* (ITV, 2003); Maggie in Owen McCafferty's *Scenes from the Big Picture* at the National (Peter Gill, Cottesloe, 2003); Hitler's doomed niece in *Uncle Adolf* (ITV, 2005); Maud in *Fingersmith* (BBC, 2005); Amy Harris in *The Ghost Squad* (Channel Four, 2005); Abigail in *The Crucible* at the RSC (Dominic Cooke, RST, 2006); Candy in *The Truth* (2006); Sandra in *And When Did You Last See Your Father?* (Anand Tucker, 2007); Louise in Frank McGuinness's *There Came a Gypsy Riding* at the Almeida (Michael Attenborough, 2007); and a beautiful realisation of E.M. Forster's Lucy in *A Room With a View* (ITV, 2007).

Ian Charleson (1949-1990, b. Edinburgh). The son of an Edinburgh printer, Ian Charleson grew up in a working-class district of the city. He studied architecture at Edinburgh University, but found his forte as a member of the drama society. He won a place on the acting course at the London Academy of Music and Dramatic Art and began his career as a member of Frank Dunlop's Young Vic company (1972-74). He played Hamlet at Cambridge (1975) and a Glaswegian thug in Simon Gray's *Otherwise Engaged* in the West End (Queen's, 1976). He first appeared at the National in 1977, as Octavius in *Julius Caesar*

(John Schlesinger) and Peregrine in *Volpone* (Peter Hall). His first film was Derek Jarman's *Jubilee* (1977).

He had quality, was an actor to watch. He went to the RSC and played disparate roles: a tough, 'human' Ariel in *The Tempest* (Clifford Williams, RST, 1978); Tranio in *The Taming of the Shrew* (Michael Bogdanov, RST, 1978); Longaville in *Love's Labour's Lost* (John Barton, RST, 1978); Man at Rehearsal/Pierre in Pam Gems's *Piaf* (Howard Davies, TOP, 1978); Joe Maguire in Tom McGrath's *The Innocent* (Davies, Warehouse, 1979); and Lawrence Vail in *Once in a Lifetime* (Trevor Nunn, Aldwych, 1979).

He left the RSC to play Eric Liddell in *Chariots of Fire* (Hugh Hudson); the success of the picture, released in 1981, led him to hope for a major career in films. He played supporting roles in *Gandhi* (Richard Attenborough, 1982), *Ascendancy* (1982) and *Greystoke* (Hudson, 1984), and starred in *Car Trouble* (1986) and *Opera* (Dario Argento, 1987). He was in three American television productions broadcast in 1984, *The Sun Also Rises*, as Mike Campbell, *Master of the Game* and *Louisiana*. For the BBC Shakespeare he played Bertram in *All's Well That Ends Well* (1980), Fortinbras in *Hamlet* (1980), and Octavius Caesar in *Antony and Cleopatra* (1981).

His final stage performances, all of them memorable, were at the National: Sky Masterson in *Guys and Dolls* (Richard Eyre, Olivier, 1982); Eddie in Sam Shepard's *Fool for Love* (Peter Gill, Cottesloe, 1984); Brick in *Cat on a Hot Tin Roof* (Davies, Lyttelton, 1988); and the title role, succeeding Daniel Day-Lewis, in *Hamlet* (Eyre, Olivier, 1989). The latter performance stilled the vast auditorium with its sadness and rage. It was not known at the time, but he had AIDS. He died a few months later in January 1990.

The Ian Charleson Awards, established by the National and *The Sunday Times*, are awarded annually to the best actors under thirty.

Nick Chelton (b. London) started out as an assistant to Richard Pilbrow at Theatre Projects. He established his reputation at the Greenwich Theatre and the Royal Court, where his work included Edward Bond's *Bingo* (Jane Howell/John Dove, 1974) and Lindsay Anderson's productions of David Storey's *The Farm* (1973) and *Life Class* (1974) and Joe Orton's *What the Butler Saw* (1975). For the RSC he lit productions by Trevor Nunn (*Macbeth*, RST, 1974), Richard Eyre (*Jingo*, Aldwych, 1975), John Barton (*The Way of the World*, Aldwych, 1978; *Love's Labour's Lost*, RST, 1978) and Peter Brook (*Antony and Cleopatra*, RST, 1978).

During the 1980s and 90s he worked most prominently in opera, designing beautiful and tellingly dramatic lighting for David Pountney, Graham Vick, Patrick Mason, Elijah Moshinsky, Richard Jones, Nicholas Hytner and Matthew Warchus: *The Valkyrie* (Pountney, ENO, 1983); *The Mastersingers* (Moshinsky, ENO, 1984); *The Bartered Bride* (Moshinsky, ENO, 1985); *The Midsummer Marriage* (Pountney, ENO, 1985); *Katya Kabanova* (Pountney, ENO, 1985); *Carmen* (Vick, Scottish Opera, 1986); *Rusalka* (Pountney, ENO, 1986); *Doctor Faust* (Pountney, ENO, 1986); *The Magic Flute* (Hytner, ENO, 1988); *The Cunning Little Vixen* (Pountney, ENO, 1988); *The Love for Three Oranges* (Jones, ENO, 1989); *Eugene Onegin* (Vick, ENO, 1989); *Un re in ascolto* (Vick, Royal Opera, 1989); *Ariane and Bluebeard* (Mason, Opera North, 1990); *The Ring* (Vick, The City of Birmingham Touring Opera, 1990); *Caritas* (Mason, Opera North, 1991); *The Marriage of Figaro* (Vick, ENO, 1991); *Mitridate* (Vick, Royal Opera, 1991); *Billy Budd* (Vick, Opera North, 1992); *Troilus and Cressida* (Warchus, Opera North, 1995); *Il trittico* (Mason, ENO, 1998); *Samson et Dalila* (Moshinsky, Royal Opera, 2004).

Chelton's theatre productions since 1980: at the RSC, Ron Daniels's *Julius Caesar* (Barbican, 1984), Ian Judge's *The Wizard of Oz* (Barbican, 1987) and Robin Lefevre's *Curse of the Starving Class* (Pit, 1991); at the Royal Exchange, Manchester, Hytner's *Don Carlos* (1987); at the Hampstead Theatre, Lefevre's *Someone*

Who'll Watch Over Me (1992); and at the Abbey, Dublin, Mason's *Chamber Music* (1994), *Angels in America* (1995), *Observe the Sons of Ulster Marching Towards the Somme* (1995), *She Stoops to Folly* (1996), *By the Bog of Cats* (1998), *The Secret Fall of Constance Wilde* (1998) and *Dolly West's Kitchen* (1999).

Alison Chitty (b. 1948) studied at St Martin's School of Art and the Central School of Art and Design. After creating the sets and costumes for over forty shows at the Victoria Theatre, Stoke-on-Trent (1970-79), she came to prominence working with Peter Gill at the Riverside Studios (*Measure for Measure*). When Gill joined Peter Hall's directorial team at the National in 1981 Chitty followed. She stayed at the National, as resident designer, until 1988, working chiefly for Gill—*A Month in the Country* (Olivier, 1981); *Don Juan* (Cottesloe, 1981); *Much Ado About Nothing* (Olivier, 1981); *Danton's Death* (Olivier, 1982); *Major Barbara* (Lyttelton, 1982); *Tales from Hollywood* (Olivier, 1983); *Venice Preserv'd* (Lyttelton, 1984); *Antigone* (Cottesloe, 1984)—and Hall—*Antony and Cleopatra* (Olivier, 1997); and the 'Late Shakespeares', *The Winter's Tale*, *The Tempest*, *Cymbeline* (Cottesloe, 1988).

In contrast, her association with the RSC has been limited. She designed Bill Alexander's productions of *Tartuffe* (Pit) and *Volpone* (TOP, both 1983); Ron Daniels's *Breaking the Silence* (Pit, 1984); David Leveaux's *Romeo and Juliet* (RST, 1991); and Steven Pimlott's *Hamlet* (RST, 2001—her re-configured all grey RST was used for the entire season).

Although Alison Chitty works principally in the theatre (and is director of the Motley Theatre Design Course), she has successfully crossed over into films, designing, most notably, Mike Leigh's *Life is Sweet* (1991), *Naked* (1993) and *Secrets and Lies* (1995).

Tony Church (1930-2008, b. London), a contemporary of Peter Hall at Cambridge, made his first professional appearance at the

Arts Theatre, London, in Hall's production of Pirandello's *Henry IV* (1953). An actor of remarkable range and effortless authority, he was a founding member of the RSC in 1960, the beginning of twenty-six years and a myriad of roles: highlights were Cornwall in Peter Brook's *King Lear* (RST, 1962), Polonius in two productions of *Hamlet* (Hall, RST, 1965; John Barton, RST, 1980), Henry IV (Barton, RST, 1966), Sir Toby Belch in *Twelfth Night* (Barton, RST, 1971), Don Armado in two productions of *Love's Labour's Lost* (David Jones, RST, 1973; Barton, Aldwych, 1979), King Lear (Buzz Goodbody, The Place, 1974), Gloucester in *King Lear* (Trevor Nunn, RST, 1976), and Pandarus in *Troilus and Cressida* (Terry Hands, Aldwych, 1981).

Church's scope was limitless: Hortensio in *The Taming of the Shrew* (Barton, RST, 1960); Frederick in the Vanessa Redgrave *As You Like It* (Michael Elliott, RST, 1961); Peter Quince in *A Midsummer Night's Dream* (Hall, RST, 1962); Pisanio in *Cymbeline* (Gaskill, RST, 1962); Aegeon in *The Comedy of Errors* (Clifford Williams, RST, 1962); Lockit in *The Beggar's Opera* (Wood, Aldwych, 1963); Count Fontana in *The Representative* (Williams, Aldwych, 1963); Holofernes in *Love's Labour's Lost* (Barton, RST, 1965); Machiavel in *The Jew of Malta* (Williams, RST, 1965); Flavius in *Timon of Athens* (John Schlesinger, RST, 1965); Stepan in *The Proposal* (Hands, Theatregoround, 1966); Antonio in *The Merchant of Venice* (Hands, RST, 1971); Mr Badger in *Toad of Toad Hall* (Euan Smith, RST, 1972); Mikhail in Gorky's *The Lower Depths* (Jones, Aldwych, 1972); Third Tempter in *Murder in the Cathedral* (Hands, Aldwych, 1972); Friar Laurence in *Romeo and Juliet* (Hands, RST, 1973); John of Gaunt in *Richard II* (Barton, RST, 1973); Duke Senior in *As You Like It* (Buzz Goodbody, RST, 1973); Belarius in *Cymbeline* (Barton, RST, 1974); Suslov in Gorky's *Summerfolk* (Jones, Aldwych, 1974); Diderot in Snoo Wilson's *The Beast* (Howard Davies, The Place, 1974); Henry VII in John Ford's *Perkin Warbeck* (Barton, TOP, 1975); Buckingham in *Richard III* (Kyle, TOP, 1975); Ulysses in *Troilus and Cressida* (Barton/Kyle, RST, 1976); Rorlund in *Pillars of the Community* (Barton, Aldwych, 1977); Old Gobbo in *The Merchant of Venice*

143

(Barton, Warehouse, 1979); Menelaus/Odysseus in *The Greeks* (Barton, Aldwych, 1980); Duke of York in *Richard II* (Hands, RST, 1980); the Husband in *La Ronde* (Barton, Aldwych, 1982); Trelawney in David Edgar's *Maydays* (Ron Daniels, Barbican, 1983); Horsham in *Waste* (Barton, Pit, 1985); Old Kno'well in *Every Man in His Humour* (John Caird, Swan, 1986); Director of the Nuclear Plant in *Sarcophagus* (Jude Kelly, Pit, 1987); and the Wizard in *The Wizard of Oz* (Ian Judge, Barbican, 1987).

His RSC performances only tell a part of the story. He founded and ran the Northcott Theatre, Exeter, from 1967 to 1971. A longtime teacher, he was Director of Drama at the Guildhall School from 1982 to 1988, and Dean of the National Theatre Conservatory, Denver, in the 1990s. As the *éminence grise* of the Denver Center Theatre Company, one of the best regional theatres in America, he played Scrooge (1990), Malvolio (1991), Lear (1995), the Bishop in *Racing Demon* (Anthony Powell, 1997) and Jonkers in Fugard's *Valley Song* (Bruce K. Sevy, 1998).

Patience Collier (1910-1987, b. London) was educated in Paris and London. She made her debut in Komisarjevsky's *Versailles* at the Kingsway Theatre (1932). It was not until her forties that she started to come into her own as a formidable character actress. For John Gielgud, at the Lyric Hammersmith and Globe, she played Charlotte Ivanovna in *The Cherry Orchard* (1954) and Anya in Noël Coward's *Nude With Violin* (1956); for Peter Brook, at the Phoenix, Maria in Graham Greene's *The Power and the Glory* and Violet in T.S. Eliot's *The Family Reunion* (1956).

She joined the RSC in 1961, the beginning of an association that lasted until her death in 1987 (although she did not appear on stage after 1976): Charlotta Ivanovna in *The Cherry Orchard* (Michel Saint-Denis, RST, 1961); Natella Abashwili in *The Caucasian Chalk Circle* (William Gaskill, Aldwych, 1962); the Queen in *Cymbeline* (Gaskill, RST, 1962); Regan in the Paul Scofield *King Lear* (Peter Brook, RST, 1962); Aemilia in *The Comedy of Errors*

(Clifford Williams, Aldwych, 1962); Frau Lina Rose in Friedrich Dürrenmatt's *The Physicists* (Brook, Aldwych, 1963); Diana Trapes in *The Beggar's Opera* (Peter Wood, Aldwych, 1963); the Histories (RST, 1964)—Duchess of York in *Richard II*, Mistress Quickly in *Henry IV* and Mistress Quickly/Alice in *Henry V* (Hall/Barton/Williams); Lady Harriet Boscoe in David Mercer's *The Governor's Lady* (David Jones, 'Exhibitions Two', Aldwych, 1965); Emma Takinainen in Brecht's *Puntila* (Saint-Denis, Aldwych, 1965); Anna Andreyevna in Gogol's *The Government Inspector* (Hall, Aldwych, 1966); Eugenia in *Tango* (Trevor Nunn, Aldwych, 1966); Frau Nomsen in Dürrenmatt's *The Meteor* (Williams, Aldwych, 1966); Gratiana in *The Revenger's Tragedy* (Nunn, RST, 1966); Edna in Edward Albee's *A Delicate Balance* (Hall, Aldwych, 1969); Mrs Heegan in Sean O'Casey's *The Silver Tassie* (Jones, Aldwych, 1969); Dame Purecraft in Ben Jonson's *Bartholomew Fair* (Terry Hands, Aldwych, 1969); Duchess in *The Revenger's Tragedy* (Nunn, Aldwych, 1969); Nurse in Albee's *All Over* (Hall, Aldwych, 1972); Mrs Dudgeon in Shaw's *The Devil's Disciple* (Jack Gold, Aldwych, 1976); and Avdotya in Chekhov's *Ivanov* (Jones, Aldwych, 1976).

Paule Constable read English and Theatre Studies at Goldsmiths College, London. As a lighting designer, she achieved her breakthrough working for Complicite (*The Street of Crocodiles*, 1992). She has since formed important creative partnerships with Tim Supple, Katie Mitchell, David McVicar, Neil Bartlett and Michael Grandage.

At the RSC: Supple's *Spring Awakening* (Pit, 1995) and *Tales from Ovid* (Swan, 1999); Mitchell's *Beckett Shorts* (TOP, 1997), *The Mysteries* (TOP, 1997) and *Uncle Vanya* (Young Vic, 1998); Bartlett's *The Dispute* (TOP, 1999) and *The Prince of Homburg* (Swan, 2002); Adrian Noble's *The Seagull* (Swan, 2000); Dominic Cooke's *As You Like It* (RST, 2005).

Elsewhere: Supple's *Slab Boys Trilogy, More Grimm Tales, Jungle Book* and *Twelfth Night* (Young Vic, 1994-99); Mitchell's *Don*

Giovanni (Welsh National Opera, 1996), *The Country* (Royal Court, 2000), *Three Sisters* (NT Lyttelton, 2003), *The City* (Royal Court, 2008) and *...Some Trace of Her* (NT Cottesloe, 2008); Ian Rickson's *The Weir* (Royal Court, 1998); McVicar's *Sweeny Todd* (Opera North, 1998), *The Rape of Lucretia* (ENO, 2001), *Rigoletto* (Royal Opera, 2002) and *Le nozze di Figaro* (Royal Opera, 2006); Bartlett's *The Servant*, *Pericles*, *A Christmas Carol* and *Oliver* (Lyric Hammersmith, 2001-04); Matthew Bourne's *Play Without Words* (NT Lyttelton, 2002); Nicholas Hytner's *His Dark Materials* (NT Olivier, 2004); Michael Grandage's *Don Carlos* (Sheffield Crucible, 2004), *Evita* (Adelphi, 2006), *Othello* (Donmar, 2007) and *Ivanov* (Wyndam's, 2008); Marianne Elliott's *Saint Joan* and *War Horse* (NT Olivier, 2007).

Dominic Cooke (b. 1966). On graduating from Warwick University, Dominic Cooke formed a company called Pan Optic and toured productions of Beaumarchais's *The Marriage of Figaro* and Strindberg's *Miss Julie* (1990). He was an assistant director at the RSC from 1992-94, working on Peter Hall's *All's Well That Ends Well* (Swan), Michael Attenborough's *The Changeling* (Swan), and Adrian Noble's *Travesties* (Barbican). The next few years saw him directing at the Nottingham Playhouse (*Of Mice and Men*, 1994), the Gate, Notting Hill (Martin Sperr's *Hunting Scenes from Lower Bavaria*, 1995; Gerhart Hauptmann's *The Weavers*, 1996), and at Terry Hands's Theatr Clwyd (*Entertaining Mr Sloane*, 1997; Rudkin's *Afore Night Come*, 1998). His ingenious production of *The Arabian Nights* at the Young Vic, Christmas 1998/99, received glowing notices.

From 2000-03 Cooke was an associate director at the Royal Court, directing fashionable new work: Marius von Mayenburg's *Fireface* (2000); Christopher Shinn's *Other People* (2000, with Daniel Evans); Rebecca Gilman's *Spinning into Butter* (2001, with Emma Fielding); Leo Butler's *Redundant* (2001); Grae Cleugh's *Fucking Games* (2001); Vasilly Sigarev's *Plasticine* (2002); and Michael Wynne's *The People are Friendly* (2002).

In 2002 he returned to the RSC to direct Antony Sher in John Marston's *The Malcontent* (Swan). He set the play in a banana republic, a garish, style-free zone of broad, cartoon-like comedy. Great entertainment (like being trapped in the *Top of the Pops* studio circa 1974), but a less than adequate response to Marston's relentlessly moral view of the world. From 2003 to 07 he was a member of Michael Boyd's directorial team: as well as running the RSC's new writing programme, he directed Emma Fielding and Anton Lesser in *Cymbeline* (Swan, 2003); Greg Hicks in *Macbeth* (RST, 2004); Lia Williams in *As You Like It* (RST, 2005); and Iain Glen in *The Crucible* (RST, 2006). The Shakespeares played like works in progress, but the Miller was lucid and passionate, benefiting from the elegant simplicity of Hildegard Bechtler's design and Jean Kalman's lighting. Cooke's RSC 'New Work festivals' were lacklustre non-events. In 2007 he took charge of the Royal Court.

Nigel Cooke went from the Bristol Old Vic Theatre School into the Old Vic Company, and later co-founded the Little Theatre. His work at the Little Theatre included Cliff to Daniel Day-Lewis's Jimmy Porter in *Look Back in Anger* (George Costigan, 1981).

He first joined the RSC in 1983/84 to play Octavius Caesar in *Julius Caesar* (Ron Daniels, RST); Sebastian in *Twelfth Night* (John Caird, RST); Surrey in *Henry VIII* (Howard Davies, RST); Bonario in *Volpone* (Bill Alexander, TOP); and Oleg/Moloka in Charles Wood's *Red Star* (Caird, Pit). He has been a regular member, growing in prominence, since 1992: Tom Stone (Shakespeare) in Peter Whelan's *The School of Night* (Alexander, TOP, 1992); Nym/Montjoy in the Iain Glen *Henry V* (Matthew Warchus, RST, 1994); Wellvile in *The Wives' Excuse* (Max Stafford-Clark, Swan, 1994); Father Karolyi in David Edgar's *Pentecost* (Michael Attenborough, TOP, 1994); *Beckett Shorts* (Katie Mitchell, TOP, 1997); Macduff in the Antony Sher *Macbeth* (Gregory Doran, Swan, 1999); the 2005 'Gunpowder' season

(Swan)—the title role in *Thomas Moore* (Robert Delamere), Marcellus/Stoic in *Believe What You Will* (Josie Rourke), Arruntius in *Sejanus: His Fall* (Doran), Cecil in *Speaking Like Magpies* (Rupert Goold); and the 2006/07 Complete Works festival (Swan)—Lysimachus in *Pericles* (Dominic Cooke), Polixenes in *The Winter's Tale* (Cooke), and Lenny in Roy Williams's *Days of Significance* (Maria Aberg).

Elsewhere: Alan Bleasdale's *Having a Ball* (Lyric Hammersmith, 1981); Officer, succeeding Albie Woodington, in Adrian Noble's production of *The Duchess of Malfi* (Roundhouse, 1981); *Serious Money* (Stafford-Clark, Wyndham's, 1987); *The Recruiting Officer* and *Our Country's Good* (Stafford-Clark, Royal Court, 1989); Nick in Martin Crimp's *Getting Attention* (Jude Kelly, West Yorkshire Playhouse, 1991); the Kevin Spacey *Iceman Cometh* (Howard Davies, Almeida, 1998); and Robespierre in Pam Gems's *The Snow Palace* (Janet Suzman, Tricycle Theatre, 1998).

Richard Cordery. One of the leading all-rounders of the contemporary classical theatre, Richard Cordery trained at RADA but worked in relative obscurity until 1981, when he joined the RSC at the Aldwych to play Menelaus in *Troilus and Cressida* (Terry Hands); Chmuta in *The Love-Girl and the Innocent* (Clifford Williams); Barnardo in the Michael Pennington *Hamlet* (John Barton); and Lord Willoughby in *Richard II* (Hands). He went on to work for Alan Ayckbourn at the Stephen Joseph Theatre, Scarborough, and the National—*A View from the Bridge* (Aldwych, 1987) and Bonaventura in *'Tis Pity She's a Whore* (Olivier, 1988).

Cordery has shown a formidable talent for playing the corrupt and the duplicitous (most of the secondary roles in Shakespeare, that club of clerics, nobles and political operators, are his for the taking). Since his return in 1996 he has been one of the few exceptional regular players at the RSC: Wilbraham in Edward Bond's *In the Company of Men* (Bond, Pit, 1996); Friar

Laurence in *Romeo and Juliet* (Michael Attenborough, Pit, 1997); Corvino in *Volpone* (Lindsay Posner, Swan, 1999); Brabantio in *Othello* (Attenborough, RST, 1999); Dr Warburton in *The Family Reunion* (Adrian Noble, Swan, 1999); Humphrey Duke of Gloucester in *Henry VI* and Buckingham in *Richard III* (Michael Boyd, Swan, 2000-01); Falstaff in *The Merry Wives of Windsor* (Rachel Kavanaugh) and Menenius in *Coriolanus* (David Farr, Swan, 2002-03); Duncan in *Macbeth* (Dominic Cooke, RST, 2004); Polonius in *Hamlet* (Boyd, RST, 2004); Malvolio in *Twelfth Night* (Boyd, RST, 2005); Egeon in *The Comedy of Errors* (Nancy Meckler, RST, 2005); and multiple roles in Boyd's 2006-08 Histories at the Courtyard—reprising Humphrey (*Henry VI*) and Buckingham (*Richard III*) and adding Edmund of Langley (*Richard II*) and the Lord Chief Justice (*Henry IV*).

Brian Cox (b. Dundee, 1946). At the age of fifteen Brian Cox joined the staff of his local repertory theatre. The Dundee Rep in 1960 was run by the Royal Court's Anthony Page and the company was brimming with talent. Cox worked as an assistant stage manager while the actors (led by Nicol Williamson, Edward Fox, Glenda Jackson and Lynn Redgrave) performed a different play every two weeks. At the age of seventeen he moved to London to study at the London Academy of Music and Dramatic Art.

He appeared for a season at the Royal Lyceum, Edinburgh (1965-66), and came to notice at the Birmingham Rep (1966-68) in *As You Like It* and *Peer Gynt*. During the next decade and a half, at the Royal Court, the Manchester Royal Exchange, the National, and elsewhere, Cox engaged with the theatrical establishment very much on his own terms: Steven in David Storey's *In Celebration* (Lindsay Anderson, Royal Court, 1969); Norman in *Don't Start Without Me* (Garrick, 1971); Lovborg in *Hedda Gabler* (Anthony Page, Royal Court, 1972); Ibsen's *Brand* (Nottingham Playhouse, 1972); Proctor in Storey's *Cromwell* (Page, Royal Court, 1973); Sergius in Shaw's *Arms and the Man*

(Royal Exchange, Manchester, 1974); Reilly in T.S. Eliot's *The Cocktail Party* (Royal Exchange, Manchester, 1975); Taoridimas in *Tamburlaine the Great* (Peter Hall, NT Olivier, 1976); Brutus in *Julius Caesar* (John Schlesinger, NT Olivier, 1977); De Flores in *The Changeling* (Peter Gill, Riverside Studios, 1978); Macbeth (Cambridge Theatre Company, Tour of India, 1980); Danton in Büchner's *Danton's Death* (Gill, NT Olivier, 1982); Captain Ahab in *Moby Dick* (Michael Elliott, Royal Exchange, Manchester, 1983); Darrell opposite Glenda Jackson in Eugene O'Neill's *Strange Interlude* (Keith Hack, Duke of York's, 1984); and the RUC interrogator in Ron Hutchinson's *Rat in the Skull* (Max Stafford-Clark, Royal Court, 1984).

For years Cox considered Stratford 'posh' and avoided the RSC. When he finally took up an offer in 1986 he intended it to be a stopgap. His participation in a brief autumn/winter season at the Barbican, playing Danton in Pam Gems's *The Danton Affair* (Ron Daniels), John Tarleton in Shaw's *Misalliance* (John Caird) and Sir Timothy Bellboys in John Whiting's *A Penny for a Song* (Howard Davies), was, in fact, the beginning of two-and-a-half years of inspired work: Paul Cash in Doug Lucie's *Fashion* (TOP, 1987); the title role in Deborah Warner's production of *Titus Andronicus* (Swan, 1987); Petruchio in *The Taming of the Shrew* (Jonathan Miller, RST, 1987); and Vershinin in *Three Sisters* (John Barton, Barbican, 1988). Cox's Titus broke Lavinia's neck while tenderly cradling her on his lap. His sombre Petruchio was the opposite of the usual swaggering chauvinist.

Although best known for playing men of power in an unadorned style, Cox is a contemplative and analytical performer who strives to find some meaning in the actor's role. While working for the RSC in 1988 he taught a group of students at the Moscow Art Theatre, brought them to London to work with RSC directors, and directed their graduation production, *The Crucible* (see Cox's autobiography, *Salem to Moscow*, Methuen, 1991).

Now an associate artist, Cox looked set to play Coriolanus and Lear for Deborah Warner and Antony for Terry Hands;

however, when Cox and Warner discovered that Nicholas Hytner and John Wood were ahead of them in the 'queue' for *King Lear* they defected to the National and mounted their production in tandem with Ian McKellen's *Richard III* (Richard Eyre, Lyttelton, 1990). Cox played Buckingham in the latter. Warner's disappointing *Lear* offered poor compensation for the loss of Cox's RSC Coriolanus and Antony (this last, scheduled for the autumn of 1989 with Jane Lapotaire as Cleopatra, was even announced). It is difficult to think of roles more suited to Cox's particular brand of contained power.

If Cox hasn't said farewell to the stage—he played Solness in *The Master Builder* at Royal Lyceum, Edinburgh, in 1993; the Critic in Conor McPherson's *St Nicholas* at the Bush in 1997; John Plunkett in McPherson's *Dublin Carol* at the Royal Court in 2000; and Max in Trevor Nunn's production of Tom Stoppard's *Rock 'n' Roll* at the Royal Court in 2006—he has for some years worked primarily in Hollywood, where he must be the hardest working British actor: *Rob Roy* (Michael Caton-Jones, 1995); *Braveheart* (Mel Gibson, 1995); *Chain Reaction* (Andrew Davis, 1996); *Kiss the Girls* (Gary Fleder, 1997); *The Boxer* (Jim Sheridan, 1997); *The Minus Man* (Hampton Fancher, 1998); *Desperate Measures* (Barbet Schroeder, 1998); *For Love of the Game* (Sam Raimi, 1999); *The Rookie* (2001); *The Bourne Identity* (Doug Liman, 2002); *The Ring* (Gore Verbinski, 2002); *Adaptation* (Spike Jonze, 2002); *X2* (Bryan Singer, 2003); *Sin* (2003); *Troy* (Wolfgang Petersen, 2004); *The Bourne Supremacy* (Paul Greengrass, 2004); *Red Eye* (Wes Craven, 2005); *The Ringer* (2005); *Zodiac* (David Fincher, 2007).

Some of Cox's best screen performances were given on British television—Henry II in *The Devil's Crown* (BBC, 1978); Laurent to Kate Nelligan's Thérèse in *Thérèse Raquin* (BBC, 1980); Hogan in *Sharpe* (ITV, 1993)—and in low-budget films—Hannibal Lecktor in Michael Mann's *Manhunter* (1986); *Rushmore* (Wes Anderson, 1998); *The Reckoning* (Paul McGuigan, 2004); and *Running with Scissors* (Ryan Murphy, 2006).

Claire Cox (b. London, 1975) was a final year student at Central when Ian McDiarmid cast her in Jonathan Dove's *Siren Song* (Almeida, 1994). She next played Frederika in *A Little Night Music* (Sean Mathias, NT Olivier, 1995-96); Gilda in Noël Coward's *Design For Living* (Tim Luscombe, English Touring Theatre, 1997); and Lydia in David Bridel's *The Last Girl* (David Prescott, Riverside Studios, 1998).

She has been one of the RSC's most striking and vocally expressive young actresses since 1999. Female roles in the classical theatre, both comedic and dramatic, oscillate between joy and hurt, vitality and vulnerability, flirtatiousness and innocence, and Cox has shown herself to be a mistress of contradictions: Beatrice in *A Servant to Two Masters* (Tim Supple, TOP, 1999); Christina in William Wycherley's *Love in a Wood* (Supple, Swan, 2001); Portia in *Julius Caesar* (Edward Hall, RST, 2001); and the Spanish Golden age season (Swan, 2004)—Marcela in Lope de Vega's *The Dog in the Manger* (Laurence Boswell), Dona Ana in Sor Juana Ines de la Cruz's *House of Desires* (Nancy Meckler) and Belica in Cervantes's *Pedro, the Great Pretender* (Mike Alfreds).

Her early screen appearances included the BBC series *The Choir* (1995) and the movies *The Leading Man* (John Duigan, 1996) and *Shooting Fish* (Stefan Schwartz, 1997). She has graced such popular television shows as *The Inspector Lynley Mysteries* (BBC, 2003); *A Touch of Frost* (ITV, 2004, 2006); *Foyle's War* (ITV, 2006); and *Spooks* (BBC, 2007).

Derbhle Crotty (b. Cavan, Ireland, 1968) was educated in Dublin at University College and the Samuel Beckett Centre. She won acclaim for her work at the Abbey, the Peacock, Andrew Lane's (all Dublin), and at the Druid Theatre, Galway, in the 1990s: roles included Bella in *Gaslight*; the title role in *Katie Roche*; Julie in *Miss Julie*; Molly in *The Well of the Saints*; and the title role in *Portia Coughlan*. At the RSC in 1996/7 she played Ophelia in *Hamlet* (Matthew Warchus, RST); a haunted Asta, subtly conveying the heartache beneath the character's social grace, in Ibsen's *Little Eyolf* (Adrian Noble, Swan); and La Medrecita in Tennessee Williams's *Camino Real* (Steven Pimlott, Swan).

She has continued to divide her life between London, Dublin and Galway: Portia in *The Merchant of Venice* (Trevor Nunn), Gorky's *Summerfolk* (Nunn) and Pegeen Mike in *Playboy of the Western World* (Fiona Buffini) at the National (1999, 2001); John B Keane's *Sive* and Jane in Christian O'Reilly's *The Good Father* for the Druid Theatre Company (Garry Hynes, 2002); Maggie in Brian Friel's *Dancing at Lughnasa* (Joe Dowling) and Margaret in Friel's *The Home Place* (Noble) at the Gate (2004-05); Natalya in Friel's *A Month in the Country* at the Abbey (Jason Byrne, 2006); and Lady Macbeth in *Macbeth* (Conall Morrison), Lady Duncan in Ionesco's *Macbett* (Silviu Purcareteat) and Maid in Margaret Atwood's *The Penelopiad* (Josette Bushell-Mingo) at the RSC (Swan, 2007).

Bob Crowley (b. Cork, 1952). The son of a Cork fireman, Bob Crowley was educated at the Crawford College of Art (now part of the Cork Institute of Technology). A scholarship took him to the Bristol Old Vic, where he teamed up with Adrian Noble, the company's trainee director. Their productions of Arthur Miller's *A View from the Bridge*, Middleton and Rowley's *The Changeling*, and, especially, Shakespeare's *Titus Andronicus* and *Timon of Athens*, brought excitement to the Bristol theatres. Here was a new style of staging, derived from storyboarding and based on simplicity and the poetic use of objects and colour.

Following acclaimed revivals of *The Duchess of Malfi* and *Doctor Faustus* at the Manchester Royal Exchange, Noble and Crowley developed their form of theatre at the RSC: *The Forest* (TOP, 1981); *King Lear* (RST, 1982); *A New Way to Pay Old Debts* (TOP, 1983); *Measure for Measure* (RST, 1983); *Henry V* (RST, 1984); *The Winter's Tale* (Small-scale Tour, 1985); *As You Like It* (RST, 1985); *Macbeth* (RST, 1986); *The Plantagenets* (RST, 1988); *Henry IV* (RST, 1991); and *Hamlet* (Barbican, 1992).

During his ten years as an associate at the RSC Crowley also designed Howard Davies's *The Time of Your Life* (TOP, 1983), *Les liaisons dangereuses* (TOP, 1985) and *A Penny for a Song* (Barbican, 1986); Barry Kyle's *Love's Labour's Lost* (RST, 1984) and *The Two Noble Kinsmen* (Swan, 1986); and Trevor Nunn's *Othello* (TOP, 1989).

Elsewhere, Crowley designed Noble's *Don Giovanni* at Kent Opera (1985) and *Three Sisters* at the Gate, Dublin (1990). His work for other directors has only rarely been as striking or as integrated. At the National he formed regular partnerships with Richard Eyre and Nicholas Hytner (*Ghetto*, 1989; *Carousel*, 1992). In recent years, dividing his time between London and New York, he has worked in the musical theatre, delivering spectacular sets for *The Witches of Eastwick* (2000), Elton John's *Aida* (2000), *Sweet Smell of Success* (Hytner, 2002), and *Mary Poppins* (Eyre, 2004).

Liam Cunningham (b. Dublin, 1961). From the working-class North Wall area of Dublin, the son of a docker, Liam Cunningham worked as an electrician until his late twenties, when, returning from a three-year job in Zimbabwe, he suddenly decided to try his hand at acting. He trained part-time at the Oscar School, and found success with his first play, Dermot Bulger's *Lament for Arthur Cleary* (Wet Paint Theatre Company, 1989-90).

After Bulger's *Lament* he worked with Dublin's Passion Machine (Paul Mercier's *Studs* at the Gaiety) and made his London debut at the Royal Court in the two-hander *Goodnight Siobhan* (1990). Billy Roche's *A Handful of Stars* and *Poor Beast in the Rain* at the Bush brought him to prominence in England (1992) and led to major roles in *Roughnecks* (BBC, 1994) and *Cracker* (episode 'Best Boys', ITV, 1995). His first film was Mike Newell's *Into the West* (1992), followed by *War of the Buttons* (1994), *A Little Princess* (1995), *First Knight* (1995), and Michael Winterbottom's *Jude* (1996).

There is nothing actorly or contrived about his work; he is adept at projecting strength through silence, makes brooders sympathetic and soulful. He joined the RSC for the 1996-97 programme and played Orlando to Niamh Cusack's Rosalind in *As You Like It* (Steven Pimlott, RST) and John Hall in Peter Whelan's *The Herbal Bed* (TOP). His quietly-spoken, reflective approach made him the least typical Orlando in years, as well as the least callow.

Cunningham has continued to work most prominently on screen, creating compelling characters in *Falling for a Dancer* (BBC, 1998); Stephen Poliakoff's *Shooting the Past* (BBC, 1999); *A Likeness in Stone* (ITV, 2000); *Rebel Heart* (BBC, 2001); *Prime Suspect 6* (ITV, 2003); *The Crooked Man* (ITV, 2003); *Messiah 3: the Promise* (BBC, 2004); Neil Jordan's *Breakfast on Pluto* (2005); Ken Loach's *The Wind That Shakes the Barley* (2006); and *Murphy's Law* (BBC, 2006). In 1998 he returned to the Dublin stage to play Stanley in *A Streetcar Named Desire* (Gate).

Julian Curry (b. 1937). Julian Curry's range extends from the austere art of Samuel Beckett to the upper-class wine-loving lawyer he played for over ten years in John Mortimer's *Rumpole of the Bailey*. A wine buff himself, he created a one-man show called *Hic! or The Entire History of Wine* (2001-02).

At Cambridge he was a member of the Marlowe Society, appearing with Ian McKellen and Derek Jacobi in John Barton's production of *Henry IV* (1959). His early theatre appearances included Morrison in *The Big Contract* (Belgrade, Coventry, 1963), Ananias in *The Alchemist* (Oxford Playhouse, 1965), and David Cregan's *Three Men For Colverton* (Royal Court, 1966).

He first joined the RSC in 1968 to play the King of France in *King Lear* (Trevor Nunn); First Lord in *As You Like It* (David Jones); Bad Angel in *Doctor Faustus* (Clifford Williams); and Friar Francis in *Much Ado About Nothing* (Nunn). *Faustus* and *Much Ado* travelled to America in the New Year; on their return, at the Aldwych, Curry added the roles of Staff Wallah in Sean

O'Casey's *The Silver Tassie* (Jones), and Val Cutting in *Bartholomew Fair* (Terry Hands).

Curry's theatre roles in the 1970s included Horatio in the Ian McKellen *Hamlet* (Robert Chetwyn, Cambridge Theatre, London, 1971), and Angelo in *Measure for Measure* (Jonathan Miller, NT Old Vic, 1974). Television parts, particularly Erskine-Brown in *Rumpole* (ITV, 1978-92), dominated until he returned to the RSC in the 1980s. He played Danforth in *The Crucible* (Barry Kyle) and Polixenes in *The Winter's Tale* (Adrian Noble) for the 1984 small-scale Tour; Philippeaux in Pam Gems's *The Danton Affair* (Daniels, Barbican, 1986); the Bishop of Winchester in *The Plantagenets* (Noble, Barbican, 1989); and Pandulph in *King John* (Deborah Warner, Pit, 1989). Later, he was once again Polixenes, succeeding Paul Jesson, in *The Winter's Tale* (Noble, US Tour, 1994); Antonio in *The Merchant of Venice* (Doran, RST, 1997-98); Mabs in Stephen Poliakoff's *Talk of the City* (Swan, 1998); the lead in Bernard Shaw's *Back to Methuselah* (David Fielding, TOP, 2000); and Fabritio in *Women Beware Women* (Laurence Boswell, Swan, 2006).

Elsewhere, during the 1980s and 90s, Curry appeared in *Timon of Athens* (Nunn, Young Vic, 1991); Thomas Bernhard's *Elisabeth II* (David Fielding, Gate, 1992); the musical *Lust* (Theatre Royal Haymarket, 1993); John Osborne's *The Entertainer*, as Billy Rice (Hampstead Theatre, 1996); and Thomas Bernhard's *Eve of Retirement* (Fielding, Gate, 1997).

Niamh Cusack (b. Dublin, 1959) studied at the Royal Academy of Music and worked for a while as an orchestral flautist before following her sisters into acting. She appeared at the Gate, Dublin, in *A Woman of No Importance* and *Arr N'a Pogh*, and at the Royal Exchange, Manchester, in *Three Sisters* (Casper Wrede, 1985), then joined Sinéad and brother-in-law Jeremy Irons at the RSC. She played Desdemona to Ben Kingsley's *Othello* (Terry Hands, RST, 1985); Jess in Angela Hewins's *Mary, After the Queen* (Barry Kyle, Warehouse, Stratford, 1985); a memorable, contemporary Juliet opposite Sean Bean in Michael Bogdanov's production of *Romeo and Juliet* (RST, 1986); the eroticised Jane (writhing around on a bed in nightie and socks) in Nick Dear's Hogarth play *The Art of Success* (Adrian Noble, TOP, 1986); and Sue, dancing ecstatically, in Nigel Williams's *Country Dancing* (Bill Alexander, TOP, 1986). On leaving the RSC she was wasted in Lenz's *The Tutor* at the Old Vic (Angelika Hurwicz, 1988) and in episodes of *Poirot* and *Jeeves and Wooster*. She played a minor part in David Hare's *Paris By Night* (1988).

Two roles placed Niamh Cusack in the front rank of young classical actresses. In 1990 she returned to Dublin to play Irina alongside her sisters and father (Chebutykin) and Finbar Lynch (Tusenbach) in Adrian Noble's production of *Three Sisters* (Gate Theatre). She presented a character in transformation: at the beginning, a pretty girl celebrating her name day, full of *joie de vivre*, if a little proud; in the claustrophobic middle act throwing water at her reflection in the mirror ('I'm twenty-three... my brain's drying up. I'm getting thinner, I'm getting ugly, old, old...'); at the end with severe drawn back hair, a plain dress, and spectacles—as though all the life had been drained away. There was a genuine sense of pain in this performance, as well as a hint of fanaticism. Three years later, also at the Gate, she excelled as Nora in *A Doll's House* (Karel Reisz, 1993).

She devoted the next few years to the popular television series *Heartbeat* (ITV). She returned to the theatre as Felicity Kendal's replacement in Tom Stoppard's *Indian Ink* (1995), then rejoined the RSC. She was physically elegant as both Rosalind in *As You Like It* (Steven Pimlott, RST, 1996) and Armande in Molière's *The Learned Ladies* (Pimlott, TOP, 1996). She has since played Claire opposite Kerry Fox in Genet's *The Maids* (John Crowley, Donmar Warehouse, 1997); Fran in Peter Moffat's *Nabokov's Gloves* (Ian Brown, Hampstead Theatre, 1988); Portia in *The Merchant of Venice* (Gale Edwards, Chichester, 2003); Elaine in Laura Wade's *Breathing Corpses* (Anna Mackmin, Royal Court, 2005); Jane in Amelia Bullmore's *Mammals* (Mackmin, Bush, 2005); Mrs Alving in Ibsen's *Ghosts* (Mackmin, Gate,

2007); Millamant in Congreve's *The Way of the World* (Selina Cadell, Royal and Derngate, Northampton, 2007); and Erna in Victoria Benedictsson's *The Enchantment* (Paul Miller, NT Cottesloe, 2007).

Sinéad Cusack (b. Dalkey, Ireland, 1948). The eldest daughter of Cyril Cusack, Sinéad Cusack grew up in a famous actor's household, but one, paradoxically, where much of the end product was denied: her father would not allow a television in the house and he discouraged trips to the cinema. Although he cast his eleven-year-old daughter in the role of the Deaf Mute in *The Importance of Mr O* (Olympia, Dublin, 1960), he did not encourage her to become a professional actress. As he planned, she went to a convent school and then read English at University College, Dublin. But as a young woman she determinedly went her own way, joining the Abbey Theatre Company while still an undergraduate and crashing out of college two months before her finals.

Following leading roles at the Abbey she came to England. With her soft blonde hair and blue eyes she had the kind of looks that attracted the film industry and she played pretty girls in *Alfred the Great* (Clive Donner, 1969), the Peter Sellers vehicle *Hoffman* (Alvin Rakoff, 1970), *David Copperfield* (1970), and *Tam-Lin* (Roddy McDowall, 1971). But theatre remained at the core of her work. She played Juliet in *Romeo and Juliet* (Shaw, 1972); Laura in *The Glass Menagerie* (Gardner Centre, Brighton, 1973); Desdemona in *Othello* (Ludlow Festival, 1974); and Raina in *Arms and the Man* (Oxford Festival and Tour, 1976).

She first joined the RSC in 1975 to play Grace in *London Assurance* (Ronald Eyre, Albery). In the 1980s she became one of the Company's most admired Shakespearean actresses, bringing to beguiling life Isabella in *Measure for Measure* (Barry Kyle, Aldwych, 1979), Celia in *As You Like It* (Terry Hands, RST, 1980), Lady Anne to Alan Howard's *Richard III* (Hands, RST, 1980), Portia in *The Merchant of Venice* (John Barton, RST, 1981),

Beatrice in *Much Ado About Nothing* (Hands, RST, 1982), Kate in *The Taming of the Shrew* (Kyle, RST, 1982), and Lady Macbeth in *Macbeth* (Adrian Noble, RST, 1986). She was also Lady Amaranth in *Wild Oats* (Clifford Williams, Aldwych, 1979); Elizaveta in Gorky's *The Children of the Sun* (Hands, Aldwych, 1979); Evadne in *The Maid's Tragedy* (Kyle, TOP, 1980); Lady Alice in *The Swan Down Gloves* (Ian Judge/Hands, RST, 1981); Ingrid in *Peer Gynt* (Ron Daniels, TOP, 1982); Daisy in Nicholas Wright's *The Custom of the Country* (David Jones, Pit, 1983); Roxane, succeeding Alice Krige, in *Cyrano de Bergerac* (Hands, US Tour, 1984); and Angellica Bianca in Aphra Behn's *The Rover* (Barton, Swan, 1986).

She met her future husband Jeremy Irons in 1975 (they were playing at neighbouring theatres in the West End). They were both at the RSC in 1986/87, appearing opposite each other in *The Rover*, and they have occasionally worked together on screen — *Waterland* (Stephen Gyllenhaal, 1992), Christopher Hampton's *Tales from Hollywood* (Howard Davies, TV, 1992), and *Stealing Beauty* (Bernardo Bertolucci, 1996). In 1989 she played Masha alongside her sisters and father in an acclaimed *Three Sisters* (Noble, Gate, Dublin), but since this highpoint has worked only sporadically on the stage: Ruth in William Nicholson's *Map of the Heart* (Peter Wood, Globe, 1991); Grace in Brian Friel's *Faith Healer* (Joe Dowling, Royal Court, 1992); Marguerite in Charles Wood's *The Tower* (Howard Davies, Almeida, 1995); Mai in Sebastian Barry's *Our Lady of Sligo* (Max Stafford-Clark, NT Cottesloe, 1998); the mother in Sam Shepard's *A Lie of the Mind* (Wilson Milam, Donmar Warehouse, 2001); Abby in Neil LaBute's *The Mercy Seat* (Michael Attenborough, Almeida, 2003); and Eleanor in Tom Stoppard's *Rock 'n' Roll* (Nunn, Royal Court, 2006). In 2002 she returned to the RSC to play Cleopatra in *Antony and Cleopatra* (Attenborough, RST).

D

Janet Dale. A member of Alan Ayckbourn's company at Scarborough during the 1970s, Janet Dale created the roles of Ruth in *The Norman Conquests* (1973), Marge in *Absent Friends* (1974) and Helen in *Ten Times Table* (1976). She also wrote a series of plays for children, including *The Christmas That Nearly Wasn't* (1974) and *The Mystery of the Lost City* (in nine parts, 1976).

She joined the RSC at the end of the decade and established her reputation as a dramatic actress playing Olga in *Three Sisters* (Trevor Nunn, TOP, 1979), and Miss Knag/Mrs Wititterley in *Nicholas Nickleby* (Nunn/John Caird, Aldwych, 1980). She continued with the RSC until 1986 and returned in 1993: May in Peter Whelan's *The Accrington Pals* (Bill Alexander, Warehouse, 1981); Kristin, succeeding Marjorie Bland, in *A Doll's House* (Adrian Noble, Pit, 1982); Micky in Peter Whelan's *Clay* (Alexander, Pit, 1982); Paulina in *The Winter's Tale* (Noble) and Ann Putnam in *The Crucible* (Barry Kyle/Nick Hamm, Small-scale Tour, 1984); Mistress Page in *The Merry Wives of Windsor* (Alexander, RST, 1985); Emilia in *Othello* (Terry Hands, RST, 1985); Yvonne in *Scenes from a Marriage* (Hands, Barbican, 1986); Goneril in the Robert Stephens *King Lear* (Noble, RST, 1993); and Mrs Fidget in *The Country Wife* (Max Stafford-Clark, Swan, 1993).

At the National she played Mum in Ayckbourn's *Invisible Friends* (Ayckbourn, Cottesloe, 1991), and Queen Charlotte in Alan Bennett's *The Madness of George III* (Nicholas Hytner, Lyttelton, 1991–92); at the Greenwich Theatre, Kath in *Entertaining Mr Sloane* (Jeremy Sams, 1993).

Timothy Dalton (b. Colwyn Bay, Wales, 1946) has found it impossible to avoid a career dominated by period dramas, literary adaptations and the phoncy glamour of the American television 'mini-series' format. He has brought his own individuality to popular roles that no longer generate excitement.

He is rightly considered a stage actor despite a paucity of stage appearances.

He was born in Wales (where his father was stationed during the war) and brought up in Derbyshire. He toured with the National Youth Theatre (1964-66) while training at RADA and quickly found work in the theatre (Arthur in *A Game Called Arthur* at the Royal Court, 1966; Richard III among other roles at the Birmingham Rep, 1966), on television (the series *Sat'day While Sunday*, 1966, with Malcolm McDowell), and in features— Philip II in *The Lion in Winter* (Anthony Harvey, 1968); Heathcliff in *Wuthering Heights* (Robert Fuest, 1970); Prince Rupert in *Cromwell* (Ken Hughes, 1970); and Lord Henry Darnley in *Mary, Queen of Scots* (Charles Jarrott, 1971).

On the stage, Dalton first appeared with the RSC in 1973, as Romeo (Terry Hands) and Costard in *Love's Labour's Lost* (David Jones). He played Edmund in *King Lear*, Berowne in *Love's Labour's Lost*, Hal in *Henry IV* and Henry V for the Prospect Theatre Company (1972-74); Byron in *The Lunatic, the Lover and the Poet* at the Old Vic (1977); a fine Hotspur in the RSC's *Henry IV* at the Barbican (Trevor Nunn, 1982); Antony and Petruchio to Vanessa Redgrave's Cleopatra and Kate at the Theatr Clwyd (Toby Robertson, 1986); Cornelius to Redgrave's Nora in Eugene O'Neill's *A Touch of the Poet* at the Young Vic (David Thacker, 1988); and, ending a fifteen-year gap, Lord Asriel in *His Dark Materials* at the National (Nicholas Hytner, Olivier, 2004).

Twice approached to play James Bond in the past, Dalton finally accepted in 1986. He introduced real acting into his two films as 007, *The Living Daylights* (John Glen, 1987) and *Licence to Kill* (Glen, 1989), but they performed below expectations at the box office. He has continued to seek diversity, mixing second division American movies with quirkier work: a terminally ill patient in *Hawks* (Robert Ellis Miller, 1989); the villain in *The Rocketeer* (Joe Johnston, 1991); an English gangster under arrest, a study in arrogance and predatory charm, in Lynda La Plante's television thriller *Framed* (Geoffrey Sax, ITV, 1993); Rhett Butler in the mini-series *Scarlett* (1994); Elliot in *Naked in New York* (Daniel Algrant, 1994); Charles Darrow in Edith Wharton's *The Reef* (Robert Allan Ackerman, 1997); and Skinner in *Hot Fuzz* (Edgar Wright, 2007).

Charles Dance (b. Redditch, Worcestershire, 1946). Charles Dance's career was changed overnight by the extravagant success of the television adaptation of Paul Scott's *The Jewel in the Crown*, in which he played the leading role of Guy Peron (Christopher Morahan and Jim O'Brien, ITV, 1984).

It initiated a film career that has seen the tall and imposing Dance oscillate between arty European features and Hollywood thrillers: Raymond Brock in *Plenty* (Fred Schepisi, 1985); *The Golden Child* (Michael Ritchie, 1986); Josslyn Hay in *White Mischief* (Michael Radford, 1987); D.W. Griffith in *Good Morning, Babylon* (Taviani Brothers, 1987); *Hidden City* (Stephen Poliakoff, 1988); *Pascali's Island* (James Deardon, 1988); *La valle di Pietra* (Maurizio Zaccaro, 1992); *Alien 3* (David Fincher, 1992); *Century* (Poliakoff, 1993); *Last Action Hero* (John McTiernan, 1993); *Undertow* (Eric Red, 1996); Soames, a fine cameo, in *Michael Collins* (Neil Jordan, 1996); *The Blood Oranges* (Philip Haas, 1997); Derek Du Pré in *Hilary and Jackie* (1998); *Dark Blue World* (2001); *Gosford Park* (Robert Altman, 2001); *Ali G Indahouse* (2002); the publisher in *Swimming Pool* (François Ozon, 2003); *Labyrinth* (2003); *Scoop* (Woody Allen, 2006); *Starter for 10* (2006); *Désaccord parfait* (Antoine de Caunes, 2006); *Intervention* (2007).

The list confirms that he has worked constantly, but as a movie leading man and villain-for-hire he has yet to fulfil the potential he showed as a supporting player at the RSC in the 1970s. The young Dance stood out as Fortinbras/Reynaldo in *Hamlet* (Buzz Goodbody, TOP, 1975); Prince John of Lancaster in *Henry IV* (Terry Hands, RST, 1975); Hialas in John Ford's *Perkin Warbeck* (Barry Kyle, TOP, 1975); Catesby/Murderer in *Richard III* (Kyle, TOP, 1975); Scroop/Williams in *Henry V* (Hands, RST, 1977); Buckingham in *Henry VI Part 2* (Hands, RST, 1977); Oliver in *As You Like It* (Trevor Nunn, RST, 1977); Volscian Lieutenant in *Coriolanus* (Hands, RST, 1977); Freeman in David Edgar's *The Jail Diary of Albie Sachs* (Howard Davies, Warehouse, 1978); Vosquin in *The Woman Pirates* (Ron Daniels, Aldwych, 1978); and Tomazo in *The Changeling* (Hands, Aldwych, 1978). For the 1979 European tour of Hands's *Coriolanus* Dance played Aufidius; when Alan Howard succumbed to laryngitis in Paris he stood in as Coriolanus. He returned to the Company in 1989/90 to play the role in earnest, again for Terry Hands (RST).

Dance's other theatre work has included the roles of Wat Dreary in *The Beggar's Opera* (Chichester, 1972); Soliony in *Three Sisters* (Greenwich, 1973); Baudricourt in *Saint Joan* (Oxford Festival, 1974); Nestor in *Irma La Douce* (Shaftesbury, 1979); Townsend in *The Heiress* (Tour, 1980); Frank in Brian Thompson's *Turning Over* (Bush, 1983); Vershinin in *Three Sisters* (Bill Bryden, Birmingham Rep, 1998); Halder in C.P. Taylor's *Good* (Michael Grandage, Donmar Warehouse, 1999); the father opposite Jessica Lange in *Long Day's Journey into Night* (Robin Phillips, Lyric, 2000-01); and the 'celebrity guest' in *A Play What I Wrote* (Kenneth Branagh, West End, 2002).

2004 saw the release of Dance's first film as a director, *Ladies in Lavender*.

Alan David (b. Merthyr Tydfil, 1947) trained at Webber Douglas and gained his early experience in repertory at Coventry and Stoke. He has worked intermittently at the RSC since the late 1970s. At his sharpest and funniest he plays with a straight face and a mean streak, as well as a Welsh relish for words: his RSC performances as Touchstone in *As You Like It* (Trevor Nunn/John Caird, RST, 1977), Fluellen in *Henry V* (Ron Daniels, RST, 1997) and Polonius in *Hamlet* (Steven Pimlott, RST, 2001) are the best examples, but there have been many other pleasures: Richardetto in *'Tis Pity She's a Whore* (Daniels, TOP, 1977); Bellini in *The Lorenzaccio Story* (Daniels, TOP, 1977); Nebewohl in David Rudkin's *The Sons of Light* (Daniels, TOP, 1977); Kurt in

Strindberg's *The Dance of Death* (Caird, Warehouse, 1978); Davies in *The Women-Pirates* (Daniels, Aldwych, 1978); Sir Mortimer in *Saratoga, or, Pistols for Seven* (Ronald Eyre, Aldwych, 1978-79); Arthur Gride/Mr Mantalini/Mobbs/Mr Folair in *Nicholas Nickleby* (Nunn/Caird, RST, 1986); Dodds in Edward Bond's *In the Company of Men* (Bond, Pit, 1996); Erik in David Edgar's *The Prisoner's Dilemma* (Michael Attenborough, TOP, 2001); and Doctor/Provost in the Ralph Fiennes *Brand* (Adrian Noble, Swan, 2003).

At the Royal Court he has appeared in Andrea Dunbar's *Rita, Sue and Bob Too* (1981); Howard Brenton's *The Genius* (Danny Boyle, 1983); Jim Cartwright's *Road* (1986); and Klaus Pohl's *Karate Billy Comes Home* (Stephen Unwin, 1992). At the National he was Snake in *The School for Scandal* (Peter Wood, Olivier, 1990); Sir Hugh Evans in *The Merry Wives of Windsor* (Terry Hands, Olivier, 1995); Mr Pugh/Mr Pritchard in *Under Milk Wood* (Roger Michell, Olivier, 1995); and Sir Politic Wouldbe in *Volpone* (Matthew Warchus, Olivier, 1995).

Daniel Day-Lewis (b. London, 1958) uses the cinema for personal ends too mysterious to comprehend. He has Richard Burton's ability but one cannot imagine him making Burton's compromises. He has played markedly different characters: a homosexual punk in *My Beautiful Laundrette* (Stephen Frears, 1985); an upper-class prig, with tragic undercurrents, in *A Room With a View* (James Ivory, 1986); a Prague surgeon and libertine, tamed by the gravitas of Juliette Binoche, in *The Unbearable Lightness of Being* (Philip Kaufman, 1988); a noble warrior in *The Last of the Mohicans* (Michael Mann, 1992); and a refined New Yorker, tortured by desire for Michelle Pfeiffer, in *The Age of Innocence* (Martin Scorsese, 1993). The method of acting interests him as much as the art: when he played Christy Brown he stayed uncomfortably in character between takes (*My Left Foot*, Jim Sheridan, 1989). With the unsubtle *In the Name of the Father* (Sheridan, 1993) it looked as if he had turned his back on his own country for good; his need to be Irish is as mysterious as his breakdown while playing Hamlet at the National in 1989.

He is the son of the poet Cecil Day-Lewis and the actress Jill Balcon, the grandson of the great movie producer, Sir Michael Balcon. His early years were spent with the Bristol Old Vic Company: Townsperson/Soldier in Adrian Noble's production of *The Recruiting Officer* (1979); Deiphobus in *Troilus and Cressida* (Richard Cottrell, 1979); Stanley in Mike Stott's *Funny Peculiar* (Pete Postlethwaite, Little Theatre, 1979); The Amazing Fez in Ken Campbell's *Old King Cole* (Bob Crowley, New Vic, 1979); Iron in Nigel Williams's *Class Enemy* (David Rome, New Vic, 1980); Leicester in *Edward II* (Cottrell, New Vic, 1980); Philostrate in *A Midsummer Night's Dream* (Cottrell, 1980); Jimmy Porter in *Look Back in Anger* (George Costigan, Little Theatre, 1981); and the title role in *Dracula* (Costigan, Little Theatre, 1981). He succeeded Rupert Everett in *Another Country* (Stuart Burge, Queen's, 1982), and then was briefly at the RSC playing the title role in *Romeo and Juliet* and Flute in *A Midsummer Night's Dream* (John Caird and Sheila Hancock respectively, Small-scale Tour, 1983-84). He was outstanding as Mayakovsky in *Futurists* at the National (Richard Eyre, Cottesloe, 1986).

Film successes continue. He played John Proctor in Hollywood's version of *The Crucible* (Nicholas Hytner, 1996); teamed up once more with Jim Sheridan for *The Boxer* (1998); ended a five year silence in bravura form as Bill the Butcher in Martin Scorsese's *Gangs of New York* (2002, Bafta for Best Actor); and starred in his wife's *The Ballad of Jack and Rose* (Rebecca Miller, 2005). Regrettably, he has ceased to work on the stage. His performance as Hamlet (Richard Eyre, NT Olivier, 1989) had the rare classical virtues of poetry and character, as well as presence and volatility.

Frances de la Tour (b. Bovingdon, Hertfordshire, 1944) is one of the most individual actresses of her generation. Educated in London at the Lycée français and the Drama Centre, she joined the RSC at the very beginning of her career in 1965 and trained under Michel Saint-Denis while walking-on as a Townsperson in *Timon of Athens* (John Schlesinger, RST) and a Servant in the David Warner *Hamlet* (Peter Hall, RST). It took only a year for her distinctive talent, particularly as a comedienne, to be revealed: Natalyia in Chekhov's *The Proposal* (Terry Hands, Theatregoround, 1966); the Widow in *The Taming of the Shrew* (Trevor Nunn, RST, 1967); Audrey in *As You Like It* (David Jones, RST, Aldwych, 1967); Miss Hoyden in John Vanbrugh's *The Relapse* (Nunn, Aldwych, 1967); Doris in Simon Gray's *Dutch Uncle* (Hall, Aldwych, 1969); Lechery in Marlowe's *Doctor Faustus* (Gareth Morgan, Theatregoround and RST, 1970); the Player Queen in *Hamlet* (Nunn, RST, 1970); Helena in *A Midsummer Night's Dream* (Peter Brook, RST, 1970); Belinda in George Etherege's *The Man of Mode* (Hands, Aldwych, 1971); and the Bishop's Girl in Jean Genet's *The Balcony* (Hands, Aldwych, 1971).

Frances de la Tour's performance as Helena in *A Midsummer Night's Dream* was in keeping with Brook's revisionist approach. Previous Stratford Helenas had been conventionally glamorous. De la Tour presented the character as written: plain, needy and doggedly refusing to take no for an answer ('Use me but as your spaniel, spurn me, strike me, neglect me, lose me; only give me leave, unworthy as I am, to follow you'). Her ability to create self-deluding fantasists reached its summation four years later in the situation comedy *Rising Damp* (ITV, 1974-78), a spin off from Eric Chappell's stage play *The Banana Box* (Hampstead Theatre, 1973). Holding her own against Leonard Rossiter, she made Miss Jones one of the iconic figures of British television comedy.

Refusing to be restricted by memories of Miss Jones, she has continued to work on the stage in both classical and modern plays: Rosalind in *As You Like It* (Oxford Playhouse, 1975); Isabella in *The White Devil* (Old Vic, 1976); the title role in *Hamlet* (New Half Moon, 1979); the violinist with MS, a great success, in her husband Tom Kempinski's *Duet for One* (Bush, 1980); Jean in

Catherine Hayes's *Skirmishes* (Hampstead Theatre, 1982); Sonya in *Uncle Vanya* (Theatre Royal Haymarket, 1982); Josie in Eugene O'Neill's *A Moon for the Misbegotten* (Riverside, 1983); the title role in *Saint Joan* (Ronald Eyre, NT Olivier, 1984); *Brighton Beach Memoirs* (Michael Rudman, NT Lyttelton, 1986); Miss Belzer in Martin Sherman's *When She Danced* (Globe, 1991); Leo in *Les parents terribles* (Sean Mathias, NT Lyttelton, 1994); Edward Albee's *Three Tall Women* (Wyndham's, 1994); Elinor in Stephen Poliakoff's *Blinded by the Sun* (Ron Daniels, NT Cottesloe, 1996); wry, poised and delightfully boastful opposite her old RSC colleague Alan Howard in Albee's *The Play About the Baby* (Howard Davies, Almeida, 1998); Raissa Pavlovna Goormizhskaya in *The Forest* (Anthony Page, NT Lyttelton, 1999); and Mrs Lintott in Alan Bennett's *The History Boys* (Nicholas Hytner, NT Lyttelton, 2004). In 1999 she made a long overdue return to the RSC to play Cleopatra opposite Alan Bates in *Antony and Cleopatra* (Steven Pimlott, RST).

Robert Demeger. With his blunt, unaffected style, Robert Demeger is an out-of-the-ordinary player of classical roles. He trained at the Central School and came to notice as a member of Deborah Warner's short-lived but acclaimed troupe Kick Theatre, playing Prospero in *The Tempest* (Edinburgh Festival, 1983), the Duke in *Measure for Measure* (Edinburgh Festival, 1984) and Lear in *King Lear* (Edinburgh Festival and Almeida, 1985). At the RSC he has given depth to supporting roles, most memorably the Gaoler in *The Two Noble Kinsmen* (Barry Kyle, Swan, 1986), a working-class Friar Laurence in Michael Bogdanov's modern-dress production of *Romeo and Juliet* (RST, 1986), and three roles in Adrian Noble's *The Plantagenets* (RST, 1988)—Lord Talbot, Dick the Butcher and Lord Stanley. He was also the Bishop of Carlisle in *Richard II* (Kyle, RST, 1986); Egeus in *A Midsummer Night's Dream* (Bill Alexander, RST, 1986); the General in Jean Genet's *The Balcony* (Terry Hands, Barbican, 1987); Charley in Tony Marchant's *Speculators* (Kyle, Pit, 1987); Don

John in *Much Ado About Nothing* (Di Trevis, RST, 1988); Hubert in *King John* (Deborah Warner, TOP, 1988); Judge in Stephen Poliakoff's *Playing With Trains* (Ron Daniels, Pit, 1989); Pig/Father in Frank McGuinness's *Mary and Lizzie* (Sarah Pia Anderson, Pit, 1989); Diego di Harana in Richard Nelson's *Columbus and the Discovery of Japan* (John Caird, Barbican, 1992); Anselme Debureau in Simon Callow's adaptation of *Les enfants du paradis* (Barbican, 1996); Duke Senior in *As You Like It* (Steven Pimlott, RST, 1996); Ross in *Macbeth* (Tim Albery, RST, 1996); and Ariste in Molière's *The Learned Ladies* (Pimlott, TOP, 1996).

Demeger played Camillo in *The Winter's Tale* and Junius Brutus in *Coriolanus* for the English Shakespeare Company (International Tour and Aldwych, 1990-91); the fencing instructor in Pirandello's *The Rules of the Game* and Aegeus in *Medea* at the Almeida (Jonathan Kent, 1992, 1993); Shamrayev in *The Seagull* at the National (John Caird, Olivier, 1994); the Cardinal in *The Duchess of Malfi* at the Greenwich Theatre (Philip Franks, 1995); the Earl of Warwick in the Joseph Fiennes *Edward II* and Derby in the Kenneth Branagh *Richard III* at the Sheffield Crucible (Michael Grandage, 2001, 2002); Gremio in *The Taming of the Shrew* at the Theatre Royal, Brighton (Mark Rosenblatt, 2003); the Psychiatrist in Pirandello's *Henry IV* at the Donmar Warehouse (Grandage, 2004); and Polonius in Yukio Ninagawa's *Hamlet* at the Barbican (2004).

Jeffery Dench (b. Tyldesly, Lancashire). One of the RSC's most committed and dependable character actors, Jeffery Dench has spent nearly all of his working life with the Company. The older brother of Judi Dench, he trained at Central and gained his early experience on regional stages. He made his London debut as Buckingham in *The Rehearsal*, a transfer from the Bristol Old Vic (1959/60).

Dench's RSC work was a huge quilt made up of relatively small moments, each created with exemplary care and craftsmanship. He joined the Company in 1963 and his first roles were Ligarius in *Julius Caesar* (John Blatchley) and Bassett in *The Wars of the Roses* (Peter Hall). The following selection indicates Dench's versatility: Scroop in *Henry IV* (Hall, RST, 1964); Gratiano in *The Merchant of Venice* (Clifford Williams, RST, 1965); Antonio in *The Revenger's Tragedy* (Trevor Nunn, RST, 1966); Page in *The Merry Wives of Windsor* (Terry Hands, RST, 1968); Henry IV/Pistol in *When Thou Art King* (John Barton, Theatregoround, 1969); Norfolk in *Henry VIII* (Nunn, RST, 1969); Harkaway in *London Assurance* (Ronald Eyre, Aldwych, 1970); Sir Andrew Aguecheek in *Twelfth Night* (Barton, RST, 1971); Capulet in *Romeo and Juliet* (Hands, RST, 1973); Gloucester in *King Lear* (Buzz Goodbody, TOP, 1974); Lucifer in *Doctor Faustus* (Barton, Aldwych, 1974); Sir Nathaniel in *Love's Labour's Lost* (David Jones, Aldwych, 1975); Pistol in *Henry V* (Hands, RST, 1977); the title role in *Cymbeline* (Jones, RST, 1979); Mr Cutler in *Nicholas Nickleby* (Nunn/John Caird, Aldwych, 1980); Sebastian in *The Tempest* (Ron Daniels, RST, 1982); Harry Trevor in *Kiss Me Kate* (Adrian Noble, RST, 1987); Old Shepherd in *The Winter's Tale* (Noble, RST, 1992); Vermandero in *The Changeling* (Michael Attenborough, Swan, 1992); Montague in *Romeo and Juliet* (Noble, RST, 1995); and Shallow in *The Merry Wives of Windsor* (Gregory Doran, RST, 2006-07).

Judi Dench (b. York, 1934) studied art in her hometown of York before moving to London to take up a place at the Central School of Speech and Drama. Her talent was recognised by Michael Benthall, who cast her as Ophelia in *Hamlet* and Maria in *Twelfth Night* at the Old Vic (1957). It was a prodigious beginning, consolidated by her return in 1960 to play Katherine in *Henry V* (John Neville); a famous Juliet, opposite John Stride, in *Romeo and Juliet* (Franco Zeffirelli); Kate in Goldsmith's *She Stoops to Conquer* (Douglas Seale); and Hermia in *A Midsummer Night's Dream* (Michael Langham).

Peter Hall brought her to the RSC in 1961, initially to play Anya alongside Peggy Ashcroft, John Gielgud and Ian Holm in

Michel Saint-Denis's production of *The Cherry Orchard* (RST). In comparison with her nearest rivals, Judi Dench was petite, pretty and seemingly malleable. In her twenties she was viewed as a better than average ingénue whereas Vanessa Redgrave, Maggie Smith and Glenda Jackson were potential movie stars. At the RSC in 1962 she played a young Isabella in *Measure for Measure* (John Blatchley, RST), Titania in *A Midsummer Night's Dream* (Hall, RST), and sexy Dorcas Bellboys in *A Penny for a Song* (Colin Graham, Aldwych), but it was Vanessa Redgrave who received all the publicity as Rosalind in *As You Like It*.

The years 1964 to 66 saw her continue an orthodox classical career at the Oxford Playhouse (Lika in *The Promise*) and the Nottingham Playhouse (Joan in *Saint Joan*). She first truly startled London audiences playing against type as Sally Bowles in *Cabaret* (Palace, 1968). It was the first indication of the range of emotion at her disposal, and of her boldness (she was not a natural singer).

The next year, 1969, she returned to the RSC and to Shakespeare. Trevor Nunn, planning his first season, asked her to play both Hermione and Perdita in his own production of *The Winter's Tale*, Bianca in *Women Beware Women* (Terry Hands) and Viola in *Twelfth Night* (John Barton). She won acclaim for the quality she brought to Shakespeare's heroines, a blend of tenderness and vivacity all her own. The expressiveness of her voice and her ability to time lines and looks were at the heart of it. *Twelfth Night* travelled the world and stayed in the repertoire for three years. The next ten years witnessed remarkable combinations across Stratford seasons: in 1971, Portia in *The Merchant of Venice* (Hands, RST) and the Duchess in *The Duchess of Malfi* (Clifford Williams, RST); in 1976/77, Beatrice in *Much Ado About Nothing* (Barton, RST), Lady Macbeth in *Macbeth* (Nunn, TOP), Adriana in *The Comedy of Errors* (Nunn, RST), Regan in *King Lear* (Nunn with Barton, RST) and Lona Hessel in *Pillars of the Community* (Barton, Aldwych); and, in 1979/80, Imogen in *Cymbeline* (David Jones, RST) and Juno in *Juno and the Paycock* (Nunn, Aldwych). 1976 was the most memorable of Trevor Nunn's

Stratford seasons. Judi Dench was deeply affecting as Beatrice, opposite Donald Sinden, sublimely funny as the exasperated Adriana, and shockingly severe as Lady Macbeth, encapsulating the character's decline in a single silent scream. In 1984/85, at the Barbican, she played the title role in *Mother Courage* (Howard Davies) and Amy in Harley Granville-Barker's *Waste* (Barton, Pit). She met her husband Michael Williams at the RSC and played opposite him in the situation comedy *A Fine Romance* (ITV, 1981-84).

In the 1980s Judi Dench joined Peter Hall at the National to play Lady Bracknell in *The Importance of Being Earnest* (Lyttelton, 1982), Deborah in Harold Pinter's *A Kind of Alaska* (Cottesloe, 1982) and Cleopatra opposite Anthony Hopkins in *Antony and Cleopatra* (Olivier, 1987). She continued on the South Bank after Hall's departure, but the work around her was second-rate— Richard Eyre's *Hamlet* (1989), John Caird's *The Seagull* (1994) and David Hare's *Amy's View* (1997). Her star turn as a contemporary Arkadina in *Amy's View* delighted audiences in London and New York. It coincided with a sudden and unexpected success in the medium that had confined her to supporting roles for years. A small BBC film about Queen Victoria called *Mrs Brown* brought her an Oscar nomination and the adulation of the Hollywood elite. She has since played Elizabeth I in *Shakespeare in Love* (John Madden, 1998, Oscar for Best Supporting Actress); Armande in *Chocolat* (Lasse Hallström, 2000); Agnis in *The Shipping News* (Hallström, 2001); and the title role in *Iris* (Richard Eyre, 2001). In movies like these, desperately seeking Academy Awards, she seems self-consciously the great actress. In contrast, her cameo as M in the Brosnan Bonds was effortless and pleasurable, equalling her earlier performances in *Wetherby* (David Hare, 1985), *A Room with a View* (James Ivory, 1986), *84 Charing Cross Road* (Jones, 1987), *A Handful of Dust* (Charles Sturridge, 1988), and *Jack and Sarah* (Tim Sullivan, 1995).

In 2001 Judi Dench opposed the demolition of the Royal Shakespeare Theatre. In 2003 she returned to Stratford to play the Countess in *All's Well That Ends Well* (Gregory Doran,

171

Swan); and again in 2006/07 to star in Doran's musical version of *The Merry Wives of Windsor* (RST).

Es Devlin (b. Kingston-upon-Thames, 1971). After reading English at Bristol University, Es Devlin studied art at Central St Martins in London. From there, in 1995, she won a place on the prestigious Motley Design Course, and was awarded the Linbury Prize (*Edward II* at the Bolton Octagon). She was an associate artist at the Bush Theatre from 1997 to 99.

Devlin's approach is conceptual and architectural. Her designs often feature the deflection and reflection of light, solid planes that glow with colour. She has worked at the highest level: Joe Penhall's *Love and Understanding* (Bush, 1997); *Snake in the Grass* (Peter Hall Company, Old Vic, 1997); Trevor Nunn's production of Pinter's *Betrayal* (NT, 1998); Christopher Bruce's *Four Scenes* and *Gods Plenty* (Rambert, 1998, 2000); Mark O'Rowe's *Howie the Rookie* (Bush, 1999); *Hamlet* (Laurence Boswell, Young Vic, 1999); the Pet Shop Boys' *Closer to Heaven* (Arts, 2001); *A Day in the Death of Joe Egg* (Boswell, Comedy, 2001); Sebastian Barry's *Hinterland* (Max Stafford-Clark, Out of Joint, NT, 2001-02); *A Streetcar Named Desire* (Northern Ballet Theatre, 2002); *Five Gold Rings* (Michael Attenborough, Almeida, 2003); Britten's *A Midsummer Night's Dream* (Hamburg Staatsoper, 2006); Bizet's *Carmen* (Sally Potter, ENO, 2007); and Strauss's *Salome* (David McVicar, Royal Opera, 2008).

At the RSC: Michael Attenborough's *Henry IV* (Swan, 2000), *The Prisoner's Dilemma* (TOP, 2001) and *Antony and Cleopatra* (RST, 2002); Steven Pimlott's *The Dog in the Manger* (Swan, 2004) and *Hecuba* (Albery, 2005).

Mark Dignam (1909-1989, b. London) grew up in Sheffield (his father worked in the steel industry). Dignam's potential as a performer was recognised by one of the priests at his school, the Mount St Mary's College. He played the leading female roles in school productions of Shakespeare, and received elocution lessons from Chris Castor, an actress in the company of the Sheffield Repertory Theatre.

Dignam learnt his craft as a classical actor touring England and America with Ben Greet's Shakespeare company in 1931, and the following year made his London debut as the Bloody Sergeant in *Macbeth* (Kingsway Theatre). He was a supporting player at the Westminster Theatre and the Old Vic in the years before the war (roles at the latter included Colonel Pickering in *Pygmalion*, the Provost in *Measure for Measure*, and Buckingham in *Richard III*). From 1941 he served as a signaller in the Royal Artillery; wounded at Anzio, he was invalided out in 1944. He resumed his career at the Arts Theatre (1945-46), and confirmed his growing reputation as a Shakespearean actor, adept at both comedic and dramatic roles, with the Old Vic company at the New (1947-50): Baptista in *The Taming of the Shrew* (John Burrell); John of Gaunt in *Richard II* (Ralph Richardson); Sicinius in *Coriolanus* (E. Martin Browne); Malvolio in *Twelfth Night* (Alec Guinness); Holofernes in *Love's Labour's Lost* (Hugh Hunt); and a formidable Claudius in the Michael Redgrave *Hamlet* (Hunt). During the 1950/51 Old Vic homecoming season he played Sir Hugh Evans in *The Merry Wives of Windsor* (Hunt), and Exeter in *Henry V* (Glen Byam Shaw).

Dignam was a redoubtable member of the RSC in the 1950s, 70s and 80s. First at Stratford between 1956 and 58, as well as returning to three favourite parts, Holofernes in *Love's Labour's Lost* (Peter Hall, 1956), Malvolio in *Twelfth Night* (Hall), and Claudius—again opposite Redgrave—in *Hamlet* (Glen Byam Shaw, both 1958), he played the Ghost in *Hamlet* (Michael Langham); the Prince of Morocco in *The Merchant of Venice* (Margaret Webster); the Duke of Venice in *Othello* (Shaw); the Provost in *Measure for Measure* (Anthony Quayle); Mr Badger in *Toad of Toad Hall* (Patrick Donnell); Duke Frederick in *As You Like It* (Shaw); Cardinal Pandulph in *King John* (Douglas Seale); Casca in *Julius Caesar* (Shaw); Pisanio in *Cymbeline* (Hall); Antonio in *The Tempest* (Peter Brook); Capulet in *Romeo and Juliet* (Shaw); and Simonides in *Pericles* (Tony Richardson). Then, ending an absence of fourteen years, he led the 1972/73 'Romans' company as Menenius in *Coriolanus*, the title role in *Julius Caesar*, Marcus Andronicus in *Titus Andronicus* (Trevor Nunn/Buzz Goodbody), and went on to create the roles of Maurice Shanklin in David Mercer's *Duck Song* (David Jones, Aldwych, 1974), Valladares/Phillip IV in Peter Barnes's *The Bewitched* (Terry Hands, Aldwych, 1974), and Vladimir in Mercer's *Cousin Vladimir* (Jane Howell, Aldwych, 1978). Finally, as an elder statesman, he played Father Barre in John Whiting's *The Devils* (John Barton, Pit, 1984); Russell Blackborough in Harley Granville-Barker's *Waste* (Barton, Pit, 1985); Perchikhin in Gorky's *Philistines* (John Caird, TOP, 1985); Adam in *As You Like It* (Adrian Noble, RST, 1985); Nestor in *Troilus and Cressida* (Howard Davies, RST, 1985); Voice 3 in Harold Pinter's *Family Voices* (Paul Marcus, RSC fringe festival, TOP, 1985); Thomas Bruckner in *Mephisto* (Noble, Barbican, 1986); Igor Gertzmann in John Berger's *A Question of Geography* (Caird, TOP, 1987); Escalus in *Measure for Measure* (Nicholas Hytner, RST, 1987); and Homer in Howard Barker's *The Bite of the Night* (Danny Boyle, Pit, 1988).

Prominent work elsewhere: Kroll in *Rosmersholm* (Royal Court, 1959-60); Auda Abu Tayek in Rattigan's *Ross* (Theatre Royal Haymarket, 1960); Polonius in the Nicol Williamson *Hamlet* (Roundhouse, 1969); the Father in John Mortimer's *A Voyage Round My Father* (Greenwich Theatre, 1970); and Cardinal Bellarmin in Brecht's *The Life of Galileo* (John Dexter, NT Olivier, 1980).

Dignam played supporting roles in the films *Beau Brummell* (1954); *Doctor in the House* (1954); *Sink the Bismarck!* (Lewis Gilbert, 1960); *The Pure Hell of St Trinian's* (1960); *Tom Jones* (Tony Richardson, 1963); *The Taming of the Shrew* (Franco Zeffirelli, 1967); and *The Charge of the Light Brigade* (Richardson, 1968).

Stephen Dillane (b. London, 1956) studied history and politics at Exeter University and initially worked as a journalist. He trained at the Bristol Old Vic Theatre School and emerged as one of his generation's most promising actors in the late 1980s. His thoughtful approach suggests an ambition for the theatre that is increasingly rare.

Dillane's early successes on the stage included Archer in *The Beaux' Stratagem* at the Belgrade, Coventry (Peter Wood, 1989); Gerry in *Dancing at Lughnasa* at the Abbey Theatre, Dublin (Patrick Mason, 1990); Edmund in *Long Day's Journey into Night* at the Bristol Old Vic (Howard Davies, 1991); and Prior in *Angels in America* at the National (Declan Donnellan, Cottesloe, 1993). He was an exceptional Hamlet, tense and anguished, in Peter Hall's acclaimed production (Peter Hall Company, Gielgud Theatre, 1994), and his Uncle Vanya, at the RSC, was wracked by despair, longing and resentment—both the pursuit of Yelena and the attempted murder of Serebryakov had real intent (Katie Mitchell, Young Vic, 1998). Overall, his theatre work has been consistently of interest: Clov—a brooding hunchback in a caretaker's coat, slave to Alun Armstrong's Hamm—in Beckett's *Endgame* (Katie Mitchell, Donmar Warehouse, 1996); Artie in *Hurlyburly* (Peter Hall Company, Old Vic, 1997); Henry in Tom Stoppard's *The Real Thing* (David Leveaux, Donmar Warehouse, 1999); Peter George in Hannie Rayson's *Life After George* (Michael Blakemore, Duchess, 2002); Herzen in Stoppard's epic *The Coast of Utopia* (Trevor Nunn, NT Olivier, 2002); Martin Crimp's *Advice to Iraqi Women* (Royal Court, 2003); a one-man version of *Macbeth* (Travis Preston, Almeida, 2005); and Jack in Caryl Churchill's *Drunk Enough to Say I Love You?* (James Macdonald, Royal Court, 2006).

An admired film actor, Dillane starred in Michael Winterbottom's *Welcome to Sarajevo* (1997); opposite Sophie Moreau in *Firelight* (William Nicholson, 1997); and as Leonard Woolf in *The Hours* (Stephen Daldry, 2002). For Hollywood, he has enlivened such mainstream product as *Stolen Hearts* (1996); *Spy Game* (Tony Scott, 2001); and *King Arthur* (Antoine Fuqua, 2004).

Joe Dixon (b. Birmingham, 1965) grew up in Birmingham and first acted with the Birmingham Youth Theatre. After RADA, his early progress included Mercutio in the Temba Theatre Company's Cuban *Romeo and Juliet* (Alby James, Young Vic, 1988); winning the Ian Charleson Award as a dandyish Jaques in Declan Donnellan's Cheek By Jowl all-male *As You Like It* (Lyric Hammersmith, 1991-92); Romeo in *Romeo and Juliet* (Michael Bogdanov, ESC, Lyric Hammersmith, 1993); and Antonio in the Juliet Stevenson *Duchess of Malfi* (Philip Franks, Greenwich Theatre, 1995).

Dixon spent the rest of the 1990s working as a screen actor. He returned to the stage in 2001, cast as Camillo in *The Winter's Tale* at the National (Nicholas Hytner, Olivier). Since 2002 he has been based at the RSC: the 'Jacobethans' (Swan, 2002)—Paris in *The Roman Actor* (Sean Holmes), King of Bakam in *The Island Princess* (Gregory Doran) and Mendoza in *The Malcontent* (Dominic Cooke); RST, 2003—Aron in *Titus Andronicus* (Bill Alexander); 'The Comedies' (RST, 2005)—Oberon in *A Midsummer Night's Dream* (Doran) and Antipholus of Syracuse in *The Comedy of Errors* (Nancy Meckler); and Courtyard, 2008—Bottom in *A Midsummer Night's Dream* and Armado in *Love's Labour's Lost* (Doran).

Elsewhere: Hercules opposite Kerry Fox in Martin Crimp's reworking of Sophocles's *Women of Trachis, Cruel and Tender* (Luc Bondy, Young Vic, 2004).

Monica Dolan (b. Middlesbrough) trained at the Guildhall School and gained her early experience at the Northcott Theatre, Ipswich, and the Theatre Royal, York, playing the Gaoler's Daughter in *The Two Noble Kinsmen*, Queen Anne in *The Three Musketeers*, Scout in *To Kill a Mockingbird*, Jessica in *The Merchant of Venice*, and the title role in *Jane Eyre*.

Her RSC career started in 1993 with the part of Feebs in Michael Hastings's *Unfinished Business* (Steven Pimlott, Pit). Already an intense, vocally expressive performer, she went on play Katherine in the Iain Glen *Henry V* (Matthew Warchus, RST, 1994); Virgilia in the Toby Stephens *Coriolanus* (David Thacker, Swan, 1994); Juliet in *Measure for Measure* (Steven Pimlott, RST, 1994); Hermia, succeeding Emma Fielding, in *A Midsummer Night's Dream* (Adrian Noble, Barbican, 1995); and Kate in *The Taming of the Shrew* (Lindsay Posner, Small-scale Tour, 2000).

Following important work with Max Stafford-Clark's Out of Joint company, including Suzanne in Judy Upton's *Sliding With Suzanne* (Royal Court, 2001), Kate in Oliver Goldsmith's *She Stoops to Conquer* (NT Lyttelton, 2002-03) and Lady Macbeth in *Macbeth* (Wilton's Music Hall, 2004), she returned to the RSC to play Regan in *King Lear* and Masha in *The Seagull* (Trevor Nunn, Courtyard, 2007).

Roy Dotrice (b. Guernsey, 1923) served with Bomber Command as an air gunner until his Lancaster was shot down over Germany. During his three years as a prisoner of war he performed in revues (thereby discovering his vocation) and played baseball with the Americans. After the war he worked in provincial repertory before forming his own troupe, the Guernsey Theatre Company (1955).

He went to Stratford in 1958. In his first seasons he played small supporting roles and organised a theatre baseball team (the 1959 team, which played the local US airbases, included Paul Robeson, Sam Wanamaker, Laurence Olivier and Albert Finney). His ability to play old men brought him the role of Firs in Michel Saint-Denis's production of *The Cherry Orchard* (RST, 1961). It was a turning point, leading to Caliban in *The Tempest* (Clifford Williams, RST, 1963), Julius Caesar (John Blatchley, RST, 1963), Edward IV in Peter Hall's *The Wars of the Roses* (RST, 1963) and the title role in Brecht's *Puntila* (Saint-Denis, Aldwych, 1965).

John Dougall (b. Dunoon, Argyll) should be better known. He has, after all, worked at the highest level, succeeding Kenneth Branagh as Judd in Adrian Mitchell's *Another Country* (Stuart Burge, Queen's, 1982); sharing Hal with Michael Pennington in the ESC's *Henry IV* and *Henry V* (Michael Bogdanov, 1989); and performing such varied characters as Yasha in *The Cherry Orchard* (Sam Mendes, Aldwych, 1989); Curley in *Of Mice and Men* (Anthony Clark, Birmingham Rep, 1990); Lucifer in *Doctor Faustus* (Philip Franks, Greenwich Theatre, 1993); Bluebeard in *Saint Joan* (Gale Edwards, Strand, 1993); Richard in Noël Coward's *Hay Fever* (Dominic Dromgoole, Oxford Stage Company, 2002); Bernard Nightingale in Tom Stoppard's *Arcadia* (Rupert Goold, Royal Theatre, Northampton, 2002); Pishchik in *The Cherry Orchard* (Dromgoole, Oxford Stage Company, 2003); the Reverend Parris in *The Crucible* (Anna Mackmin, Sheffield Crucible, 2004); and Pompey in *Measure for Measure* (John Dove, Globe, 2004).

At the RSC, Dougall has played Florizel in *The Winter's Tale* (Adrian Noble, Small-scale Tour, 1984); Pug in Ben Jonson's *The Devil is an Ass* (Matthew Warchus, Swan, 1995); the tavern thug Siebel, reinvented as a Glaswegian skinhead, in Howard Brenton's unsubtle *Faust* (Bogdanov, Swan, 1995); Yepikhodov—tragically, poignantly ridiculous—in *The Cherry Orchard* (Noble, Swan, 1995); Gratiano in *The Merchant of Venice* (Gregory Doran, RST, 1997); Speed in *The Two Gentlemen of Verona* (Edmund Hall, Swan, 1998); Elbow in *Measure for Measure* (Michael Boyd, RST, 1998); Malcolm in *Macbeth* (Doran, Swan, 1999); Horatio in *Hamlet* (Steven Pimlott, RST, 2001); and Vincent in William Wycherley's *Love in a Wood* (Tim Supple, Swan, 2001).

Penny Downie (b. Australia). A chance meeting with Sheila Hancock and John Caird in the bar of the Bush Theatre initiated Penny Downie's RSC career. Hancock tells the story in her autobiography *Ramblings of an Actress*. They were in the process of assembling the RSC's 1983 small-scale touring troupe and a sixth sense told them that Downie was an actress (she had, in fact, achieved some success in her native Australia). As Titania in *A Midsummer Night's Dream* and a very young and sensual Lady Capulet in *Romeo and Juliet*, Downie revealed a natural affinity for classical roles.

She went on to play Lady Anne in the Antony Sher *Richard III* (Bill Alexander, RST, 1984); Peggy Smith in Robert Holman's *Today* (Alexander, TOP, 1984); Agnes in Strindberg's *Dreamplay* (John Barton, Pit, 1985); Anne in Howard Barker's *The Castle* (Nick Hamm, Pit, 1985); Struggle in Barker's *Crimes in Hot Countries* (Alexander, Pit, 1985); both Hermione and Perdita in *The Winter's Tale* (Terry Hands, RST, 1986); Sarah Sprackling in Nick Dear's *The Art of Success* (Adrian Noble, TOP, 1986); a moving Lady Macduff in *Macbeth* (Noble, RST, 1986); a fierce Queen Margaret in *The Plantagenets* (Noble, RST, 1988); a refined and unfashionably sympathetic Portia in *The Merchant of Venice* (David Thacker, RST, 1993); the title role in Nick Dear's *Zenobia* (Mike Ockrent, Young Vic, 1995); Gina in David Edgar's *The Prisoner's Dilemma* (Michael Attenborough, TOP, 2001); Penelope in Margaret Atwood's *The Penelopiad* (Josette Bushell-Mingo, Swan, 2007); and Gertrude in *Hamlet* (Gregory Doran, Courtyard, 2008).

Elsewhere, she was Marianne opposite Alan Howard in Ingmar Bergman's *Scenes From a Marriage* (Rita Russek, Chichester, 1990); Paulina in *Death and the Maiden* (Lindsay Posner, Duke of York's, 1992); Alice in *Berlin Bertie* (Danny Boyle, Royal Court, 1992); Katherine in *An Enemy of the People* (Trevor Nunn, NT Olivier, 1997); Sophie in Hanif Kureshi's *Sleep With Me* (Antony Page, NT Cottesloe, 1999); Wynne in Moira Buffini's *Dinner* (Fiona Buffini, NT Loft, 2002); and the Chorus in *Henry V* (Nicholas Hytner, NT Olivier, 2003).

Amanda Drew (b. Boston, Lincolnshire, 1969) graduated from RADA in 1992. In an intriguing and varied list of credits in the theatre, she has comfortably crossed the divide between drama and comedy. She made her name at the Royal Court playing the contrasting figures of Rochester's wife (abused by her husband) in Stephen Jeffreys's *The Libertine*, and Harriet (vivacious and witty, pursued by the Rochester-inspired Dorimant) in *The Man of Mode* (Max Stafford-Clark, Out of Joint, 1994-95). At the National's Lyttelton, 1995-96, she was Mincing, woman to Fiona Shaw's Mistress Millamant, in *The Way of the World* (Phyllida Lloyd), and the sullen maid in the Paul Scofield/Vanessa Redgrave *John Gabriel Borkman* (Richard Eyre). At the Almeida, the following year, she appeared in Phyllida Lloyd's production of García Lorca's *Dona Rosita, the Spinster*, and at the Young Vic in 1999 she played the young lead in *The House of Bernarda Alba* (Polly Teale, Shared Experience).

Her work in contemporary writing has been of equal note: Mary in Stewart Harcourt's *The Good Times Will Come* (Old Red Lion, Islington, 1994); the lonely heroine of Kara Miller's *Tamagotchi Heaven* (Edinburgh Festival, 1998); Peter Whelan's *The School of Night* (Jack Shepherd, Minerva Theatre, Chichester, 1999); Sarah in David Gieselmann's *Mr Kolpert* (Richard Wilson, Royal Court, 2000); and Marlene in *Top Girls* (Roxana Silbert, New Vic, Newcastle-under-Lyme, 2000).

She joined the RSC in 2001, cast as Lydia in William Wycherley's *Love in a Wood* (Tim Supple, Swan) and Lydia in Peter Barnes's *Jubilee* (Gregory Doran, Swan). The following year she returned to Stratford's Swan to perform leading roles in a trio of plays rarely seen since the 17th century: Gertrude, a bravura display, in Jonson, Marston and Chapman's *Eastward Ho!* (Lucy Pitman-Wallace); Domitilla in *The Roman Actor* (Sean Holmes); and Aurelia, dangerously alluring, in Marston's *The Malcontent* (Dominic Cooke).

Elsewhere, since 2003, Amanda Drew has played the title role in *Madame Bovary* (Polly Teale, Shared Experience, Lyric Hammersmith, 2003); Abigail in Steve Thompson's *Damages* (Roxana Silbert, Bush, 2004); Elvira in Noël Coward's *Blithe Spirit* (Thea Sharrock, Peter Hall Company, Theatre Royal, Bath, 2004); Beth in Simon Gray's *Otherwise Engaged* (Simon Curtis, Criterion, 2005); Tatyana in Gorky's *Enemies* (Michael Attenborough,

Almeida, 2006); and Fanny in Marius von Mayenburg's *The Ugly One* (Ramin Gray, Royal Court, 2007).

Kate Duchêne was a member of the Footlights while studying at Trinity College, Cambridge, and gained her early experience at the Octagon Theatre, Bolton, and the Traverse Theatre, Edinburgh, where she played Lucy in John Clifford's *Lucy's Play* (1986). She came to notice in productions directed by Sam Mendes: the Princess of France in *Love's Labour's Lost* and Kaleria in Gorky's *Summerfolk* at Chichester (Minerva, 1989); Carlotta in *The Cherry Orchard* at the Aldwych (1989); and Amy in Sartre's *Kean* at the Old Vic (1990). In 1991 she joined the National to play Elise in *The Miser* (Steven Pimlott, Olivier) and Dockdaisy in *The Resistible Rise of Arturo Ui* (Di Trevis, Olivier).

It was because of Mendes that Kate Duchêne first came to the RSC, cast as Queen Elizabeth in his revival of *Richard III* (TOP and Small-scale Tour, 1992). Kate Duchêne and the production's star, Simon Russell Beale, had been at Cambridge together. She continued with the Company as Chorus in T.S. Eliot's *Murder in the Cathedral* (Steven Pimlott, Swan, 1993); a highly-strung Jessica in *The Merchant of Venice* (David Thacker, RST, 1993); Alithea in William Wycherley's *The Country Wife* (Max Stafford-Clark, Swan, 1993); Amanda in John Vanbrugh's *The Relapse* (Ian Judge, Swan, 1995); a deeply affecting Varya in *The Cherry Orchard* (Adrian Noble, Swan, 1995); Earth Spirit/Martha/Helen of Troy in *Faust* (Michael Bogdanov, Swan, 1995); Marie in Georg Büchner's *Woyzeck* (Sean Holmes, TOP, 1996); and Susanna, succeeding Teresa Banham, in Peter Whelan's *The Herbal Bed* (Michael Attenborough, Duchess Theatre, 1997).

Elsewhere, Kate Duchêne has played Simone in Naomi Wallace's *The Inland Sea* (Dominic Dromgoole, Oxford Stage Company, 2002); and the mother in Lucy Prebble's *The Sugar Syndrome* (Marianne Elliott, Royal Court, 2003). At the National, directed by Katie Mitchell, she was an intensely enigmatic presence in *Iphigenia at Aulis* (Lyttelton, 2004), Virginia Woolf's

Waves (Cottesloe, 2006-07), Martin Crimp's *Attempts on Her Life* (Lyttelton, 2007), and *Women of Troy* (Lyttelton, 2008).

William Dudley (b. London, 1947) studied at St Martin's School of Art and made his name working with Bill Bryden on *The Passion* at the National in 1977. A designer who favours naturalism over abstraction, he has nevertheless always been technically innovative, exploiting the Olivier Theatre's stage machinery to the full (*The Shaughraun*, 1988), and pioneering the use of 3D computer-generated images (Trevor Nunn's production of Tom Stoppard's *The Coast of Utopia* at the Olivier, 2002; Terry Johnson's *Hitchcock Blonde* at the Royal Court, 2003).

Work at the RSC: Peter Gill's *Twelfth Night* (RST, 1974); David Jones's *Ivanov* (Aldwych, 1976); Barry Kyle's *That Good Between Us* (Warehouse, 1977) and *Richard II* (RST, 1986); Bill Alexander's *Richard III* (RST, 1984), *Today* (TOP, 1984), *The Merry Wives of Windsor* (RST, 1985), *A Midsummer Night's Dream* (RST, 1986) and *Country Dancing* (TOP, 1986); Howard Davies's *The Party* (TOP, 1984) and *The General from America* (Swan, 1997); Adrian Noble's *Kiss Me Kate* (RST, 1987); and David Thacker's *The Merry Wives of Windsor* (RST, 1992).

Susan Dury (b. Bristol, 1946) trained at the Guildford School of Acting and began her career working with experimental theatre groups in Edinburgh, Amsterdam and Paris. She appeared in the film *The Assistant* (1968), and during the early 1970s lived in Los Angeles (Clea in *Black Comedy*). Her work on the fringe included *High in Vietnam* (Almost Free); *Morituri* (King's Head); *A Voyage Round My Father* (Windsor); and *Love Story* (King's Head). She appeared in the television serial *The Cedar Tree* (ITV, 1976), and in the film *Return of a Man Called Horse* (1976).

She joined the RSC in 1976 and gave fine performances as Witch/Lady Macduff in the Ian McKellen *Macbeth* (Trevor Nunn, TOP); Luce in the musical *The Comedy of Errors* (Nunn, RST); Joan in Edward Bond's *Bingo* (Howard Davies, TOP); and

Hermione, replacing the indisposed Marilyn Taylerson, in *The Winter's Tale* (Nunn/John Barton, RST). She was next a suburb Doll Common in *The Alchemist* (Nunn, TOP, 1977). She decided against transferring with *Macbeth* to the Young Vic and turned down the role of Natasha in Nunn's touring *Three Sisters* so that she could play Jean in Tony and Nick Bicât's musical version of *All's Well That Ends Well* (Oxford Playhouse, 1978). She resumed her RSC career as Miss Leigh's Maid in *Once in a Lifetime* (Nunn, Aldwych, 1979); Efimia in *The Children of the Sun* (Terry Hands, Aldwych, 1979); and Chorus in *The Greeks* (Barton, Aldwych, 1980). Almost twenty years would elapse before her return to Stratford to lead the Eumenides in *The Family Reunion* (Adrian Noble, Swan, 1999), and to play Dorothy in *A Warwickshire Testimony* (Alison Sutcliffe, TOP, 1999).

Chris Dyer studied at the Ravensbourne College of Art and Design and began his career in 1968 as an assistant designer at the Marlowe Theatre, Canterbury. For the next three years he worked as a scene painter at the Bristol Old Vic. He was then given an opportunity in the Bristol Old Vic Studio, as resident designer. For Howard Davies, the studio's director, he designed productions of Edward Bond's *Early Morning* and Edward Albee's *Who's Afraid of Virginia Woolf?*

Howard Davies joined the RSC in 1974 and Dyer followed. As one of the RSC's house designers (1974-86) he was highly versatile: changing his style from job to job, he worked for all the associate directors and designed some of the Company's finest productions, including Buzz Goodbody's *Hamlet* (TOP, 1975), Trevor Nunn's *The Alchemist* (TOP, 1977) and Michael Bogdanov's *Taming of the Shrew* (RST, 1978). He was centrally involved in the development of The Other Place. He designed the Company's first portable auditorium (small-scale tour, 1979) and the Pit Theatre. With John Napier he designed the 1976 RST stage configuration—a wooden, Jacobean-style arena with balconies.

Among Dyer's other RSC assignments were: *The Beast* (Howard Davies, The Place, 1974); *Perkin Warbeck* (John Barton/Barry Kyle, TOP, 1975); *Romeo and Juliet* (Trevor Nunn, RST, 1976); *The Iceman Cometh* (Davies, Aldwych, 1976); *Troilus and Cressida* (Barton/Kyle, RST, 1976); *'Tis Pity She's a Whore* (Ron Daniels, TOP, 1977); *Days of the Commune* (Davies, Aldwych, 1977); *Savage Amusement* (John Caird, Warehouse, 1978); *Pericles* (Daniels, TOP, 1979); *Much Ado About Nothing* (Davies) and *The Caucasian Chalk Circle* (Caird, Small-scale Tour, 1979); *The Children of the Sun* (Terry Hands, Aldwych, 1979); *The Shadow of a Gunman* (Bogdanov, TOP, 1980); *The Fool* (Davies, TOP, 1980); *Timon of Athens* (Daniels, TOP, 1980); *The Knight of the Burning Pestle* (Bogdanov, Aldwych, 1981); *Macbeth* (Davies, RST, 1982); *Peer Gynt* (Daniels, TOP, 1982); *The Roaring Girl* (Kyle, Barbican, 1983); *The Dillen* (Kyle, TOP, 1983); *The Desert Air* (Adrian Noble, TOP, 1984); *Romeo and Juliet* (Bogdanov, RST, 1986); *All's Well That Ends Well* (Kyle, RST, 1989); *King Lear* (Cicely Berry, Almeida, 1989); and *Faust* (Bogdanov, Swan, 1995).

He has been less visible at the RSC since the mid-1980s. Most prominently he has worked with Michael Bogdanov, designing productions of *The Henries* (1986-88), *Coriolanus* (1990), *The Winter's Tale* (1991), *The Tempest* (1992) and *Romeo and Juliet* (1993) for the English Shakespeare Company; *Julius Caesar, Reineke Fuchs, Romeo and Juliet, The Tempest, Dancing at Lughnasa* and *The Ginger Man* at the Deutsches Schauspeilhaus, Hamburg; and *The Merry Wives of Windsor, The Merchant of Venice* and *The Winter's Tale* at the Ludlow Festival (2002-03). He designed Peter Hall's 1989 production of *The Merchant of Venice* (Phoenix Theatre).

E

Richard Easton (b. Montreal, 1933). A veteran of topflight theatre on both sides of the Atlantic, Richard Easton finally became a Broadway star in his late sixties—his Tony-winning performance as the older Housman in Tom Stoppard's *The Invention of Love* (Richard Eyre, 2001) was followed by Mowbray in Michael Frayn's *Noises Off* (Jeremy Sams, Brooks Atkinson, 2001-02); Pyper in Frank McGuinness's *Observe the Sons of Ulster Marching Towards the Somme* (Lincoln Center, 2003); and the title role, alongside Kevin Kline (Falstaff) and Ethan Hawke (Hotspur), in *Henry IV* (Jack O'Brien, Lincoln Center, 2003).

A native of Montreal, he acted with a children's theatre group before moving, at the age of seventeen, to Ottawa to work in weekly rep. A scholarship took him to London, and during the first English phase of his career he joined the Shakespeare Memorial Theatre Company at the Palace to play Claudio in *Much Ado About Nothing* (John Gielgud) and Edgar in the Gielgud *King Lear* (George Devine, 1955). During the 1960s he was a member of the New York troupe APA-Phoenix. The 1970s saw him back in England. He played Fagan in *Oliver!* on tour, and starred in the BBC's popular drama series *The Brothers* (1972-76).

For four years from 1984 he was one of the RSC's most authoritative figures. In 1984/85 he played the Constable of France in the Kenneth Branagh *Henry V* (Adrian Noble, RST), the Duke of Venice in *The Merchant of Venice* (John Caird, RST), the Ghost in the Roger Rees *Hamlet* (Ron Daniels, RST), Don Armado, succeeding Edward Petherbridge, in *Love's Labour's Lost* (Barry Kyle, Barbican), and Rochfort in Peter Barnes's *Red Noses* (Terry Hands, Barbican); in 1986/87, Camillo in *The Winter's Tale* (Hands, RST), Theseus in *A Midsummer Night's Dream* (Bill Alexander, RST), Northumberland in the Jeremy Irons *Richard II* (Kyle, RST), Cecil Sharp in Nigel Williamson's *Country Dancing* (Alexander, TOP), Radio Voice in *Sarcophagus* (Jude Kelly, Pit), and Envoy in *The Balcony* (Hands).

The next few years saw him supporting Kenneth Branagh's new venture, Renaissance. He was the backbone of the season at the Birmingham Rep and the Phoenix, playing Jaques in *As You Like It* (Geraldine McEwan), Leonato in *Much Ado About Nothing* (Judi Dench) and Claudius in *Hamlet* (Derek Jacobi), and appeared in Branagh's first two films, *Henry V* (1989) and *Dead Again* (1991).

In 1989 Easton returned to America and began ten years with the Old Globe Theatre in San Diego.

David Edgar (b. Birmingham, 1948). David Edgar's early plays were staged by politicised fringe touring groups. He worked as a journalist and a university teacher, and these activities, particularly the reporting, bled into his writing. He writes about contemporary events in a documentary style, while occasionally injecting a stream of fantasy—in *Dick Deterred*, about Watergate, Nixon meets Richard III. He was writer in residence at the Birmingham Rep in 1974, but first achieved wide recognition when the RSC premiered his play *Destiny* in 1976. A study of British fascism, *Destiny* remains pre-eminent in a body of work that examines the motives and ethics of contemporary politics.

Chief among his subsequent RSC plays were *Maydays*, a history of post-war protest and dissent; *The Prisoner's Dilemma*, an account of a regional war in post-Communist eastern Europe, from the fighters on the ground to the UN peace-makers; and the eight-hour *Nicholas Nickleby*, based on Dickens's novel. *Maydays* was the first new drama to occupy the vast Barbican stage. The *Nickleby* project saw Edgar working as a company playwright, responding on a daily basis to the work of the actors in the rehearsal room.

Increasingly he has written plays of discourse in which the moments of action illustrate a hypothesis. *The Prisoner's Dilemma* was intellectually compelling and strikingly topical, but some of the writing belonged in the lecture hall or on *Newsnight*. At his considerable best Edgar is passionate without being sentimental and committed without being polemical.

During the 1980s Edgar served on the RSC's new play committee, and since 1989 he has taught playwriting at Birmingham University.

Rob Edwards (b. Lincoln). A graduate of Oxford University and the Bristol Old Vic Theatre School, Rob Edwards was first at the RSC in 1980/81, playing Amintor in *The Maid's Tragedy* (Barry Kyle, TOP); Wadlow/Governor in Edward Bond's *The Fool* (Howard Davies, TOP); Lucullus in *Timon of Athens* (Ron Daniels, TOP); Lord Grey in *Richard III* (Terry Hands, RST); Lancelot Gobbo in *The Merchant of Venice* (John Barton, RST); and Khomich in *The Love-Girl and the Innocent* (Clifford Williams, Aldwych).

Following acclaimed work for David Thacker at the Young Vic—Lucio in *Measure for Measure* (1987), and the Duke in *Measure for Measure* (1989)—he returned to Stratford: Lysimachus, then the title role, in Thacker's production of *Pericles* (David Thacker, Swan, 1989); Dumaine the Younger in *All's Well That Ends Well* (Kyle, RST, 1989); First Citizen in *Coriolanus* (Hands, RST, 1989); Pritykin in *Barbarians* (David Jones, Barbican, 1990); a moody, dangerous Poins in *Henry IV* (Adrian Noble, RST, 1991); Polynices/Chorus in *The Thebans* (Noble, Swan, 1991); Messenger in *The Dybbuk* (Katie Mitchell, Pit, 1992); Bakin in *Artists and Admirers* (Phyllida Lloyd, Pit, 1992); a fine Horatio, wearing (at court) a borrowed evening suit one size too small, in the Kenneth Branagh *Hamlet* (Noble, Barbican, 1992); Cassius in *Julius Caesar* (Thacker, Small-scale Tour, 1993); Antonio in *Twelfth Night* (Noble, RST, 1997); Quarlous in *Bartholomew Fair* (Laurence Boswell, Swan, 1997); Walt Disney in Stephen Poliakoff's *Talk and the City* (Poliakoff, Swan, 1998); Hippolito in *Women Beware Women* (Boswell, Swan, 2006); and Page in *The Merry Wives of Windsor* (Gregory Doran, RST, 2006-07).

At the Open Air Theatre, Regent's Park, in 1997 he was Oberon to Serena Evans's Titania in *A Midsummer Night's Dream* (Rachel Kavanagh), and a gangster in *Kiss Me Kate* (Ian Talbot). From 1999 to 2005 he played Scar in Disney's hit musical *The Lion King* (Julie Taymor, Lyceum).

Peter Egan (b. London, 1946) flirted with Penelope Wilton over four series of *Ever Decreasing Circles* (BBC, 1984-87), played Henry Simcox in John Mortimer's *Paradise Postponed* (1986) and the haunted Pym in John le Carré's *The Perfect Spy* (BBC, 1987). If he is best known for these and other television roles, he has given some memorable performances on the stage, in the West End, at Chichester and at the RSC. Also a theatre director, his credits include *Uncle Vanya* for Renaissance (Tour and Lyric Hammersmith, 1991).

Egan's television career began when he played a London gangster in the controversial series *Big Breadwinner Hogg* (1969), and continued in the 70s with appearances in *Elizabeth R* (1971) as Southampton; in *Callan* (1974); and in *Lillie* (1978) as Oscar Wilde. He first joined the RSC in 1970 and played Osric in the Alan Howard *Hamlet* (Trevor Nunn, RST), Froth in *Measure for Measure* (John Barton, RST), and, most memorably, Valentine in Robin Phillips's modern-dress production of *The Two Gentlemen of Verona* (RST). Almost twenty years elapsed before he rejoined the Company to play Tsyganov in Gorky's *Barbarians* (David Jones, Barbican, 1990). Then, in 1997/98, Egan gave his best RSC performance, and one of the best of his career, as the ageing Casanova, exhausted and at the end of his tether, in Tennessee Williams's *Camino Real* (Steven Pimlott, Swan).

Other highlights of Egan's stage career: Stanhope in *Journey's End* (West End, 1972); Astrov in the already mentioned *Uncle Vanya*; Jimmy Porter in Osborne's *Déjà Vu* (Tony Palmer, Comedy Theatre, 1992); the director in Michael Frayn's *Noises Off* (Jeremy Sams, NT Lyttelton, 2000); and Tom in *The Secret Rapture* (Guy Retallack, Lyric, 2003-04). On the big screen, he played Cantrip in Joseph Losey's *The Hireling* (1973), and the Duke of Sutherland in *Chariots of Fire* (Hugh Hudson, 1981).

Susan Engel (b. Vienna, 1935) read French and Drama at Bristol University before training for the stage in Bristol and Paris (under Henri Rollan). She went from the Bristol Old Vic School into the Old Vic Company (1959).

She was first at the RSC from 1962 to 65. Although still in her twenties, she possessed the character actor's ability to play different ages and styles: Ludovica in *The Caucasian Chalk Circle* (William Gaskill, Aldwych, 1962); Constance in *Curtmantle* (Stuart Burge, Aldwych, 1962); Ninon in *The Devils* (Peter Wood, Aldwych, 1962); Juno in *The Tempest* (Clifford Williams, RST, 1963); Calphurnia in *Julius Caesar* (John Blatchley, RST, 1963); a Courtezan in *The Comedy Errors* (Williams, RST, 1963); Queen Elizabeth in *The Wars of the Roses* (Peter Hall with John Barton, RST, 1963); Doll Tearsheet to Hugh Griffith's Falstaff in *Henry IV Part 2* (Hall/Barton/Williams, RST, 1964); Adriana in *The Comedy of Errors* (Williams, RST, 1965); and Manda in Brecht's *Squire Puntila and His Servant Matti* (Michel Saint-Denis, Aldwych, 1965).

She did not return to the RSC until the late 1980s, and has maintained a distinguished, if occasional, association in the years since: Constance in *King John* (Deborah Warner, TOP, 1988); Frade in *The Dybbuk* (Katie Mitchell, Pit, 1992); Agnes in Robert Holman's *Bad Weather* (Steven Pimlott, TOP, 1998); Margaret in Nick Stafford's *Luminosity* (Gemma Bodinetz) and Stella in *Epitaph for the Official Secrets Act* (Simon Reade, Pit, 2001); a chillingly grave mother to Ralph Fiennes's *Brand* (Adrian Noble, Swan, 2003); and the Widow in *Women Beware Women* (Laurence Boswell, Swan, 2006). At the National, and elsewhere, she has been just as formidable: *Watch on the Rhine* (Mike Ockrent, NT Lyttelton, 1980); Kate in Neil Simon's *Brighton Beach Memoirs* (Michael Rudman, NT Aldwych, 1986); *The Good Person of Sichuan* (Warner, NT Olivier, 1989); Goneril in *King Lear* (Warner) and Queen Margaret in *Richard III* (Richard Eyre, NT Lyttelton, 1990); Meg in Brian Phelan's *Himself* (Paul Unwin, Richmond, 1993); Hannah Pitt and Ethel Rosenburg in *Angels in America* (Declan Donnellan, NT Cottesloe, 1993); the mother in Beckett's *Footfalls* (Warner, Garrick, 1994); Mrs Heidelberg in *The Clandestine Marriage* (Nigel Hawthorne, Queen's, 1994-95); Sybil Birling in *An Inspector Calls* (Stephen Daldry, Garrick, 1995); Sarah in Sebastian Barry's *Prayers of Sherkin* (John Dove, Old Vic, 1997); Mrs Rafi in Edward Bond's *The Sea* (Sean Holmes, Minerva, Chichester, 2000); the dean in Rebecca Gilman's *Spinning into Butter* (Dominic Cooke, Royal Court, 2001); Marie in *After the Gods* (Gemma Bodinetz, Hampstead Theatre, 2002); and Mrs Moore in *A Passage to India* (Nancy Meckler, Shared Experience, 2002).

She delivered expert cameos in the films *Charlie Bubbles* (Albert Finney, 1968); *Inspector Clouseau* (1968); *King Lear* (Peter Brook, 1970), as Regan; *Butley* (Harold Pinter, 1974); *Hopscotch* (1980); *Ascendancy* (1982); and *Damage* (Louis Malle, 1993).

Daniel Evans (b. Cwmparc, South Wales, 1973). Growing up in the Rhondda Valley, Daniel Evans won prizes for acting (including the Richard Burton award at the 1990 National Eisteddfod) and appeared in children's programmes on Welsh-language television. From the Guildhall School in London he joined the RSC's 1994 Stratford company, cast as Boy in *Henry V* (Matthew Warchus, RST), Citizen in *Coriolanus* (David Thacker, Swan) and Flute in *A Midsummer Night's Dream* (Adrian Noble, RST). After the transfer to London in 1995 he succeeded Toby Stephens as Lysander. The following year he travelled with the production to New York.

In 1997 he joined the National to play Neil in Peter Gill's *Cardiff East* (Cottesloe) and the title role in *Peter Pan* (John Caird, Olivier). As a member of Trevor Nunn's 1999 NT Ensemble, he was Patroclus in *Troilus and Cressida* (Nunn, Olivier), Lorenzo in *The Merchant of Venice* (Nunn, Cottesloe), and the title role in *Candide* (Caird, Olivier).

Another singing role, Charley in *Merrily We Roll Along*, directed by Michael Grandage at the Donmar Warehouse, brought him an Olivier award. At the Royal Court, alongside Jo McInnes and Madeleine Potter, he performed Sarah Kane's poetic *4:48 Psychosis* (James Macdonald, 2000, 2001), and appeared in two plays by Christopher Shinn, *Other People* (Dominic Cooke, 2000) and *Where Do We Live* (Richard Wilson, 2002). He toured as Osvald in Ibsen's *Ghosts* (English Touring Theatre, 2002), and was Ariel to Derek Jacobi's Prospero in *The Tempest* at the Sheffield Crucible and the Old Vic (Grandage, 2002-03).

In 2003 he returned to the RSC to play Angelo opposite Emma Fielding in *Measure for Measure* (Sean Holmes, RST) and Posthumous in *Cymbeline* (Cooke, Swan). In 2004, at the Sheffield Crucible and the Donmar Warehouse respectively, he was Betty in Caryl Churchill's *Cloud Nine* (Anna Mackmin) and Kringelein, the dying bookkeeper, in *Grand Hotel* (Grandage).

On television, Evans has played leading roles in Tony Marchant's version of *Great Expectations* (BBC, 1999), *Love in a Cold Climate* (BBC, 2001), and *Daniel Deronda* (BBC, 2002).

F

Lynn Farleigh (b. Bristol, 1942) trained at the Guildhall School. At the beginning of her career she appeared in repertory at Salisbury and Canterbury, and toured with Anna Neagle. She was in James Saunders's *Triangle* at the Close Theatre, Glasgow (1965), and played a telephone receptionist in twenty episodes of *Z Cars* (BBC).

She joined the RSC in 1966, and during that first year toured with Theatregoround (John Barton's *The Battle of Agincourt*) and played Castiza in Trevor Nunn's production of *The Revenger's Tragedy* (RST). Peter Hall cast her in the pivotal role of Ruth for the New York transfer of Harold Pinter's *The Homecoming* (1967). At the Aldwych in 1968 she succeeded Estelle Kohler as Helena in *All's Well That Ends Well* and Elizabeth Spriggs as Portia in *Julius Caesar* (both Barton), and played Amanda opposite her first husband Michael Jayston in *The Relapse* (Nunn). She co-starred in Peter Hall's film *Three Into Two Won't Go* (1969).

Her subsequent RSC work has been separated by long intervals: Monique in Marguerite Duras's *Suzanna Andler* (Howard Sackler, Aldwych, 1973); Mrs Forsythe in Stephen Poliakoff's *Shout Across the River* (Bill Alexander, Warehouse, 1978); Jane in Howard Barker's *The Hang of the Gaol* (Alexander, Warehouse, 1978-79); Elizabeth Proctor in *The Crucible* (Barry Kyle) and Hermione in *The Winter's Tale* (Adrian Noble, Small-scale Tour, 1984); Agatha in *The Family Reunion* (Noble, Swan, 1999); and Elizabeth in *The Prince of Homburg* (Neil Bartlett, Swan, 2002).

Lynn Farleigh's work elsewhere has included: *Brand* (Christopher Morahan, NT Olivier, 1978); Simon Gray's *Close of Play* (Harold Pinter, NT Lyttelton, 1979); Kate in *All My Sons* (Gregory Hersov, Royal Exchange Manchester, 1988); Peter Nichols's *Forget Me Not Lane* (Greenwich Theatre, 1990); *Black Angel* (Rob Mulholland, King's Head, 1990); *Coriolanus* (ESC, Tour, 1990); Hermione in *The Winter's Tale* (Bogdanov, ESC, Tour, 1991); the women in John Osborne's *Inadmissible Evidence* (Di Trevis, NT Lyttelton, 1993); *Machinal* (Stephen Daldry, NT Lyttelton, 1993); Mrs Gascoigne in D.H. Lawrence's *The Daughter-in-Law* (Trevis, Theatr Clwyd, 1995); Margaret in *The Wax King*, adapted from Shakespeare's *Henry VI Part 3* (Bruce Wall, London Shakespeare Workout Prison Project, Pentonville Prison chapel, 2003); and Bernarda in García Lorca's *The House of Bernarda Alba* (Auriol Smith, Orange Tree, 2003).

David Farr (b. Guildford, 1969). It was during the 1991 Edinburgh Fringe Festival that David Farr emerged as one of the bright new hopes of the British theatre. Just down from Trinity Hall, Cambridge, with a first in English, Farr arrived in Edinburgh with two devised plays, one performed by his own company, Talking Tongues, the other by the Cambridge Mummers. Talking Tongues' show, *Slight Possession*, a duet for two girls performed on and around stepladders, was raw and erotic (one of the girls was Rachel Weisz). The Mummers' surreal *Glue*

Wedding consisted of silent action performed to music by Murray Gold. The style of both shows was hauntingly oblique.

Stephen Daldry invited Talking Tongues to perform *Slight Possession*, along with another short piece called *The Detour*, at the Gate in London (1992). Weisz left to make a television series, but Farr kept the company going for another year, devising and directing *Hove* (NT Cottesloe, 1993) and *Liars, Fakers and People Being Honest* (BAC, 1993). He continued to work at the Gate, first as an associate and then (from 1995) as artistic director: Botho Strauss's *Seven Doors* (1992); Strindberg's *The Great Highway* (1993); Gil Vicente's *The Boat Plays* (1994 — the auditorium was transformed into a wooden boat); Ramón del Valle-Inclán's *Silverface* and *Ballad of Wolves* (1995); Stig Larsson's *Sisters, Brothers* (1996); Voltaire's *Candide* (1997); and Büchner's *Danton's Death* (1997).

Farr's plays of the 1990s were *Max Klapper: a Life in Pictures* (Electric Cinema, 1996); the humane and humorous *Elton John's Glasses* (Terry Johnson, Palace Theatre, Watford, 1997); *The Nativity* (Young Vic, 1999-00); and a modern, east London retelling of Dostoyevsky, *Crime and Punishment in Dalston* (Arcola Theatre, 2002). In 2001 he worked at the RSC for the first time, directing Jody Watson in his own dramatic monologue *The Thoughts of Joan of Arc on the English as She Burns at the Stake* (Young Vic, 2001). This was followed by *Night of the Soul* — a businessman staying in a modern hotel encounters the ghost of a young woman, a plague victim (Farr directed Tom Mannion and Zoë Waites, Pit, 2002); a stylish Kurosawa-inspired *Coriolanus* (Swan and Small-scale Tour, 2003-04); and a modern dress *Julius Caesar* (Swan and Small-scale Tour, 2004-05).

Shakespeare has become a passion. As joint Artistic Director of the Bristol Old Vic (2003-05), he directed first-rate productions of *A Midsummer Night's Dream* (2003), *The Comedy of Errors* (2003) and *Twelfth Night* (2004), as well as his own versions of *Paradise Lost* (2004) and *The Odyssey* (2005). He succeeded Neil Bartlett at the Lyric Hammersmith in 2005, and returned to the RSC as an associate director in 2009.

Farrah (1926-2005, b. Ksar El Bokhari, Algeria). Abd'Elkader Farrah studied in Paris and established his reputation working for Michel Saint-Denis. He was Saint-Denis's head of design at the Centre National Dramatique de l'Est (Strasbourg) from 1952 and went with him to the RSC in 1961 to design *The Cherry Orchard*. The Algerian War was at its height and Farrah's RSC contract enabled him to settle in England at a time when life in France was difficult. He would remain an associate artist of the Company until his retirement thirty years later.

Farrah loved the height and depth of the Stratford stage, always thought in three dimensions, loved emptiness, swathes of light and the abstraction of pure colour. His great partnership with Terry Hands in the 1970s and 80s brought this highly distinctive style of stagecraft to the fore: *Richard III* (RST, 1970); *The Balcony* (Aldwych, 1971); *Murder in the Cathedral* (Aldwych, 1972); *Romeo and Juliet* (RST, 1973); *The Bewitched* (Aldwych, 1974); *Henry IV* (RST, 1975); *Henry V* (RST, 1975); *Henry VI* (RST, 1977); *Coriolanus* (RST, 1977); *As You Like It* (RST, 1980); *Richard II* (RST, 1980); *Richard III* (RST, 1980); *Troilus and Cressida* (Aldwych, 1981); *Poppy* (Barbican, 1982); *Red Noses* (Barbican, 1985); *Julius Caesar* (RST, 1987); *The Balcony* (Barbican, 1987); and *Romeo and Juliet* (Swan, 1989).

Mia Farrow (b. Los Angeles, 1945). The daughter of the Australian movie director John Farrow and the Irish actress Maureen O'Sullivan, Mia Farrow was brought up in the Hollywood of the 1940s and 50s. At the age of nine she contracted polio and entered the public's consciousness.

She was still a teenager when her father gave her a small part in *John Paul Jones* (1959). She appeared in *The Importance of Being Earnest* on the New York stage (1963). She made her name in the television soap *Peyton Place* (1964), and became an international celebrity when Frank Sinatra married her.

She travelled to London to replace Britt Ekland in *Guns at Batasi* (1964), a minor British classic starring Richard Attenborough and Jack Hawkins. Her marriage to Sinatra was over by 1968. She was one of the stars who joined the Beatles at the court of the Maharishi Mahesh Yogi in India. She returned to London to play a disturbed character in *Secret Ceremony* (Joseph Losey, 1968). In *Rosemary's Baby* (1969) Roman Polanski made intrusive but compelling use of her fragile beauty.

She played opposite Dustin Hoffman in *John and Mary* (Peter Yates, 1970) and Robert Redford in *The Great Gatsby* (Jack Clayton, 1974). The other films of her twenties and early thirties were *A Dandy in Aspic* (1968); *See No Evil* (Richard Fleischer, 1971); *Follow Me* (Carol Reed, 1972); *Docteur Popaul* (Claude Chabrol, 1972); *Full Circle* (Richard Loncraine, 1976), *Death on the Nile* (1978); *Avalanche* (1978); *A Wedding* (1978); and *Hurricane* (1980).

From 1970 to 79 she was married to André Previn, and it was during this period, when she lived in England (Previn was running the LSO), that she appeared on the English stage. A member of the RSC for two years, she played Ann Leete in Granville-Barker's *The Marrying of Ann Leete* (David Jones, Aldwych, 1975), Pavla in Gorky's *The Zykovs* (Jones, Aldwych, 1976), and Sasha in Chekhov's *Ivanov* (Jones, Aldwych, 1976). She had previously appeared at the Shaw Theatre in *Mary Rose* (1973), and at the Greenwich Theatre in *Three Sisters* and Tom Stoppard's version of García Lorca's *The House of Bernarda Alba* (1974). She subsequently played Titania in *A Midsummer Night's Dream* at the Leicester Haymarket (1976).

From 1982 she was Woody Allen's leading actress and partner, until finally their lives disintegrated into a very public domestic tragedy. She was scrutinised by Allen's camera in thirteen movies: *A Midsummer Night's Sex Comedy* (1982); *Zelig* (1983); *Broadway Danny Rose* (1984); *The Purple Rose of Cairo* (1985); *Hannah and Her Sisters* (1986); *Radio Days* (1987); *September* (1988); *Another Woman* (1989); *New York Stories* (1989); *Crimes and Misdemeanours* (1990); *Alice* (1990); *Husbands and Wives* (1992); and *Shadows and Fog* (1992).

Ray Fearon (b. London, 1967) played tennis at junior level for Great Britain, sponsored by the Greater London Council. When the Thatcher government abolished the GLC he took up acting, appearing with the Brent-based company Alton Kumato's Theatre Troop and the Royal Court Youth Theatre—this led to a small part in Caryl Churchill's *Serious Money* (Max Stafford-Clark, 1987)—before training at Rose Bruford. He left before the end of the course to play Ferdinand in an Oxford Stage Company production of *The Tempest* (International Tour). Among his other early roles were Othello (Liverpool Everyman), and Hugo/Fred in *Ring Round the Moon* (Lilian Baylis).

He joined the RSC in 1993 to play First Knight/First Murderer in *Murder in the Cathedral* (Steven Pimlott, Swan), the Prince of Morocco in *The Merchant of Venice* (David Thacker, RST), and Stubb in *Moby Dick* (Gerry Mulgrew, TOP). After his starring role, as Pierre, in Ian McDiarmid's production of *Venice Preserv'd* at the Almeida (1995), Fearon returned to the RSC to play Brachiano—callous virility in action—in Webster's *The White Devil* (Gale Edwards, Swan) and Paris in *Troilus and Cressida* (Ian Judge, RST, 1996). His Romeo (Michael Attenborough, Pit, 1997) and Othello (Attenborough, RST, 1999) were the most powerful in years. Alongside Othello he played Posa in Schiller's *Don Carlos* (Edwards, TOP). His beautifully spoken and subtly shaded performance as Pericles in Adrian Noble's production at the Roundhouse (2002) confirmed his growing reputation as one of the best Shakespearean actors of his generation.

Since Pericles Fearon has played Oberon/Theseus in *A Midsummer Night's Dream* at the Sheffield Crucible (Michael Grandage, 2003); Kiyabe in Steve Waters's *World Music* at the Donmar Warehouse (Josie Rourke, 2004); Mark in Roy Williams's *Sing Yer Heart Out for the Lads* at the National (Paul Miller, Cottesloe, 2004); a regular role in *Coronation Street* (ITV,

2005-06); himself in *Strictly Come Dancing* (BBC, 2006); and Beaugard in Thomas Otway's *The Soldiers' Fortune* at the Young Vic (David Lan, 2007).

Michael Feast (b. Brighton, 1946). The young Michael Feast played Woof in the London production of *Hair* (Tom O'Horgan, Shaftesbury, 1968) and looked destined for a career in the musical theatre. But he was too good and too charismatic an actor. At the National Peter Hall cast him as an androgynous, flying Ariel to Gielgud's Prospero in *The Tempest* (1974), and as the enigmatic Foster in Harold Pinter's *No Man's Land* (1975). Also on the South Bank, he was Raymond in John Osborne's *Watch It Come Down* (Bill Bryden, Lyttelton, 1976); Bobby in David Mamet's *American Buffalo* (Bryden, Cottesloe, 1978); and Mayhew in *Dispatches* (Bryden, Cottesloe, 1979).

Feast's other stage appearances during the 1970s and 80s included, at the Manchester Royal Exchange, Nicholas in *What the Butler Saw* (Braham Murray, 1976), Henry in Thornton Wilder's *The Skin of Our Teeth* (Richard Negri/James Maxwell, 1977), Telegin in *Uncle Vanya* (Michael Elliott, 1977), Roland in *Present Laughter* (Maxwell, 1977), Billy Bigelow in *Carousel* (Steven Pimlott, 1984), and Subtle in *The Alchemist* (Gregory Hersov, 1987); at the Royal Court, Joe Conran in Ann Devlin's *Ourselves Alone* (1985), the Card Player in Mamet's *Prairie du Chien* (1986), and John in Mamet's *The Shawl* (1986); and at the Almeida, Verkhovensky in Dostoevsky's *The Possessed* (Yuri Lyubimov, 1985).

At the RSC in the 1990s he played Becket in *Murder in the Cathedral* (Steven Pimlott, Swan, 1993), the Duke in *Measure for Measure* (Pimlott, RST, 1994) and the title role in *Faust* (Michael Bogdanov, Swan, 1995)—gaunt and fanatical, three variations on a theme. Since leaving the Company he has played Ian/Fitzroy in Timberlake Wertenbaker's *After Darwin* (Hampstead Theatre, 1998); Neschastlivtsev in *The Forest* (Anthony Page, NT Lyttelton, 1999); the title role in *The Servant* (Neil Bartlett, Lyric Hammersmith, 2001); four parts for Steven Pimlott at

Chichester 2003/04—Dorn in *The Seagull*, Nathan in *Nathan the Wise*, the Devil in Mikhail Bulgakov's *The Master and Margarita*, Mephistopheles in Marlowe's *Doctor Faustus*; and Chichester 2007—a manic if musically melancholy Feste in *Twelfth Night* (Philip Franks). On screen, he created compelling characters in Stephen Poliakoff's *The Tribe* (BBC, 1998), Paul Greengrass's *The Murder of Stephen Lawrence* (ITV, 1999), and Paul Abbott's *State of Play* (BBC, 2003).

Emma Fielding (b. Yorkshire, 1966) abandoned a law degree at Cambridge to study acting at the Royal Scottish Academy of Music and Drama, a decision vindicated by her performances at the National, the Almeida and the RSC. The daughter of a soldier, much of her childhood was spent abroad in Malaya and Nigeria. Before she became an actress she worked briefly as an usherette at the Oxford Apollo.

Slight and dark-eyed, with an expressive, instantly recognisable voice, she was the heroine of the thriller *Tell-Tale Hearts* (Thaddeus O'Sullivan, BBC, 1992); the first Thomasina in Tom Stoppard's *Arcadia* (Trevor Nunn, NT Lyttelton, 1993); a fresh and moving Agnes in *The School for Wives* (Jonathan Kent, Almeida, 1994); and, at the RSC (1994/95), a perfect Viola in an otherwise bland *Twelfth Night* (Ian Judge, RST), a touching Hermia to Toby Stephens's Lysander in *A Midsummer Night's Dream* (Adrian Noble, RST), and the doomed Penthea, giving up on Iain Glen and life, in John Ford's *The Broken Heart* (Michael Boyd, Swan). She won the Ian Charleson Award for *The School for Wives*, the London Critics' Circle Most Promising Newcomer Award for *Arcadia*, and the Dame Peggy Ashcroft Best Actress Award for her RSC work.

She returned to the Almeida to play Ira in Craig Raine's *1953* (Patrick Marber, 1995), and Ellie Dunn in *Heartbreak House* (David Hare, 1997). Increasingly in demand on television, she starred in *Kavanagh* (ITV, 1995); *Drovers' Gold* (Lesley Manning/Tristram Powell, BBC, 1997); *A Dance to the Music of Time*

(Channel Four, 1997); *A Respectable Trade* (Suri Krishnamma, BBC, 1998); *Big Bad World* (ITV, 1999); *Other People's Children* (BBC, 2000); *Green-Eyed Monster* (2001); *Birthday Girl* (ITV, 2002); and *My Uncle Silas* (ITV, 2003).

She remains first and foremost a theatre actress: Lady Teazle—Irish accent, frizzy blonde wig, lightly powdered skin—in the RSC's *The School for Scandal* (Declan Donnellan, RST, 1998); an academic in Rebecca Gilman's *Spinning into Butter* (Dominic Cooke, Royal Court, 2001); Sybil in *Private Lives* (Howard Davies, Albery, 2001); the RSC's 2003 Stratford season—Isabella in *Measure for Measure* (Sean Holmes, RST) and Imogen in *Cymbeline* (Cooke, Swan); and Lady Macbeth opposite Simon Russell Beale in *Macbeth* (John Caird, Almeida, 2005).

Joseph Fiennes (b. Salisbury, 1970). The younger brother of Ralph Fiennes, Joseph Fiennes has followed a similar path, moving from the RSC to leading roles in major films. He was a member of the Young Vic Youth Theatre, and worked backstage at the National as a dresser before going to the Guildhall School. He made an impression in his first productions: *The Woman in Black* (Fortune, 1993); Belyaev in *A Month in the Country* (Bill Bryden, Albery, 1994); and Rodolpho in *A View from the Bridge* (David Thacker, Bristol Old Vic, 1995). On television he starred opposite Tara Fitzgerald in *The Vacillations of Poppy Carew* (James Cellan Jones, 1995). His first films were Bertolucci's *Stealing Beauty* (1996) and *Martha—Meet Frank, Daniel and Laurence* (Nick Hamm, 1998).

He joined the RSC in London in 1995 to play a young, charismatic Jesus in Dennis Potter's *Son of Man* (Bryden, Pit). He was in Simon Callow's disastrous *Les enfants du paradis* (Barbican, 1996), playing Lacenaire, before moving to Stratford for Silvius in *As You Like It* (Steven Pimlott, RST), Rafe Smith opposite Teresa Banham in Peter Whelan's *The Herbal Bed* (Michael Attenborough, TOP), and Troilus opposite Victoria Hamilton in *Troilus and Cressida* (Ian Judge, RST).

The roles that made his name in the cinema—Robert Dudley opposite Cate Blanchett in *Elizabeth I* (Shekhar Kapur, 1998) and Shakespeare opposite Gwyneth Paltrow in *Shakespeare in Love* (John Madden, 1998)—were a natural continuation of this theatre work.

Fiennes returns to the stage at intervals: the title role in *Edward II* (Michael Grandage, Sheffield Crucible, 2001); Berowne in Trevor Nunn's *Love's Labour's Lost* (NT Olivier, 2003); Dillon in John Osborne's *Epitaph for George Dillon* (Peter Gill, Comedy, 2005).

Ralph Fiennes (b. Suffolk, 1962) trained at RADA, along with Imogen Stubbs, Iain Glen and Jane Horrocks, and gained his early experience in provincial repertory—*Night and Day, See How They Run* (Theatr Clwyd), *Me Mam Sez, Don Quixote* and *Cloud Nine* (Oldham). He came to notice playing Romeo opposite Sarah Woodward in *Romeo and Juliet* (Declan Donnellan) and Lysander in *A Midsummer Night's Dream* at the Open Air Theatre, Regent's Park (1985). At the National in 1987 he played The Son in *Six Characters in Search of an Author* (Olivier), Arkady in *Fathers and Sons* (Lyttelton) and Lisha Ball in Nick Darke's *Ting Tang Mine* (Cottesloe), all directed by Michael Rudman.

He joined the RSC in 1988. In his first season he played Claudio in *Much Ado About Nothing* (Di Travis, RST); Lewis the Dauphin in Deborah Warner's studio version of *King John* (TOP); a grave and edgy Henry VI in Adrian Noble's *The Plantagenets* (RST); Bert in *The Man Who Came To Dinner* (Gene Saks, Barbican); and Gant in Stephen Poliakoff's *Playing With Trains* (Ron Daniels, Pit). A member of Terry Hands's last company (1990/91) he was outstanding as Troilus in *Troilus and Cressida* (Sam Mendes, Swan), as a stylish Edmund in *King Lear* (Nicholas Hytner, RST), and as Berowne in *Love's Labour's Lost* (Terry Hands, RST). Few of Fiennes's contemporaries speak Shakespeare's verse with such assurance.

On the screen, the early 1990s saw him playing T.E. Lawrence in the made-for-television *Dangerous Man* (1990); Heathcliff to Juliette Binoche's Cathy in a disappointing version of *Wuthering Heights* (Peter Kosminsky, 1992); the Bishop's Son in Peter Greenaway's *Baby of Mâcon* (1993); and Amon Goeth in *Schindler's List* (Steven Spielberg, 1993)—Fiennes's remarkable performance brought an Oscar nomination and international fame.

He followed *Schindler's List* with two very different American films, *Quiz Show* (Robert Redford, 1994) and Kathryn Bigolow's thriller *Strange Days* (1995). He then returned to the stage to play a Broadway-bound Hamlet, an interpretation of verve and intelligence let down by Jonathan Kent's truncated production (Almeida Company, Hackney Empire, 1995). His performance as Almásy in Anthony Minghella's *The English Patient* (1996) revealed a style of enigmatic reserve. His serious approach to acting has made him seem, to the press, as moody in real life as in the flashback scenes of *The English Patient*. Since this film he has sought to extend his screen persona: the red-headed oddball opposite Cate Blanchett in *Oscar and Lucinda* (Gillian Armstrong, 1997); Steed in *The Avengers* (Jeremiah Chechik, 1998); the title role in *Onegin* (Martha Fiennes, 1999); *Sunshine* (István Szabó, 1999); Bendrix opposite Julianne Moore in *The End of the Affair* (Neil Jordan, 1999); the title role in *Spider* (David Cronenberg, 2002); the serial killer in *Red Dragon* (2002); *The Good Thief* (Jordan, 2002); exuding old Hollywood charm opposite Jennifer Lopez in *Maid in Manhattan* (Wayne Wang, 2002); Justin Quayle in John le Carré's *The Constant Gardener* (Fernando Meirelles, 2005); *The White Countess* (James Ivory, 2005); *Chromophobia* (Martha Fiennes, 2005); Lord Voldemort in *Harry Potter and the Goblet of Fire* (Mike Newell, 2005); *Land of the Blind* (2006); *Harry Potter and the Order of the Phoenix* (David Yates, 2007); *Bernard and Doris* (2007); the crime boss in *In Bruges* (Martin McDonagh, 2008).

Fiennes remains committed to the theatre. He worked at the Almeida during the 1990s and has since returned to the national companies: the title role in *Ivanov* (Jonathan Kent, Almeida, 1997); the title roles in *Richard II* and *Coriolanus* (Kent, Almeida at the Gainsborough Film Studios, Shoreditch, 2000); Jung in Christopher Hampton's *The Talking Cure* (Howard Davies, NT Cottesloe, 2002-03); the title role in Ibsen's *Brand* (Adrian Noble, RSC Swan, 2003); Mark Antony in *Julius Caesar* (Deborah Warner, Barbican, 2005); Frank Hardy in Brian Friel's *Faith Healer* (Kent, Gate, Dublin, 2006); Alain in Yasmina Reza's *God of Carnage* (Matthew Warchus, Gielgud, 2008); and the title role in *Oedipus* (Kent, NT Olivier, 2008).

Susan Fleetwood (1944-1995) was born in St Andrews, where her father, an officer in the RAF, was temporarily stationed. An unorthodox and unsettling childhood—among the ports of call were Egypt and Norway—gave her a rich experience but a fragmentary primary education. Returning to England the family set up residence on a Thames barge. Fleetwood attended a convent school.

At the age of sixteen she won a scholarship to RADA. She led a RADA tour to Arizona, playing Rosalind in *As You Like It* and Lady Macbeth in *Macbeth* (1964), and received the Bancroft Gold Medal. She also met Terry Hands, who played opposite her as Orlando. After RADA she was one of the actors who went with Hands to form the Liverpool Everyman (1964). At the Everyman, between 1965 and 67, she played Lady Percy in *Henry IV*; Gwendolen in *The Importance of Being Earnest*; Alison in *Look Back in Anger*; Liz in *Fando and Liz*; Margaret in *The Great God Brown*; Chorus Leader in *Murder in the Cathedral*; the Woman in *The Four Seasons*; and Lady Macbeth in *Macbeth*.

When Hands went to the RSC Fleetwood followed. She was only in her early twenties but as a classical actress she had remarkable maturity. She first made a bold impression as a very young Regan in *King Lear* (Trevor Nunn, RST, 1968), and confirmed her promise as Marina and Thaisa in *Pericles* (Hands, RST, 1969), Portia, succeeding Judi Dench, in *The Merchant of*

Venice (Hands, Aldwych, 1972), Kate to Alan Bates's Petruchio in *The Taming of the Shrew* (Clifford Williams, RST, 1973), and Imogen in *Cymbeline* (Barton/Williams, RST, 1974). Her other RSC roles to 1975 were: Amanda in *The Relapse* (Trevor Nunn, Aldwych, 1967); Beba in *Criminals* (Terry Hands, Aldwych, 1967); Audrey, succeeding Frances de la Tour, in *As You Like It* (David Jones, RST, 1968); Cassandra in *Troilus and Cressida* (John Barton, RST, 1968); Margaret in *Much Ado About Nothing* (Nunn, RST, 1968); Isabella in *Women Beware Women* (Hands, RST, 1969); Julia in *Two Gentlemen of Verona* (Gareth Morgan, Theatregoround, 1969); Chorus Leader in *Murder in the Cathedral* (Hands, Aldwych, 1972); the Bondwoman in *The Island of the Mighty* (Jones, Aldwych, 1972); Princess of France in *Love's Labour's Lost* (Jones, RST, 1973); Kaleria in *Summerfolk* (Jones, Aldwych, 1974); and Bertha in Strindberg's *Comrades* (Kyle, The Place, 1974).

When, in 1973, Peter Hall offered Susan Fleetwood the role of Barbara in John Hopkins's *Next of Kin* at the National, Trevor Nunn and John Barton reacted badly (see *Peter Hall's Diaries*) — but this had more to do with the turmoil caused by Hall's move to the opposition than with the actress, who found her own compromise, remaining with the Company for another two years and then joining the National to play Pegeen Mike in *Playboy of the Western World* (Bill Bryden, Old Vic, 1975); Ophelia in the Albert Finney *Hamlet* (Hall, Old Vic, 1975); Jo in John Osborne's *Watch it Come Down* (Bryden, Old Vic, 1976); Zenocrate in *Tamburlaine the Great* (Hall, Olivier, 1976); Nora in *The Plough and the Stars* (Bryden, Olivier, 1977); Clare in John Mackendrick's *Lavender Blue* (Sebastian Graham-Jones, Cottesloe, 1977); Varya in *The Cherry Orchard* (Hall, Olivier, 1978); and Ismene in Edward Bond's *The Woman* (Bond, Olivier, 1978).

She returned to the RSC for the 1980/81 cycle and gave one of her finest performances as Rosalind in *As You Like It* (Hands, RST). She also performed *Pleasure and Repentance* (Hands, Fortune, 1981), and played the Wife in *La Ronde* (Barton, Aldwych, 1982). Then, back on the South Bank, she was June Taylor in

Way Upstream (Alan Ayckbourn, Lyttelton, 1982), Titania in *A Midsummer Night's Dream* (Bryden, Cottesloe, 1982), and Laura in Osborne's version of Strindberg's *The Father* (David Leveaux, Cottesloe, 1988).

Her final seasons with the RSC were the last Terry Hands planned as artistic director. She played Beatrice in *Much Ado About Nothing* (Alexander, RST, 1990), Madame Arkadina in *The Seagull* (Hands, Swan, 1990), and Ella in *Curse of the Starving Class* (Robin Lefevre, Pit, 1991). Unbeknown to almost everyone, she was fighting cancer.

Susan Fleetwood played important supporting roles in the films *Heat and Dust* (James Ivory, 1982); *The Sacrifice* (Andrei Tarkovsky, 1986); *White Mischief* (Michael Radford, 1987); and *The Krays* (Peter Medak, 1990). On television she appeared in *The Good Soldier* (ITV, 1981); John Mortimer's *Summer's Lease* (BBC, 1989); *The Buddha of Suburbia* (Roger Michell, BBC, 1993); *Chandler and Co* (BBC, 1994); and *Persuasion* (Michell, BBC, 1995).

Oliver Ford Davies (b. 1939) was a leading member of the Oxford University Dramatic Society while studying at Merton College—he played Falstaff in *Henry IV* (Peter Dew, 1962) and the title role in *Othello* (1963)—but on graduating he initially pursued a career as an academic historian (and part-time dramatist). He has acted (and occasionally directed) professionally since 1967. Early roles included John of Gaunt in *Richard II* (Birmingham Rep, 1967); the Bishop of Caerleon in *Hadrian VII* (Mermaid, 1968); Colonel Pickering in *Pygmalion* (Birmingham Rep, 1970); Friar Laurence in *Romeo and Juliet* (Oxford Playhouse, 1972); and Horatio in *Hamlet* (Cambridge Theatre Company, 1973).

From 1975 to 1986 he was a popular player at the RSC. His ability to give life to supporting roles was particularly evident in Terry Hands's productions of the Histories (RST, 1975-77)— Montjoy in *Henry V*; Sir Michael etc. in *Henry IV*; Somerset in *Henry VI*. Also: Earl of Huntly in John Ford's *Perkin Warbeck*

(Barry Kyle, TOP, 1975); Duke Senior in *As You Like It* (Trevor Nunn, RST, 1977); Junius Brutus in *Coriolanus* (Hands, RST, 1977); Boyet, succeeding Alan Rickman, in *Love's Labour's Lost* (John Barton, Aldwych, 1979); Priam/Polymestor/Peleus in *The Greeks* (Barton, Aldwych, 1980); Milonov in Alexander Ostrovsky's *The Forest* (Adrian Noble, TOP, 1981); Nestor in *Troilus and Cressida* (Hands, Aldwych, 1981); Mulligan in Sean O'Casey's *The Shadow of a Gunman* (Michael Bogdanov, Warehouse, 1981); the doctor in Alexander Solzhenitsyn's *The Love-Girl and the Innocent* (Clifford Williams, Aldwych, 1981); Senator in *Timon of Athens* (Daniels, Warehouse, 1981); Marullus/Titinius in *Julius Caesar* (Ron Daniels, RST, 1983); Gardiner in *Henry VIII* (Howard Davies, RST, 1983); Provost in *Measure for Measure* (Noble, RST, 1983); Jean D'Armagnac in John Whiting's *The Devils* (Barton, Pit, 1984); Gilbert Wedgecroft in Granville-Barker's *Waste* (Barton, Pit, 1985); Scaramuré in Giordano Bruno's *Il Candelaio* (Williams, Pit, 1986); Fouquier-Tinville in Pam Gems's *The Danton Affair* (Daniels, Barbican, 1986); and Norton Quinn in Richard Nelson's *Principia Scriptoriae* (David Jones, Pit, 1986).

Oliver Ford Davies's career has been based around an ability to play figures of minor authority—he looks and sounds instantly right as a cleric, lawyer, civil servant or schoolmaster. His Olivier Award winning performance in David Hare's *Racing Demon* at the National (Eyre, Cottesloe, 1990) is the best example. Other work on the South Bank: *The Saughraun* (Howard Davies, Olivier, 1989); Player King in the Daniel Day-Lewis *Hamlet* (Richard Eyre, Olivier, 1989); David Edgar's *The Shape of the Table* (Jenny Killick, Cottesloe, 1990); the David Hare Trilogy—*Racing Demon*, *Murmuring Judges* and *The Absence of War* (Eyre, Olivier, 1993); the Cardinal Inquisitor in Bertolt Brecht's *The Life of Galileo* (Davies, Olivier); and the Inquisitor in Bernard Shaw's *Saint Joan* (Marianne Elliot, Olivier, 2007).

In the late 1990s he joined the Almeida for two high-profile productions directed by Jonathan Kent—the Ralph Fiennes *Ivanov* (1997) and Luigi Pirandello's *Naked* (1998), in which he played Ludovico Nota to Juliette Binoche's Ersilia. He returned in 2002 to play the title role in *King Lear* (Kent, Almeida at King's Cross). In 2003 he was at his dry, sardonic best as Lamberto Laudisi in Franco Zeffirelli's production of Pirandello's *Absolutely! (Perhaps)* at the Wyndham's, before playing the title role in his own play *King Cromwell* at the Orange Tree (Sam Walters). In 2008 he finally returned to the RSC to play Polonius in *Hamlet* (Gregory Doran, Courtyard).

Philip Franks (b. London). After student roles at Oxford University, including Timon in *Timon of Athens*, Philip Franks played Romeo at Coventry and appeared in Doug Lucie's *Heroes* (New End). For most of the 1980s he worked at the RSC: Lysander in *A Midsummer Night's Dream* (Ron Daniels, RST, 1981); Bassanius in *Titus Andronicus* and Outlaw in *The Two Gentlemen of Verona* (John Barton, RST, 1981); Dumaine in *All's Well That End's Well* (Trevor Nunn, RST, 1981); Prince Humphrey of Gloucester in *Henry IV* (Nunn, Barbican, 1982); Florizel in *The Winter's Tale* (Ronald Eyre, Barbican, 1982); Bertram, succeeding Mike Gwilym, in *All's Well* (Nunn, Barbican, 1982); John in *Peter Pan* (Nunn/John Caird, Barbican, 1982, 1984); Matthew in Jonson's *Every Man in His Humour* (Caird, Swan, 1986); Fielding in Nick Dear's *The Art of Success* (Adrian Noble, TOP, 1986); Gaston in *World's Apart* (Nick Hamm, TOP, 1986); Tikhon in Ostrovsky's *The Storm* (Hamm, Pit, 1987); and, for the 1987 Small-scale Tour, First Merchant in *The Comedy of Errors* (Hamm) and the title role in *Hamlet* (Roger Michell). Elsewhere, he played Octavius Caesar in *Antony and Cleopatra* (Robin Phillips, Chichester, 1985), and Claudio in the Alan Bates/Felicity Kendall *Much Ado About Nothing* (Elijah Moshinsky, Strand Theatre, 1989).

During the 1990s Franks acted in popular television productions—most prominently *The Darling Buds of May* (ITV) and *Heartbeat* (ITV), but also *The Buddha of Suburbia* (Roger Michell, BBC, 1993), and *Martin Chuzzlewit* (BBC, 1995). Since his return to live performing he has played Lloyd Dallas in Michael

Frayn's *Noises Off* (Jeremy Sams, NT Piccadilly, 2003), and Alan Turing in *Breaking the Code* (Philip Wilson, Theatre Royal, Northampton, 2003). He has worked more often on the other side of the footlights, directing Juliet Stevenson and Simon Russell Beale in *The Duchess of Malfi* (Greenwich Theatre, 1995); Michael Maloney and Zoë Waites in an admired *Hamlet* (Greenwich Theatre, 1996); T.S. Eliot's *The Cocktail Party* (Lyceum Theatre Company, Edinburgh Festival, 1997); Juliet Stevenson and Anton Lesser in Noël Coward's *Private Lives* (NT Lyttelton, 1999); Zoë Waites in *The White Devil* (Lyric Hammersmith, 2000); and Patrick Stewart in *Twelfth Night* (Chichester, 2007).

Paul Freeman (b. Barnet, Hertfordshire, 1943) has had an unusual international career. Although he began in the politicised fringe theatre of the 1970s, for some years he has excelled at providing American film producers with their idea of a suave European villain. He was especially convincing as Rene Belloq, Indiana Jones's rival, in Spielberg's *Raiders of the Lost Ark* (1981). Other American assignments were less rewarding: they included *Shanghai Surprise* (Jim Goddard, 1986), and appearances in *Cagney and Lacey*, *Perry Mason* and the soap *Falcon Crest* (1984-85). He had a prime part as the villain in *Mighty Morphin Power Rangers* (1995), a box-office success, but was totally hidden by the make-up. Despite working in America, and occasionally on the continent—he turns up at the end of *Le hussard sur le toit* (Jean-Paul Rappeneau, 1995) in a non-speaking part—Freeman has never abandoned the English stage. In 1997 he committed himself to a full RSC season.

He broke into professional acting relatively late, having worked in advertising and teaching. He appeared in provincial repertory and at the Royal Court (Jim Sharman's production of Sam Shepard's *Tooth of Crime*, 1974). He first came to notice as a founding member of the radical fringe company Joint Stock, appearing in the premiere productions of David Hare's *Fanshen*

(1975) and Howard Brenton's *Epsom Downs* (1977). When Hare went to the National to stage his play *Plenty* (Lyttelton, 1978) he cast Freeman as the enigmatic agent Lazar. Also at the National Freeman played The Man in Edward Bond's *The Woman* (Bond, Olivier, 1978) and Limber in Middleton and Rowley's *A Fair Quarrel* (William Gaskill, Olivier, 1979). For the Oxford Playhouse Company he played the lead role in Howard Barker's *No End of Blame* (Nicolas Kent, 1981).

It was therefore from a springboard of left-wing new drama that Freeman leapt into commercial movies as a character player. During gaps between films he returned to the stage to play both classical and modern roles: Jabe Torrance in Peter Hall's production of *Orpheus Descending* (Theatre Royal Haymarket, 1988); Oberon in *A Midsummer Night's Dream* and Claudius in *Hamlet* (Regent's Park, 1994); Alec in *The Cutting* (Dominic Dromgoole, Bush, 1992); Geraldo in *Death and the Maiden* (Lindsay Posner, Duke of York's, 1992); Prospero in *The Tempest* (Ron Daniels, American Repertory Theatre, 1995); and *Art* (Matthew Warchus, Wyndham's, 2000).

Freeman first joined the RSC in 1985 to take part in a short season of Howard Barker plays staged in the Pit. He played Toplis in *Crimes in Hot Countries* (Bill Alexander), Krak in *The Castle* (Nick Hamm), and Wilson in *Downchild* (Alexander and Hamm). More than ten years elapsed before he returned, this time to classical roles in Stratford (RST, 1997). He was a splendidly shifty Iachimo—a small neat figure with hawkish eyes and a ponytail—in *Cymbeline* (Adrian Noble), and played Claudius in *Hamlet* (Matthew Warchus) as a smooth politician.

Geoffrey Freshwater. A distinguished character actor, in both classical and new work, Geoffrey Freshwater has been a stalwart of the RSC since 1978. At one extreme he played the sadistic sergeant in Howard Brenton's *The Churchill Play* (Barry Kyle, Barbican, 1988); at the other, Mr Beaver in *The Lion, the Witch and the Wardrobe* (Adrian Noble, RST, 1998). Overall, his contribution has been splendidly diverse: Elbow in *Measure for Measure* (Kyle, RST, 1978); Mr Meterstein in *Once in a Lifetime* (Trevor Nunn, Aldwych, 1979); Borachio in *Much Ado About Nothing* (Terry Hands, Barbican, 1983); Vidocq in Caryl Churchill's *Softcops* (Howard Davies, Pit, 1984); Grumio in *The Taming of the Shrew* and Bill Cracker in *Happy End* (Di Trevis, Small-scale Tour, 1985); Casca in *Julius Caesar* (Hands, RST, 1987); Gratiano in *The Merchant of Venice* (Bill Alexander, RST, 1987); Lavache in *All's Well That Ends Well* (Kyle, RST, 1989); Techelles in *Tamburlaine the Great* (Hands, Swan, 1992); Lollio in *The Changeling* (Michael Attenborough, Swan, 1992); Lenin in Tom Stoppard's *Travesties* (Adrian Noble, Barbican, 1993); Ragueneau in *Cyrano de Bergerac* (Gregory Doran, Swan, 1997); Camillo in *The Winter's Tale* (Doran, RST, 1998); Philip of France in *King John* (Doran, Swan, 2001); Ben Jonson in Peter Barnes's *Jubilee* (Doran, Swan, 2001); the 'Jacobethans' ensemble (Swan, 2002)—Touchstone in *Eastward Ho!* (Lucy Pitman-Wallace), Sura in *The Roman Actor* (Sean Holmes), the unknowing fool Bilioso (stained white uniform; ill-fitting toupee) in *The Malcontent* (Dominic Cooke, Swan, 2002); the 'Gunpowder' ensemble (Swan, 2005)—Sir Robert Cholmley/Erasmus in *Thomas Moore* (Robert Delamere), Creon in Middleton and Rowley's *A New Way to Please You* (Sean Holmes), Silius in Jonson's *Sejanus: His Fall* (Doran); and the Histories (Michael Boyd, Courtyard, 2006-08)—Winchester/Cardinal Beaufort in *Henry VI*, Scrivenor in *Richard III* (Boyd) and Shallow in *Henry IV*.

G

Mariah Gale (b. London) was educated at Birmingham University and the Guildhall School of Music and Drama. The RSC's most promising young actress of the last few years, she was a haunted Ophelia in *Hamlet* and the Princess of France in *Love's Labour's Lost* at the Courtyard (Gregory Doran, 2008) having previously played Octavia in *Antony and Cleopatra* (Doran, Swan), Portia in *Julius Caesar* (Sean Holmes, RST) and Miranda in *The Tempest* (Rupert Goold, RST) during the Complete Works season (2006).

Her earlier work included Emily in Phil Porter's *Stealing Sweets and Punching People* (Crispin Bonham-Carter, Latchmere, 2003); *The Lost Child* (Andy Brereton, Minerva, Chichester, 2003-04); Hero in *Much Ado About Nothing* (Tamara Harvey, Globe, 2004); Anna in James MacMillan's music-theatre piece *Parthenogenesis* (Guildhall School, 2005); 'The Last Waltz' season—Klara in Frank Wedekind's *Musik* (Deborah Bruce) and the nurse in Arthur Schnitzler's *Professor Bernhardi* (Mark Rosenblatt, Dumbfounded/Oxford Stage Company, Arcola Theatre, 2005); Viola in *Twelfth Night* (Timothy Sheader, Regent's Park, 2005); and Annabella in *'Tis Pity She's a Whore* (Edward Dick, Southwark Playhouse, 2005). She received the Ian Charleson Award for Viola, Annabella and The Last Waltz season.

Michael Gambon (b. Dublin, 1940). An untypical leading actor, who started in the theatre after a long apprenticeship in engineering, Michael Gambon was christened 'the great Gambon' by Ralph Richardson—the tough authenticity of his presence comes, in part, from a working-class background, but he is a subtle artist in plays that range from Shakespeare to Ayckbourn, able to express the inner life of a character without revealing the technique. Puffy-faced, often melancholic, he is a master of morose modern comedy.

He began his career with the Edwards/MácLiammoir Company in Dublin, playing the Second Gentleman in *Othello* (Gaiety and European Tour, 1962). He was still working in a factory in Islington when, later that year, he successfully auditioned to join the first National Theatre ensemble at the Old Vic: *Hamlet* (Olivier, 1963); *Saint Joan* (John Dexter, 1963); Coster Pearmain in *The Recruiting Officer* (William Gaskill, 1963); Max Frisch's *Andorra* (Lindsay Anderson, 1964); *Philoctetes* (Gaskill,

1964); *Othello* (Dexter, 1964); Diego in *The Royal Hunt of the Sun* (Dexter, 1964); Herrick in *The Crucible* (Olivier, 1965); Eilif in *Mother Courage* (Gaskill, 1965); Snap in *Love for Love* (Peter Wood, 1965); *Juno and the Paycock* (Olivier, 1966); and *The Storm* (Dexter, 1966).

Gambon left the National to star on regional stages: the title role in *Othello*, Patrick in *The Doctor's Dilemma*, Cauchon in *Saint Joan* and The Button Moulder in *Peer Gynt* at the Birmingham Rep (1967-68); the title role in *Macbeth* at the Forum Theatre, Billingham (1968); Andrew in David Storey's *In Celebration* and the title role in *Coriolanus* at the Liverpool Playhouse (1969). He broke into the front rank as Tom in Alan Ayckbourn's *The Norman Conquests* (Greenwich, 1974), Simon in Simon Gray's *Otherwise Engaged* (Queen's, 1976) and Neil in Ayckbourn's *Just Between Ourselves* (Queen's, 1977).

Gambon rejoined the National in 1978. Pinter, Ayckbourn and Shakespeare have been his constant companions: Jerry in Pinter's *Betrayal* (Peter Hall, Lyttelton, 1978); Henry in Gray's *Close of Play* (Harold Pinter, Lyttelton, 1979); Buckingham in *Richard III* (Christopher Morahan, Olivier, 1979); Roderigo in *Othello* (Hall, Olivier, 1980); Ayckbourn's *Sisterly Feelings* (Morahan, Olivier, 1980); Galileo, a great triumph, in Brecht's *The Life of Galileo* (John Dexter, Olivier, 1980); Benedick to Penelope Wilton's Beatrice in *Much Ado About Nothing* (Peter Gill, Olivier, 1981); Horváth in Christopher Hampton's *Tales From Hollywood* (Gill, Olivier, 1983); Dafydd in Ayckbourn's *A Chorus of Disapproval* (Ayckbourn, Olivier, 1985); Sprules, the butler, in *Tons of Money* (Ayckbourn, Lyttelton, 1986); Eddie in *A View from the Bridge* (Ayckbourn, Cottesloe, 1987); Jack in Ayckbourn's *A Small Family Business* (Ayckbourn, Olivier, 1987); Sergeant in Pinter's *Mountain Language* (Pinter, Lyttelton, 1988); Tom in *Skylight* (Richard Eyre, Cottesloe, 1995); the title role in *Volpone* (Matthew Warchus, Olivier, 1995); and Falstaff in both parts of *Henry IV* (Hytner, Olivier, 2005).

He first appeared with the RSC in London in 1970: Hotspur/Warwick/Ralph/Fluellen in John Barton's *When Thou Art*

King (Theatregoround, Roundhouse); Charles Lomax in *Major Barbara* (Clifford Williams, Aldwych); and Surrey, succeeding John Forgeham, in *Henry VIII* (Trevor Nunn, Aldwych). Returning in 1982/83 he gave powerful performances as Lear, ferocious but movingly perplexed, in *King Lear* (Adrian Noble, RST), and Antony opposite Helen Mirren in *Antony and Cleopatra* (Noble, TOP). His one subsequent RSC play was Yasmina Reza's *The Unexpected Man* (Matthew Warchus, Pit, 1998).

Elsewhere: Deeley in Pinter's *Old Times* (Theatre Royal Haymarket, 1985); the title role in *Uncle Vanya* (Michael Blakemore, Vaudeville, 1988); Douglas in Ayckbourn's *Man of the Moment* (Globe, 1990); the title role in *Othello* (Ayckbourn, Scarborough, 1990); Shank in Nicholas Wright's *Cressida* (Nicholas Hytner, Almeida, 2000); Davies in Pinter's *The Caretaker* (Patrick Marber, Comedy, 2000); Salter in Caryl Churchill's *A Number* (Stephen Daldry, Royal Court, 2002); Hamm in Samuel Beckett's *Endgame* (Matthew Warchus, Albery, 2004); and, at the Gate, Dublin, the title role in Beckett's *Eh Joe* (Atom Egoyan, 2006) and Hirst in Pinter's *No Man's Land* (Rupert Goold, 2008).

Since his extraordinary depiction of pain, rage and fantasy in Dennis Potter's *The Singing Detective* (BBC, 1986) he has appeared regularly on screen, for both British and American producers (he delivers a convincing gangster): *Turtle Diary* (John Irvin, 1985); *The Cook, the Thief, His Wife and Her Lover* (Peter Greenaway, 1989); *The Heat of the Day* (1989); *Paris By Night* (David Hare, 1989); *A Dry White Season* (1990); *Mobsters* (1992); *Toys* (1992); *The Browning Version* (Mike Figgis, 1993); *A Man of No Importance* (1994); *Mary Reilly* (Stephen Frears, 1994); *The Wings of the Dove* (Iain Softley, 1997); *The Gambler* (Károly Makk, 1997); *Plunkett and MaCleane* (1998); *Dancing at Lughnasa* (Pat O'Connor, 1998); outstanding as the tobacco company magnate in *The Insider* (Michael Mann, 1999); *Sleepy Hollow* (Tim Burton, 1999); *High Heels and Low Lifes* (Mel Smith, 2001); the patriarch in *Gosford Park* (Robert Altman, 2001); pretending to be French with more skill than his co-stars in *Charlotte Gray* (Gillian Armstrong, 2001); alongside Michael Caine in *The Actors* (Conor

McPherson, 2003); the villain in Kevin Costner's Western *Open Range* (2003); *Sylvia* (2003); succeeding Richard Harris in *Harry Potter and the Prisoner of Azkaban* (Alfonso Cuarón, 2004); *Being Julia* (István Szabó, 2004); *Sky Captain and the World of Tomorrow* (2004); *Layer Cake* (2004); *The Life Aquatic with Steve Zissou* (Wes Anderson, 2004); *Harry Potter and the Goblet of Fire* (Mike Newell, 2005); *Amazing Grace* (Michael Apted, 2006); *The Good Shepherd* (Robert De Niro, 2006); *Harry Potter and the Order of the Phoenix* (David Yates, 2007); *Brideshead Revisited* (Julian Jarrold, 2008).

Television: the title roles in *Oscar* (BBC, 1986) and *Maigret* (ITV, 1992); Squire Hamley in *Wives and Daughters* (BBC, 1999); John Harrison in *Longitude* (Charles Sturridge, 2000); Pinter's *Celebration* (Channel Four, 2006); *Cranford* (BBC, 2007); and three pieces by Stephen Poliakoff, *Perfect Strangers* (BBC, 2001), *The Lost Prince* (BBC, 2003) and *Joe's Palace* (2007).

Romola Garai (b. London, 1982). The daughter of a banker, Romola Garai spent her early childhood in Hong Kong and Singapore. On returning to England the family settled in Wiltshire. While studying for her A levels at the City of London School for Girls Garai won the roles of Young Elizabeth in *The Last of the Blonde Bombshells* (Gillies MacKinnon, BBC, 2000) and Zoë in *Attachments* (BBC, 2000). She read English Literature at London University but was soon in demand as an actress.

Her performance as watchful young Cassandra in *I Capture the Castle* (Tim Fywell, 2003) was pitch-perfect. However, the BBC's adaptation of George Eliot's *Daniel Deronda* (Tom Hooper, 2002) gave a more precise measure of her ability. Moody, conflicted and denied a happy ending, Gwendolen is not a typical 19th century heroine and Garai found the character's complexity: her youthful vulnerability added to the fascination of a story that was half melodrama, half tragedy.

She made her stage debut in 2004, starring movingly as James Joyce's mentally ill daughter in Michael Hastings's *Calico* at the Duke of York's. Three years later she joined the RSC to play Cordelia in *King Lear* and Nina in *The Seagull*, both directed by Trevor Nunn at the Courtyard. Her enigmatic Nina began as an egotistical theatre groupie with a hopeless crush on a boring second rate writer. The defeated young woman of the final scene was beautifully portrayed (both her mental disquiet and her unthinking cruelty towards Konstantin).

In the cinema: Kate in *Nicholas Nickleby* (2002); Amelia in *Vanity Fair* (Mira Nair, 2004); *Inside I'm Dancing* (2004); Barbara Wilberforce in *Amazing Grace* (Michael Apted, 2006); Vivian in *Scoop* (Woody Allen, 2006); Celia in *As You Like It* (Kenneth Branagh, 2006); the title role in *Angel* (François Ozon, 2007); Briony in *Atonement* (Joe Wright, 2007).

Alexandra Gilbreath (b. Buckinghamshire, 1969) has followed a path dominated by Ibsen, Shakespeare and García Lorca. She trained at the London Academy of Music and Dramatic Art and gained her early experience at the Harrogate Theatre (Cecily in *The Importance of Being Earnest*, Ophelia in *Hamlet*); the Northcott Theatre, Exeter (Jane in *Wild Oats*, Susan in *Company*); and the Palace Theatre, Watford (Ann in *The Complaisant Lover*). In 1992 she had her first break when Katie Mitchell cast her as Adela in García Lorca's *The House of Bernada Alba* at the Gate.

It was Katie Mitchell who brought her into the RSC for the 1993-94 cycle. She played a sullen but sexy Regina alongside Jane Lapotaire and Simon Russell Beale in Mitchell's production of Ibsen's *Ghosts* (TOP), a delightfully knowing servant girl in Wycherley's *The Country Wife* (Max Stafford-Clark, Swan), and Maria in *Love's Labour's Lost* (Ian Judge, RST).

In 1995 she played Regan in *King Lear* (Jude Kelly, West Yorkshire Playhouse), and Sarah Casey in Phyllis Nagy's *Disappeared* (Nagy, Royal Court Theatre Upstairs). She made her name as a young Hedda, startlingly cold, predatory and vengeful, in *Hedda Gabler* (Stephen Unwin, English Touring Theatre, Donmar Warehouse, 1996). The performance brought her the

Ian Charleson Award. Also in 1996 she appeared at the Young Vic as the Bride in García Lorca's *Blood Wedding* (Tim Supple).

Since 1997 she has been back at the RSC. Working with Gregory Doran and Antony Sher, she was Roxane in *Cyrano de Bergerac* (Swan, 1997) and Hermione in *The Winter's Tale* (RST, 1998). In the latter play's trial scene she wore a filthy prison smock, her hair shorn: a harrowing image and a powerful realisation of character. She was a deep-voiced Rosalind in *As You Like It* (Doran), but seemed too much of the sophisticated middle-class woman to convince as Juliet in *Romeo and Juliet* (Michael Boyd, RST, 2000). She dazzled as Kate and Maria in Doran's pairing of Shakespeare's *The Taming of the Shrew* (RST) with Fletcher's *The Tamer Tamed* (Swan, 2003), and played Mistress Ford in his musical version of *The Merry Wives of Windsor* (RST, 2006-07).

John Gielgud (1904-2000) was born into a well-to-do London family. His father, of Lithuanian descent, was a stockbroker. His maternal great-aunt was the actress Ellen Terry. Theatre-obsessed from an early age, Gielgud enrolled at Lady Benson's private drama academy as soon as his schooldays (at Westminster) came to an end in 1921, the year he made his unpaid debut as the Herald in *Henry V* at the Old Vic. Two years later he won a scholarship to RADA. Although tall, distinguished-looking and immaculately dressed, Gielgud was, as his first teachers noted, physically uncomfortable on the stage, which was not to say that he lacked style or presence, only that he was unconvincing as a man of action. This limitation would have damaged his prospects had he not been blessed with the century's most magisterial voice, and had he not been a member of the clique that ran West End theatre from the 1930s to the 50s.

Gielgud's early progress included *Charley's Aunt* at the Comedy Theatre (1923); a season at the Oxford Playhouse (1924); Romeo to Gwen Ffrangcon-Davies's Juliet for Barry Jackson at the Regent (1924); Nicky in Noël Coward's controversial *The*

Vortex at the Little Theatre (1925); and leading roles in the English theatre's first significant productions of Chekhov— Trofimov in *The Cherry Orchard* (J.B. Fagan, Oxford Playhouse and Lyric Hammersmith, 1925), Konstantin in *The Seagull* (A.E. Filmer, Little Theatre, 1925), and Tusenbach in *Three Sisters* (Theodore Komisarjevsky, Barnes Theatre, 1926). Performing in these plays the young Gielgud discovered a naturalistic style of acting. In contrast, as a Shakespearean, Gielgud's awareness of the musicality of his voice initially encouraged a declamatory style that, although matchlessly lyrical and of wide appeal (his 1930 Hamlet at the Old Vic was considered to be the deepest and most intelligently-spoken of the era), made him seem a more traditional classical actor than Ralph Richardson, Michael Redgrave or Laurence Olivier. Gielgud's 1935 production of *Romeo and Juliet* at the New, in which he alternated the leading roles with Olivier, allowed playgoers to compare his asexual romanticism with Olivier's physical approach. The majority of reviewers favoured Gielgud because Olivier's verse-speaking was unpolished. They never shared a stage again and their rivalry became a constant subtext of British theatrical life, with Olivier, somewhat maliciously, scoring points at every opportunity.

While Olivier travelled to Hollywood, Gielgud moved further into direction and management, forming a company to perform an ambitious programme of classical work at the Queen's Theatre (1937-38). Here was a prototype national theatre, an ensemble of actors working on a common project under the direction of artists of the calibre of Michel Saint-Denis and Tyrone Guthrie. After the war, both stars appeared at Stratford, but Gielgud was the more prominent, transformed by the young Peter Brook into a darker, more edgy and less rhetorical performer than was felt possible (Angelo in *Measure for Measure*, 1950; Prospero in *The Tempest*, 1957), and regularly directing— *Much Ado About Nothing* (1949-55, Gielgud's Benedict was partnered by Peggy Ashcroft and Diana Wynyard), his own *King Lear* (1950), Ralph Richardson in *Macbeth* (1952), and, traumatically, Olivier and Vivien Leigh in *Twelfth Night* (1955). However, it was Olivier, on the back of his movie versions of *Henry V* and *Richard III*, who was chosen to lead the National Theatre. He had embraced the new theatre of the late 1950s, creating the role of Archie Rice in John Osborne's *The Entertainer* at the Royal Court (1957), whereas Gielgud, slower to adapt, was tied to those declining giants Binkie Beaumont, Terence Rattigan and Noël Coward. Gielgud accepted Peter Hall's invitation to join the new RSC but acted (both on the stage and in the rehearsal room) as if the 1950s had never ended. The old hierarchies that separated stars from the rest were breaking down, at least at the RSC, and Gielgud, living in a Cotswold cottage with his valet, found the process difficult. Hall had been so determined to bring Gielgud into the RSC that he had allowed him to choose the play (*Othello*) and the director (Franco Zeffirelli), and to approve the casting of Iago (Ian Bannen). Recollection of Gielgud's success as the jealous Leontes in Brook's *The Winter's Tale* at the Phoenix (1951) gave Hall reason to think that he would similarly defy expectations as Othello. Zeffirelli, not unreasonably, thought that a master Shakespearean would perform without direction. He was no Brook and left the actors floundering within the grand folly of his operatic staging. In public Gielgud responded with typical dignity, but his letters reveal that he blamed the director and particularly Bannen for the debacle. Although the same season's *Cherry Orchard* (RST, Aldwych), reuniting the 1930s team of Michel Saint-Denis, Gielgud (Gaev) and Peggy Ashcroft, was a happier experience, Gielgud never returned to an RSC theatre. He continued to work as a critically-underrated director, responsible for at least one landmark premiere—Benjamin Britten's opera *A Midsummer Night's Dream* at Covent Garden (1961).

Olivier, of course, decided who worked at the National. Gielgud was excluded until 1967/68, and then miscast as Orgon in Molière's *Tartuffe* (Guthrie), and wasted in Brook's disappointing *Oedipus*. When Peter Hall replaced Olivier as director, Gielgud was at the centre of his first season, playing Prospero in

The Tempest (1974) and Spooner in Harold Pinter's *No Man's Land* (1975). This last was the culmination of Gielgud's belated acceptance of the avant-garde, a final phase of theatre appearances that included the premieres of David Storey's *Home* (1970), Charles Wood's *Veterans* (1972) and Edward Bond's *Bingo* (1974) at the Royal Court, and which amounted to his most daring, original and relevant work since the early 1950s.

Peter Gill (b. Cardiff, 1939). Peter Gill's early life as an actor included appearances at the Royal Court (Arnold Wesker's *The Kitchen*, 1959) and the RSC (1962). It was at the Royal Court in the years that followed that he made his name as a playwright and director. Of particular interest were his productions of the plays of D.H. Lawrence. In the late 1970s he ran the Riverside Studios, and from 1980 to 97 he was an associate director at the National. He founded and directed the influential NT Studio while staging revivals in the main theatres.

His association with the RSC has been patchy but noteworthy. As a member of the 1962 acting company at the Aldwych he succeeded Peter McEnery as Silvius in the Vanessa Redgrave *As You Like It* (Michael Elliott), and played Kazbeki in *The Caucasian Chalk Circle* (William Gaskill). In 1974 he directed his first RSC production, *Twelfth Night* (RST). Conceived with originality as a study in narcissism, and performed on a bare stage, it initiated a new phase for Gill of precise, elegant versions of the classics (*The Cherry Orchard*, *The Changeling* and *Measure for Measure* at the Riverside Studios were all admired). For Adrian Noble he staged Richard Nelson's *New England* (Pit, 1994) and John Osborne's *A Patriot For Me* (Barbican, 1995), and provided translations of *The Cherry Orchard* (1995) and *The Seagull* (2000). He returned in 2004, Michael Boyd's inaugural season, to direct a traditional-looking *Romeo and Juliet* in the RST: it was like a ballet production without the dance.

Gill's first play, *The Sleepers' Den*, was produced at the Royal Court in 1965. It was followed by *Over Gardens Out* (1969), *Small*

Change (1976), *Kick For Touch* (1983), *In the Blue* (1985), *Mean Tears* (1987), *Boys Talk* (1990), *Certain Young Men* (1993), and *Cardiff East* (1997).

Iain Glen (b. Edinburgh, 1961) left RADA with the Bancroft Gold Medal in 1985. He started superbly as a menacing north London villain, a Pinkie of the 80s, in *The Fear* (ITV, 1988), and as a young businessman, spending a night with Charlotte Rampling, in *Paris By Night* (David Hare, 1988). After his small part in *Gorillas in the Mist* (Michael Apted, 1988), he won the key role of John Hanning Speke in Bob Rafelson's handsome epic *Mountains of the Moon* (1990). Also in 1990 he played Hamlet in Tom Stoppard's film of *Rosencrantz and Guildenstern Are Dead* and appeared alongside Julie Christie in *Fools of Fortune* (Pat O'Connor). These were quiet projects, far removed from his harrowing performance as Larry Winters in *Silent Scream* (David Hayman, 1990).

It was a watershed. Glen has turned increasingly to the classical theatre to find roles as stretching as Winters. Previous work on the stage had included Brazen in *The Recruiting Officer*, Ekdal in *The Wild Duck* (Birmingham Rep), Spencer the Younger in *Edward II* (Nicholas Hytner, Manchester Royal Exchange, 1986), and Ridley in Tom Stoppard's *Hapgood* (West End, 1988). He now brought danger, intelligence and subtlety to *Hamlet* (Paul Unwin, Bristol Old Vic, 1991); Aufidius opposite Kenneth Branagh's *Coriolanus* (Tim Supple, Chichester, 1992); the title role in *Macbeth* (Michael Boyd, Tron, Glasgow, 1993); and Edgar in *King Lear* (Max Stafford-Clark, Royal Court, 1993). At the RSC, in 1994/95, his Henry V (Matthew Warchus, RST) was thoughtful, troubled, quick-witted—but ruthless in politics and battle. In the same season, reunited with the Tron's Michael Boyd, he played Orgilus in John Ford's *The Broken Heart* (Swan).

This last performance revealed a fine singing voice but it was still a surprise when Glen signed with Cameron MacKintosh to sing the lead in the Boublil and Schönberg musical *Martin*

Guerre (Declan Donnellan, Prince Edward, 1996). He has since partnered Nicole Kidman in *The Blue Room* (Sam Mendes, Donmar Warehouse, 1998); played Stanley in *A Streetcar Named Desire* (Trevor Nunn, NT Lyttelton, 2002); Trigorin in *The Seagull* (Peter Stein, King's Theatre, Edinburgh Festival, 2003); Judge Brack in *Hedda Gabler* (Richard Eyre, Almeida, 2005); and, returning to the RSC, John Proctor to Elaine Cassidy's Abigail in *The Crucible* (Dominic Cooke, RST, 2006).

His screen career continues to be remarkably diverse, mixing character and leading roles in all genres: the title role in *Adam Bede* (BBC, 1991); *Frankie's House* (ITV, 1992); *Black and Blue* (TV, 1992); *The Young Americans* (1993); *Painted Lady* (ITV, 1997); Mr Preston in *Wives and Daughters* (BBC, 1999); *The Wyvern Mystery* (BBC, 2000); *Paranoid* (John Duigan, 2000); *Beautiful Creatures* (2000); *Glasgow Kiss* (BBC, 2000); *Lara Croft: Tomb Raider* (2001); *Jimmy Spud* (2001); Lee Hall's *Gabriel and Me* (2001); *Darkness* (Jaume Balagueró, 2002); Jung in *Prendimi l'anima* (Roberto Faenza, 2003); *Resident Evil: Apocalypse* (2004); *Man to Man* (Régis Wargnier, 2005); *Kidnapped* (BBC, 2005); *Kingdom of Heaven* (Ridley Scott, 2005); *Tara Road* (Gillies MacKinnon, 2005); *Small Engine Repair* (2006); *The Last Legion* (2007); *Mrs Ratcliffe's Revolution* (2007); *Resident Evil: Extinction* (2007).

Robert Glenister (b. Harrow). A graduate of the National Youth Theatre and provincial repertory, Robert Glenister emerged without fanfare as a gifted and versatile leading actor during the 1990s: Barnet in Beth Henley's *Crimes of the Heart* (Bush, 1983); Edward Voysey in *The Voysey Inheritance* (Gregory Hersov, Manchester Royal Exchange, 1989); Shigeo in *Tango at the End of Winter* (Yukio Ninagawa, Edinburgh Festival, 1991); Boxler in Naomi Wallace's *In the Heart of America* (Bush, 1994); Micky in William Gaminara's *According to Hoyle* (Hampstead Theatre, 1995); Bosola opposite Juliet Stevenson in *The Duchess of Malfi* (Philip Franks, Greenwich Theatre, 1995); and, at the National, Stanley in *Brighton Beach Memoirs* (Michael Rudman,

Lyttelton, 1986), Bazarov in *Fathers and Sons* (Rudman, Lyttelton, 1987), Jan in Nick Darke's *Ting Tang Mine* (Rudman, Cottesloe, 1987), and Donald in Dennis Potter's *Blue Remembered Hills* (Patrick Marber, Lyttelton, 1996).

He was at the RSC from 1996 to 98, playing, with originality, Alfred to Joanne Pearce's Rita in the astonishing *Little Eyolf* (Adrian Noble, Swan); a sadistic Lorenzo in *The Spanish Tragedy* (Michael Boyd, Swan); a dirt-black Caliban in *The Tempest* (Noble, RST); and a paranoid, mentally unstable Vincentio in *Measure for Measure* (Boyd, RST). Subsequent theatre: Astrov in *Uncle Vanya* (Gregory Hersov, Manchester Royal Exchange, 2001); West in Jez Butterworth's *The Winterling* (Ian Rickson, Royal Court, 2006).

On the screen: the situation comedies *Sink or Swim* (BBC, 1981) and *The Lonelyheart Kid* (ITV, 1984); Keith in Kingsley Amis's *Ending Up* (Peter Sasdy, ITV, 1989); Jeremy in the film of David Hare's *The Secret Rapture* (Howard Davies, 1993); Captain Harvile, a fine cameo, in *Persuasion* (Roger Michell, BBC, 1995); Chris Hughes, the prime suspect, in *Prime Suspect 4*, 'The Lost Child' (John Madden, ITV, 1996); Dr Markby in *Drovers' Gold* (Lesley Manning/Tristram Powell, BBC, 1997); David Jason's sergeant in *Frost* (ITV, 2001); *Laissez-passer* (Bertrand Tavernier, 2002); Nick Dear's *Eroica* (Simon Cellan Jones, BBC, 2003); *Between the Sheets* (ITV, 2003); *Hustle* (BBC, 2004-06); *Spooks* (BBC, 2007).

Jamie Glover (b. 1969). A graduate of the Central School, Jamie Glover first made his mark playing Jack Hunter in Tennessee Williams's *The Rose Tattoo* and Valerie in Molière's *Tartuffe* for Peter Hall at the Playhouse (1991). Followed by: Jeremy in Alan Franks's *The Mother Tongue* (Richard Cottrell, Greenwich, 1992); Trofimov in *The Cherry Orchard* (Misha Mokeiev, Leicester Haymarket, 1994); Bengt in Ronald Hayman's play about August Strindberg (Derek Jacobi), *Playing the Wife* (Richard Clifford, Minerva, Chichester, 1995); the title role in *Hamlet*

(Norwich Playhouse, 1996, working with his father, Julian Glover, who directed and played the Ghost, and his mother, Isla Blair, who played Gertrude); the title role in *Henry V* (Edward Hall, Watermill Theatre, Newbury, 1997); Dominic in David Bridel's *The Last Girl* (David Prescott, Riverside Studios, 1998); Tom in *The Glass Menagerie* (Mark Clements, Derby Playhouse, 1998); Moses Jackson in Tom Stoppard's *The Invention of Love* (Richard Eyre, NT Theatre Royal Haymarket, 1998-99); Hugo, the Hamlet-like assassin, in *The Novice* (Richard Eyre, Almeida, 2000, adapted from Jean-Paul Sartre's *Les mains salles*); and, at the Sheffield Crucible, David (the title role) opposite Charlotte Randle in Arthur Miller's *The Man Who Had All the Luck* (David Hunt, 2001), and Charles, alongside Michael Pennington and Teresa Banham, in David Mamet's *The Shawl* (Angus Jackson, 2001).

After a decade, then, of skilfully performed leading roles, Glover joined the RSC: Gregory Doran's 'Jacobethans' season at the Swan and Garrick (2002-03)—Edward Prince of Wales in *Edward III* (Anthony Clark), First Tribune in *The Roman Actor* (Sean Holmes), and Armusia in *The Island Princess* (Gregory Doran); then Bertram in *All's Well That Ends Well* (Doran, Swan, 2003-04).

Screen work: *Cadfael* (ITV, 1994); *Joseph* (TV, 1995); *A Dance to the Music of Time* (Channel Four, 1997); *Dalziel and Pascoe* (BBC, 1998); *The Reef* (1999); *The Thing About Vince* (ITV, 2000); Brian Epstein in *In His Life* (TV, 2000); *Men Only* (Peter Webber, Channel Four, 2001); *New Tricks* (BBC, 2004); *Waterloo Road* (BBC, 2006).

Julian Glover (b. London, 1935). One of the talented actors produced by Stratford in the late 1950s, Julian Glover was effectively an apprentice for three seasons, playing small roles in such shows as Peter Brook's *Tempest* (1957) and Peter Hall's *Cymbeline* (1957), *Twelfth Night* (1958) and *A Midsummer Night's Dream* (1959). He went on to appear at the Royal Court in John

Osborne's *Luther* (Tony Richardson, 1961), George Devine's *Twelfth Night* (1962) and Ann Jellicoe's *The Knack* (Keith Johnstone, 1962).

Glover has always been an all-rounder, less a theatre star than a highly regarded character actor in motion pictures and television dramas. That he has grown in stature with age is demonstrated by his RSC career. Starting with the Baron in Gorki's *The Lower Depths* (Toby Robertson, Arts Theatre, 1962), he returned only at long intervals, but the work was first-rate: Mr Medley in *The Man of Mode* (Terry Hands, Aldwych, 1971); Brian Leary in *The Oz Trial* (Buzz Goodbody, The Place, 1971); the Earl of Warwick in the three parts of *Henry VI* and Aufidius to Alan Howard's *Coriolanus* (Hands, RST, 1977); Gordon in David Mercer's *Cousin Vladimir* (Jane Howell) and Alonzo in *The Changeling* (Hands, Aldwych, 1978); Henry—a poignant depiction of a strong man in decline—in the two parts of *Henry IV* (Adrian Noble) and the Chorus in *Romeo and Juliet* (David Leveaux, RST, 1991); Friar Laurence in *Romeo and Juliet* (Noble) and, reunited with Peter Hall at Stratford after thirty-six years, Cassius in *Julius Caesar* (RST, 1995).

Among Julian Glover's other commanding performances of the 1990s and 2000s were the Wing Commander in Arnold Wesker's *Chips With Everything* at the National (Howard Davies, Lyttelton, 1997); Theseus in Racine's *Phèdre* at the Almeida (Jonathan Kent, Albery, 1998); Prospero in *The Tempest* at the Nuffield Theatre, Southampton (Patrick Sandford, 2000); the title role in *King Lear* at the Globe (Barry Kyle, 2001); Duncan in the Sean Bean *Macbeth* at the Albery (Edward Hall, 2002); and, for Peter Hall, Vladimir in *Waiting for Godot* at the Old Vic (1997), Galileo in Timberlake Wertenbaker's *Galileo's Daughter* and Mr Malone in Shaw's *Man and Superman* at the Theatre Royal, Bath (2004), and Sir in Ronald Harwood's *The Dresser* at the Duke of York's (2005).

Glover's movies: *Tom Jones* (Tony Richardson, 1963); *Quartermass and the Pit* (Roy Ward Baker, 1967); *The Magus* (Guy Green, 1968); *Nicholas and Alexandra* (Franklin Schaffner, 1971);

The Internecine Project (Ken Hughes, 1974); *The Empire Strikes Back* (Irvin Kershner, 1980); *For Your Eyes Only* (John Glen, 1981); *Heat and Dust* (James Ivory, 1982); *Cry Freedom* (Richard Attenborough, 1987); *Indiana Jones and the Last Crusade* (Spielberg, 1989); *In the Mouth of Madness* (John Carpenter, 1994); *Vatel* (Roland Joffé, 2000); *Two Men Went to War* (2002); *Harry Potter and the Chamber of Secrets* (2002); and *Troy* (Wolfgang Petersen, 2004).

Derek Godfrey (1924-1983, b. London). Derek Godfrey has almost faded from the theatrical record. Today it is difficult to find an obituary, let alone a full account of his life and work. And yet Godfrey was a charismatic leading actor who attained the highest level of achievement on the stage, not least at the RSC where, during the early 1960s, he played both leading and character parts. At the time of his death he was enjoying a new phase of work with the Company. Godfrey was not a celebrity actor, and never became a screen star: the best of his career, therefore, is sadly hidden away in clippings and photographs.

He first worked with the Stratford company in 1953, cast as Peto in *Henry IV Part One* (Anthony Quayle, New Zealand Tour). It was at the Old Vic in 1956-57 that he made his name as a Shakespearean actor playing the title role in *Titus Andronicus* (Walter Hudd); Iachimo in *Cymbeline* (Michael Benthall); Enobarbus in *Antony and Cleopatra* (Robert Helpmann); and the Duke of Milan in *The Two Gentlemen of Verona* (Michael Langham). He became a pivotal actor for Peter Hall at the RSC during the early 1960s, starring in a body of work that included Christopher Fry and John Whiting as well as Shakespeare: Proteus in *The Two Gentlemen of Verona* (Hall, RST, 1960); Orsino to Dorothy Tutin's Viola in *Twelfth Night* (Hall, RST, 1960); Hector in *Troilus and Cressida* (Hall, RST, 1960); Antonio in the Peggy Ashcroft *Duchess of Malfi* (Donald McWhinnie, RST, 1960); King of Ondines in *Ondine* (Hall, Aldwych, 1961); De la Rochepozay/Henri de Conde in *The Devils* (Peter Wood, Aldwych, 1961);

Petruchio to Vanessa Redgrave's Kate in *The Taming of the Shrew* (Maurice Daniels, Aldwych 1961); Henry in Christopher Fry's *Curtmantle* (Stuart Burge, Aldwych, 1962); Bernard in *Everything in the Garden* (McWhinnie, Arts Theatre, 1962); Macheath in *The Beggar's Opera* (Wood, Aldwych, 1963); Charles in Roger Vitrac's *Victor* (Robin Midgley, Aldwych, 1964); and Machevil in *The Jew of Malta* (Clifford Williams, Aldwych, 1964). At the RST in 1971 he succeeded Donald Sinden as Malvolio in John Barton's famous production of *Twelfth Night* and starred opposite Elizabeth Spriggs in *Much Ado About Nothing* (Ronald Eyre).

Screen work dominated Godfrey's career during his forties. He appeared in the horror films *The Vengeance of She* (1968), *The Abominable Dr Phibes* (1971) and *Hands of the Ripper* (1971), and on television in the BBC's *The Pallisers* (1974) and *The Tempest* (1980).

From 1980 he was back at the RSC, effortlessly authoritative as Jaques in *As You Like It* (Terry Hands, RST 1980); Claudius in the Michael Pennington *Hamlet* (Barton, RST 1980); Buckingham in the Alan Howard *Richard III* (Hands, RST, 1980); Henry in Howard Brenton's *Thirteenth Night* (Barry Kyle, Warehouse, 1981); Don Pedro in *Much Ado About Nothing* (Hands, RST, 1982); Solveig's Father/Button-Moulder/The Strange Passenger in *Peer Gynt* (Ron Daniels, TOP, 1982); Louis XIV in *Molière* (Bill Alexander, TOP, 1982); and the Rector in Nick Darke's *The Body* (Nick Hamm, Pit, 1983).

Patrick Godfrey. A supporting actor at the RSC for ten years from 1971, Patrick Godfrey was a master of pointed characterisations. He was particularly fine in David Jones's productions of Gorky and Chekhov at the Aldwych, and in Trevor Nunn's 'The Romans', *Three Sisters* (the first small-scale tour, 1978) and *Nicholas Nickleby*. In 1989/90 he returned to the Company to play, with typical precision, Polonius in *Hamlet*, Friar Laurence in *Romeo and Juliet*, and Pavlin in Gorky's *Barbarians*.

His RSC career began and ended with Gorky: First Worker in Gorky's *Enemies* (David Jones, Aldwych, 1971); Mr Smirk in *The Man of Mode* (Terry Hands, Aldwych, 1971); Servant in *Miss Julie* (Robin Phillips, The Place, 1971); Louis in Jean Genet's *The Balcony* (Hands, Aldwych, 1971); Maecenas in *Antony and Cleopatra* (Nunn/Goodbody, RST, 1972); Sempronius in *Titus Andronicus* (Nunn/Goodbody, RST, 1972); Somerset Swayze in *Section Nine* (Charles Marowitz, The Place, 1973); Sir Edward Leighton in *Sherlock Holmes* (Frank Dunlop, Aldwych, 1974); Torres in Peter Barnes's *The Bewitched* (Hands, Aldwych, 1974); Kirill in Gorky's *Summerfolk* (Jones, Aldwych, 1974); Gendarme Snoo Wilson's *The Beast* (Howard Davies, The Place, 1974); Boyet, succeeding Sebastian Shaw, in *Love's Labour's Lost* (Jones, Aldwych, 1975); Mr Tetgeen in *The Marrying of Ann Leete* (Jones, Aldwych, 1975); The Doctor in *Too True to be Good* (Clifford Williams, Aldwych, 1975); Tarakanov in Gorky's *The Zykovs* (Jones, Aldwych, 1976); Hugo Kalmar in O'Neill's *The Iceman Cometh* (Davies, Aldwych, 1976); Major Swindon in Shaw's *The Devil's Disciple* (Jack Gold, Aldwych, 1976); Kosych in *Ivanov* (Jones, Aldwych, 1976); Smooth in *Wild Oats* (Williams, Aldwych, 1976); Kulighin in *Three Sisters* (Nunn) and Antonio in *Twelfth Night* (John Amiel, Small-scale Tour, 1978); Shallow in *The Merry Wives of Windsor* (Nunn/John Caird, RST, 1979); Belarius in *Cymbeline* (Jones, RST, 1979); Watzmann in Brecht's *Baal* (Jones, TOP, 1979); Kulighin in *Three Sisters* (Nunn, TOP, 1979); Mr Kenwigs in *Nicholas Nickleby* (Nunn/Caird, Aldwych, 1980); Polonius in the Mark Rylance *Hamlet* (Ron Daniels, RST, 1989); Friar Laurence in *Romeo and Juliet* (Hands, Swan, 1989); and Pavlin in Gorky's *Barbarians* (Jones, Barbican, 1990).

In features, his ability to deliver a vivid cameo is best seen in four films by James Ivory — *Heat and Dust* (1983), *A Room With a View* (1986, as the Reverend Mr Eager), *Maurice* (1987), and *The Remains of the Day* (1993).

Stella Gonet (b. Greenock, 1963). With her fair, Polish features, Stella Gonet has been a striking actress at the RSC and elsewhere since the mid-1980s. A vibrant, intelligent interpreter of classical and modern roles on the stage, she has had few major opportunities on screen, although her surprisingly long commitment to the BBC series *House of Elliott* (1991-93) brought her to the attention of a large audience.

Brought up in Greenock, she trained at the Royal Scottish Academy of Music and Drama in Glasgow and gained her early experience at the Dundee Rep, the Traverse Theatre, Edinburgh, and the Liverpool Playhouse. At the RSC she has played Bridie in Deborah Levy's *Heresies* (Susan Todd, Pit, 1986); Irina in Arthur Miller's *The Archbishop's Ceiling* (Nick Hamm, Pit, 1986); Liz in Doug Lucie's *Fashion* (Hamm, TOP, 1987); Bellamira in the *Jew of Malta* (Barry Kyle, Swan, 1987); Castiza in *The Revenger's Tragedy* (Di Trevis, Swan, 1987); Irina, alongside Harriet Walter and Deborah Findlay, in *Three Sisters* (John Barton, Barbican, 1988); Angelique in Stephen Lowe's *Divine Gossip* (Kyle, Pit, 1988); Greta in Ann Devlin's *After Easter* (Michael Attenborough, TOP, 1994); a cool Hippolyta and highly-sexed Titania in *A Midsummer Night's Dream* (Adrian Noble, RST, 1994); and a grave, fascinating Isabella in a monochrome *Measure for Measure* (Steven Pimlott, RST, 1994).

Other theatre work: Roxane in the Robert Lindsay *Cyrano de Bergerac* (Elijah Moshinsky, Theatre Royal Haymarket, 1992-93); Shelagh Stephenson's *The Memory of Water* (Vaudeville, 1999); and, at the National, Debbie Horsfield's *True Dare Kiss* and *Command or Promise* (John Burgess, Cottesloe, 1985), Ophelia to Daniel Day-Lewis's prince in *Hamlet* (Richard Eyre, Olivier, 1989), *The Shaughraun* (Howard Davies, Olivier, 1989), and David Hare's *Racing Demon* (Eyre, Cottesloe, 1990) and *Skylight* (Eyre, West End, 1997).

Television: *Heading Home* (BBC, 1991); Zina in *Stalin* (Ivan Passer, 1992); Marigold in Simon Gray's *The Common Pursuit* (Christopher Morahan, 1992); *The Crow Road* (Gavin Millar, BBC,

1996); the abused wife in Lucy Gannon's *Trip Trap* (Danny Hiller, BBC, 1996); the female lead in Lynda La Plante's *Supply and Demand* (Waris Hussein, ITV, 1998); *The Secret* (BBC, 2002); *Foyle's War* (ITV, 2004); *The Inspector Lynley Mysteries* (BBC, 2005); and *Holby City* (BBC, 2007).

Henry Goodman (b. London, 1950). Of Russian and Polish Jewish heritage, Henry Goodman was brought up in Whitechapel, east London. At the age of ten he appeared in the film *Conspiracy of Hearts* (1960). He went to RADA and was taught by Steven Berkoff. There is a connection to be made between his early life working in Petticoat Lane market and the roles—fast-talking, streetwise New Yorkers—that made his name in the 1990s.

After RADA he married a South African and spent ten years teaching and acting in her country (he ran his own theatre). On their return he had to begin again. He started to make his mark as a supporting player at the RSC: Harry in *The Time of Your Life* (Howard Davies, TOP, 1983); Sir Thomas Lovell/Cranmer in *Henry VIII* (Davies, RST, 1983); Dromio of Ephesus in *The Comedy of Errors* (Adrian Noble, RST, 1983); Voltore in *Volpone* (Bill Alexander, TOP, 1983); Azhog/Stalin in *Red Star* (John Caird, Pit, 1984); Prince Henri DeConde in *The Devils* (John Barton, Pit, 1984); Grandpre/Le Fer in *Henry V* (Noble, RST, 1985); Paulina's Steward in *The Winter's Tale* (Terry Hands, RST, 1986); Thomas Kitely in *Every Man in His Humour* (Caird, Swan, 1986); Fernando in *Worlds Apart* (Nick Hamm, TOP, 1986); and Rocky Gravo in *They Shoot Horses Don't They?* (Ron Daniels, Mermaid, 1987).

On leaving the Company he was in Gregory Motton's *Downfall* (Lindsay Posner, Royal Court Theatre Upstairs, 1988); Caryl Phillips's *All or Nothing at All* (Tricycle Theatre, 1989); and Berkoff's *Kvetch* (King's Head, 1991). When Sam Mendes's production of Stephen Sondheim's *Assassins* opened at the Donmar Warehouse in 1992 Goodman finally stepped forward as a virtuosic leading actor. Other leading American roles in musicals and modern classics followed—Buddy Fidler, the movie producer, in *City of Angels* (Michael Blakemore, Prince of Wales, 1993); Roy Cohn in Tony Kushner's *Angels in America* (Declan Donnellan, NT Cottesloe, 1993); Philip Gellburg in Arthur Miller's *Broken Glass* (David Thacker, NT Lyttelton, 1994); Nathan Detroit in *Guys and Dolls* (Richard Eyre, NT Olivier, 1996); and Billy Flynn, the bent lawyer, in *Chicago* (1997). In 1999/2000, as a member of Trevor Nunn's NT Ensemble, he played a famous Shylock in *The Merchant of Venice* (Cottesloe) and appeared in *Summerfolk* (Olivier). He also devised a late night cabaret called *Metropolis Kabarett* (Terrace Café, 2000). In 2003 he returned to the RSC to play the title role in *Richard III* (Sean Holmes, RST). Inspired by Victorian music hall and melodrama, Goodman's lunatic comedian had all the subtlety of the Joker in *Batman*. Other theatre work since 1990: Freud in Terry Johnson's *Hysteria* (Phyllida Lloyd, Royal Court, 1993); *Art* on Broadway (Matthew Warchus, 1998); Pinter's *The Birthday Party* (Posner, Birmingham Rep, 2005).

Screen work: Strauss in Simon Gray's *Old Flames* (Christopher Morahan, BBC, 1989); *The Gravy Train Goes East* (ITV, 1991); *Son of the Pink Panther* (1993); *Cold Lazarus* (BBC, 1996); Haffinger in *Mary Reilly* (Stephen Frears, 1996); *Private Parts* (1997); Dr Lev Botvin in *The Saint* (Philip Noyce, 1997); the situation comedy *Unfinished Business* (BBC, 1998); the concierge in *Notting Hill* (Roger Michell, 1999); *Dirty Tricks* (ITV, 2000); Joshua Jopp in *The Mayor of Casterbridge* (David Thacker, ITV, 2003); *Foyle's War* (ITV, 2003); and *The Life and Death of Peter Sellers* (Stephen Hopkins, 2004).

Rupert Goold (b. London, 1972) read English at Trinity College, Cambridge, and then attended New York University on a Fulbright Scholarship. There are few training opportunities for young directors, but the high flying Goold bagged most of them—programmes at the Donmar and the NT Studio (1995), followed by the Regional Theatre Young Director Scheme at the Salisbury Playhouse. He made his name on regional stages, first as an associate at Salisbury—Graham Greene's *Travels With My Aunt* (1997); Brian Friel's *Dancing at Lughnasa* (1998); P.G. Woodhouse's *Summer Lightning* (1998); Alan Bennett's *Habeus Corpus* (1999); *Scaramouche Jones* (2003)—and then as Artistic Director of the Northampton Theatre Royal—Tom Stoppard's *Arcadia* (2002); Harold Pinter's *Betrayal* (2002); Conor McPherson's *The Weir* (2003); *Waiting for Godot* (2003); *Othello* (2003); *Paradise Lost* (2004); Terry Johnson's *Insignificance* (2004); *Faustus* (2004); and *Hamlet* (2005). Elsewhere: *The End of the Affair* (Bridewell, 1997); *Romeo and Juliet* (Greenwich Theatre, 1998); Hristo Boytchev's *The Colonel Bird* (Gate, 1999); Alan Bennett's *The Wind in the Willows* (Birmingham Rep, 2001); Rossini's *Le comte Ory* (Garsington Opera, 2005).

At the RSC he has directed Frank McGuinness's *Speaking Like Magpies* (Swan, 2005), and *The Tempest* (RST, 2006). *The Tempest*, starring an authoritative Patrick Stewart, was an inventive and thought-provoking main house debut. If the polar concept was a negation of the text's metaphors, its continuously shifting, dreamlike landscapes, it created a number of atmospheric moments, suggesting—with originality—that Prospero's island was a place of hardship and austerity.

In 2005 Goold took charge of the Oxford Stage Company. In 2007 he continued his partnership with Patrick Stewart with a powerful studio *Macbeth* at Chichester (Minerva).

Marius Goring (1912-1988, b. Newport, Isle of Wight). A graduate of the pre-war Old Vic, Marius Goring worked prolifically in films without adapting his theatrical style of acting. A skilled linguist, he played Hitler on radio as part of the war effort (*The Shadow of the Swastika*, 1939) and subsequently became typecast as a German of one kind or another. But when given the opportunity, as in the films of Powell and Pressburger, he was memorable: his wryly humorous French fop in *A Matter of*

Life or Death (1946) is the best example. Goring had a continental European outlook and saw theatre within a wider context of culture and society.

His father was a Home Office criminologist. His mother, a pianist, had studied under Clara Schumann. He first appeared on the stage at the age of thirteen in Cambridge (the show was called *Crossings*), and made his London debut as Harlequin at the Rudolph Steiner Hall (1927). He attended the universities of Frankfurt, Munich, Vienna and Paris before training under Harcourt Williams at the Old Vic school (1929-32). On graduating he went straight into the Old Vic company and made his name playing opposite Peggy Ashcroft in *Romeo and Juliet* (Harcourt Williams, 1933). The following year he joined Michel Saint-Denis's La Compagnie des Quinze and toured Europe performing Hamlet in French. His association with Saint-Denis, the most important of his career, continued with productions of *Noah* at the New (1935), *The Witch of Edmonton* at the Old Vic (1936) and *The White Guard* at the Phoenix (1938). Other significant roles, all at the Old Vic, were Feste in *Twelfth Night* (1937), the Chorus in the Laurence Olivier *Henry V* (1937) and Ariel in the John Gielgud *Tempest*, a show he co-directed with George Devine (1940).

At the outbreak of the war Goring joined the Queen's Royal Regiment but was seconded to the Foreign Office to supervise radio broadcasts to Germany (working with Dick Crossman and Hugh Greene at the BBC, he used the pseudonym Charles Richardson). In 1941 he married a refugee German actress, Lucie Mannheim. In the immediate post-war period he led a number of tours to Berlin.

In 1953 he appeared at Stratford for the first time, a rich repertory of Richard III (Glen Byam Shaw); Octavius Caesar in *Antony and Cleopatra* (Shaw); Petruchio in *The Taming of the Shrew* (George Devine); and the Fool in the Michael Redgrave *King Lear* (Devine). He returned in 1962 to play Angelo in *Measure for Measure* (John Blatchley, RST) and Sir Timothy Bellboys in *A Penny for a Song* (Colin Graham, Aldwych).

He worked constantly in the theatre during the 1970s and 80s but only Peter Shaffer's *Sleuth* (St Martin's, 1970-73) brought him before a wide public. He was best known for his starring roles in the television drama serials *The Scarlet Pimpernel* (1955) and *The Expert* (1968-70). A founding member of Equity (1929), he served as the union's vice-president from 1963-65 and again from 1975-82, and fought a battle against left-wing militants (such as the Redgraves) who were politicising Equity against the wishes of the majority. He took the union to court because it was passing resolutions in support of the Ayatollah Khomeini and Irish republicanism.

Goring's body of work in movies included Michael Powell's *The Spy in Black* (1939), *The Red Shoes* (1948) and *Ill Met by Moonlight* (1957); Jacques Tourneur's *Circle of Danger* (1951); Joseph L. Mankiewicz's *The Barefoot Contessa* (1954); John Guillermin's *I Was Monty's Double* (1958); Robert Aldrich's *The Angry Hills* (1959); Otto Preminger's *Exodus* (1960); Jack Cardiff's *Girl on a Motorcycle* (1968); and Peter Brook's *Meetings with Remarkable Men* (1979).

Richard Griffiths (b. Thornaby-on-Tees, Yorkshire, 1947) left school at fifteen and worked for a time in the same firm as his father, making steel piles for the building industry. He then studied art and drama in Manchester.

His early theatre work included Salinas in Peter Shaffer's *The Royal Hunt of the Sun* (Harrogate, 1970); Doolittle in *Pygmalion* and the Chaplain in *Mother Courage* (Orchard Theatre, Dartford, 1973); Macduff in *Macbeth* (Belfast, 1973); York in *Richard II* (Library Theatre, Manchester, 1974); and The Jew in *Woyzek* (Newcastle, 1975).

He came to prominence during ten years with the RSC. As Bottom in *A Midsummer Night's Dream* (John Barton, RST, 1977) and Trinculo in *The Tempest* (Clifford Williams, RST, 1978) he made comedic use of his physique, then subverted the image through the subtlety and aplomb of his acting. Also: Sailor in

Twelfth Night (Peter Gill, RST, 1974); Gonzalo in *The Tempest* (Keith Hack, TOP, 1974); Tiny in *Afore Night Come* (Ron Daniels, TOP, 1974); Peter in *Romeo and Juliet* (Trevor Nunn, RST, 1976); Tanky in Charles Wood's *Dingo* (Barry Kyle, TOP, 1976); an Officer in *The Comedy of Errors* (Nunn, RST, 1976); Thiers in Brecht's *Days of the Commune* (Howard Davies, Aldwych, 1977); Dr Gordon in *A Miserable and Lonely Death* (Walter Donohue, Warehouse, 1978); Pompey in *Measure for Measure* (Kyle, RST, 1978); Navarre in *Love's Labour's Lost* (Barton, RST, 1978); Messenger in *Antony and Cleopatra* (Peter Brook, RST, 1978); Larion in *The White Guard* (Kyle, Aldwych, 1979); George Lewis in *Once in a Lifetime* (Nunn, Aldwych, 1979); the title role in *Henry VIII* (Davies, RST, 1983); the title role in *Volpone* (Bill Alexander, TOP, 1983); and Mikhailovich in Charles Wood's *Red Star* (John Caird, Pit, 1984).

In the years since he has become a well-known screen actor. He played Allardyce, the pig-obsessed accountant, in Alan Bennett's *A Private Function* (Malcolm Mowbray, 1985) and the repulsive Uncle Monty in *Withnail and I* (Bruce Robinson, 1987), and both ITV and the BBC created series based around him, respectively *Ffizz* (1987-89) and *Pie in the Sky* (1993-98). Other credits: *The French Lieutenant's Woman* (Karel Reisz, 1981); *Chariots of Fire* (Hugh Hudson, 1981); *Gandhi* (Richard Attenborough, 1982); *Britannia Hospital* (Lindsay Anderson, 1982); *Gorky Park* (Michael Apted, 1983); *Greystoke* (Hudson, 1984); *Sleepy Hollow* (Tim Burton, 1999); *Harry Potter* (2001); *The History Boys* (Nicholas Hytner, 2006).

He returns to the stage at intervals: *Lady in the Dark* (concert performance, Usher Hall, Edinburgh Festival, 1988); the husband in Pirandello's *Rules of the Game* (Jonathan Kent, Almeida, 1992); the title role in *The Life of Galileo* (Jonathan Kent, Almeida, 1994); Captain Shotover in *Heartbreak House* (Almeida, 1997); Marc in *Art* (Matthew Warchus, Wyndham's, 1998); Henry VIII in William Nicholson's *Katherine Howard* (Robin Lefèvre, Chichester, 1998); Yvan in *Art* (Warchus, Wyndham's, 2001); Tetzel in John Osborne's *Luther* (Peter Gill, NT Olivier, 2001); and Hector in Alan Bennett's *The History Boys* (Nicholas Hytner, NT Lyttelton, 2004).

Pippa Guard (b. Edinburgh, 1952). Brought up in Canada, Pippa Guard returned to Britain to take up a place at RADA. On leaving the academy, she joined the RSC's exceptional 1976 Stratford company. Initially seen in minor parts—a Lady in *Romeo and Juliet* (Trevor Nunn/Barry Kyle); a Maid in the Donald Sinden/Judi Dench *Much Ado About Nothing* (John Barton); Mopsa in *The Winter's Tale* (Barton/Nunn); a Lady in *Troilus and Cressida* (Barton/Kyle); and Girl at the Porpentine in *The Comedy of Errors* (Nunn)—she quickly progressed to Luciana, succeeding Francesca Annis, in *The Comedy of Errors* (RST, 1977); Ursula in *Much Ado* (Aldwych, 1977); Hermia in *A Midsummer Night's Dream* (Barton/Gillian Lynne, RST, 1977); and Evie in James Robson's *Factory Birds* (Bill Alexander, Warehouse, 1977).

A good foundation for a classical stage career, but Guard worked mostly in television for the next ten years: Maggie in *The Mill on the Floss* (1978); Barbara in *The Mallens* (ITV, 1978); Ava alongside Peter Firth and Caroline Langrishe in the memorable oddity *The Flipside of Dominick Hide* (Alan Gibson, BBC, 1981) and its sequel *Another Flip for Dominick* (1982); Prue in a high-class adaptation of *To the Lighthouse* (Colin Gregg, BBC, 1983); Edith Holden in *The Country Diary of an Edwardian Lady* (ITV, 1984); and, for the BBC Shakespeare, Miranda to Michael Hordern's Prospero in *The Tempest* (John Gorrie, 1979), Diana in *All's Well That Ends Well* (Elijah Moshinsky, 1980) and Hermia in *A Midsummer Night's Dream* (Moshinsky, 1981). She played the lead, a young private investigator thrown into the deep end of a mystery, with some style in Christopher Petit's *An Unsuitable Job for a Woman* (1981), but this was, and remains, an isolated role in features. At the National she played the title role in *Antigone* (Peter Gill, Cottesloe, 1984) and Fay in Ayckbourn's *A Chorus of Disapproval* (Lyric, 1986).

She returned to the RSC for the 1987/88 season: Mistress Bonavent in *Hyde Park* (Barry Kyle, Swan); Nerissa in *The Merchant of Venice* (Bill Alexander, RST); Maria in *Twelfth Night* (Alexander, RST); and Natasha in John Barton's production of *Three Sisters* (Barbican). She was unfortunate to miss out on the leading roles of Portia, Olivia and Olga. She was next Rose in Doris Lessing's *In Pursuit of the English* (Matthew Francis, Lyric Studio, 1990), and Katherine Uruhart in the RSC's adaptation of *The Strange Case of Dr Jekyll and Mr Hyde* (Peter Wood, Barbican, 1991).

Screen appearances since 1990: Ronald Pickup's American secretary, an exceptional black comedy performance, in *The Riff Raff Element* (BBC, 1993); India Wilkes in *Scarlett* (1994); *Daisies in December* (Mark Haber, ITV, 1995); *All or Nothing At All* (ITV, 1993); John Sullivan's *Roger Roger* (BBC, 1996, 1998); *Gobble* (BBC, 1997); the situation comedy *The Creatives* (BBC, 1998); *Hope and Glory* (BBC, 1999); *Hearts and Bones* (BBC, 2000); and *Dalziel and Pascoe* (BBC, 2002).

Peter Guinness. Peter Guinness's career began with seasons at Dundee and Southampton. A number of incisive performances in classical roles at the major provincial and fringe theatres brought him to notice: Tybalt in *Romeo and Juliet* at the Bristol Old Vic; De Flores in *The Changeling* at the Contact Theatre, Manchester; Aston in *The Caretaker* at the Greenwich Theatre; Edgar in *King Lear* (Sam Walters, 1982), a servant in Ostrovsky's *The Diary of a Scoundrel* (Peter Rowe, 1985), and the title role in *Hamlet, the First Quarto* (Walters, 1985) at the Orange Tree; the Duke in *Measure for Measure* (David Thacker, 1985) and the title role in *Doctor Faustus* (Anthony Clark, 1988) at the Young Vic. He joined the RSC for the 1986/87 season and played Gideon Sachs in David Lan's *Flight* (Howard Davies, TOP); Theseus in *The Two Noble Kinsmen* (Barry Kyle, Swan); Frederick in *The Rover* (John Barton, Swan); a formidable Macduff in the Jonathan Pryce *Macbeth* (Adrian Noble, RST); the Investigator in

Vladimir Gubaryev's Chernobyl play *Sarcophagus* (Jude Kelly, Pit); and James Reilly in *They Shoot Horses Don't They?* (Ron Daniels, Mermaid).

Subsequent theatre roles: Goroudolin in *Too Clever By Half* (David Jones) and Sebastian in *The Tempest* (Miller) at the Old Vic (1989); Trigorin in *The Seagull* (Anthony Clark) at the Birmingham Rep Studio (1990); Xuthus in *Ion* (Nicholas Wright) at the RSC (Pit, 1994); the professor opposite Lorna McDevitt in David Mamet's *Oleana* (Robert David MacDonald) and George in *Who's Afraid of Virginia Woolf* (Giles Havergal) at the Glasgow Citizens' (1998-99); Jaques in *As You Like It* (Marianne Elliott) at the Manchester Royal Exchange (2000); Horace in *The Little Foxes* (Marianne Elliott) at the Donmar Warehouse (2001); King Thoas in Goethe's *Under the Curse* (Joe Hill-Gibbins) at the Gate (2003, Catherine McCormack as Iphigenia); Rank in *A Doll's House* (Rachel Kavanaugh) at the Birmingham Rep (2004); and Guardiano in *Women Beware Women* (Laurence Boswell) at the RSC (Swan, 2006).

For many years the charismatic, effortlessly imposing Guinness has been luxury casting as a heavy or policeman on television: *Smiley's People* (BBC, 1982); *By the Sword Divided* (BBC, 1983); *Blackeyes* (Dennis Potter, BBC, 1989); *Old Flames* (Christopher Morahan, BBC, 1989); *The Widowmaker* (John Madden, ITV, 1990); *The Cloning of Joanna May* (Philip Saville, ITV, 1992); *Spender* (BBC, 1992-93); *Heartbeat* (ITV, 1993); *Smokescreen* (BBC, 1994); *The Bill* (ITV, 1996); *Hostile Waters* (1997); *Ivanhoe* (BBC, 1997); *Cadfael* (ITV, 1997); *Casualty* (BBC, 1997-98); *C15* (1998); *Rhodes* (BBC, 1998); *Arabian Nights* (2000); *Harbour Lights* (BBC, 2000); *Coronation Street* (ITV, 2000-02); *The Bill* (ITV, 2002); *Red Cap* (BBC, 2001, 2003); *Sea of Souls* (BBC, 2004-06); *Bleak House* (BBC, 2005).

Films: *The Keep* (Michael Mann, 1983); *Alien 3* (David Fincher, 1992); *Christopher Columbus* (John Glen, 1992); *The Saint* (Philip Noyce, 1997); *Sleepy Hollow* (Tim Burton, 1999); and *Greenfingers* (2000).

Mike Gwilym (b. Wales, 1949). A leading actor at the RSC from 1974 to 1982, whose fiery, agitated style was highly distinctive, Mike Gwilym has mysteriously dropped from sight in recent years, although he remains an associate artist of the Company.

After roles for the Oxford University Dramatic Society, including Romeo (1969), Gwilym joined the Glasgow Citizens', where he played Estragon in *Waiting for Godot* (Keith Hack, 1971); Malvolio in *Twelfth Night* (Giles Havergal, 1971); Robespierre in *Danton's Death* (Philip Prowse, 1971); Octavius in *Antony and Cleopatra* (Havergal, 1972); the title role in *Tartuffe* (Havergal, 1972); the title role in *Tamburlaine* (Hack, 1973); and Achilles in *Troilus and Cressida* (Prowse, 1973).

An impressive body of work which led naturally to Stratford. At the RSC Gwilym brought to his classical characters a tense physicality, making them seem perpetually on the edge of an outburst: Peter of Pomfret in *King John* (John Barton/Barry Kyle, TOP, 1974); Edgar in the Tony Church *King Lear* (Buzz Goodbody, TOP, 1974); Stanley Dibble in *I Was Shakespeare's Double* (Howard Davies, TOP, 1974); Vlass in *Summerfolk* (David Jones, Aldwych, 1974); Raspe in Wedekind's *The Marquis of Keith* (Ronald Eyre, Aldwych, 1974); Death in *King John* (Barton/Kyle, Aldwych, 1975); Costard in *Love's Labour's Lost* (Jones, Aldwych, 1975); George Leete opposite Mia Farrow in *The Marrying of Ann Leete* (Jones, Aldwych, 1975); *He That Plays the King* (US Tour, 1975); Mikhail in *The Zykovs* (Jones, Aldwych, 1976); Troilus opposite Francesca Annis in *Troilus and Cressida* (Barton/Kyle, RST, 1976); Antipholus of Ephesus in *The Comedy of Errors* (Trevor Nunn, RST, 1976); Surly in *The Alchemist* (Nunn, TOP and Aldwych, 1977); Johann Tonnesen in *Pillars of the Community* (Barton, Aldwych, 1977); François in Brecht's *Days of the Commune* (Davies, Aldwych, 1977); Wang in Edward Bond's *The Bundle* (Davies, Warehouse, 1977); Achilles/Orestes in John Barton's trilogy *The Greeks* (Aldwych, 1980); Benjamin Wouldbe, an electrifying performance of angst-ridden malevolence, in Farquhar's *The Twin Rivals* (John Caird, TOP, 1981); a sinister Oberon, doubled with Theseus, in *A Midsummer Night's Dream* (Ron Daniels, RST, 1981); a cruel Bertram in *All's Well That End's Well* (Nunn, RST, 1981); and a hilariously paranoid, scene-stealing Pistol in *Henry IV* (Nunn, Barbican, 1982)—he turned the simple act of forcing a place beside Falstaff on an over-crowded bench into a comic *tour de force*.

He took part in John Barton's RSC series *Playing Shakespeare* (LWT, 1984), but soon after left the Company. His screen credits make for a surprisingly dull list: Ronald Wilson in *How Green Was My Valley* (BBC, 1975); *Ice Age* (BBC, 1978); the lead in Dick Francis's *The Racing Game* (ITV, 1979); Alfie in the spy film *Hopscotch* (Ronald Neame, 1980); John Middleton Murray in *Priest of Love* (Christopher Miles, 1981); the British horror film *Venom* (Piers Haggard, 1982); Aufidius to Alan Howard's *Coriolanus* (Elijah Moshinsky, 1983), the title role in *Pericles* (David Hugh Jones, 1983) and Berowne opposite Jenny Agutter in *Love's Labour's Lost* (Elijah Moshinsky, 1986) for the BBC Shakespeare; Haemon in *Antigone* (Don Taylor, BBC, 1984); Paul in *A.D.* (Stuart Cooper, 1985); the American mini series *Peter the Great* (Marvin Chomsky, 1986); *On the Black Hill* (Andrew Grieve, 1987); Herzfelde in *Enemy of the State* (Andrew Piddington, 1987); and Hitler in *The Plot to Kill Hitler* (Lawrence Schiller, 1990).

Gwilym's other theatre appearances: Angelo in *Measure for Measure* (Guildford, 1973), the title role in *Macbeth* (Bristol Old Vic, 1976), and Ferdinand alongside Helen Mirren and Bob Hoskins in Adrian Noble's production of *The Duchess of Malfi* (Royal Exchange, Manchester, 1980).

H

Mark Hadfield made his name on the London stage playing Linus in *Snoopy* (Kay Cole, Duchess, 1983); a soulful Stan Laurel in *Blockheads* (Cole, Mermaid, 1984); Benny South-street in *Guys and Dolls* (Richard Eyre, NT Prince of Wales, 1985); and both Mercutio and Friar Laurence in his friend Kenneth Branagh's production of *Romeo and Juliet* (Lyric Hammersmith Studio, 1986). He later co-starred in Branagh's film *In the Bleak Midwinter* (1995).

He has been a member of the RSC since 1987, when he played Dromio of Syracuse in *The Comedy of Errors* (Nick Hamm) and Osric/Reynaldo in *Hamlet* (Roger Michell, Small-scale Tour). An admired actor of all-round ability, he has moved between comedic and dramatic roles: Novel in *The Plain Dealer* (Ron Daniels, Swan, 1988); Young Talbot/Young Clifford/Simpcox/Lovel in *The Plantagenets* (Adrian Noble, RST, 1988); Sanchez in Nick Darke's *Kissing the Pope* (Michell, Almeida, 1989); Autolycus, succeeding Richard McCabe, in *The Winter's Tale* (Noble, US Tour, 1994); Lantern Leatherhead in *Bartholomew Fair* (Laurence Boswell, Swan, 1997); Launce in *The Two Gentlemen of Verona* (Edward Hall, Swan, 1998); Bernard in *Talk of the City* (Stephen Poliakoff, Swan, 1998); Medvedenko in *The Seagull* (Noble, Swan, 2000); Feste, played brilliantly as a sad clown in a Buster Keaton hat, in *Twelfth Night* (Lindsay Posner, RST, 2001); Ackers Brother in Peter Barnes's *Jubilee* (Gregory Doran, Swan, 2001); Verino in Lope de Vega's *Madness in Valencia* (Jonathan Munby, TOP, 2001); Chaucer in *The Canterbury Tales* (Doran, Swan and Small-scale Tour, 2005-06); and Puck in *A Midsummer Night's Dream*, the Gravedigger in *Hamlet* and Boyet in *Love's Labour's Lost* (Doran, Courtyard, 2008).

Elsewhere: Grumio in *The Taming of the Shrew* (Mark Brickman, Sheffield Crucible, 1990); Little Monk in *Becket* (Theatre Royal Haymarket, 1991); Dancing Master in *Le bourgeois gentilhomme* (Richard Jones, NT Lyttelton, 1992); Starveling in *A Midsummer Night's Dream* (Robert Lepage, NT Olivier, 1992); Young Covey in *The Plough and the Stars* (Matthew Warchus, West Yorkshire Playhouse, 1993); Borachio in *Much Ado About Nothing* (Warchus, Queen's, 1993); La Flèche in *The Miser* (Nicholas Broadhurst, Chichester, 1995); Smee in *Peter Pan*

(Warchus, West Yorkshire Playhouse, 1996); Davies in Daniel Hill's Gulf War play *Cracked* (Terry Johnson, Hampstead, 1997); Rob Stein in *Twilight of the Golds* (Arts Theatre, 1997); Timon in *The Lion King* (Julie Taymor, Lyceum, 2003-04); Sganarelle in Molière's *Don Juan* (Thea Sharrock) and Henry Straker, the chauffeur, in Shaw's *Man and Superman* (Peter Hall, Theatre Royal, Bath, 2004); Lee Hall's monologues *Two's Company* and *Child of the Snow* (Simon Reade, Bristol Old Vic Studio, 2005); and Matt Charman's *A Night at the Dogs* (Abigail Morris, Soho Theatre, 2005).

David Haig (b. 1955) trained at the London Academy of Music and Dramatic Art and came to notice at the Royal Court in the late 1970s and early 80s: D.H. Lawrence's *Touch and Go* (Gordon McDougall, 1979); Andrea Dunbar's *The Arbor* (Max Stafford-Clark, 1980); and Maurice in the premiere production of Michael Hastings's *Tom and Viv* (Stafford-Clark, 1984).

He joined the RSC in London in 1984 to succeed Miles Anderson as Dudley in *The Time of Your Life* (Howard Davies, Pit), and John Dicks as Corvino in *Volpone* (Bill Alexander, Pit). Then, in 1986, he was Peter Quince—a spot-on parody of a certain type of theatre director—in *A Midsummer Night's Dream* (Alexander, RST); Joaquin in *Worlds Apart* (Nick Hamm, TOP); and Brainworm in Ben Jonson's *Every Man in His Humour* (John Caird, Swan). When Alexander's *Dream* reached London Haig was cast as Bottom (Barbican, 1987). He returned in 1991 to play Angelo in *Measure for Measure* (Nunn, TOP). He powerfully conveyed the psychological darkness lurking beneath the ordinary exterior of his Angelo (sniffing Claire Skinner's hair as a prelude to attempted rape).

Since the late 1980s he has been a busy television actor, only occasionally appearing on the stage, but these appearances have been fascinating: Farquhar's *The Recruiting Officer* and Timberlake Wertenbaker's *Our Country's Good* (Stafford-Clark, Royal Court, 1988), played in repertory; Antiochus opposite Lindsay

Duncan in Racine's *Berenice* (Tim Albery, NT Cottesloe, 1990); Richard in Terry Johnson's *Dead Funny* (Hampstead, 1994); Lord Morotaka in Peter Oswald's adaptation of the Japanese play *Fair Ladies at a Game of Poem Cards* (John Crowley, NT Cottesloe, 1996); Yasmina Reza's *Art* (Matthew Warchus, Wyndham's, 1997); Teddy in Alan Ayckbourn's *House/Garden* (NT Lyttelton/Olivier, 2000); Henri in Yasmina Reza's *Life x 3* (Birmingham Rep, 2001); Alex in Terry Johnson's *Hitchcock Blonde* (Royal Court, 2003); Osborne in R.C. Sherriff's *Journey's End* (David Grindley, Comedy, 2004); and Mr Banks in *Mary Poppins* (Richard Eyre, Prince Edward, 2004-05).

Haig's screen roles, mostly comedies, show his versatility—in particular, he plays earnest, opinionated little men with relish. His performances in *Cracker* (ITV, 1993), *Four Weddings and a Funeral* (Mike Newell, 1994) and the situation comedies *Nice Day At The Office* (BBC, 1994) and *The Thin Blue Line* (BBC, 1995) are good examples. Dramatic roles have included Harold Nicolson in *Portrait of a Marriage* (BBC, 1990) and Luzhin in *Crime and Punishment* (BBC, 2002).

David Haig has written two plays for the Hampstead Theatre: *My Boy Jack* (1988), about Rudyard Kipling at the start of the Great War; and *The Good Samaritan* (2000).

Victoria Hamilton (b. Wimbledon, London, 1971) made a terrific splash as Hilde in Peter Hall's production of *The Master Builder* (Peter Hall Company, West End, 1995), playing opposite Alan Bates. Dark-eyed and petite, she has a refreshingly natural way of speaking dialogue, an expressiveness that sets her apart. Before *The Master Builder* she received the Critics' Circle Best Newcomer Award for her performances as Hannah in *Retreat* and Maria in *The Memorandum* at the Orange Tree (1995). She trained at the London Academy of Music and Dramatic Art.

At the RSC in 1996/97 she played Phebe in *As You Like It* (Steven Pimlott) and Cressida in *Troilus and Cressida* (Ian Judge, RST), both in partnership with Joseph Fiennes. Her Cressida was physically unguarded and tragically fallible (by confronting the character's contradictions she rejected the feminist reading favoured by actresses of the previous generation such as Juliet Stevenson). Reunited with Peter Hall as a member of his company at the Old Vic (1997) she won acclaim as Nina in *The Seagull*, Lady Brute in *The Provok'd Wife* and Cordelia in the Alan Howard *King Lear*. Her tender and touching Rosalind in Michael Grandage's Sheffield *As You Like It* (2000) was the finest of its time. Other theatre: Shaw's *The Doctor's Dilemma* (Grandage, Almeida, 1998); Clara in Edward Bulwer-Lytton's *Money* (John Caird, NT Olivier, 1999); slightly cloying (the adverse side of emotive acting) as Sheila in Peter Nichols's *A Day in the Life of Joe Egg* (Laurence Boswell, Comedy, 2001); Victoria in Somerset Maugham's *Home and Beauty* (Christopher Luscombe, Lyric, 2002); Clare in Stephen Poliakoff's *Sweet Panic* (Duke of York's, 2003); and Catherine in Tennessee Williams's *Suddenly Last Summer* (Grandage, Lyceum, Sheffield, 2004).

Amanda Harris (b. Adelaide, 1963) has been a leading actress at the RSC since 1986 when she played Emilia in the Swan's inaugural production, *The Two Noble Kinsmen* (Barry Kyle). In a 1985 BBC adaptation of *Oliver Twist* she was a very young Nancy, and she brought the same quality—toughness masking vulnerability—to the Shakespeare.

She was born in Australia, where her English father, a quantity surveyor, was working for the government. She was still a student when Declan Donnellan cast her as Desdemona in his Cheek By Jowl production of *Othello* (1982). She remained with the troupe for two years, playing, on tour and in repertory at the Donmar Warehouse, Amelia Sedley/Mrs Raggles in *Vanity Fair* (1983), Marina in *Pericles* (1984), and the title role in *Andromache* (1984). During her first RSC season, alongside Emilia, she played a bossy upper-class Hermia, first in a silk cocktail dress then tomboyish in a blue shirt and baggy trousers, in *A Midsummer Night's Dream* (Bill Alexander, RST); Gracielita alongside

Janet McTeer, Joely Richardson and Geraldine Fitzgerald in the Cuba of José Triana's *Worlds Apart* (Nick Hamm, TOP); Anne in Nigel Williamson's *Country Dancing* (Bill Alexander, TOP); Faith in Vladimir Gubaryev's *Sarcophagus* (Jude Kelly, Pit); and Sarah in Tony Marchant's *Speculators* (Kyle, Pit).

She returned in 1989/90 to play Ruby in Peter Flannery's *Singer* (Terry Hands, Swan) and Virgilia in the Charles Dance *Coriolanus* (Hands and John Barton, RST). Continuing, she was exceptional as Anna in *Barbarians* (David Jones, Barbican, 1990); as a wounded Kate, amazed to find love, in *The Taming of the Shrew* (Bill Alexander, RST, 1992); Penelope in Derek Walcott's version of *The Odyssey* (Gregory Doran, TOP, 1992); Meriel in *A Jovial Crew* (Max Stafford-Clark, Pit, 1993); and as the sexy librarian Cecily in Stoppard's *Travesties* (Adrian Noble, Barbican, 1993).

Following work at the Birmingham Rep (*The Servant*, Lady Macduff in *Macbeth* and Mrs Marwood in *The Way of the World*, all directed by Bill Alexander, 1994-95) and the Bristol Old Vic (the Countess in Terence Rattigan's *Flare Path*, 1995), she succeeded Lindsay Duncan as Hippolyta/Titania in Adrian Noble's RSC production of *A Midsummer Night's Dream* (Tour). In 1998 she played the lead—a woman who takes a young lover and is put on trial for the murder of her husband—in Neil Bartlett's production of Rattigan's *Cause Célèbre* (Lyric Hammersmith): her sensual performance was one of the hits of the season.

Her next projects were Gregory Doran's double-bill of Stoppard's *The Real Inspector Hound* and Shaffer's *Black Comedy* (Comedy, 1998); and four monologues by Jean Cocteau, *Take the Fire* (Paul Garrington, Lyric Hammersmith Studio, 1999). The first years of the new millennium saw her playing Lady Macbeth to Corin Redgrave's *Macbeth* (Tom Morris, Battersea Arts Centre, 2000); Regan to Bill Wallis's *King Lear* (Jan Sargent, Bristol Old Vic, 2000); the rapacious Lady Driver in Michael Frayn's *Donkeys' Years* (Salisbury Playhouse, 2002); and the mistress in Marivaux's *The Island of Slaves* (Neil Bartlett, Lyric Hammersmith, 2002). Back at the RSC, she was a tragic, drink-dependent

Emilia to Anthony Sher's Iago in Doran's *Othello* (Swan, 2004, Olivier Award); a decadent Titania in *A Midsummer Night's Dream* (Doran, RST, 2005); and Celia in *As You Like It* (Dominic Cooke, RST, 2005).

Howard Harrison (b. London) studied at the Central School of Speech and Drama. One of the contemporary theatre's outstanding lighting designers, Harrison creates effects that are eerily natural as well as breathtakingly beautiful—for example, it is impossible to forget the watery, pre-thunderstorm ambience of Adrian Noble's 1998 production of *The Tempest* conjured by Harrison and designer Anthony Ward.

Other RSC productions: Elijah Moshinsky's *The Lord of the Flies* (TOP, 1995); Gregory Doran's *Henry VIII* (Swan, 1996), *Cyrano de Bergerac* (Swan, 1997), *The Merchant of Venice* (RST, 1997), *Timon of Athens* (RST, 1999) and *As You Like It* (RST, 2000); Stephen Poliakoff's *Talk of the City* (Swan, 1998); Michael Attenborough's *The Prisoner's Dilemma* (TOP, 2001).

Lisa Harrow (b. Auckland, New Zealand, 1943) trained at RADA and was a member of the BBC Drama Repertory Company before joining the RSC for the 1969 Stratford season. She was cast straight away in good roles—Diana in *Pericles* (Terry Hands), Dorcas in *The Winter's Tale* (Trevor Nunn), and Olivia to Judi Dench's Viola in *Twelfth Night* (John Barton). At the Aldwych, the following year, she repeated Dorcas and Olivia and added The Hairdresser in Günter Grass's *The Plebeians Rehearse the Uprising* (David Jones), Sarah Undershaft in *Major Barbara* (Clifford Williams), and Anne Bullen in *Henry VIII* (Nunn).

She then played Queen Isobel in *Richard II* (Barton, RST and Theatregoround, 1971); Desdemona opposite Brewster Mason in *Othello* (Barton, RST, 1971); Natasha in *The Lower Depths* (Jones, Aldwych, 1972); Lady Amaranth in *Wild Oats* (Williams, Aldwych, 1976); and Portia to Patrick Stewart's Shylock in *The*

Merchant of Venice (Barton, Warehouse, 1979). She took part in Barton's *Playing Shakespeare* (Channel Four, 1984), and returned briefly in 1990 to play Glynis in Paula Milne's *Earwig* (Ron Daniels, Pit). She has appeared in such disparate movies as *All Creatures Great and Small* (1974); *Omen III: The Final Conflict* (1981); *Other Halves* (John Laing, 1984); *Shaker Run* (1985); *Always Afternoon* (1987); Gillian Armstrong's *The Last Days of Chez Nous* (1992); *That Eye, the Sky* (1994); and *Sunday* (1997).

Nigel Hawthorne (1929-2001). Born in Coventry but brought up in Cape Town, Nigel Hawthorne returned to England in his early twenties to pursue a career as an actor. For twenty years his progress was frustratingly devoid of real opportunities. Then, suddenly, one masterly creation—the Whitehall mandarin Sir Humphrey in *Yes, Minister* and *Yes, Prime Minister* (BBC, 1980-87)—placed him among the elite of British character actors. The following few years saw his finest work on the stage—Blair in Tom Stoppard's *Hapgood* (Peter Wood, Aldwych, 1988), C.S. Lewis opposite Jane Lapotaire in William Nicholson's *Shadowlands* (Elijah Moshinsky, Queen's, 1989), and George III in Alan Bennett's *The Madness of George III* (Nicholas Hytner, NT, 1992).

He first worked at the RSC in London in 1977/78, cast as Major Flack in Peter Nichols's *Privates on Parade* (Michael Blakemore, Aldwych), and Prins in *A Miserable and Lonely Death* (Walter Donohue, Warehouse). Then, in 1983/84, in the Barbican Pit, he played Solveig's Father in *Peer Gynt* (Ron Daniels), and Orgon in *Tartuffe* (Bill Alexander). His final return, in 1999, for *King Lear* (Barbican, RST) was wrecked by difficulties. It is clear from Hawthorne's autobiography that he was struggling with the culture shock of working with a Japanese director (Yukio Ninagawa) and opening in Tokyo.

James Hayes (b. Limerick, Ireland). A versatile character actor, James Hayes was for many years one of the National Theatre's small band of regular players, appearing in productions by John

Dexter—*The Good Natured Man* (Old Vic, 1971), *The Misanthrope* (Old Vic, 1973), *The Life of Galileo* (Olivier, 1980); Michael Blakemore—*Macbeth* (Old Vic, 1972), *The Front Page* (Old Vic, 1972), *Grand Manoeuvres* (Old Vic, 1974); Peter Hall—*Amadeus* (Olivier, 1979), *The Oresteia* (Olivier, 1981), *Coriolanus* (Olivier, 1984); Alan Ayckbourn—*A Chorus of Disapproval* (Olivier, 1985), *A View from the Bridge* (Cottesloe, 1987); and Michael Bogdanov—*The Romans in Britain* (Olivier, 1980), *The Spanish Tragedy* (Cottesloe, 1982), *Strider, the Story of a Horse* (Cottesloe, 1984). He was also in *The White Devil* (Frank Dunlop, Old Vic, 1969); *The Fawn* (Giles Block, Cottesloe, 1983); Peter Gill's *As I Lay Dying* (Gill, Cottesloe, 1985); *Othello* (Sam Mendes, Cottesloe and Salzburg Festival, 1997); *The Relapse* (Trevor Nunn, Olivier, 2001); and Shelagh Stephenson's *Mappa Mundi* (Bill Alexander, Cottesloe, 2002).

In the early 1990s Hayes joined Bogdanov's English Shakespeare Company to play an Irish Autolycus in *The Winter's Tale* (1991) and Sir Andrew Aguecheek in *Twelfth Night* (Michael Pennington, 1992). It was through Bogdanov that he formed his long association with the RSC: Brighella in Bogdanov's riotous production of Goldoni's *The Venetian Twins* (Swan, 1993); Antonio in *The Tempest* (Sam Mendes, RST, 1993); George Bernard Shaw in *Elgar's Rondo* (Di Trevis, Swan, 1993); Mr Mulleady in *The Hostage* (Bogdanov, Barbican, 1994); Gremio in *The Taming of the Shrew* (Gale Edwards, RST, 1995); Semyonov-Pishchik in *The Cherry Orchard* (Adrian Noble, Swan, 1995); Director/Chancellor in *Faust* (Bogdanov, Swan, 1995); Doctor in *Woyzeck* (Sean Holmes, TOP, 1996); Father Christmas/Air-raid Warden in *The Lion, the Witch and the Wardrobe* (Noble, RST, 1998); Old Shepherd in *The Winter's Tale* (Gregory Doran, RST, 1998); Escalus in *Measure for Measure* (Sean Holmes, RST, 2003); Stanley in *Richard III* (Holmes, RST, 2003); the 'Gunpowder' season (Swan, 2005)—Lisander in *A New Way to Please You* (Holmes), Sir Thomas Palmer in *Thomas Moore* (Robert Delamere), Sabinus in *Sejanus: His Fall* (Doran, Swan); and the Complete Works season (2006)—Lepidus in *Antony and Cleopatra* (Doran, Swan), the title role in *Julius Caesar* (Holmes, RST), Gonzalo in *The Tempest* (Rupert Gould, RST).

Guy Henry. An important member of the RSC since the beginning of the 1990s, the very tall Guy Henry is an original and incisive actor, with a gift for unexpected comedy.

He trained at RADA and gained wide theatre experience in provincial repertory (Windsor, Leeds, Salisbury, early 1980s): roles included Paris in *Romeo and Juliet*, Sergey in *Wild Honey*, Algernon in *The Importance of Being Earnest*, Alec in *Tess of the d'Urbervilles*, and Denis in *Loot*. His West End debut was as Delahay in Adrian Mitchell's *Another Country* (Queen's). He first came to notice at the National alongside three other future players of Adrian Noble's RSC—Paul Jesson, Mark Lockyer and Hugh Bonneville: Franciscus in *The Changeling* (Howard Davies, Lyttelton, 1988); Bartholomew Cokes in *Bartholomew Fair* (Richard Eyre, Olivier, 1988); Guildenstern in the Daniel Day-Lewis *Hamlet* (Eyre, Olivier, 1989); Denis Tregoning in *The Voysey Inheritance* (Richard Eyre, Cottesloe, 1989); and Sir Benjamin Backbite in *The School for Scandal* (Peter Wood, Olivier, 1990).

Henry moved to the RSC in 1991. He has given intelligent, finely-tuned performances as Sir Formal Trifle in *The Virtuoso* (Phyllida Lloyd, Swan, 1991); Thurio in *The Two Gentlemen of Verona* (David Thacker, Swan, 1991); Poggio in *'Tis Pity She's a Whore* (David Leveaux, Swan, 1991); Ananias in *The Alchemist* (Sam Mendes, Swan, 1991); a dignified Osric in the Branagh *Hamlet* (Adrian Noble, Barbican, 1992); Knight/Tempter in *Murder in the Cathedral* (Steven Pimlott, Swan, 1993); Lelio in *The Venetian Twins* (Michael Bogdanov, Swan, 1993); Longaville in *Love's Labour's Lost* (Ian Judge, RST, 1993); Sir Andrew Aguecheek in *Twelfth Night* (Ian Judge, Barbican, 1996); Lord Chamberlain in *Henry VIII* (Gregory Doran, Swan, 1996); Dr Caius in *The Merry Wives of Windsor* (Ian Judge, RST, 1996); a hilariously dim and over-confident Cloten in *Cymbeline* (Adrian Noble, RST, 1997); the title role in *King John* (Doran, Swan, 2001);

Malvolio in *Twelfth Night* (Lindsay Posner, RST, 2001); and Parolles/King John in *All's Well That Ends Well* (Doran, Swan, 2003-04).

Nicky Henson (b. London, 1945). The son of the great comedy actor and manager Leslie Henson, Nicky Henson was initially a pop singer and songwriter. While still at Charterhouse he formed a band called The Wombats with two friends from Eton, Ian Ogilvy and Michael Reeves (Reeves would later direct Henson and Ogilvy in the horror film *The Witchfinder General*), and released a single called 'Till I See You Cry' (1960).

The band never progressed beyond debutantes' balls and Henson moved into cabaret and musical theatre. He made his London debut in the revue *All Square*, alongside Beryl Reid (Vaudeville, 1963). He was next in the musicals *Camelot* (Drury Lane, 1964), *Passion Flower Hotel*, with Francesca Annis and Jane Birkin (Prince of Wales, 1965), and *The Canterbury Tales* (Phoenix, 1968-69). At the same time he worked prolifically in British sex comedies and horror films. In 1968 he married the *Till Death Us Do Part* actress Una Stubbs.

His career changed direction in 1970. He was one of a number of popular young stars recruited by Frank Dunlop to lead the first NT satellite company at the Young Vic (the aim was to attract a young audience to the classics). Over a two-year period he played leading roles in Molière's *Scapino* (the inaugural production, Dunlop, 1970); *Waiting for Godot*; *She Stoops to Conquer*; *The Taming of the Shrew*; *Measure for Measure*; *The Soldier's Tale*; *Oedipus*; *Romeo and Juliet*; Jean Genet's *The Maids* (Dunlop, 1972); *Look Back in Anger*; *Rosencrantz and Guildenstern are Dead*; and *Charley's Aunt*. He enhanced his theatre reputation elsewhere in the capital—*Ride Across Lake Constance* (Mayfair, 1973), *Hamlet* (Greenwich, 1973), *A Midsummer Night's Dream* (Regent's Park, 1973)—, returned to musicals—*Cinderella* (Casino, 1973), *Mardi Gras* (Prince of Wales, 1976)—, then began three years with the NT's South Bank company: Yepikhodov in *The Cherry Orchard*

(Peter Hall, Olivier, 1978); Malcolm in *Macbeth* (Hall, Olivier, 1978); Edward Bond's *The Woman* (Bond, Olivier, 1978); *The Double Dealer* (Peter Wood, Olivier, 1978); Middleton and Rowley's *A Fair Quarrel* (William Gaskill, Olivier, 1979); *The Browning Version* (Michael Rudman, Lyttelton, 1980); *The Elephant Man* (Roland Rees, Lyttelton, 1980); and Constant in *The Provok'd Wife* (Wood, Lyttelton, 1980).

In the decades since he has continued to show versatility in the theatre, alternating roles in the classics with light comedies and musicals: *Rookery Nook* (Her Majesty's, 1980); Michael Frayn's *Noises Off* (Savoy, 1982); *The Relapse* (Lyric, 1983); Dennis Potter's *Sufficient Carbohydrate* (Nancy Meckler, Hampstead, 1983); Niccolo Machiavelli's *Mandragola* (David Gilmore, NT Olivier, 1984); *Journey's End* (Whitehall, 1986); *Ivanov* and *Much Ado About Nothing* (Elijah Moshinsky, Strand, 1989); Vershinin, succeeding Michael Pennington, in *Three Sisters* (Adrian Noble, Royal Court, 1990); Roger Hall's *Conjugal Rites* (Palace Theatre, Watford, 1991); Panama in *Matador* (Elijah Moshinsky, Queen's, 1991); the actor in Ronald Harwood's *Reflected Glory* (Moshinsky, Vaudeville, 1992); the surgeon in Frayn's *Donkeys' Years* (Michael Rudman, Sheffield Crucible, 1993); Lord Goring, succeeding Martin Shaw, in *An Ideal Husband* (Hall, Globe, 1993); Dr Ellis in Richard Zajdlic's *Rage* (Mike Bradwell, Bush, 1994); Peter Kyle in Terence Rattigan's *Flare Path* (Andrew Hay, Bristol Old Vic, 1995); Craig Bohmler in Marion Adler's *Enter the Guardsman* (Jeremy Sams, Donmar Warehouse, 1997); Michael Frayn's *Alarms and Excursions* (Michael Blakemore, Gielgud, 1998); Pozzo in *Waiting for Godot* (Matthew Lloyd, Manchester Royal Exchange, 1999); Peter Nichols's *Passion Play* (Michael Grandage, Comedy, 2000); Keith Reddin's *Frame 312* (Josie Rourke, Donmar Warehouse, 2002); *One for the Pot* (Ray Cooney, Theatre Royal, Windsor, 2002); and the vice-chancellor, succeeding Jonathan Hyde, in Tom Stoppard's *Jumpers* (David Leveaux, Piccadilly, 2003).

He first appeared with the RSC in 1977, cast as Henry Straker in *Man and Superman* (Clifford Williams, Malvern Festival). He returned in 1985/86—Frank Ford in *The Merry Wives of Windsor* (Bill Alexander, RST); Touchstone in *As You Like It* (Adrian Noble, RST)—and again in 2005—Sir Toby Belch in *Twelfth Night* (Michael Boyd, RST).

Greg Hicks (b. Leicester, 1953) began his crowded theatre career with the fringe group Community Egg in Manchester. His early progress included such dissimilar roles as the Narrator in *Under Milk Wood* (London Theatre Company, 1974), Brandon in *Rope* (Derby Playhouse), Bosola in *The Duchess of Malfi* (Oval Theatre, Kennington, 1975), and Bernard in *Death of a Salesman* (Queen's Theatre, Hornchurch, 1975).

He was first at the RSC from 1976 to 1978, playing Balthazar in *Romeo and Juliet* (Trevor Nunn, RST); the Leader of the Watch in *Much Ado About Nothing* (John Barton, RST); Paris's Servant in *Troilus and Cressida* (Barton/Barry Kyle, RST); the Duke of Burgundy in *King Lear* (Nunn, RST); Doctor/Second Blonde in Charles Wood's *Dingo* (Kyle, TOP); Paul in David Edgar's *Destiny* (Ron Daniels, TOP); Donalbain/Seyton in the Ian McKellen *Macbeth* (Nunn, Warehouse); Roy/Phil in C.P. Taylor's *Bandits* (Howard Davies, Warehouse); Jean in Brecht's *Days of the Commune* (Davies, Aldwych); and Kaka/Water Seller 2 in Edward Bond's *The Bundle* (Davies, Warehouse).

He appeared in Arnold Wesker's *The Merchant* at the Birmingham Rep (1978), and then began an eight-year association with the National that saw him emerge as a leading actor: Mr Brisk in *The Double Dealer* (Peter Wood, 1978); Semyon in Tolstoy's *The Fruits of Enlightenment* (Christopher Morahan, Olivier, 1979); Otto in *Undiscovered Country* (Wood, Olivier, 1979); Silvius in *As You Like It* (John Dexter, Olivier, 1979); the Marquis of Dorset in *Richard III* (Morahan, Olivier, 1979); Venticelli in *Amadeus* (Peter Hall, Olivier, 1979); Melvyn in *Sisterly Feelings* (Ayckbourn, Olivier, 1980); Marban, the raped Druid, in Howard Brenton's *The Romans in Britain* (Michael Bogdanov, Olivier, 1980); Hector Malone in *Man and Superman* (Morahan, Olivier,

1981); Simon Chachava in *The Caucasian Chalk Circle* (Bogdanov, Cottesloe, 1982); Lorenzo in *The Spanish Tragedy* (Bogdanov, Cottesloe, 1982); the title role in Alfred de Mussett's *Lorenzaccio* (Bogdanov, Olivier, 1983); Malcolm in *Macbeth* (Bogdanov, Cottesloe, 1983); Tony Kirby in *You Can't Take It With You* (Bogdanov, Lyttelton, 1983); Snowball in *Animal Farm* (Hall, Cottesloe, 1984); Aufidius in *Coriolanus* (Hall, Olivier, 1984); Antonio in *The Duchess of Malfi* (Philip Prowse, Lyttelton, 1985); Simon Gascoyne in *The Real Inspector Hound* (Tom Stoppard, Olivier, 1985); Master of Horse/Beefeater in Sheridan's *The Critic* (Sheila Hancock, Olivier, 1985); and Yepikhodov in *The Cherry Orchard* (Mike Alfreds, Cottesloe, 1985).

Hicks succeeded Sean Bean as Romeo at the end of the London run of Bogdanov's RSC production of *Romeo and Juliet* (Barbican, 1987), and the following year played Valmont in *Les liaisons dangereuses* (Howard Davies, Ambassadors). His most significant performances of the 1990s were given for Philip Prowse at the Glasgow Citizens' and Peter Hall at the Old Vic. His Glasgow work included the title role in Luigi Pirandello's *Enrico IV* (1990); Otto in *Design for Living* (1991); Orestes in *1953* (1992); Eliot in *Private Lives* (1994); Flanders in *The Milk Train Doesn't Stop Here Anymore* (1994); and Loveless in *The Relapse* (1998). At the Old Vic (1997) he played Justin O'Connell in *Waste* (Hall); Medvedenko in *The Seagull* (Hall); Lucky in *Waiting for Godot* (Hall); Edgar in *King Lear* (Hall); and Carshalton in *Snake in the Grass* (Dominic Dromgoole). Elsewhere: the title role in *Macbeth* (Battersea Arts Centre, 1989); Gardel in *The Day You'll Love Me* (Lisa Forrell, Hampstead, 1990); *Vanilla* (Harold Pinter, Lyric, 1990); Teddy in *The Homecoming* (Hall, Comedy, 1991); Harry in Sarah Miles's *Charlemagne* (Old Fire Station, Oxford, 1992); Inspector Egan in *Murder by Misadventure* (Val May, Vaudeville, 1992); Paul Verlaine in *Total Eclipse* (Lisa Forrell, Greenwich Theatre, 1993); Vershinin in *Three Sisters* (Chichester, 1994); Hugh Marriner in *Absolute Hell* (Anthony Page, NT Lyttelton, 1995); Tiresias/Polynices in *The Oedipus Plays* (Hall, NT Olivier, 1996); Herod to Emily Woof's *Salomé* (Mick Gordon,

Riverside Studios, 1998); and Skelton in Peter Barnes's *Dreaming* (Matthew Lloyd, Manchester Royal Exchange, 1999).

Back at the RSC since the turn of the century Hicks has played—with typical style and consideration—Harry in T.S. Eliot's *The Family Reunion* (Adrian Noble, Swan, 1999); Agamemnon in John Barton's *Tantalus* (Peter Hall/Edward Hall, Denver Center for the Performing Arts, 2000); Brutus in *Julius Caesar* (Edward Hall, RST, 2001); Dr Caius in *The Merry Wives of Windsor* (Rachel Kavanaugh) paired with the title role in *Coriolanus* (David Farr, Swan and Small-scale Tour, 2002-03); and, leading Michael Boyd's first season (2004-05), the title role in *Macbeth* (Dominic Cooke), Ghost/Player King/Gravedigger in *Hamlet* (Boyd, RST), and Cinyras in Joanna Laurens's *Poor Beck* (Daniel Fish, TOP).

Anastasia Hille (b. London) has concentrated on the classics. Her first leading roles were Lady Macbeth opposite Alan Howard in *Macbeth* (Richard Eyre, NT Olivier, 1993); the youngest of Edward Albee's *Three Tall Women* (Wyndham's, 1994); an aristocratic but vulnerable Duchess, chain-smoking cigarettes, in Declan Donnellan's 1930s *The Duchess of Malfi* (Cheek By Jowl, Tour, 1995); an elegant Silvia to Mark Rylance's Proteus in *The Two Gentlemen of Verona*, the Globe's opening production (Jack Shepherd, 1996); Charlotte Corday in *Marat/Sade* (Jeremy Sams, NT Olivier, 1997); Beatrice in Giorgio Battistelli's fusion of music and drama *The Cenci* (Almeida, 1997); and a fine Rosalind in *As You Like It* (Lucy Bailey, Globe, 1998).

In 1998 she joined the RSC to play Yelena in Katie Mitchell's *Uncle Vanya* (Young Vic). As lithe and body-conscious as a model, she conveyed the paradox of a woman who needs to be watched and desired but who finds such scrutiny oppressive. Her subsequent work has included four productions by Mitchell: Claire in Genet's *The Maids* (Mitchell, Young Vic, 1999); Clytemnestra in *The Oresteia* (Mitchell, NT Cottesloe, 1999); Louisa in Charlotte Jones's *The Dark* (Anna Mackmin,

Donmar Warehouse, 2004); Diana in Kevin Elyot's *Forty Winks* (Mitchell, Royal Court, 2004); and Christine in Strindberg's *A Dream Play* (Mitchell, NT Cottesloe, 2005). The role of Hermione in *The Winter's Tale* enticed her back to the RSC in 2002 (Matthew Warchus, Roundhouse).

Anastasia Hille's work on screen has included Andy Hamilton's football satire *Eleven Men Against Eleven* (Channel Four, 1995); *Drovers' Gold* (Lesley Manning/Tristram Powell, BBC, 1997); Lynda La Plante's *Trial and Retribution* (ITV, 1997); *A Dance to the Music of Time* (Channel Four, 1997); Fay Weldon's *Big Women* (Renny Rye, Channel Four, 1998); *The Wisdom of Crocodiles* (Po-Chih Leong, 1998); one of Daniel Auteuil's clients in *Mauvaise passe* (Michel Blanc, 1999); Carole Lombard in *RKO 281* (Benjamin Ross, 1999); and *The Cazalets* (BBC, 2001).

Louis Hilyer (b. Coventry) appeared with the Belgrade Youth Theatre before training for the stage at RADA. His early work in provincial repertory included Nicholas Hytner's *Edward II* at the Manchester Royal Exchange (1986), and Stephen Daldry's *Of Mice and Men* at the Library Theatre, Manchester (1988). His performance as Curley in the latter led to further work with Daldry: a season at the Gate in Notting Hill—Genesius in *The Great Pretenders* (Laurence Boswell, 1991); Juan Pedro in Griselda Gambaro's *Bad Blood* (Kate Rowland, 1992)—and the role of Gerald Croft in *An Inspector Calls* at the National (Lyttelton, 1992).

In 1988 he joined the cast of the RSC's production of *Les liaisons dangereuses* (Howard Davies, Ambassadors)—he played Danceny, and then (1990) the leading role of Valmont. He has worked regularly with the Company since 1996: Hector in *Troilus and Cressida* (Ian Judge, RST, 1996); Tranio in *The Taming of the Shrew* (Lindsay Posner, Small-scale Tour, 2000); Fraser Cullen in Peter Whelan's *A Russian in the Woods* (Robert Delamere, TOP, 2001); Sir Simon Addleplot in *Love in a Wood* (Tim Supple, Swan, 2001—his wife, Matilda Ziegler, played Olivia in that season's *Twelfth Night*); and a leading member of Michael Boyd's first 'core' company (2004/05)—Banquo in *Macbeth* (Dominic Cooke) and Kent in *King Lear* (Bill Alexander, RST).

Other theatre: Archer in *The Beaux' Stratagem* (Stephen Unwin, English Touring Theatre, 1994); Alan in *French Without Tears* (Christopher Luscombe, Palace Theatre, Watford, 1995); Harcourt in *The Country Wife* (Boswell, The Touring Partnership, 1997); Golovan in *Flight* (Howard Davies, NT Lyttelton, 1998); Danton in Pam Gems's *The Snow Palace* (Janet Suzman, Tour and Tricycle Theatre, 1998); and Caliban in the Derek Jacobi *Tempest* (Michael Grandage, Sheffield Crucible, 2002).

Ian Hogg (b. Newcastle, 1937) trained at the Central School of Speech and Drama and the Drama Centre, London. His RSC career began in 1964 with an unnamed part in Marlowe's *The Jew of Malta* (Clifford Williams, RST). He became a member of the RSC's experimental wing under Peter Brook, appearing in *Marat/Sade* (Aldwych, 1964), *The Investigation* (Aldwych, 1965), and the controversial anti-Vietnam war piece *US* (Aldwych, 1966). Between and after the Brook work he was cast in Shakespeare productions at the RST and new plays at the Aldwych: Rugby in *The Merry Wives of Windsor* (John Blatchley, Aldwych, 1964); Jammy in *Henry V* (John Barton/Trevor Nunn, Aldwych, 1965); Major Friedli in Friedrich Dürrenmatt's *The Meteor* (Williams, Aldwych, 1966); Sea Captain in Robert Bolt's *The Thwarting of Baron Bolligrew* (Nunn, Aldwych, 1966); Adrian in *Coriolanus* (Barton, RST, 1967); Lavache in *All's Well That Ends Well* (Barton, RST, 1967); Seyton in the Scofield *Macbeth* (Peter Hall, RST, 1967); Tybalt in the Holm/Kohler *Romeo and Juliet* (Karolos Koun, RST, 1967); Lester in *The Latent Heterosexual* (Terry Hands, Aldwych, 1968); James Ames in Jules Feiffer's *God Bless* (Geoffrey Reeves, Aldwych, 1968); Edmund in Brook's film of his 1962 *King Lear* (1970); the title role in *Coriolanus* (Nunn/Buzz Goodbody, RST, 1972); and Lucius in *Titus Andronicus* (Goodbody/Nunn, RST, 1972). Hogg left the RSC in

1972 and did not play Coriolanus in London (Nicol Williamson replaced him).

In the 1970s, 80s and 90s he followed a screen career, delivering expert cameo performances in *The Hireling* (Joseph Losey, 1973); *Dead Cert* (1974); *Hennessy* (1975); *Meetings with Remarkable Men* (Brook, 1979); *Lady Jane* (Nunn, 1986); *The Pleasure Principle* (1991); *Rasputin* (1996); and *Forgotten* (Ben Bolt, ITV, 1999). His most prominent role was Rockcliffe in the television series *Rockcliffe's Babies* (1987). On the stage, he played Howard in Somerset Maugham's *For Services Rendered* (Michael Rudman, NT Lyttelton, 1979); Kent in *King Lear* (Jonathan Miller, Old Vic, 1989); the Senator in *Insignificance* (Terry Johnson, Donmar Warehouse, 1995); and Talbot in *Mary Stuart* (Howard Davies, NT Lyttelton, 1996).

From 1996 to 2002, back at the RSC, Hogg was in powerful form playing Wolsey in *Henry VIII* (Gregory Doran, Swan, 1996); Belarius in *Cymbeline* (Noble, RST, 1997); Duke Senior/Duke Frederick in *As You Like It* (Doran, RST, 2000); Capulet in *Romeo and Juliet* (Michael Boyd, RST, 2000); and the title role in *Julius Caesar* (Edward Hall, RST, 2001).

Theatre work since 2002: the French King in *Henry V* (Nicholas Hytner, NT Olivier, 2003); the Duke of Alba in *Don Carlos* (Grandage, Sheffield Crucible, 2004).

Ian Holm (b. Goodmayes, Ilford, 1931) had been absent from the classical stage for nearly twenty years when he joined the National to play King Lear in Richard Eyre's studio production (Cottesloe, 1997). His masterly account of the role was greeted by many as a landmark, the return of a great classical actor. But Holm had never been away, just in another medium. Constantly in demand, he worked for filmmakers as distinguished as Ridley Scott, Terry Gilliam, Woody Allen, David Cronenberg, Steven Soderbergh, Atom Egoyan, Danny Boyle and Luc Besson.

Holm's association with Stratford began in the 1950s. He was the product of five seasons of supporting roles: a soldier in *Othello* (1954); Harold Rabbit in *Toad of Toad Hall* (a rare London production for the SMT company, Princes Theatre, 1954); Page in *All's Well That Ends Well* (Noel Willman, 1955); Donalbain in the Laurence Olivier *Macbeth* (Glen Byam Shaw, 1955); Mutius in the Olivier *Titus Andronicus* (Peter Brook, 1955); Sebastian in *Twelfth Night* (Peter Hall, 1958); Peter in *Romeo and Juliet* (Shaw, 1958); Second Player in the Michael Redgrave *Hamlet* (Shaw, 1958); Verges in *Much Ado About Nothing* (Douglas Seale, 1958); Duke of Venice in the Paul Robeson/Mary Ure/Sam Wanamaker *Othello* (Tony Richardson, 1959); Puck in *A Midsummer Night's Dream* (Hall, 1959); Fourth Roman Citizen in the Olivier *Coriolanus* (Hall, 1959); and Fool in the Charles Laughton *King Lear* (Shaw, RST, 1959).

By 1960 Holm was ready to lead a generational change in the acting of Shakespeare. His performances as Richard of Gloucester/Richard III in *The Wars of the Roses* (Hall, 1963-64) and as the first non-heroic Hal/Henry V in the 1964 history cycle, classical in technique but contemporary in style, helped to define Peter Hall's RSC. He was also Lorenzo in *The Merchant of Venice* (Michael Langham, 1960); Sebastian in *Twelfth Night* (Hall, 1960); Gremio in the Peggy Ashcroft/Peter O'Toole *The Taming of the Shrew* (John Barton, 1960); First Judge in *Ondine* (Hall, RST, 1961); Mannoury in John Whiting's *The Devils* (Peter Wood, Aldwych, 1961); Little Monk in *Becket* (Hall, Aldwych, 1961); Trofimov in *The Cherry Orchard*, alongside Ashcroft, Gielgud, Dorothy Tutin and Judi Dench (Michel Saint-Denis, RST, 1961); Claudio in *Measure for Measure* (John Blatchley, RST, 1962); Troilus in *Troilus and Cressida* (Hall, Aldwych, 1962); Ariel in *The Tempest* (Clifford Williams with Peter Brook, RST, 1963); Lenny in Harold Pinter's *The Homecoming* (Hall, Aldwych, 1965-66); Witness 8 in Peter Weiss's *The Investigation* (Brook and David Jones, 1965); Malvolio in *Twelfth Night* (Williams, RST, 1966); and Romeo opposite Estelle Kohler in *Romeo and Juliet* (Karolos Koun, RST, 1967).

Holm played Puck in Peter Hall's RSC film of *A Midsummer Night's Dream* (1968) and then left Stratford. His next stage appearances were in contemporary plays: Manfred in Arnold Wesker's *The Friends* (Roundhouse, 1970); Nelson in Terence Rattigan's *A Bequest to the Nation* (Theatre Royal Haymarket, 1970); Hatch in Edward Bond's *The Sea* (William Gaskill, Royal Court, 1973); and Dave in Mike Stott's *Other People* (Hampstead, 1974). In 1976, back at the RSC, he dried badly during a performance of *The Iceman Cometh* (Howard Davies, Aldwych) and, his confidence shattered, withdrew from the production. His only stage appearance for almost two decades was as Astrov in Pam Gems's version of *Uncle Vanya* (Nancy Meckler, Hampstead, 1979). He ended his exile in 1993 to create the role of Andy in Harold Pinter's short play *Moonlight* (David Leveaux, Almeida). Then came the acclaimed Lear. In the years since only Pinter has been able to persuade Holm to pause one of the most prolific and richly diverse bodies of work in movies. He played Duff in *Landscape* (Pinter, Gate, Dublin, and NT Cottesloe, 1994) and Max in *The Homecoming* (Robin Lefevre, Gate, Dublin, and Comedy, 2001). Some writers creep into an actor's psyche and Holm can claim both Shakespeare and Pinter. As imagined by Holm, Richard III and Lenny, Lear and Max, merge into one another across the centuries.

Clare Holman (b. 1964) has appeared in major stage productions, television dramas and films—there are few routine or forgettable pieces in her list of credits. Her early roles included the Player Queen in *Hamlet* and Ophelia in Tom Stoppard's *Rosencrantz and Guildenstern are Dead* for the Oxford Stage Company; Cécile, alongside Jonathan Hyde and Samantha Bond, in Howard Davies's RSC production of *Les liaisons dangereuses* in the West End (Ambassadors, 1987); and Mabel in Brian Friel's *Making History* for Field Day (Simon Curtis, Irish Tour and NT Cottesloe, 1988). She joined the National proper in 1990 to play a fiery, sensual Abigail in Arthur Miller's *The Crucible* (Davies, Olivier).

At the RSC, during the 1990s, she brought to life four of Shakespeare's young heroines: Julia in *The Two Gentlemen of Verona* (David Thacker, Swan, 1991); Juliet opposite Michael Maloney in *Romeo and Juliet* (David Leveaux, RST, 1991); a bespectacled Olivia in *Twelfth Night* (Adrian Noble, RST, 1997); and Isabella in *Measure for Measure* (Michael Boyd, RST, 1998). Between RSC seasons she played Greta in Klaus Pohl's *Karate Billy Comes Home* (Stephen Unwin, Royal Court, 1992); Steph in Meredith Oakes's *The Neighbour* (John Burgess, NT Cottesloe, 1993); Harper in Tony Kushner's *Angels in America* (Declan Donnellan, NT Cottesloe, 1993); Honey in the David Suchet/Diana Rigg *Who's Afraid of Virginia Woolf?* (Davies, Almeida, 1996); Elisa in Yasmina Reza's *Conversations after a Burial* (Davies, Almeida, 2000); Magda in David Farr's *The Danny Crowe Show* (Bush, 2001); Elmire in *Tartuffe* (Lindsay Posner, NT Lyttelton, 2002); the Wife in Carlo Gébler's *Ten Rounds* (Nicolas Kent, Tricycle, 2002); and Margarita in *The Master and Margarita* (Steven Pimlott, Chichester, 2004).

She has had some good opportunities in British films: the sister in *Let Him Have It* (Peter Medak, 1991); Rose in *Afraid of the Dark* (Mark Peploe, 1991); Louise Purdon in *Tom and Viv* (Brian Gilbert, 1994); and *Dot.Kill* (John Irvin, 2004).

Television: Gudrun to Imogen Stubbs's Ursula in Ann Devlin's adaptation of *The Rainbow* (Stuart Burge, BBC, 1988); *The Woman in Black* (Herbert Wise, 1989); *Close Relations* (Adrian Shergold, 1990); the plum role, beautifully executed, of a feisty MP, determined to ban fox hunting, in *Giving Tongue* (1996); an adulterous wife in Jimmy McGovern's *The Lakes* (BBC, 1997); *Big Women* (Channel Four, 1988); the pathologist in *Morse* and *Lewis* (ITV, 1995-08); *David Copperfield* (BBC, 1999); Ruth Rendell's *Harm Done* (ITV, 2000); Catherine Parr in *Henry VIII* (ITV, 2003); *Prime Suspect 6* (ITV, 2003); *Island at War* (Thaddeus O'Sullivan, ITV, 2004); *Messiah 3* (BBC, 2004); *The Ghost Squad* (Channel Four, 2005); *New Tricks* (BBC, 2006); *Fallen Angel* (ITV, 2007).

John Hopkins (b. London, 1974) read English at Leeds University and joined the RSC soon after graduating from RADA in 2001. His potential became clear at once: the Dauphin in *King John* (Gregory Doran, Swan), Vincent's Man in *Love in a Wood* (Tim Supple, Swan) and Octavius Caesar in *Julius Caesar* (Edward Hall, RST); followed by Claudio in *Much Ado About Nothing* (Doran) and Dolabella in *Antony and Cleopatra* (Michael Attenborough, RST, 2002).

He worked in television for a few years (most prominently as John Nettles's sidekick in *Midsomer Murders*, ITV, 2004-05) and then returned to the RSC to play Octavius Caesar in *Antony and Cleopatra* (Doran) and Sebastian in *The Tempest* (Rupert Goold, RST, 2006). Hopkins brings to the stage the kind of individuality and presence that creates an illusion of unpredictability. His Claudio in *Much Ado About Nothing* had no redeeming features, treating Kirsten Parker's Hero with contempt and cruelty; and he made Octavius in *Antony and Cleopatra* a young man wracked by emotional conflict over his treatment of his sister and his destruction of Antony.

Michael Hordern (1911-1995, b. Berkhamsted, Hertfordshire) possessed one of the great Shakespearean voices of the 20th century, along with wisdom, imagination and, when appropriate, a glorious eccentricity. In real life he looked like a country squire; on the stage, as King Lear, as Don Armado, he existed in a melancholy realm of the imagination all his own.

As a young man he was first a schoolmaster and then a travelling salesman, although he acted as an amateur with the St Pancras People's Theatre. He made his professional debut in 1937 at the People's Palace, east London, playing Lodovico in *Othello*, and later in the year joined the repertory company of the Little Theatre in Bristol. It was here that he met his future wife, the actress Eve Mortimer. After the hiatus of the war years—he served in the Royal Navy—he resumed his career on

the stage, quickly winning the important role of Bottom in Pur-
cell's *The Fairy Queen* at Covent Garden (1946).

It was now, playing Toad in *Toad of Toad Hall*, his Stratford
debut (John Franklyn, 1948-49, John Kidd, 1949-50), the title role
in Chekhov's *Ivanov* (Arts, 1950), and, especially, Paul South-
man in John Whiting's *Saint's Day* (Arts, 1951), that Hordern
started to build his reputation as a performer whose formidable
range included a singular talent for inhabiting any degree of
mental disquiet, from the dotty to the deranged. As he grew
older, his face, full of character, looked as if it had been crum-
pled up and creased out as best as possible. Much of his work of
the 1950s belonged to the classics, particularly Shakespeare. At
Stratford, 1952, he played Menenius Agrippa in *Coriolanus* (Glen
Byam Shaw), Caliban in *The Tempest* (Michael Benthall), an acclaimed Jaques in *As You Like It* (Shaw), and Sir Politick in
Volpone (George Devine). Moving to the Old Vic (1953-54; 1958-
59), he was Polonius in the Richard Burton *Hamlet* (Benthall),
Parolles in *All's Well That Ends Well* (Benthall), King John (De-
vine), Malvolio in *Twelfth Night* (Denis Carey), Prospero in *The
Tempest* (Robert Helpmann), Cassius in *Julius Caesar*, Pastor
Manders in Ibsen's *Ghosts*, Macbeth, and Mr Posket in Pinero's
The Magistrate (Douglas Seale).

But Hordern kept half an eye on new writing. For the RSC, at
the Aldwych, as well as playing Ulysses in *Troilus and Cressida*
(Peter Hall, 1962) and the Father in Strindberg's *Playing With
Fire* (John Blatchley, 1962), he was Harry in Harold Pinter's *The
Collection* (Hall/Pinter, 1962), Herbert Beutler in Friedrich Dürrenmatt's *The Physicists* (Peter Brook, 1963), and Tobias in
Edward Albee's *A Delicate Balance* (Hall, 1969). Elsewhere, he
created roles for Alan Ayckbourn (Philip in *Relatively Speaking*,
Duke of York's, 1967), David Mercer (the vicar in *Flint*, Criterion, 1970), Howard Barker (the judge in *Stripwell*, Royal Court,
1975), and Tom Stoppard (George in *Enter a Free Man*, St Martin's, 1968; George Moore in *Jumpers*, NT Old Vic, 1972).

Hordern's fine Lear—his compassionate understanding of
the character was evident throughout—was directed by Jona-

than Miller, at the Nottingham Playhouse in 1970, and for the BBC in 1982. In 1978 he returned to Stratford to play a wise, caring Prospero in *The Tempest* (Williams), and, lost in the fantasy, Don Armado in *Love's Labour's Lost* (John Barton). In 1983, at the National, he was in brilliant comic form as the lecherous, cane-wielding Sir Anthony Absolute in Sheridan's *The Rivals* (Peter Wood, Olivier).

Hordern worked prolifically in movies. The following selection includes the best known (he supported Richard Burton on eight occasions): *Passport to Pimlico* (1949); Graham Greene's *The Heart of the Matter* (1953); *The Beachcomber* (1954); *Storm Over the Nile* (1955); *Alexander the Great* (1956); *I Was Monty's Double* (1958); *Sink the Bismark!* (Lewis Gilbert, 1960); *El Cid* (Anthony Mann, 1961); *Cleopatra* (Joseph L. Mankiewicz, 1963); Terence Rattigan's *The V.I.P.s* (Anthony Asquith, 1963); Rattigan's *The Yellow Rolls-Royce* (Asquith, 1964); *The Spy Who Came in from the Cold* (Martin Ritt, 1965); *Khartoum* (1966); *A Funny Thing Happened on the Way to the Forum* (Richard Lester, 1966); Baptista in *The Taming of the Shrew* (Franco Zeffirelli, 1967); *How I Won the War* (Lester, 1967); *Where Eagles Dare* (1968); *The Bed-Sitting Room* (Lester, 1969); *Anne of the Thousand Days* (1969); *Up Pompeii* (1971); *Theatre of Blood* (1973); *The MacKintosh Man* (John Huston, 1973); Graham Greene's *England Made Me* (1973); the narrator of Stanley Kubrick's *Barry Lyndon* (1975); *Lucky Lady* (Stanley Donen, 1975); *Joseph Andrews* (Tony Richardson, 1977); *The Medusa Touch* (Jack Gold, 1978); *The Missionary* (1982); *Gandhi* (Richard Attenborough, 1982); *Lady Jane* (Trevor Nunn, 1986); *Comrades* (Bill Douglas, 1987); *The Fool* (Christine Edzard, 1990).

Television: the narrator of *Paddington* (BBC, 1975); Capulet in *Romeo and Juliet* (BBC, 1978); Prospero in *The Tempest* (BBC, 1980); *Shogun* (1980); *The History Man* (BBC, 1981); Lafeu in *All's Well That Ends Well* (BBC, 1981); Simeon Simcox in John Mortimer's *Paradise Postponed* (ITV, 1986); Evelyn Waugh's *Scoop* (Gavin Millar, ITV, 1987); *Inspector Morse* (ITV, 1987); Stoppard's *The Dog It Was That Died* (Peter Wood, ITV, 1988); Kingsley Amis's *Ending Up* (ITV, 1989); *Danny, the Champion of the World*

(Millar, ITV, 1989); *The Green Man* (Elijah Moshinsky, BBC, 1990); and Peter Featherstone in *Middlemarch* (BBC, 1994).

William Houston (b. Sussex, 1968). One of the finds of Adrian Noble's regime, William Houston was the first RSC actor since Alan Howard to play Hal in both parts of *Henry IV* (Michael Attenborough, Swan) and *Henry V* (Edward Hall, RST, 2000-01).

The son of Northern Irish Protestants, he was born in Sussex but lived in Ulster from the age of six. He trained at Central and initially appeared at the Salisbury Playhouse (Belyaev in *A Month in the Country*; *Abel versus Cain*). At the Bush Theatre in 1993 he played Pierce in Helen Edmundson's *The Clearing*. He joined the RSC in 1994. Following the small roles of Manus in Ann Devlin's *After Easter* (Attenborough, TOP), Wilding's Footman in *The Wives' Excuse* (Max Stafford-Clark, Swan), and Prophilus in John Ford's *The Broken Heart* (Michael Boyd, Swan), he came into his own as Laertes in the Alex Jennings *Hamlet* (Matthew Warchus, RST, 1997) and Troilus in *Troilus and Cressida* (Boyd, Pit, 1998). Since Henry V, Houston has played Titus Flaminius in Philip Massinger's *Believe What You Will* (Josie Rourke), the title role in Ben Jonson's *Sejanus* (Gregory Doran) and King James in Frank McGuinness's *Speaking Like Magpies* (Rupert Goold, all Swan, 2005); and the title role in *Coriolanus* (Doran, RST, 2007).

Alan Howard (b. London, 1937). Even if Alan Howard never performs at Stratford again he will always be considered first and foremost an RSC actor, the result of almost twenty years of continuous work (1966-85). He is particularly identified with Shakespeare's kings, but was also the central figure in some of the finest work of Trevor Nunn (*The Revenger's Tragedy*), Peter Brook (*A Midsummer Night's Dream*) and Adrian Noble (*The Forest*). He reinvented main house Shakespearean acting for a new age, sardonic, ambiguous and questioning.

Howard comes from a family of achievers in the arts. His great-grandfather was the actor-manager Edward Compton, a Stratford player from 1879, the inaugural year, to 1882, and director of the 1881 and 1882 festivals. His great-uncle was the novelist Compton Mackenzie, and his uncle the film star Leslie Howard. He gained his initial experience at the Belgrade Theatre, Coventry (1958-59), where his roles included Frankie Bryant in Arnold Wesker's *Roots*. He went with the Belgrade Company to the Royal Court to perform the whole of Wesker's Trilogy— *Roots* (1959), *Chicken Soup with Barley* (1960) and *I'm Talking About Jerusalem* (1960), all directed by John Dexter—and then stayed on to play de Piraquo in *The Changeling* (Tony Richardson, 1961). A member of Laurence Olivier's prototype National Theatre company at the first Chichester Festival in 1962 he played the Duke of Ferrara in John Fletcher's *The Chances*, Nearchis in John Ford's *The Broken Heart* and Loveless in Vanbrugh's *Virtue in Danger*. His affinity for Shakespeare was revealed in 1964 when he toured Europe as Lysander in *A Midsummer Night's Dream* and Bassanio in *The Merchant of Venice*. In 1965 he played Simon in Julian Mitchell's *A Heritage and its History* (Phoenix) and appeared at the Nottingham Playhouse as Angelo in *Measure for Measure* and Bolingbroke in *Richard II*.

Howard's RSC career can be divided into two phases. The first revealed an impressive range: Orsino opposite Diana Rigg (Viola) and Estelle Kohler (Olivia) in *Twelfth Night* (Clifford Williams, RST, 1966); the Duke of Burgundy in the Ian Holm *Henry V* (John Barton/Trevor Nunn, RST, 1966); Lussurioso in *The Revenger's Tragedy* (Nunn, RST, 1966); Jaques in *As You Like It* (David Jones, RST, 1967); Young Fashion in John Vanbrugh's *The Relapse* (Nunn, Aldwych, 1967); Edgar in the Eric Porter *King Lear* (Nunn, RST, 1968); Achilles in *Troilus and Cressida* (Barton, RST, 1968); Benedick to Janet Suzman's Beatrice in *Much Ado About Nothing* (Nunn, RST, 1968); Bartholomew Cokes in Ben Jonson's *Bartholomew Fair* (Terry Hands, Aldwych, 1969); Mephostophiles in Marlowe's *Doctor Faustus* (Gareth Morgan, Theatregoround and RST, 1970); the title role in *Hamlet* (Nunn,

RST, 1970); Theseus/Oberon in *A Midsummer Night's Dream* (Peter Brook, RST, 1970); Ceres in *The Tempest* (Barton, RST, 1970); Nikolai in Gorky's *Enemies* (Jones, Aldwych, 1971); Dorimant in George Etherege's *The Man of Mode* (Hands, Aldwych, 1971); the Envoy in Jean Genet's *The Balcony* (Hands, Aldwych, 1971); and Carlos II in Peter Barnes's *The Bewitched* (Hands, Aldwych, 1974).

The second phase was dominated by his psychologically astute performances in Terry Hands's productions of the Histories: Hal in *Henry IV* and *Henry V* (RST, 1975); Jack Rover in John O'Keeffe's *Wild Oats* (Williams, Aldwych, 1976); *Henry VI* (RST, 1977); *Coriolanus* (RST, 1977); Antony in *Antony and Cleopatra* (Brook, RST, 1978); Boris in Gorky's *The Children of the Sun* (Hands, Aldwych, 1979); *Richard II* and *Richard III* (RST, 1980); Neschastlivsev in Ostrovsky's *The Forest* (Adrian Noble, TOP, 1981); Halder in C.P. Taylor's *Good* (Howard Davies, Warehouse, 1981); and Nikolai, succeeding Daniel Massey, in Stephen Poliakoff's *Breaking the Silence* (Ron Daniels, Mermaid, 1985).

In 1990 he starred in *The Silver King* and *Scenes From a Marriage* at Chichester. Since 1992 he has worked most prominently at National, the Almeida, and for Peter Hall at the Old Vic: Professor Higgins in *Pygmalion* (Davies, Olivier, 1992); Christopher Logue's version of Homer's *Iliad* called *Kings* (Liane Aukin, Cottesloe, 1992); the title role in *Macbeth* (Richard Eyre, Olivier, 1993); *Les parents terribles* (Sean Mathias, Lyttelton, 1994); Calogero in *La grande magia* (Eyre, Lyttelton, 1995); Vladimir to Ben Kingsley's Estragon in *Waiting for Godot*, and the title role in *King Lear* (Peter Hall, Old Vic, 1997); *Flight* (Davies, Lyttelton, 1998); Man in Edward Albee's *The Play About the Baby* (Davies, Almeida, 1998); the father in *The Heiress* (Philip Franks, Lyttelton, 2000); Schoning in *Lulu* (Jonathan Kent, Almeida at King's Cross, 2001); and Gabriel in Frank McGuinness's *Gates of Gold* (Gate, Dublin, 2002). The 2000s saw two brief returns to the RSC: the right-wing poet in Sean O'Brien's verse drama *Keepers of the Flame* (Max Roberts, Live Theatre, Newcastle, 2003); and *The Hollow Crown* (Barton, RST, 2005).

His best screen work was filmed during the 1980s: the title role in *Coriolanus* (BBC, 1984); Maurice Wilkins alongside Juliet Stevenson and Jeff Goldblum in *Life Story* (Mick Jackson, BBC, 1987); Jack Brotherhood in John le Carré's *A Perfect Spy* (BBC, 1987); and Richard opposite Helen Mirren in *The Cook, the Thief, His Wife and Her Lover* (Peter Greenaway, 1989).

Richard Hudson (b. Zimbabwe, 1954). A graduate of the Wimbledon School of Art, Richard Hudson first came to prominence as Jonathan Miller's resident designer at the Old Vic, where he produced striking abstract sets (geometric structures and angled walls) for *Too Clever By Half* (Richard Jones) and *King Lear* (Miller, 1988).

At the RSC he worked with Adrian Noble on three acclaimed productions: *The Master Builder* (Barbican, 1989), *Travesties* (Barbican, 1993) and *The Cherry Orchard* (Swan, 1995). Also: Ron Daniels's *A Clockwork Orange* (Barbican, 1990); Laurence Boswell's *Women Beware Women* (Swan, 2006); and Gregory Doran's *Coriolanus* (RST, 2007).

Elsewhere: Graham Rick's *The Queen of Spades* and *Eugene Onegin* at Glyndebourne (1992, 1994); the multi-award winning success of *The Lion King* (Julie Taymor, 1997); and Kim Brandstrup's *Rushes* at the Royal Ballet (2008), for which Hudson created a beautifully simple monochrome setting of two aluminium bead curtains that were lit (by Jean Kalman) to seem solid one moment, transparent the next.

Ian Hughes (b. Merthyr Tydfil) was a member of the National Youth Theatre of Wales. On graduating from Birmingham University, he gained his early experience on provincial stages (Cardiff, York, Manchester and Coventry): roles included Dennis in *Habeas Corpus*, John Darling in *Peter Pan*, Razor in *The Provok'd Wife*, Frank in *Mrs Warren's Profession*, and Buttons in

Cinderella. On tour he played the title role in *The Fool* (East Midlands/Southern Arts), Mercutio in *Romeo and Juliet* (Wales Actors' Company), and Eros in *Antony and Cleopatra* (British Actors' Company). At the Soho Poly in 1989 he was Charlie in Daniel Scott's *Below the Belt* (Ruth Garnault), Tassi in Dei Treanor's *Redefining the Whore* (Mark Ravenhill), and Evans in Rufus Orishayomi's *Wush Way* (Orishayomi).

It was his Ian Charleson Award-winning performance in *Tasso* (ATC, Lyric Hammersmith, 1990) that brought him to the attention of the RSC. As a member of Adrian Noble's first company, 1991-92, he played John of Lancaster in *Henry IV* (Noble, RST); Sebastian in *Twelfth Night* (Griff Rhys Jones, RST); Messenger in *The Thebans* (Noble, Swan); Tybalt in *Romeo and Juliet* (David Leveaux, Barbican); and Reynaldo/Fortinbras in the Kenneth Branagh *Hamlet* (Noble, Barbican). Noble next cast him as the Fool in his production of *King Lear* (RST, 1993). Some of the RSC's most important actors have come to prominence playing this role (Ian Holm, Alec McCowen, Michael Williams, David Suchet and Antony Sher), and Hughes's performance lived up to that history. Dressed in 18th century livery (yellow waistcoat, cravat, wig), his face powdered, Hughes created a forlorn, acutely sensitive, musical Fool, a faithful servant to Robert Stephens's Lear. Subsequent roles: Arlecchino in *The Venetian Twins* (Michael Bogdanov, Swan, 1993); a young priest, alongside Alec McCowen's Sir Edward, in *Elgar's Rondo* (Di Trevis, Swan); Puck in *A Midsummer Night's Dream* (Noble, RST, 1996); Mr Tumnus in *The Lion, the Witch and the Wardrobe* (Noble, RST, 1998); Autolycus in *The Winter's Tale* (Gregory Doran, RST, 1998); Faulkland in *The Rivals* (Lindsay Posner, Swan, 2000); Dromio of Syracuse in *The Comedy of Errors* (Lynne Parker, RST, 2000); and Evans in *The Merry Wives of Windsor* (Doran, RST, 2006-07).

Geoffrey Hutchings (b. Dorchester, Dorset, 1939) studied French and Physical Education at Birmingham University before training for the stage at RADA. His early theatre work included the musical *No Strings* (1963). His long RSC career began in 1968, when, among other roles, he played Simple in *The Merry Wives of Windsor* (Terry Hands) and Dr Serringe in *The Relapse* (Trevor Nunn). This work set the pattern for the next twenty years, for he remained, primarily, an exponent of comedic roles. The imaginative use of character detail (the right accent or physical mannerism) has often been a feature of his performances. He unlocked, and made accessible, the humour in Shakespeare's clowns, achieving a different character, a different mood, each time: Cleon/Pandar in *Pericles* (Hands, RST, 1969); the Young Shepherd in *The Winter's Tale* (Nunn, RST, 1969); Launce in *The Two Gentlemen of Verona* (Gareth Morgan, Theatregoround, 1969); Dromio of Syracuse in *The Comedy of Errors* (Clifford Williams, RST, 1972); Dr Caius in *The Merry Wives of Windsor* (Nunn/John Caird, RST, 1979); Feste in *Twelfth Night* (Hands, RST, 1979); Autolycus in *The Winter's Tale* (Ronald Eyre, RST, 1981); Bottom in *A Midsummer Night's Dream* (Ron Daniels, RST, 1981); Launce in *The Two Gentlemen of Verona* (John Barton, RST, 1981); and Lavache in *All's Well That Ends Well* (Nunn, RST, 1981).

But there we many other pleasures: Octavius in *Julius Caesar* (Barton, RST, 1968); Cromwell in *Henry VIII* (Nunn, RST, 1969); Podulla in Günter Grass's *The Plebeians Rehearse the Uprising* (David Jones, Aldwych, 1970); Black Will in *Arden of Faversham* (Buzz Goodbody, Theatregoround, 1970); Gratiano in *The Merchant of Venice* (Hands, RST, 1971); Bosola in *The Duchess of Malfi* (Williams, RST, 1971); Demetrius in *Titus Andronicus* (Nunn/Goodbody, RST, 1972); David Rudkin's *Cries from the Casement* (Hands, The Place, 1973); Jasper 906 in Philip Magdalany's *Section Nine* (Charles Marowitz, The Place, 1973); the Dauphin in *Henry V* (Hands, RST, 1975); Cicely Berry's *The Mouth Organ* (TOP, 1975); Galy Gay in Brecht's *Man is Man* (Howard Davies, TOP, 1975); Vasques in *'Tis Pity She's a Whore* (Daniels, TOP, 1977); Somerset in *Henry VI Part Three* (Hands, RST, 1977); Yescanab, succeeding Peter McEnery, in Rudkin's

The Sons of Light (Daniels, Warehouse, 1978); Pisanio in *Cymbeline* (Jones, RST, 1979); Lady Dodo in Peter Nichols's *Poppy* (Hands, Barbican, 1982); Colonel Gore in Nicholas Wright's *The Desert Air* (Adrian Noble, TOP, 1984); and Cap'n Andy Hawks in *Showboat* (Ian Judge, Tour, 1990).

Since the mid-1980s Hutchings has worked regularly at the National and in the West End: Jacobowski in Wersel and Behrman's *Jacobowski and the Colonel* (Jonathan Lynn, Olivier, 1986); Erwin Trowbridge in *Three Men on a Horse* (Lynn, Cottesloe, 1987); the musical *Ziegfeld* (Palladium, 1988); Peter Hall's production of Feydeau's *An Absolute Turkey* (Globe Theatre, 1994); the cook in *Mother Courage* (Jonathan Kent, Olivier, 1995); Sid, replacing Antony Sher, in Terry Johnson's *Cleo, Camping, Emmanuelle and Dick* (Lyttelton, 1998); the mayor in Nick Darke's *The Riot* (Mike Shepherd, Kneehigh Theatre, Cottesloe, 1999); Luther's father in *Luther* (Peter Gill, Olivier, 2001); *The Lady from the Sea* (Nunn, Almeida, 2003); Lucien in *See You Next Tuesday* (Robin Lefevre, Albery, 2003); and *Endgame* (Matthew Warchus, Albery, 2004).

Notable screen work: Alan Clarke's *Made in Britain* (ITV, 1982); *Clockwise* (Christopher Morahan, 1986); *Wish You Were Here* (David Leland, 1987); Nym in *Henry V* (Kenneth Branagh, 1989); Alec Laing in *White Hunter, Black Heart* (Clint Eastwood, 1990); *Inspector Maigret* (ITV, 1992); *Heart of Darkness* (Nicolas Roeg, 1994); John Edwards in *Our Friends in the North* (BBC, 1996); *Witness Against Hitler* (BBC, 1996); *Topsy-Turvy* (Mike Leigh, 1999); *Mike Bassett, England Manager* (2001); *It's All About Love* (Thomas Vinterberg, 2003).

Jonathan Hyde (b. Brisbane, Australia, 1947) came to notice at the Glasgow Citizens' during the golden era of Giles Havergal, Philip Prowse and Robert David MacDonald. In tune with the decadent pomp and high theatricality of the Prowse style, he played Casanova in Tennessee Williams's *Camino Real* (1974); Aufidius in *Coriolanus* (1974); Mr President in *Indians* (1974);

Slift in *Saint Joan of the Stockyards* (1974); De Sade in *The De Sade Show* (1975); the Cardinal in *The Duchess of Malfi* (1975); the Superintendent of Schools in *The Government Inspector* (1975); Polonius in *Hamlet* (1975); Capulet in *Romeo and Juliet* (1975); the Doctor in *Woyzeck* (1976); Rance in *What the Butler Saw* (1976); the Mother in *Seven Deadly Sins* (1976); Forlipopoli in *Mirandolina* (1976); Sprich in *Masquerade* (1976); Levka/Gabriel in *Chinchilla* (1977); Dorilant in *The Country Wife* (1977); Bartolo in *Figaro* (1977); Lady Bracknell in *The Importance of Being Earnest* (1977); and Silvestra in *Good Humoured Ladies* (1979).

That the saturnine Hyde had something of the manner of the young Ian Richardson became clear when he joined the RSC. Essentially anti-heroic, he made characters arrogant and chilly at will, although he could play comedy and goodness too. In his first season (1980/81) he was a Caravaggio-like Mercutio, relishing the hard drinking and the threat of violence, in *Romeo and Juliet* (Ron Daniels, RST); in his second (1982/83), directed by Adrian Noble, a fine Edgar in the Michael Gambon *King Lear* (RST) and an unusually sympathetic Octavius in the Gambon/Helen Mirren *Antony and Cleopatra* (TOP). Around these high points he was a versatile company actor: Oliver in *As You Like It* (Terry Hands, RST, 1980); Richmond in *Richard III* (Hands, RST, 1980); Aumerle in *Richard II* (Hands, RST, 1980); Tom Nightwork in *The Swan Down Gloves* (Ian Judge/Hands, RST, 1981); Bassanio in *The Merchant of Venice* (John Barton, RST, 1981); the Porter in *Macbeth* (Howard Davies, RST, 1982); and Laxton in *The Roaring Girl* (Barry Kyle, Barbican, 1983).

In 1987 Hyde succeeded Alan Rickman as Valmont in *Les liaisons dangereuses* (Davies, Ambassadors). In 1991 he returned to Stratford as an associate artist: Vasques in *'Tis Pity She's a Whore* (David Leveaux, Swan); Face in *The Alchemist* (Sam Mendes, Swan); Brutus in *Julius Caesar* (Steven Pimlott, RST); and Columbus in Richard Nelson's *Columbus and the Discovery of Japan* (John Caird, Barbican, 1992). Disappointed by the critical failure of *Julius Caesar* Hyde waited fifteen years before rejoining the

Company to play a curiously low-key Kent in *King Lear* and Dorn in *The Seagull* (Trevor Nunn, Courtyard, 2007).

Hyde's other work in the theatre has included seasons at the National, the Almeida and the Old Vic: Ferdinand in *The Duchess of Malfi* (Philip Prowse, NT Lyttelton, 1985); Muldoon in *The Real Inspector Hound* (Tom Stoppard, NT Olivier, 1985); Mr Sneer in *The Critic* (Sheila Hancock, NT Olivier, 1985); Yasha in *The Cherry Orchard* (Mike Alfreds, NT Cottesloe, 1985); the Doge of Venice in Howard Barker's *Scenes from an Execution* (Ian McDiarmid, Almeida, 1990); the Count in Anouilh's *The Rehearsal* (McDiarmid, Almeida, 1990); Charles in Hanif Kureishi's *Sleep With Me* (NT Cottesloe, 1999); Creon opposite Tara Fitzgerald in Sophocles's *Antigone* (Declan Donnellan, Old Vic, 1999); and Archie in Stoppard's *Jumpers* (David Leveaux, NT Lyttelton, 2003).

Hyde's work in film has included Derek Jarman's *Caravaggio* (1986); Hollywood's *Titanic* (1997) and *The Mummy* (1999); and John Boorman's *The Taylor of Panama* (2001).

Nicholas Hytner (b. Manchester, 1956). Like his father, Benet Hytner QC, Nicholas Hytner was educated at Manchester Grammar School and Trinity Hall, Cambridge. The first phase of his career saw him directing at the Northcott Theatre, Exeter, and the Leeds Playhouse. He made his name with a visually striking production of Handel's *Xerxes* at English National Opera (1985). During the next few years, at the Manchester Royal Exchange and the RSC, he brought considerable flare to his productions of classic texts. At Manchester, where he was an associate, he directed Janet McTeer in *As You Like It* (1986), Ian McDiarmid in *Edward II* (1986), Gary Oldman and Cheryl Campbell in *The Country Wife* (1986-87), and Michael Grandage in *Don Carlos* (1987). At the RSC, his main house productions of *Measure for Measure* (1987), *The Tempest* (1988) and *King Lear* (1990) were modish exhibits of theatrical art. The set of *The Tempest* looked like a spacecraft, and *King Lear*'s huge spinning cube belonged in the Tate, but the acting of John Wood as Prospero and Lear was unforgettable. At the end of Hytner's fascinating *Measure for Measure* Josette Simon's Isabella calmly rejected Roger Allam's Duke: the claustrophobic set opened to reveal a new world, a landscape of cypress trees.

Hytner was the first young pretender to walk through the door opened by Trevor Nunn. In 1989 he directed the Holocaust drama *Ghetto* (NT Olivier) and the pop musical *Miss Saigon* (Drury Lane) as though they were masterpieces by Shakespeare and Verdi. As an associate director at the National, he staged Alan Bennett's hit shows *The Wind in the Willows* (1990) and *The Madness of George III* (1991). He made a movie of the latter (1994) and for the next few years worked in Hollywood. Uninspired with the camera, he directed Daniel Day-Lewis in *The Crucible* (1996) and Jennifer Aniston in *The Object of My Affection* (1998). Neither film performed at the box office, so Hytner returned, perhaps reluctantly, to the theatre, directing *Twelfth Night* (New York, 1998); Bennett's *The Lady in the Van* (Queen's, 1999); Michael Gambon in Nicholas Wright's *Cressida* (Almeida, 2000); Helen Mirren in *Orpheus Descending* (Donmar Warehouse, 2000); and Alex Jennings in *The Winter's Tale* (NT Olivier, 2001). In 2003 he succeeded Trevor Nunn as Director of the National. After his 'Glastonbury' *Winter's Tale* and contemporary musical *Mother Clap's Molly House* (NT, 2001) it remained to be seen whether he could re-capture the quality of his early work. *Henry V* (Olivier, 2003) was excitingly staged, but the ideas were surprisingly derivative in their lack of subtlety (it was Michael Bogdanov who, back in the 1980s, first dressed the English soldiers in football shirts and flak jackets). *Henry IV* (Olivier, 2005) was shrouded in Brechtian gloom and seemed worthy rather than inspired. Hytner's National, though, buzzes with ideas and possibilities.

I

Jeremy Irons (b. Cowes, Isle of Wight, 1948) came to sudden prominence in 1981 playing staid middle-class characters in *Brideshead Revisited* (Charles Sturridge/Michael Lindsay-Hogg) and *The French Lieutenant's Woman* (Karel Reisz). For a time these roles, immaculately executed, seemed to represent the actor himself, but his languorous performance as Charles Ryder in *Brideshead* was not typical of his apprentice work and he has since gone to lengths to reveal other aspects of his ability.

He worked for ten years on the stage before breaking into films. Following his training at the Bristol Old Vic Theatre School he stayed for three years with the Bristol Old Vic Company (1968-71): *Major Barbara*, Goldoni's *The Servant to Two Masters*, *The Boyfriend*, *As You Like It*, Florizel in *The Winter's Tale*, Nick in *What the Butler Saw* and Simon in *Hay Fever*. He moved to London and worked as a builder and gardener (busking in Leicester Square at night) before landing the part of John the Baptist in the hit musical *Godspell* (Roundhouse and Wyndham's, 1971-73). He then played Mick in Harold Pinter's *The Caretaker* at the Young Vic (1974) and Petruchio in *The Taming of the Shrew* for the New Shakespeare Company (Roundhouse, 1975). He first joined the RSC in London in 1976 to play Harry Thunder in John O'Keeffe's *Wild Oats* (Clifford Williams, Aldwych), a hit production that transferred briefly to Stratford and then to the West End.

He did not stay with the RSC but instead began his screen career with roles in the television dramas *Love for Lydia*, the Pinter scripted *Langrishe Go Down* (David Jones, BBC, 1978), and *The Voysey Inheritance* (Robert Knights, 1979). He made his film debut as Mikhail Fokhine in *Nijinsky* (Herbert Ross, 1980). Following his success in *Brideshead* he set out to become a star in international films, and while he has revisited Charles Ryder a number of times one has constantly been struck by both his perfectionist technique and his adventurousness. Performances of particular interest: the exiled Pole in *Moonlighting* (Jerzy Skolimowski, 1982); Jerry in Pinter's *Betrayal* (David Jones, 1983); Charles Swann in *Swann in Love* (Volker Schlöndorff, 1984); Gabriel in *The Mission* (Roland Joffé, 1986); Beverly Mantle/Elliot Mantle in *Dead Ringers* (David Cronenberg, 1988); Claus von Bülow in *Reversal of Fortune* (Barbet Schroeder, 1990); the villain—cropped blonde hair and sunglasses—in *Die Hard with a Vengeance* (John McTiernan, 1995); the dying writer in *Stealing Beauty* (Bernardo Bertolucci, 1996); Humbert Humbert in *Lolita* (Adrian Lyne, 1997); and Antonio in *The Merchant of Venice* (Michael Radford, 2005). If there is a pattern to his choice of characters it is a fascination with figures, often of authority, who keep beneath a surface of strict etiquette a brooding immorality. But this is the gaunt, faded elegance that constantly needs to be shattered by movies such as *Dead Ringers* and *Die Hard*.

In 1984 he played Henry in Tom Stoppard's *The Real Thing* on Broadway. His connection with the RSC was maintained through his wife Sinéad Cusack, an associate artist of the Company. In 1986 he made a surprise return for a full two-year cycle. He played contrasting roles with great success: Leontes in *The Winter's Tale* (Terry Hands, RST); Willmore, a performance of Errol Flynn dash and swagger filtered through irony, in *The Rover* (John Barton, Swan); and the title role, world-weary and elegiac, in *Richard II* (Barry Kyle, RST).

J

Glenda Jackson (b. Birkenhead, 1936). The Member of Parliament for Hampstead and Highgate (Labour, since 1992) was in the 1960s one of the RSC's most challenging performers, and in the 1970s one of the cinema's most acclaimed stars, winning the Best Actress Oscar for both *Women in Love* (Ken Russell, 1970) and *A Touch of Class* (Melvin Frank, 1972). Her profile as a politician is surprisingly dour and uncharismatic—deliberately untheatrical. As an actress she was no less serious, but she was also adventurous and self-mocking, equally at ease playing Hedda Gabler or appearing on the *Morecambe and Wise* TV show.

If never conventionally beautiful, she was striking in her youth, an antidote to the bland beauty of contemporaries such as Julie Christie. Her intense stare, high cheekbones and helmet of dark hair made her seem severe—it was a look which suggested an uncompromising intelligence.

The daughter of a builder, she was educated at West Kirby County Grammar School for Girls and RADA. Her early theatre appearances included *Separate Tables* (Worthing, 1957), *All Kinds of Men* (Arts, 1957), *The Idiot* (Lyric, 1962), and *Alfie* (Mermaid and Duchess, 1963). She also worked as a stage manager for the Crewe Repertory Company. In 1963 she joined the RSC as a member of Peter Brook's experimental group, taking part in the *Theatre of Cruelty* seasons at the LAMDA Theatre Studio and the Donmar Rehearsal Theatre (1963-64). She was suddenly thrown into the spotlight by the short piece *The Public Bath*, in which she stripped and took a bath on stage. In Genet's *The Screens*, the second season's main production, she played Kadidja. Staying with Brook's group, at the Aldwych, she made a lasting impression as Charlotte Corday in Peter Weiss's *Marat/Sade* (1964), and was the leading actress in the rehearsed reading of Weiss's *The Investigation* (1965) and the protest piece *US* (1966).

The intention of Brook's programme was that it should influence the RSC's mainstream work. Glenda Jackson, like many of the *Theatre of Cruelty* actors, was also cast in classical roles: Bellamira in *The Jew of Malta* (Clifford Williams, Aldwych, 1964); the Princess of France in *Love's Labour's Lost* (John Barton, RST, 1965); Eva in Brecht's *Puntila* (Michel Saint-Denis, Aldwych, 1965); and Ophelia in the David Warner *Hamlet* (Peter Hall, RST, 1965).

She only returned to the RSC twice during the remainder of her life as an actress: in 1975 she played an admired Hedda in Trevor Nunn's production of *Hedda Gabler* (Aldwych); and in

1978-79, reunited with Brook, she was an abrasive, volatile, un-romantic Cleopatra to Alan Howard's Antony in *Antony and Cleopatra* (RST).

Elsewhere, her choices were fascinatingly diverse: Masha in *Three Sisters* (William Gaskill, Royal Court, 1967); Tamara in David Pinner's *Fanghorn* (Fortune, 1967); Katherine in John Mortimer's *The Collaborators* (Duchess, 1973); Solange in Genet's *The Maids* (Greenwich, 1974); Vittoria in *The White Devil* (Old Vic, 1975); Stevie Smith in Hugh Whitemore's *Stevie* (Vaude-ville, 1977); the title role in Andrew Davies's *Rose* (Duke of York's, 1980); Eva Braun in Robert David MacDonald's *Summit Conference* (Philip Prowse, Glasgow Citizens', 1982); Lotte in Botho Strauss's five hour *Great and Small* (Keith Hack, Vaude-ville, 1983); Nina in Eugene O'Neill's *Strange Interlude* (Duke of York's, 1984); the title role in Racine's *Phèdre* (Philip Prowse, Old Vic, 1984); Bernarda in *The House of Bernarda Alba* (Núria Espert, Lyric Hammersmith, 1986); Lady Macbeth in *Macbeth* (New York, 1988); Galactia in Howard Barker's *Scenes from an Execution* (Almeida, 1990); and the title role in *Mother Courage* (Mermaid, 1990).

Strong, unconventional characters featured prominently in her work for the cinema. She was at her most enigmatic in John Schlesinger's *Sunday Bloody Sunday* (1971) and Joseph Losey's *The Romantic Englishwoman* (1974). Predictably enough, she played a militant *Elizabeth R* (BBC, 1971) and her tragic adver-sary *Mary Queen of Scots* (Charles Jarrott, 1972); Emma Hamilton in *Bequest to the Nation* (James Cellan Jones, 1973); and Sarah Bernhardt in *The Incredible Sarah* (Richard Fleischer, 1976). Her remorseless realisation of D.H. Lawrence's Gudrun in Ken Rus-sell's *Women in Love* remains her most powerful work. Her admiration for Russell resulted in five further collaborations: *The Music Lovers* (1971); *The Boyfriend* (1972); *Salome's Last Dance* (1988); *The Rainbow* (1989); and *The Secret Life of Arnold Bax* (1992).

Derek Jacobi was born in Leytonstone, east London (1938). His ability was recognised early on. At the National Youth Theatre he played the title role in *Hamlet*. At Cambridge (he studied at St John's College) his performances as Edward in Marlowe's *Edward II* (Toby Robertson) and Hal in *Henry IV* made him the star actor of a generation that also included Ian McKellen and Corin Redgrave.

After Cambridge, he worked for two years at the Birmingham Rep, cast, most notably, as Honeybone in N.F. Simpson's *One Way Pendulum* (1960); Marlow in *She Stoops to Conquer* (John Harrison, 1961); Henry VIII in Robert Bolt's *A Man For All Seasons* (Bernard Hepton/David Buxton, 1961); and Ferdinand in *The Tempest* (John Harrison, 1962).

In 1963 Jacobi joined Laurence Olivier's company at Chichester (Brother Martin in *Saint Joan*; Liversedge in John Arden's *The Workhouse Donkey*), and for the rest of the decade he was a member of Olivier's National Theatre at the Old Vic. One of only a handful of great actors developed by Olivier's regime, he played Laertes in *Hamlet* (Olivier, 1963); Cassius in *Othello* (1964); Simon in Noël Coward's *Hay Fever* (Coward, 1964); Felipillo in Peter Shaffer's *The Royal Hunt of the Sun* (John Dexter, 1964); Don Pedro in Franco Zeffirelli's *Much Ado About Nothing* (1965); Brindsley Miller in Shaffer's *Black Comedy* (Dexter, 1966); Tusenbach in *Three Sisters* (Olivier, 1967); Touchstone to Anthony Hopkins's Audrey in Clifford Williams's all-male *As You Like It* (1967); Navarre in *Love's Labour's Lost* (Olivier, 1968); Adam in Shaw's *Back to Methuselah* (Williams, 1969); Lodovico in *The White Devil* (Frank Dunlop, 1970); and Charles Mountford in *A Woman Killed With Kindness* (Dexter, 1971).

He left the National to play leading roles with the Prospect Theatre Company: the title role in *Ivanov* (1972); Buckingham in *Richard III* (1972); Sir Andrew Aguecheek in *Twelfth Night* (1973); the title role in *Pericles* (1973); Raketin in *A Month in the Country* (Toby Robertson, Albery, 1974); the title role in *Hamlet* (Robertson, Old Vic, 1977); and Mendip in *The Lady's Not for Burning*

(Old Vic, 1978). His exciting Hamlet was less quirky but more rounded than most of the 1970s and 80s. He repeated the role for the BBC Shakespeare in 1980.

Jacobi was first at the RSC in 1975, touring America with *The Hollow Crown* (John Barton) and *Pleasure and Repentance* (Terry Hands). His entry into the RSC proper in 1982 was long overdue. He was seen at his most astute as Benedick in *Much Ado About Nothing* (Terry Hands, RST); the title role in *Peer Gynt* (Ron Daniels, TOP); Prospero in *The Tempest* (Daniels, RST); and the title role in *Cyrano de Bergerac* (Hands, Barbican).

His RSC work was the climax of almost twenty-five years spent with theatre troupes. He has since appeared in the West End and at Chichester, often in old fashioned star vehicles such as *Kean* (Sam Mendes, Old Vic, 1990), *Becket* (Theatre Royal Haymarket, 1991), *Mad, Bad and Dangerous to Know* (Ambassadors, 1992), and *Hadrian VII* (Hands, Chichester, 1995). He was outstanding as Alan Turing in *Breaking the Code* (Theatre Royal Haymarket, 1986); the title role in *Uncle Vanya* (Bill Bryden, Chichester, 1996); Prospero in *The Tempest* (Michael Grandage, Sheffield Crucible, 2002); Philip II in *Don Carlos* (Grandage, Sheffield Crucible, 2004); and the Father in John Mortimer's *A Voyage Round My Father* (Thea Sharrock, Donmar Warehouse, 2006). His RSC Macbeth (Adrian Noble, Barbican, 1993) was underrated. In 2002 he returned to Barton's *Hollow Crown* (Tour and RST).

Jacobi has maintained a popular if patchy screen career since the mid-1970s when he played Claudius in *I, Claudius* (Herbert Wise, 1976), Burgess in *Philby, Burgess and Maclean* (ITV, 1977), and the title role in *Richard II* (1978). He portrayed Hitler in *Inside the Third Reich* (1982); revisited Turing in *Breaking the Code* (Herbert Wise, BBC, 1996); and starred in *Cadfael* (ITV, 1994-99).

Jacobi has always been good at playing cerebral characters such as Cadfael, but his capacity for depicting pain, anger and despair in roles such as Hamlet, Cyrano and Turing has been unfairly undervalued. Underused by the cinema, he nevertheless produced some of his best work in the features *Little Dorrit*

(Christine Edzard, 1988), *Henry V* (Kenneth Branagh, 1989), *The Fool* (Christine Edzard, 1990), and *Hamlet* (Branagh, 1996). His extraordinary performance as Francis Bacon in *Love is the Devil* (John Maybury, 1998) led to a burst of activity—*Up at the Villa* (Philip Haas, 1999); Gracchus in *Gladiator* (Ridley Scott, 1999); *Gosford Park* (Robert Altman, 2001); Stanley Baldwin in *The Gathering Storm* (Richard Loncraine, BBC, 2002); *A Revenger's Tragedy* (Alex Cox, 2002); *Two Men Went to War* (2002); and *The Long Firm* (BBC, 2004).

Sally Jacobs (b. London, 1932) studied at the Central School of Art and Design. She first worked at the RSC in 1961, assisting Jocelyn Herbert on *Richard III* (William Gaskill, RST). She then designed David Jones's *The Empire Builders* and Anthony Page's *Women Beware Women* at the Arts (1962). Now one of the Company's associate artists, Peter Brook chose her to design his 'Theatre of Cruelty' productions, including *The Screens* (Donmar Rehearsal Theatre, 1964), and their collaboration continued: *Marat/Sade* (Aldwych, 1964); *US* (Aldwych, 1966); *A Midsummer Night's Dream* (RST, 1970); and *Antony and Cleopatra* (RST, 1978). Her other RSC productions were John Barton's *Love's Labour's Lost* (RST, 1965), and Clifford Williams's *Twelfth Night* (RST, 1966).

Emrys James (1930-1989, b. Machynlleth, Wales). The son of a miner, Emrys James went to RADA and began his career as a member of Peter Hall and John Barton's Elizabethan Theatre Company (1953). At Stratford, in 1956, he played Guildenstern in the Alan Badel *Hamlet* (Michael Langham), Salerio in *The Merchant of Venice* (Margaret Webster), and Claudio in *Measure for Measure* (Anthony Quayle). He was then with the Bristol Old Vic company as Touchstone in *As You Like It* and the Narrator in *Under Milk Wood* (1958). From 1959 he established his reputation in the capital: Evans in Willis Hall's *The Long and the Short and the Tall* (Lindsay Anderson, New, 1959); Malcolm in *Macbeth*

(Oliver Neville), Richmond in *Richard III* (Colin George), Caesar/Octavius in *Julius Caesar* (Minos Volanakis, all Old Vic, 1961-62); and Juryman No. 9 in *Twelve Angry Men* (1964).

He was a leading figure at the RSC from 1968. With his bullish style he was an intimidating actor—and not only when playing intimidating roles. His prickly personality provoked disputes in the rehearsal room but gave an edge to his acting. Among his achievements were a melancholy Feste in *Twelfth Night* (John Barton, RST, 1969); a chilling Iago in *Othello* (Barton, RST, 1971); a formidable Henry in *Henry IV* (Terry Hands, RST, 1975); and a narcissistic York in *Henry VI* (Hands, RST, 1977). Also: *Under Milk Wood* (Hands, Theatregoround, 1968); Decius Brutus in *Julius Caesar* (Barton, RST, 1968); Sir Hugh Evans in *The Merry Wives of Windsor* (Hands, RST, 1968); Sitting Bull in Arthur Kopit's *Indians* (Jack Gelber, Aldwych, 1968); Worthy in *The Relapse* (Trevor Nunn, Aldwych, 1968); a Welsh-accented Gower in *Pericles* (Hands, RST, 1969); Cranmer in *Henry VIII* (Nunn, RST, 1969); the Boss in Günter Grass's *The Plebeians Rehearse the Uprising* (David Jones, Aldwych, 1970); Thomas Arden in *Arden of Faversham* (Buzz Goodbody, Theatregoround, 1970); Shylock in *The Merchant of Venice* (Hands, RST, 1971); Cardinal in *The Duchess of Malfi* (Clifford Williams, RST, 1971); Merlin in *The Island of the Mighty* (David Jones, Aldwych, 1972); the title role in *King John* (Barton/Barry Kyle, RST, 1974); Mephostophiles to Ian McKellen's *Doctor Faustus* (Aldwych, 1974); Chorus in the Alan Howard *Henry V* (Hands, RST, 1975); Sir Hugh Evans in *The Merry Wives of Windsor* (Hands, RST, 1975); Jaques in *As You Like It* (Nunn, RST, 1977); Edgar in *The Dance of Death* (John Caird, Warehouse, 1978); De Flores in *The Changeling* (Hands, Aldwych, 1978); Cassius in *Julius Caesar* (Ron Daniels, RST, 1983); Malvolio in *Twelfth Night* (Caird, RST, 1983); and Sir Giles Overreach in *A New Way to Pay Old Debts* (Adrian Noble, TOP, 1983).

Michael Jayston (b. Nottingham, 1935) worked as a trainee accountant before enrolling at the Guildhall School. Seasons at the Salisbury Playhouse (1962-63) and the Bristol Old Vic (1963-65) led to his entry into the RSC. He met and married Lynn Farleigh and played such disparate roles as Exeter in *Henry V* (John Barton/Trevor Nunn, Aldwych, 1965); Red-Haired Workman in Brecht's *Puntilla* (Michel Saint-Denis, Aldwych, 1965); Witness 2 in Peter Weiss's *The Investigation* (Peter Brook/David Jones, Aldwych, 1965); the Storyteller in Robert Bolt's *The Thwarting of Baron Bolligrew* (Nunn, Aldwych, 1965); Exeter in both parts of *Henry IV* and *Henry V* (Barton/Nunn, RST, 1966); the Chorus in *Romeo and Juliet* (Karolos Koun, RST, 1967); and Custer/Logan in Arthur Kopit's *Indians* (Jack Gelber, Aldwych, 1968). Jayston's growing reputation as an actor of range and interpretative subtlety was confirmed by his performances as Laertes in the David Warner *Hamlet* (Peter Hall, RST, 1966); Lenny, succeeding Ian Holm, in Harold Pinter's *The Homecoming* (Hall, New York, 1967); Oswald in Ibsen's *Ghosts* (Alan Bridges, Aldwych, 1967); Bertram, succeeding Ian Richardson, in *All's Well That Ends Well* (Barton, Aldwych, 1968); and Young Fashion in John Vanbrugh's *The Relapse* (Nunn, Aldwych, 1968). Before leaving the RSC he played Demetrius in Hall's film of *A Midsummer Night's Dream* (1968).

The cinema occupied most of Jayston's working life for the next ten years. He starred, impressively, opposite his RSC contemporary Janet Suzman in *Nicholas and Alexandra* (Franklin Schaffner, 1971), but the relative failure of the film nullified his achievement. It was at the centre of a body of work typical for the period: Henry Ireton in *Cromwell* (Ken Hughes, 1970); Charles opposite Mia Farrow in *Follow Me* (Carol Reed, 1972); Lewis Carroll in *Alice's Adventures in Wonderland* (1972); Captain Hardy in *A Bequest to the Nation* (1973); *Tales That Witness Madness* (1973); Teddy in *The Homecoming* (Hall, 1973); *Craze* (1973); *The Internecine Project* (Ken Hughes, 1974); *Dominique* (1978); and *Zulu Dawn* (1979). On television he played Gratiano in the Laurence Olivier *The Merchant of Venice* (Jonathan Miller, 1973); Rochester in *Jane Eyre* (BBC, 1973); the title role in *Quiller* (BBC, 1975); and Alec Guinness's diligent and loyal enforcer in John le Carré's *Tinker, Tailor, Soldier, Spy* (BBC, 1979).

In 1974 Jayston played Dysart in Peter Shaffer's *Equus* at the Old Vic. Since returning to live performance at the beginning of the 1980s he has chosen to appear in well-made plays in the West End and at Chichester—Noël Coward's *Private Lives* (Duchess, 1980); *The Sound of Music* (Apollo, 1981); William Congreve's *The Way of the World* (Chichester, 1984); Alan Ayckbourn's *Woman in Mind* (Vaudeville, 1987); Brian Friel's *Dancing at Lughnasa* (Garrick, 1992); Alan Bennett's *The Wind in the Willows* (NT Olivier, 1994); Coward's *Easy Virtue* (Maria Aitken, Chichester, 1999); and Roger Crane's *The Last Confession* (Jones, Chichester, 2007).

Barbara Jefford (b. Plymstock, Devon, 1930) was nineteen when Peter Brook cast her as Isabella in his Stratford production of *Measure for Measure* (1950). She had only been working for a year since leaving RADA with the Bancroft Gold Medal—Viola in *Twelfth Night* at the Dolphin Theatre, Brighton (1949); Bertha in *Frenzy* at the Q Theatre (1949); Lydia in *The Rivals* and Janet in *The Gioconda Smile* at the Dundee Rep (1949-50). Suddenly she found herself playing one of Shakespeare's most taxing female roles opposite John Gielgud (Angelo) and Harry Andrews (Vincentio). She stayed at Stratford for the next four years: Anne Bullen in *Henry VIII* (Tyrone Guthrie, RST, 1950); Calphurnia in *Julius Caesar* (Anthony Quayle/Michael Langham, RST, 1950); Hero in the John Gielgud/Peggy Ashcroft *Much Ado About Nothing* (Gielgud, RST, 1950); Lady Percy in *Henry IV* (John Kidd/Quayle/Michael Redgrave, RST, 1951); Isabel in the Richard Burton *Henry V* (Quayle, RST, 1951); Desdemona to Anthony Quayle's *Othello* (Quayle, RST, 1952); Rosalind in *As You Like It* (Glen Byam Shaw, New Zealand Tour, 1953); Helena in *A Midsummer Night's Dream* (George Devine, RST, 1954); Kate to Keith Michell's Petruchio in *The Taming of the Shrew* (Devine, RST, 1954); and Helen in *Troilus and Cressida* (Shaw, RST, 1954). It was a remarkable beginning.

She consolidated her reputation at the Old Vic, 1956-62: Portia in *The Merchant of Venice* (Michael Benthall); Imogen in *Cymbeline* (Benthall); Beatrice in *Much Ado About Nothing* (Denis Carey); Julia in *The Two Gentlemen of Verona* (Michael Langham); Tamora in *Titus Andronicus* (Walter Hudd); Lady Anne in *Richard III* (Douglas Seale); Viola in *Twelfth Night* (Benthall); Queen Margaret in *Henry VI 1-3* (Seale); Isabella in *Measure for Measure* (Margaret Webster); Regan in *King Lear* (Seale); Rosalind in *As You Like It* (Wendy Toye); and Viola in *Twelfth Night* (Colin Craham).

Despite the stature of her early work she never achieved celebrity status. She continued to work quietly, but with great authority, on the stage: *Tiger at the Gates* (Apollo, 1955); Lina in *Misalliance* (Royal Court, 1963); the step-daughter in *Six Characters in Search of an Author* (Mayfair, 1963); Nan in *Ride a Cock Horse* (Piccadilly, 1965); Mother Vauzou in *Mistress of Novices* (Piccadilly, 1973); Gertrude in *Hamlet* (Hall, NT Lyttelton, 1976); Zabina in *Tamburlaine the Great* (Hall, NT Olivier, 1976); Gertrude in *Hamlet*, Cleopatra in *All for Love*, Cleopatra in *Antony and Cleopatra*, Nurse in *Romeo and Juliet* and Anna in *The Government Inspector* (Prospect, Old Vic, 1977-79); the title role in *Filumena* (Lyric, 1979); the mother in *Six Characters in Search of an Author* (Michael Rudman, NT Lyttelton, 1987); Arina Bazarov in *Fathers and Sons* (Rudman, NT Lyttelton, 1987); Salathiel in Nick Darke's *Ting Tang Mine* (Rudman, NT Cottesloe, 1987); the Duchess of York in *Richard II* and Queen Margaret in *Richard III* (Phoenix, 1988-89); the mother in D.H. Lawrence's *A Collier's Friday Night* (John Dove, Hampstead Theatre, 1994); Lady Sneerwell in *The School for Scandal* (UK Tour, 1995); Somerset Maugham's *Our Betters* (Rudman, Chichester, 1997); Mrs Railton Bell in Terence Rattigan's *Table Number Seven/Harlequinade* (Colin Ellwood, King's Head, 1998); Racine's *Phèdre* and *Britannicus* (Jonathan Kent, Almeida at the Albery, 1998); Volumnia to

Ralph Fiennes's *Coriolanus* (Kent, Almeida at the Gainsborough Studios, 2000); and Anne of Austria in Nick Dear's *Power* (Lindsay Posner, NT Cottesloe, 2003).

At the RSC she played Patsy in Jules Feiffer's *Little Murders* (Christopher Morahan, Aldwych, 1967), Hippolyta in Peter Hall's film of *A Midsummer Night's Dream* (1968), and Mistress Quickly in the small-scale touring production of *Henry IV* (Bill Alexander, 1980). It was not until the end of the 1980s that she returned in earnest: Volumnia to Charles Dance's *Coriolanus* (Terry Hands/John Barton, RST, 1989); Tatyana in Gorky's *Barbarians* (David Jones, Barbican, 1990); the Countess, replacing Rosemary Harris, in Peter Hall's production of *All's Well That Ends Well* (Swan, 1992); Mistress Quickly in *The Merry Wives of Windsor* (David Thacker, RST, 1992); Katia in Richard Nelson and Alexander Gelman's *Misha's Party* (David Jones, Pit, 1993); and Countess Terzky in Schiller's *Wallenstein* (Tim Albery, Pit, 1993-94).

Peter Jeffrey (1929-1999, b. Bristol). After making his debut with the Chorlton-cum-Hardy repertory company in 1951, Peter Jeffrey joined the Elizabethan Theatre Company, a troupe co-directed by John Barton and Peter Hall, his Cambridge contemporaries. He played the title role in the ETC's *Julius Caesar* at the Westminster Theatre (1953) and toured with the company until 1955. For a season he played an inspector in the BBC's *Dixon of Dock Green*, his wise lived-in face becoming familiar to thousands. He was then at the Bristol Old Vic for two years before joining Hall's new RSC in 1960. During his first, and longest, period with the Company he was luxury casting in supporting roles, including Lucentio in the Peter O'Toole/Peggy Ashcroft *Taming of the Shrew* (Barton, RST, 1960); Agamemnon in *Troilus and Cressida* (Hall, RST, 1960); Delio in *The Duchess of Malfi* (Donald McWinnie, RST, 1960); De Cerisay in John Whiting's *The Devils* (Peter Wood, Aldwych, 1961); Gilbert Folliot in *Becket* (Hall, Aldwych, 1961); Banquo in *Macbeth* (McWhinnie, RST,

1962); Angelo, the goldsmith, in *The Comedy of Errors* (Clifford Williams, RST, 1962); Albany in the Brook/Scofield *King Lear* (RST, 1962); and Stomil in *Tango* (Trevor Nunn, Aldwych, 1966).

The next few years saw him make his mark as one of the most trusted and versatile supporting players in features and on television. He was an actor without false notes who liked to play public servants and officials (as well as impostors in public school ties)—his creations were sometimes flawed and severe, sometimes upstanding and honourable, but always commanding and, in his subtle characterisations, recognisable as people. Of particular note: two roles for Lindsay Anderson, the headmaster in *If* (1968) and the prison governor in *Oh Lucky Man!* (1973); Berezhinsky in *The Fixer* (John Frankenheimer, 1968); Philip II in *Elizabeth R* (BBC, 1971); Mr Peabody in *The Jewel in the Crown* (Christopher Morahan and Jim O'Brien, ITV, 1984); Colonel Bernwood in Denis Potter's *Lipstick on Your Collar* (Channel Four, 1993); Bulstrode in *Middlemarch* (BBC, 1994); and Sir Colin Blamire in *Our Friends in the North* (BBC, 1996).

On the stage, he continued to deliver beautifully crafted and spoken performances: the title role in *Macbeth* (Prospect Productions, 1966); Malvolio to Vanessa Redgrave's Viola in *Twelfth Night* (Shaw Theatre, 1972); Buckle in Michael Frayn's *Donkey's Years* (West End, 1976); Wilfred Cedar in Somerset Maugham's *For Services Rendered* (Michael Rudman, NT Lyttelton, 1979); Henry Ormonroyd in J.B. Priestley's *When We Are Married* (Robin Lefevre, NT Lyttelton, 1979-80); Frank opposite Penelope Keith in Stanley Price's *Moving* (Queen's, 1981); Gloucester in *King Lear* (Deborah Warner, NT Lyttelton, 1990); Clarence in *Richard III* (Richard Eyre, NT Lyttelton, 1990); and the Inquisitor in *Saint Joan* (Gale Edwards, Strand, 1994).

He made two returns to the RSC. In 1975 he created the role of Percy in Charles Wood's *Jingo* (Richard Eyre, Aldwych). In 1985/86, at the RST and Barbican, he played Falstaff in *The Merry Wives of Windsor* (Bill Alexander), and Ulysses in *Troilus and Cressida* (Howard Davies). Strong directorial concepts—1950s suburbia and the Crimean War—forced Jeffrey (whose Falstaff wore plus-fours and a canary yellow waistcoat) into a realm of caricature.

Alex Jennings (b. 1957) has excelled at comedic, character and leading dramatic roles. His rise to prominence owed much to Nicholas Hytner, who cast him as Robespierre in *The Scarlet Pimpernel* (Chichester, 1985), Mr Sparkish in *The Country Wife* (Manchester Royal Exchange, 1986/87), and, at the RSC, Lucio in *Measure for Measure* (RST, 1987). That season he was also Fairfield in James Shirley's *Hyde Park* (Barry Kyle, Swan) and Lucentio in the Brian Cox/Fiona Shaw *The Taming of the Shrew* (Jonathan Miller, RST). He played Gloumov in Ostrovsky's *Too Clever By Half* (Richard Jones) and Dorante in Corneille's *The Liar* (Miller) at the Old Vic (1988-89), then, reunited with Hytner at the National, showed a new side to his ability as the music-loving SS Officer in Joshua Sobol's *Ghetto* (Olivier, 1989). He was a fine Ekdal in Peter Hall's *The Wild Duck* (Peter Hall Company, 1990).

Back with the RSC from 1990, Jennings was an unusual Richard II, strong and sardonic, in Ron Daniels's expressionistic production (RST); an inspired Peer Gynt (John Barton, Swan, 1994); Theseus/Oberon in *A Midsummer Night's Dream* (Adrian Noble, RST, 1994); Angelo in *Measure for Measure* (Steven Pimlott, RST, 1994); Benedick in *Much Ado About Nothing* (Michael Boyd, RST, 1996); and Hamlet (Matthew Warchus, RST, 1997).

He started the new millennium at the National: the title role in David Edgar's *Albert Speer* (Trevor Nunn, Lyttelton, 2000); Leontes to Claire Skinner's Hermione in *The Winter's Tale* (Hytner, Olivier, 2001); Lord Foppington in *The Relapse* (Nunn, Olivier, 2001); Higgins, succeeding Jonathan Pryce, in *My Fair Lady* (Nunn, Theatre Royal, Drury Lane, 2002); Walter Burns opposite Zoë Wanamaker in *His Girl Friday* (Jack O'Brien, Olivier, 2003); Bush in David Hare's *Stuff Happens* (Hytner, Olivier, 2004); Subtle in *The Alchemist* (Hytner, Olivier, 2006); Gary Essendine in Noël Coward's *Present Laughter* (Howard Davies, Lyttelton, 2007).

Less well known as a screen actor, Alex Jennings starred in *Ashenden* (Christopher Morahan, BBC, 1991), and portrayed Sergei Diaghilev in *Riot at the Rite* (BBC, 2005) and Prince Charles in *The Queen* (Stephen Frears, 2006).

Paul Jesson (b. 1946) studied at Manchester Polytechnic and the Guildhall School. His early work included seasons at the Library Theatre, Manchester, and the role of Wally in Edward Bond's *Bingo* at the Royal Court (1974). He emerged as an important actor in London during the 1980s. It was a phase of his career dominated by new plays: Wallace Shawn's *Marie and Bruce* (1979), Louise Page's *Falkland Sound* (1983), and Sam Shepard's *A Lie of the Mind* (Simon Curtis, 1987) at the Royal Court; *Rents* (1979) at the Lyric Hammersmith; and Mike Leigh's *Goose Pimples* (1981) at the Hampstead Theatre. His performance as Felix in *The Normal Heart* (David Hayman, Royal Court, 1986) brought him the Olivier for Best Supporting Actor.

He has subsequently concentrated on classical roles. At the National, 1988-89, he played Gooper in *Cat on a Hot Tin Roof* (Howard Davies, Lyttelton); Alsemero in *The Changeling* (Richard Eyre, Lyttelton); Lovborg in the Juliet Stevenson *Hedda Gabler* (Davies, Olivier); Kruk in *Ghetto* (Nicholas Hytner, Olivier); and Horatio in *Hamlet* (Eyre, Olivier). He returned to play Anderson in *The Devil's Disciple* (Christopher Morahan, Olivier, 1994), and Lord Burleigh in *Mary Stuart* (Davies, Lyttelton, 1996).

For much of the 1990s Jesson worked at the RSC. Good use was made of his direct, conversational style: Ulysses in *Troilus and Cressida* (Sam Mendes, Swan, 1990); John Ryder in Richard Nelson's *Two Shakespearean Actors* (Roger Michell, Swan, 1990); Earl of Northumberland in *Richard II* (Ron Daniels, RST, 1990); Peachum in *The Beggar's Opera* (John Caird, Swan, 1992); Oldrents in *A Jovial Crew* (Max Stafford-Clark, Swan, 1992);

Polixenes in *The Winter's Tale* (Adrian Noble, RST, 1992); Enobarbus in *Antony and Cleopatra* (Caird, RST, 1992); Prospero in *The Tempest* and Shakespeare in *Bingo* (both David Thacker, Swan and Small-scale Tour, 1995); the title role in *Henry VIII* (Gregory Doran, Swan, 1996); and First Gravedigger in *Hamlet* (Matthew Warchus, RST, 1997). Since leaving the RSC he has played Mr Braddock in *The Graduate* (Terry Johnson, Gielgud, 2000); Kent in *King Lear* (Jonathan Kent, Almeida at King's Cross, 2002); Sir Toby Belch in *Twelfth Night* (Mendes, Donmar Warehouse, 2002); Sorin in Peter Stein's *The Seagull* (King's Theatre, Edinburgh Festival, 2003); and Willy Loman in *Death of a Salesman* (John Dove, Royal Lyceum, Edinburgh, 2004).

Darlene Johnson was a regular supporting player at the RSC from 1978 to 1995. Among her many roles were Marlene in Pam Gems's *Piaf* (Howard Davies, TOP, 1978); Mistress Overdone in *Measure for Measure* (Barry Kyle, RST, 1978); Julia in Howard Brenton's *The Churchill Play* (Kyle, TOP, 1978); Hippolyta in *The Two Noble Kinsmen* (Kyle, Swan, 1986); Carmen in José Triana's *Worlds Apart* (Nick Hamm, TOP, 1986); Feklusha in Alexander Ostrovsky's *The Storm* (Hamm, Pit, 1987); Creusa in Howard Barker's *The Bite of the Night* (Danny Boyle, Pit, 1988); Chorus in *Electra* (Deborah Warner, Pit, 1988); Iris in *The Tempest* (Nicholas Hytner, Barbican, 1989); the Queen in Timberlake Wertenbaker's *The Love of the Nightingale* (Garry Hynes, Pit, 1989); Anticleia in *The Odyssey* (Gregory Doran, TOP, 1992); Zabina in *Tamburlaine the Great* (Terry Hands, Swan, 1992); Nadya in Tom Stoppard's *Travesties* (Adrian Noble, Barbican, 1993); Charlotte in *The Cherry Orchard* (Noble, Swan, 1995); and Delphina in *The Phoenician Women* (Katie Mitchell, TOP, 1995). She returned in 2006/07 to play Rebecca Nurse in *The Crucible* (Dominic Cooke, RST) and Valeria in *Coriolanus* (Gregory Doran, RST).

Richard Johnson (b. Upminster, Essex, 1927) trained at RADA and at the age of seventeen was given his first job by John Gielgud. As a member of Gielgud's repertory company at the Haymarket he played minor roles in *Hamlet, Love for Love* and *The Duchess of Malfi* (1944-45). National Service in the Royal Navy (1945-48) interrupted his career. He returned to the stage in Perth, and then began to build his reputation in the West End: Pierre in *The Madwoman of Chaillot* (St James's, 1951); Demetrius in *A Midsummer Night's Dream* (Regent's Park, 1951); Beauchamp in Jean Anouilh's *The Lark* (Peter Brook, Lyric Hammersmith, 1955); and Laertes in the Brook/Scofield *Hamlet* (Moscow and Phoenix, 1955). The last two shows in particular revealed Johnson's star-quality, his dark good looks and resonant voice.

In successive seasons at Stratford he played romantic leads and character parts: Orlando to Peggy Ashcroft's Rosalind in *As You Like It* (Glen Byam Shaw, 1957); Mark Antony in *Julius Caesar* (Shaw, 1957); Posthumus to Ashcroft's Imogen in *Cymbeline* (Peter Hall, 1957); Ferdinand in the John Gielgud *The Tempest* (Peter Brook, 1957); Romeo opposite Dorothy Tutin in *Romeo and Juliet* (Shaw, 1958); Aguecheek in *Twelfth Night* (Hall, 1958); the title role in *Pericles* (Tony Richardson, 1958); and Don John in *Much Ado About Nothing* (Douglas Seale, 1958). As a member of Peter Hall's first RSC company he played Aguecheek (Hall, RST, 1960), Hans in Giraudoux's *Ondine* (Hall, Aldwych, 1961), and Urbain Grandier in *The Devils* (Peter Wood, Aldwych, 1961). From the late 1950s, Johnson worked most prominently in movies, co-starring in the Frank Sinatra war film *Never So Few* (John Sturges, 1959), *The Haunting* (Robert Wise, 1963), Harold Pinter's *The Pumpkin Eater* (Jack Clayton, 1964), *The Amorous Adventures of Moll Flanders* (Terence Young, 1965), and *Khartoum* (Basil Dearden, 1966).

Trevor Nunn's offer of the role of Marc Antony in both *Julius Caesar* and *Antony and Cleopatra* brought Johnson back to the RSC in 1972. His performance as a virile, charismatic, increasingly sombre and world-weary Antony threw into sharp relief the banality of his casting in movies. It was a critically acclaimed return, but Johnson remained an occasional theatre actor. A burst of activity at the National in the late 1970s—Charles in Coward's *Blithe Spirit* (Harold Pinter, Lyttelton, 1976), Pontius Pilate in *The Passion* (Bill Bryden, Cottesloe, 1977), Pinchwife in *The Country Wife* (Hall, Olivier, 1977), and Nandor in Ferenc Molnár's *The Guardsman* (Wood, Lyttelton, 1978)—was followed by a long silence.

In the 1990s he was seen in *The War That Still Goes On* (Young Vic, 1991), *An Inspector Calls* (Stephen Daldry, Aldwych, 1994), and *The Rivals* (Albery, 1994-95). Most notably he rejoined the RSC to play—uniquely—his second Antony in *Antony and Cleopatra* (John Caird, RST, 1992), the King of France in Peter Hall's *All's Well That Ends Well* (Swan, 1992), and Dorn in Adrian Noble's *The Seagull* (Swan, 2000). Chekhov's country doctor and ageing womaniser provoked a performance of sublime skill from an actor who in his time has been both a great Shakespearean and a heartthrob. His subsequent appearances have included Heinrich Mann in *Tales From Hollywood* (John Crowley, Donmar Warehouse, 2001); Harry in John Mortimer's *Hock and Soda Water* (Christopher Morahan, Minerva, Chichester, 2001); Conrad in Frank McGuinness's *Gates of Gold* (Gate, Dublin, 2002); Sir George in Shaw's *Mrs Warren's Profession* (Hall, Strand, 2002-03); and the RSC's *Hollow Crown* (Barton, RST, 2005).

Gemma Jones (b. London, 1942). One of the best actresses of her generation, Gemma Jones has drifted in and out of a major career. The daughter of Griffith Jones, she grew up surrounded by the theatre. As a young woman she played Madeleine in Ken Russell's controversial *The Devils* (1971). This was a memorable performance, but she did not act again in major features until *On the Black Hill* (Andrew Grieve, 1987). Soon after *The Devils* she joined the RSC to play Titania in Peter Brook's *A Midsummer Night's Dream*, one of the cast changes for the production's international tour. She had to wait ten years for her next RSC role.

Her biggest moment during these years came with the television series *The Duchess of Duke Street* (BBC, 1976-77).

Then in the early 1980s she won great acclaim for a string of striking performances: Hermione in *The Winter's Tale* (Ronald Eyre, RST, 1981); Lady Mortimer in *Henry IV Part 1* and Doll in *Part 2* (Trevor Nunn, Barbican, 1982); Win in Peter Whelan's *Clay* (Bill Alexander, Pit, 1982); Katharine in *Henry VIII* (Howard Davies, RST, 1983); Portia in *Julius Caesar* (Ron Daniels, RST, 1983); Maria in *Twelfth Night* (John Caird, RST, 1983); Lady Politic Would-Be in *Volpone* (Alexander, TOP, 1983); and Eugenia in Stephen Poliakoff's *Breaking the Silence* (Daniels, Pit, 1984). In 1989 she played Titania in Adrian Noble's production of *The Fairy Queen* at the Aix-en-Provence Festival (Peter Hall Company), and in his 1992 production of *The Winter's Tale* (RST) she gave a wonderfully spirited account of Paulina. In-between she played Goneril in *King Lear* (Jonathan Miller, Old Vic, 1989) and appeared in the premiere of Arthur Miller's *A Ride Down Mount Morgan* (West End, 1991).

After her perfect Mrs Dashwood in Ang Lee's movie of *Sense and Sensibility* (1995) she was suddenly in demand: Lady Queensberry in *Wilde* (Brian Gilbert, 1997); *The Theory of Flight* (Paul Greengrass, 1998); Grace Winslow in *The Winslow Boy* (David Mamet, 1999); *Captain Jack* (1999); *Cotton Mary* (Ismail Merchant, 1999); Bridget's Mum in *Bridget Jones's Diary* (Sharon Maguire, 2001) and *Bridget Jones: the Edge of Reason* (Beeban Kidron, 2004); Queen Victoria in *Shanghai Knights* (2003); *Spooks* (BBC, 2007-08).

Theatre work since 1999: Jersey in Nick Stafford's *Battle Royal* (Howard Davies, NT Lyttelton, 1999); Big Mamma to Ned Beatty's Big Daddy in the Brendan Fraser/Frances O'Connor *Cat on a Hot Tin Roof* (Anthony Page, Lyric, 2001); the Gravedigger in Fermin Cabal's *Tejas Verdes* (Thea Sharrock, Gate, 2005); *And Then There Were None* (Steven Pimlott, Gielgud, 2005); Grace in Mick Gordon and A.C. Grayling's *On Religion* (Mick Gordon, Soho Theatre, 2006); Simon Block's *Everything is Illuminated* (Rachel O'Riordan, Hampstead Theatre, 2006).

Griffith Jones (1910-2007, b. London). With his deep voice and splendid snow-white beard Griffith Jones was one of the RSC's most recognisable and admired members, and something of a figurehead. He was still working at Stratford in his late eighties. During the days when he was young, dark and clean-shaven he was a successful screen actor, appearing in more than one film a year.

He was educated at University College, London, and RADA. His most successful films, in which he supported (as second male lead) such stars as Elisabeth Bergner, Douglas Fairbanks Jnr., Robert Taylor, Vivien Leigh, Michael Redgrave, Laurence Olivier, Margaret Lockwood, James Mason, Rex Harrison, and Trevor Howard, were *Catherine the Great* (1934); *Escape Me Never* (1935); *A Yank at Oxford* (1938); *The Four Just Men* (Walter Forde, 1939); *Atlantic Ferry* (Forde, 1941); *Henry V* (Olivier, 1944); *The Wicked Lady* (1945); *The Rake's Progress* (Sidney Gilliat, 1945); and *They Made Me a Fugitive* (1947). The movies he made as the male lead were less successful: *The Wife of General Ling* (1937); *Once Upon a Dream*, opposite Googie Withers (Ralph Thomas, 1947); *Look Before You Love*, opposite Margaret Lockwood (1948); *Honeymoon Deferred* (1951); *Kill Her Gently* (1957); and *Account Rendered* (1957).

He was just as busy in the West End. He made his debut in 1930 while still at RADA (Achmed in *Carpet Slippers* at the Embassy Theatre). Before and after the war—he served in the army—there were few years when he was absent from the stage. Two Noël Coward premieres—*Operette* (His Majesty's, 1938) and *Quadrille* (Phoenix, 1952)—enliven a list dominated by forgotten plays.

He joined the RSC in 1975, the beginning of twenty-five back-to-back years. His contributions included the 1975 and 76 Other Place seasons (the Ghost in Buzz Goodbody's *Hamlet*, Duncan in Trevor Nunn's *Macbeth*); the first small-scale tour (Chebutikin in Nunn's *Three Sisters*, 1978); Tim Linkinwater/Fluggers in *Nicho-*

las Nickleby (Aldwych, 1980); Abhorson in Adrian Noble's *Measure for Measure* (RST, 1983); and Priam in Sam Mendes's *Troilus and Cressida* (Swan, 1990). Also: Glendower/Lord Chief Justice in *Henry IV* (Terry Hands, RST, 1975); Lord Stanley in *Perkin Warbeck* (Barry Kyle, TOP, 1975); Lord Stanley in *Richard III* (Kyle, TOP, 1975); Escalus in *Romeo and Juliet* (Trevor Nunn, RST, 1976); Antigonus in *The Winter's Tale* (John Barton, RST, 1976); Aegeon in *The Comedy of Errors* (Nunn, RST, 1976); Egeus in *A Midsummer Night's Dream* (Barton, RST, 1977); Gower in *Pericles* (Ron Daniels, TOP, 1979); Soothsayer/Jupiter in *Cymbeline* (David Jones, RST, 1979); the Gentleman in *All's Well That Ends Well* (Nunn, RST, 1981); Lord Chief Justice in *Henry IV* (Nunn, Barbican, 1982); Rainbow in *The Happiest Days of Your Life* (Clifford Williams, Barbican, 1984); Le Beau/Sir Oliver Martext in *As You Like It* (Noble, RST, 1985); d'Estaing in Pam Gems's *The Danton Affair* (Daniels, Barbican, 1986); Albert in *Scenes from a Marriage* (Hands, Barbican, 1986); Soothsayer in *Julius Caesar* (Hands, RST, 1987); Sir Nathaniel in *The Taming of the Shrew* (Jonathan Miller, RST, 1987); Jordan in *The New Inn* (Caird, Swan, 1987); Ferapont in *Three Sisters* (Barton, Barbican, 1988); Old Capulet/Apothecary in *Romeo and Juliet* (Hands, Swan, 1989); Old Vago in Julius Hay's *Have* (Janice Honeyman, Pit, 1990); Old Man in *King Lear* (Nicholas Hytner, RST, 1990); Marcade in *Love's Labour's Lost* (Hands, RST, 1990); Wat Dreary in *The Beggar's Opera* (Caird, Swan, 1992); Gentleman in *All's Well That Ends Well* (Peter Hall, Swan, 1992); Schoolmaster in *Antony and Cleopatra* (Caird, RST, 1992); Volscian Senator in *Coriolanus* (David Thacker, Swan, 1994); Abhorson in *Measure for Measure* (Steven Pimlott, RST, 1994); Angel in Byron's *Cain* (Barton, Pit, 1995); Old Man in *Macbeth* (Tim Albery, RST, 1996); Priam in *Troilus and Cressida* (Ian Judge, RST, 1996); Priest in *Twelfth Night* (Noble, RST, 1997); and Tubal in *The Merchant of Venice* (Gregory Doran, RST, 1997).

Emily Joyce (b. London, 1969) trained at Webber Douglas and began her career at the RSC as a member of the 1991-92 company. She was cast as a virgin in *'Tis Pity She's a Whore* (David Leveaux, Swan); a citizen in *Romeo and Juliet* (Leveaux, RST); Lady to Calpurnia in *Julius Caesar* (Steven Pimlott, RST); Isobel Motley in *A Woman Killed With Kindness* (Katie Mitchell, Pit); and Cherry in *King Baby* (Simon Usher, Pit). In early 1995 she played Maria in the revival of the 1993 *Love's Labour's Lost* (Ian Judge, Barbican). In the winter of 1995/96 she was Belle in *A Christmas Carol* (Judge, Barbican) before succeeding Emma Fielding as Viola in *Twelfth Night* (Judge, Barbican).

On television, Emily Joyce gave an eye-catching performance as the murderess—mousy lap technician by day, *femme fatale* after dark—in the *Cracker* drama 'True Romance' (Granada, 1995), and played the tender young wife in *Grafters* (ITV, 1998), and Ardal O'Hanlon's girlfriend in the BBC situation comedy *My Hero* (2000). Returning to the stage, she was seen at the Royal Court as the Wife in Debbie Tucker Green's *Stoning Mary* (Marianne Elliott, 2005), and Neighbour/Woman in Alexandra Wood's *The Eleventh Capital* (Natalie Abrahami, 2007).

Ian Judge (b. Warrington, 1946) grew up in Southport and studied at the Guildhall School. Initially an actor, he moved into full-time directing during the 1970s. He was an assistant director at the RSC from 1975 to 76, working on Terry Hands's productions of *Henry IV, Henry V* and *Merry Wives of Windsor* (RST), and later co-directed with Hands the Christmas show *The Swan Down Gloves* (RST, 1981) and the musical *Poppy* (Barbican, 1982).

Judge is an opera specialist, skilled at choreographing large casts on big stages. If, at one extreme, grand opera needs a Peter Sellars, it also, at the other, needs an Ian Judge, a director who actually likes and respects the multiple absurdities of the form. It comes as no surprise to learn that as a boy he was influenced by the old-style theatricality of seaside shows.

As a director of the classics, he worked most prominently at the RSC in the 1990s. *The Comedy of Errors* (RST, 1990) was stylish and colourful; *Love's Labour's Lost* (RST, 1993), set in an Oxbridge college just before the Great War, was both charming and melancholy; and *Troilus and Cressida* (RST, 1996), if a little too camp and old Hollywood in its spectacle, was unflinching in its cynicism and despair.

K

Jean Kalman (b. Paris). Jean Kalman's subtle artistry has given an extra dimension to the work of a select group of directors — Peter Brook (he came to notice working with Brook at the Bouffes du Nord from 1981), Hans Peter Cloos, Pierre Audi, Deborah Warner, Robert Carsen, and Adrian Noble.

Kalman's RSC designs: David Leveaux's *Romeo and Juliet* (RST, 1991); Adrian Noble's *Little Eyolf* (Swan, 1996) and *Pericles* (Roundhouse, 2002); and Dominic Cooke's *The Crucible* (RST, 2006). He lit Noble's productions of Monteverdi's *Le retour d'Ulysse* (Aix-en-Provence, 2000), Mozart's *Cosi fan tutte* and *Le nozze di Figaro* (Lyon, 2006-07) and Verdi's *Macbeth* (Met, New York, 2007).

John Kane (b. Dundee, 1945). An accomplished classical actor in both comedic and dramatic roles, John Kane spent the formative years of his career with the RSC (1966-71) — he trained under Michel Saint-Denis in the RSC Studio and played Myshkin in *The Government Inspector* (Peter Hall, Aldwych, 1966); Second Gravedigger/Francisco in *Hamlet* (Hall, RST, 1966); Francis in *Henry IV* and *Henry V* (John Barton/Trevor Nunn, RST, 1966); Supervacuo in *The Revenger's Tragedy* (Nunn, RST, 1966); Biondello/Curtis in *The Taming of the Shrew* (Nunn, RST, 1967); Silvius in *As You Like It* (David Jones, RST, 1967); La Verole in *The Relapse* (Nunn, Aldwych, 1967); Mel Delaney in

The Latent Heterosexual (Terry Hands, Aldwych, 1968); Ezekiel Edgworth in *Bartholomew Fair* (Hands, Aldwych, 1969); Pompey in *Measure for Measure* (Barton, RST, 1970); Lovell in *Richard III* (Hands, RST, 1970); Guildenstern in *Hamlet* (Nunn, RST, 1970); and, most significantly, Puck in Peter Brook's *A Midsummer Night's Dream* (RST, 1970).

Kane's second period of work with the Company began in 1984: Verkoff in Stephen Poliakoff's *Breaking the Silence* (Ron Daniels, Pit); Caliban in *The Tempest* (Nicholas Hytner, RST, 1988); Police Superintendent in *Barbarians* (Jones, Barbican, 1990); Ghost of Christmas Present in *A Christmas Carol* (Ian Judge, Barbican, 1994); Peter Quince in *A Midsummer Night's Dream* (Adrian Noble, International Tour, 1996); Duke of Norfolk in *Henry VIII* (Gregory Doran, Swan, 1996); Sir Hugh Evans in *The Merry Wives of Windsor* (Judge, RST, 1996); Soothsayer in *Cymbeline* (Noble, RST, 1997); Father Christmas/Air Raid Warden in *The Lion, the Witch and the Wardrobe* (Noble, RST, 1999-00); and Exeter/Lord Clifford/John Stanley in *Henry VI 1-3* (Michael Boyd, Swan, 2000-01).

Also a writer, particularly for television, Kane wrote the situation comedies *Happy Ever After* (BBC, 1974), *Me and My Girl* (ITV, 1984-88) and *Never the Twain* (ITV, 1981-91); and the Joss Ackland/Jean Simmons drama *Daisies in December* (Mark Haber, ITV, 1995). He adapted *The Wizard of Oz* for the RSC in 1987 (Ian Judge, Barbican).

Charles Kay (b. Coventry, 1930). After RADA, Charles Kay joined the English Stage Company at the Royal Court. He created the roles of Jimmy in Arnold Wesker's *Roots* (John Dexter, 1959) and Charles V in John Osborne's *Luther* (Tony Richardson, 1961), and was also in Stuart Holroyd's *The Tenth Chance* (Anthony Creighton, 1958), Wesker's *The Kitchen* (Dexter, 1959), *The Changeling* (Richardson, 1961), and *Twelfth Night* (George Devine, 1962).

His command of characterisation was particularly evident in the Osborne. At the RSC until 1966 he was equally impressive playing clerics in the histories and clowns in the comedies: Octavius Caesar in *Julius Caesar* (John Blatchley, RST, 1963); Sir John Hume/Clarence in *The Wars of the Roses* (Peter Hall, RST, 1963); Archbishop of Canterbury/Dauphin in *Henry V* (Hall/John Barton/Clifford Williams, RST, 1964); Navarre in *Love's Labour's Lost* (Barton, RST, 1965); Launcelot Gobbo in *The Merchant of Venice* (Williams, RST, 1965); Antipholus of Ephesus in *The Comedy of Errors* (Williams, RST, 1965); a Poet in *Timon of Athens* (John Schlesinger, RST, 1965); Player Queen/Osric in the David Warner *Hamlet* (Hall, RST, 1965); Dobchinsky in *The Government Inspector* (Hall, Aldwych, 1966); Jochen in *The Meteor* (Williams, Aldwych, 1966); and Moloch in *The Thwarting of Baron Bolligrew* (Trevor Nunn, Aldwych, 1966). He was next seen at the National in *As You Like It* (Williams, 1967) and Peter Nichols's *The National Health* (Michael Blakemore, 1969).

In the years that followed Kay continued to build a distinguished, if unspectacular, career. Screen work dominated: *A Fall of Eagles* (BBC, 1974); *Hennessy* (1975); Lord Randolph Churchill in *Jennie, Lady Randolph Churchill* (ITV, 1975); Gallus in *I, Claudius* (BBC, 1976); Louis VII in *The Devil's Crown* (BBC, 1978); *To Serve Them All My Days* (BBC, 1980); *Nijinsky* (1980); *Whoops Apocalypse* (ITV, 1982); Count Orsini-Rosenberg in *Amadeus* (Milos Forman, 1984); *Edge of Darkness* (BBC, 1986); outstanding as the calm diplomat in *Fortunes of War* (BBC, 1987); the Archbishop of Canterbury in *Henry V* (Kenneth Branagh, 1989); *Bomber Harris* (BBC, 1992); *Heart of Darkness* (Nicolas Roeg, 1994).

Since 1980 he has returned to the stage at intervals. At the RSC: Basilio in *Life's a Dream* (Barton, TOP, 1983); Charles Cantelupe in *Waste* (Barton, Pit, 1985); Oliver in David Edgar's *Pentecost* (Michael Attenborough, TOP, 1994); and Lafeu in *All's Well That Ends Well* (Gregory Doran, Swan, 2003-04). Elsewhere: *Danton's Death* (Peter Gill, NT Olivier, 1982); *The Scarlet Pimpernel* (Nicholas Hytner, Chichester, 1985); *The Woman in Black*

(Lyric Hammersmith, 1989); Harpagon in *The Miser* (Steven Pimlott, NT Olivier, 1991); Willis in Alan Bennett's *The Madness of George III* (Hytner, NT Lyttelton, 1991); Victor in Ben Travers's *The Bed Before Yesterday* (Peter Wood, Almeida, 1994); Stephen in Simon Gray's *Simply Disconnected* (Richard Wilson, Minerva, Chichester, 1996); Praed in Bernard Shaw's *Mrs Warren's Profession* (Alan Strachan, Richmond Theatre, 1997); and Sir Timothy Bellboys in *A Penny for a Song* (Paul Miller, Oxford Stage Company, 1999).

Sara Kestelman (b. London, 1944). An actress with a strong stage presence who has often played assertive women, Sara Kestelman came to prominence when, plucked from the RSC ranks, she created a proud, predatory Titania (doubled with Hippolyta) in Peter Brook's production of *A Midsummer Night's Dream* (RST, 1970). Soon after she appeared opposite Sean Connery in John Boorman's *Zardoz* (1973) and the camera revealed a photogenic face of girlish freckles.

Born in London, she trained to be a dancer and made her first professional appearance, aged sixteen, as a spirit in *The Tempest* (Robert Atkins, Open Air Theatre, Regent's Park). She then went to Central and began her career at the Liverpool Playhouse and the Library Theatre, Manchester (1965-67). She joined the RSC in 1968 and in the years leading up to Brook's *Dream* played Lechery in *Doctor Faustus* (Clifford Williams, RST, 1968); the Duchess of Vanholt in *Doctor Faustus* (US Tour, 1969); Margaret, succeeding Susan Fleetwood, in *Much Ado About Nothing* (Trevor Nunn, Aldwych, 1969); Cassandra, succeeding Susan Fleetwood, in *Troilus and Cressida* (John Barton, Aldwych, 1969); Jessie in *The Silver Tassie* (David Jones, Aldwych, 1969); Mariana in *Measure for Measure* (Barton, RST, 1970); and Jane Shore in *Richard III* (Terry Hands, RST, 1970). She followed the *Dream* with Kleopatra in *Enemies* (Jones, Aldwych, 1971), Natasha in Robert Montgomery's *Subject to Fits* (A.J. Antoon, The Place, 1971) and

Anna in Wedekind's *The Marquis of Keith* (Ronald Eyre, Aldwych, 1974).

For the rest of the 1970s she worked outside of the RSC: Lady Macbeth and Ruth in Pinter's *The Homecoming* (1972) at the Birmingham Rep; Yelena in *Uncle Vanya* (1973) at the Bristol Old Vic; Sally Bowles in *I am a Camera* (1976) for the Cambridge Theatre Company; and, at the National, Susannah in Alan Ayckbourn's *Bedroom Farce* (Peter Hall, Lyttelton, 1977), Alexandra in Robert Bolt's *State of Revolution* (Christopher Morahan, Lyttelton, 1977), Lady Touchwood in *The Double Dealer* (Peter Wood, Olivier, 1978), Enid Underwood in Galsworthy's *Strife* (Morahan, Olivier, 1978), the Lady With A Monocle in Lev Tolstoy's *The Fruits of Enlightenment* (Morahan, Olivier, 1979), Mrs Wahl in Stoppard's adaptation of Schnitzler's *Undiscovered Country* (Wood, Olivier, 1979), and Rosalind in *As You Like It* (John Dexter, Olivier, 1979).

In 1982/83, back at the RSC, she was an intimidating Lady Macbeth opposite Bob Peck (Howard Davies, RST), an icy Goneril in Adrian Noble's production of *King Lear* (RST) and Bodice in Edward Bond's *Lear* (Barry Kyle, TOP). She returned briefly in 1990 to play Raisa Gorbachev in *Moscow Gold* (Kyle, Barbican), and in 1993 to play Mary in *Misha's Party* (Jones, Pit).

Theatre work since 1995: Edward Albee's *Three Tall Women* (Wyndham's, 1995); the Duchess in Martin Sherman's *Some Sunny Day* (Roger Michell, Hampstead Theatre, 1996), alongside Corin Redgrave, Rupert Everett and Cheryl Campbell; *Sarrasine* (Neil Bartlett, Lyric Hammersmith, 1996); Liliane La Fleur, the movie producer, in the musical *Nine* (David Leveaux, Donmar Warehouse, 1997); Margrethe in Michael Frayn's *Copenhagen* (Michael Blakemore, NT Cottesloe, 1998); Gertrude in the Simon Russell Beale *Hamlet* (John Caird, NT Lyttelton, 2000); Golda/Sara in Richard Morris's *Bitter Fruit of Palestine* (David Newman, Baron's Court, 2002); and Nell in Thomas Kilroy's *The Shape of Metal* (Lynne Parker, Abbey, Dublin, 2003).

Zardoc remains the best of her films—she was also in *Lisztomania* (Ken Russell, 1975), *Break of Day* (1977) and *Lady Jane*

(Trevor Nunn, 1986). On television, she played Elena opposite Anthony Hopkins in Sartre's *Kean* (James Cellan Jones, BBC, 1978); Queenie to Ian Holm's Leavis in *The Last Romantics* (BBC, 1992); Madame Zarene in *Brazen Hussies* (Elijah Moshinsky, 1996); Mrs Wilkins in *Tom Jones* (Metin Hüseyin, BBC, 1997); and Countess Vronskaya in *Anna Karenina* (Channel Four, 2000).

Ben Kingsley (b. Snainton, Yorkshire, 1943). A single film changed the course of Ben Kingsley's career. Before winning the Best Actor Oscar for his fine performance as *Gandhi* (Richard Attenborough, 1982) he was a long-term RSC actor with only one picture to his name (the Alistair Maclean thriller *Fear is the Key*, 1972, in which he played a gangster); since, he has worked predominantly in international features. One supreme performance during this period—Itzhak Stern in *Schindler's List* (Steven Spielberg, 1993)—along with first-rate work in smaller-scale pieces—Pinter's *Betrayal* (David Jones, 1983), with Jeremy Irons; *Turtle Diary* (John Irvin, 1985); *Maurice* (James Ivory, 1987); Shostakovich in *Testimony* (Tony Palmer, 1988); *Pascali's Island* (James Dearden, 1988); *Searching for Bobby Fischer* (Steven Zaillian, 1993); *Death and the Maiden* (Roman Polanski, 1994); Feste in *Twelfth Night* (Trevor Nunn, 1996); *Photographing Fairies* (Nick Willing, 1997); Meyer Lansky in *Bugsy* (Barry Levinson, 1991); the psychotic London gangster in *Sexy Beast* (Jonathan Glazer, 2000); *House of Sand and Fog* (Vadim Perelman, 2003)—more than make up for *Harem* (Arthur Joffé, 1985), a soft-porn film with the sex left out; *Sneakers* (Phil Alden Robinson, 1992), in which he played an improbable villain; *Species* (Roger Donaldson, 1995); *The Assignment* (Christian Duguay, 1997); *Rules of Engagement* (William Friedkin, 2000); *Thunderbirds* (2004); and two biblical epics, made for television, *Joseph* (1995) and *Moses* (1996). The remarkable range of Kingsley's work is explained by his passion for acting, his technical skill and his appearance—he can play European, Middle-Eastern and Eastern characters without contrivance. His best performances have been finely detailed and deeply felt.

One senses that Ben Kingsley's heart remains in the theatre despite his long absences away. He is an RSC associate artist but has not performed with the Company since 1985-86, when he played the title role in *Othello* (Terry Hands, RST, David Suchet as Iago) and Caracol in Bernard Pomerance's *Mellons* (Alison Sutcliffe, Pit, 1986). The son of an Indian GP and an English actress, brought up in Yorkshire, his early opportunities included a spell (mid-1960s) in *Coronation Street* (Granada) and repertory at the Victoria Theatre, Stoke (Doolittle in *Pygmalion*, 1965). In 1966 he appeared in Alan Plater's *A Smashing Day* at the Arts Theatre and *Macbeth* at Chichester. He joined the RSC in 1967, and in his first season played a Huntsman in *The Taming of the Shrew* (Trevor Nunn, RST), Third Lord in *The Revenger's Tragedy* (Nunn, RST), Amiens in *As You Like It* (David Jones, RST), and a Wigmaker in *The Relapse* (Nunn, Aldwych). Over the course of the next twelve years he progressed to leading roles and, working with Buzz Goodbody, played a key role in the development of studio theatre: Oswald in *King Lear* (Nunn, RST, 1968); Aeneas in *Troilus and Cressida* (John Barton, RST, 1968); Conrade in *Much Ado About Nothing* (Nunn, RST, 1968); the Croucher in *The Silver Tassie* (Jones, Aldwych, 1969); Winwife in *Bartholomew Fair* (Terry Hands, Aldwych, 1969); Claudio in *Measure for Measure* (Barton, RST, 1970); Demetrius in Peter Brook's *A Midsummer Night's Dream* (RST, 1970); Ariel in *The Tempest* (Barton, RST, 1970); Sintsov in Gorky's *Enemies* (Jones, Aldwych, 1971); Gramsci in Trevor Griffiths's *Occupations* (Buzz Goodbody, The Place, 1971); Ippolit in Robert Montgomery's *Subject to Fits* (A.J. Antoon, The Place, 1971); *The Oz Trial* (Buzz Goodbody, The Place, 1971); Johnnie opposite Janet Suzman in Athol Fugard's *Hello and Goodbye* (Peter Stevenson, The Place, 1973); Fritz in John Wiles's *A Lesson of Blood and Roses* (Clifford Williams, The Place, 1973); the title role in Buzz Goodbody's *Hamlet* (TOP, 1975); Slender in *The Merry Wives of Windsor* (Hands, RST, 1975); Bonze Wang in *Man is Man* (Howard Davies, TOP, 1975); Frank Ford in *The Merry Wives of Windsor* (Nunn/John Caird, RST, 1979); Iachimo in *Cymbeline* (Jones, RST, 1979); the title role in Brecht's *Baal* (Jones, TOP, 1979), for which he also wrote the music; Brutus in *Julius Caesar* (Barry Kyle, RST, 1979); and Squeers/Wagstaff in *Nicholas Nickleby* (Nunn/Caird, Aldwych, 1980).

Elsewhere, he played Errol Philander in Athol Fugard's *Statements after an Arrest* (Fugard, Royal Court, 1974); the title role in Adrian Noble's production of *Doctor Faustus* (Manchester Royal Exchange, 1981); and the title role in *Kean* (Theatre Royal Haymarket, 1983). For Peter Hall at the National (Olivier), 1977-78, he was Mosca in *Volpone*, Sparkish in *The Country Wife* and Trofimov in *The Cherry Orchard*. In 1997 he made a much-anticipated return to the stage to play Estragon to Alan Howard's Vladimir in *Waiting for Godot*, the highlight of Peter Hall's season at the Old Vic.

Alex Kingston (b. London, 1963) appeared in the children's soap *Grange Hill* (BBC) when she was fifteen, playing a schoolgirl bully. She went on to RADA, where she met her future husband, Ralph Fiennes, and began her adult career in the theatre of the late 1980s. Her progress was relatively quiet, but she is an assertive performer who now works in Los Angeles.

Among her early roles were Pam in *Saved* (Birmingham Rep Studio, 1988), Fräulein Müller in Lenz's *The Tutor* (Angelika Hurwicz, Old Vic, 1988), and Diana in Terence Rattigan's *French Without Tears* (Simon Usher, Leicester Haymarket, 1988).

In 1990 she joined Ralph Fiennes at the RSC. She played Hero in *Much Ado About Nothing* (Bill Alexander, RST), Cordelia in the John Wood *King Lear* (Nicholas Hytner, RST) and a very slutty Jaquenetta (her performance consisted almost entirely of body language) in *Love's Labour's Lost* (Terry Hands, RST). On the transfer to London (Pit), she added Emma in Sam Shepard's *The Curse of the Starving Class* (Robin Lefevre) and Grace in Peter Whelan's *The Bright and Bold Design* (Alexander).

In 1992 she played Dolores in Griselda Gambaro's *Bad Blood* at the Gate (Kate Rowland), and Hippolyta/Titania in *A Midsummer Night's Dream* at the Sheffield Crucible (Michael Rudman); in 1993, Desdemona in *Othello* at the Birmingham Rep (Alexander). The publicity that accompanied the break-up of her marriage and her starring role in a glossy adaptation of *Moll Flanders* (David Attwood, ITV, 1996) raised her profile, particularly in America: in 1997 she joined the cast of the American medical series *ER*.

Michael Kitchen (b. Leicester, 1948) has been involved in some of the most fascinating television pieces of the last thirty years. Most memorably, he played the devil figure in Dennis Potter's long banned *Brimstone and Treacle* (1976); Foster, a dark shadow at the edge of Ralph Richardson and John Gielgud, in Harold Pinter's *No Man's Land* (Peter Hall, 1978); and appeared opposite Peggy Ashcroft in Stephen Poliakoff's *Caught on a Train* (Peter Duffell, 1980). These last two productions were so good that they have lasted in the memory through all the endless hours of bad TV since. But Kitchen is always good, even in indifferent dramas. Two examples: he found complexity in the character of a lawyer who rapes a secretary (Caroline Catz) in a turgid thriller called *The Guilty* (Colin Gregg, 1993); and his king in the over-cooked political satire *To Play the King* (Paul Seed, 1993) was a brilliant parody of the Prince of Wales—whatever the intention of the writer (Andrew Davies), Kitchen's characterisation could almost been seen as an act of homage.

Kitchen's film roles have been more predictable. He was in *Mrs Dalloway* (Marleen Gorris, 1997), played an MI5 man in the Bond adventure *Goldeneye* (Martin Campbell, 1995), and back in 1985 almost hit the big time in the Hollywood epic *Out of Africa* (Sydney Pollack).

For the first decade of his career Kitchen maintained a balance between theatre and television. He started as a member of the National Youth Theatre and worked as an assistant stage manager at the Belgrade, Coventry, before training at RADA. From the middle 1970s to the early 80s he was a member of the National Theatre, where his work included *Spring Awakening* (Bill Bryden, Old Vic, 1974); *Romeo and Juliet* (Bryden, Old Vic, 1974); Foster in *No Man's Land* (Peter Hall, Lyttelton, 1976); Trotsky in Robert Bolt's *State of Revolution* (Christopher Morahan, Lyttelton, 1977); Ayckbourn's *Bedroom Farce* (Hall, Lyttelton, 1977); Heartfree in *The Provok'd Wife* (Peter Wood, Lyttelton, 1980); Stoppard's *On the Razzle* (Wood, Lyttelton, 1981); Pinter's *Family Voices* (Hall, 1982); and Dvornichek in Stoppard's *Rough Crossing* (Wood, Lyttelton, 1984).

In 1986 he joined the RSC to play a bored, bitterly sarcastic Mercutio in *Romeo and Juliet* (Michael Bogdanov, RST); a sardonic, Pinteresque Bolingbroke in the Jeremy Irons *Richard II* (Barry Kyle, RST); and Hogarth in Nick Dear's *The Art of Success* (Adrian Noble, TOP). Kitchen brings to the classics a modern sense of irony and detachment. He is also, at times, very droll (his Mercutio dropped Alka-Seltzer into a glass of wine).

Estelle Kohler (b. Johannesburg, 1940) travelled from South Africa to England in 1963 to take up a scholarship at RADA. The RSC engaged her in 1965 to understudy (John Schlesinger's production of *Timon of Athens*) and immediately saw her appeal. The following year she was cast as Ophelia in the David Warner *Hamlet* (Peter Hall), Olivia in *Twelfth Night* (Clifford Williams) and Lady Percy in the first part of *Henry IV* (John Barton/Trevor Nunn/Williams).

The prettiest but least filmed RSC actress of her generation, she went on to play Virgilia in *Coriolanus* (Barton, RST, 1967); Helena in *All's Well That Ends Well* (Barton, RST, 1967); Juliet opposite Ian Holm in *Romeo and Juliet* (Karolos Koun, RST, 1967); Isabella in *Measure for Measure* (Barton, RST, 1970); Sylvia to Helen Mirren's Julia in *The Two Gentlemen of Verona* (Robin Phillips, RST, 1970); Miranda in *The Tempest* (Barton, RST, 1970); Angelica in *Occupations* (Buzz Goodbody, The Place, 1971); Beatrice in Harold Pinter's production of James Joyce's *Exiles* (Aldwych, 1971); Carmen in *The Balcony* (Terry Hands, Aldwych, 1971); Guenhwyvar in John Arden's *Island of the Mighty* (David Jones, Aldwych, 1972); Juliet opposite Timothy Dalton in *Romeo and Juliet* (Hands, RST, 1973); Voice 2 in *Sylvia Plath* (Barry Kyle, TOP, 1973); Sylvia Plath's *Three Women* (Kyle, TOP, 1973); Rosaline in *Love's Labour's Lost* (Jones, RST, 1973); Mikhailovna Varvara in *Summerfolk* (Jones, Aldwych, 1974); Judith in *The Devil's Disciple* (Jack Gold, Aldwych, 1976); Anna in Chekhov's *Ivanov* (Jones, Aldwych, 1976); and Sarah in Granville-Barker's *The Marrying of Ann Leete* (Jones, Aldwych, 1976).

She then took a long break from the RSC. Since her return she has played Sister Jeanne in *The Devils* (Barton, Pit, 1984); Amanda in Doug Lucie's *Fashion* (Nick Hamm, TOP, 1987); a sexually alluring Tamora, aroused by violence, in Deborah Warner's production of *Titus Andronicus* (Swan, 1987); Hester opposite Antony Sher in *Hello and Goodbye* (Janice Honeyman, Almeida, 1988); Lorraine Sheldon in *The Man Who Came to Dinner* (Gene Saks, Barbican, 1989); Mrs Kepes in *Have* (Janice Honeyman, Pit, 1990); Adriana in *The Comedy of Errors* (Ian Judge, RST, 1990); an unusually complicated Goneril, losing her head to Ralph Fiennes's younger Edmund, in *King Lear* (Nicholas Hytner, RST, 1990); the White Witch in *The Lion, the Witch and the Wardrobe* (Adrian Noble, RST, 1998, Barbican, 1999); and Paulina in *The Winter's Tale* (Gregory Doran, RST, 1998). Her wonderful Paulina, graceful and wise, was a reminder that her adult life can be measured out in RSC performances, particularly of Shakespeare.

Estelle Kohler's stage appearances outside of the RSC have included Mrs Birling in Stephen Daldry's *An Inspector Calls* (Garrick, 1996); a poignant Madame Ranyevskaya (renamed Rademayer) in Janet Suzman's ingenious South African version of *The Cherry Orchard* (Birmingham Rep and Market Theatre, Johannesburg, 1997); and Judith in Noël Coward's *Hay Fever* (Dominic Dromgoole, Oxford Stage Company, 2001).

Ralph Koltai (b. Berlin, 1924) studied at the Central School of Art and Design. One of the most influential designers of the post-war theatre, an innovator in the use of modern materials, Ralph Koltai worked as an associate artist at the RSC from 1962 to 1966, and again from 1976 to 1988. He designed William Gaskill's *The Caucasian Chalk Circle* (Aldwych, 1962); Clifford Williams's *The Representative* (Aldwych, 1963), *The Jew of Malta* (Aldwych, 1964), *The Merchant of Venice* (RST, 1965), *Major Barbara* (Aldwych, 1970), *Wild Oats* (Aldwych, 1976) and *The Love-Girl and the Innocent* (Aldwych, 1981); Harold Pinter's *The Birthday Party* (Aldwych, 1964); Terry Hands's *Old World* (Aldwych, 1976), *Much Ado About Nothing* (RST, 1982), *Cyrano de Bergerac* (Barbican, 1983) and *Othello* (RST, 1985); Ron Daniels's *The Sons of Light* (TOP, 1977) and *Romeo and Juliet* (RST, 1980); John Barton's *Love's Labour's Lost* (RST, 1978) and *Hamlet* (RST, 1980); David Jones's *Baal* (TOP, 1979); and Howard Davies's *Troilus and Cressida* (RST, 1985).

Alice Krige (b. Upington, South Africa, 1954) spent two years with the RSC (1982-83) before concentrating on a film career that had already begun with leading roles in *Ghost Story* (John Irving, 1981) and *Chariots of Fire* (Hugh Hudson, 1981). At the RSC she played Bianca in *The Taming of the Shrew* (Barry Kyle), an irresistible Miranda to Derek Jacobi's Prospero in *The Tempest* (Ron Daniels), and Cordelia in *King Lear* (Adrian Noble, all RST). Noble's production opened with the startling image of Alice Krige's beautiful Cordelia and Antony Sher's clown sitting on Lear's thrown, joined together at the neck by a noose. She was also the Gravedigger's Boy's Wife in Edward Bond's *Lear* (Barry Kyle, TOP) and Roxane in *Cyrano de Bergerac* (Terry Hands, Barbican, 1983).

She played Bathsheba opposite Richard Gere in *King David* (Bruce Beresford, 1985), but the film failed at the box office and subsequently she has been denied real opportunities. She was in *Barfly* (Barbet Schroeder, 1987); *Spies Inc.* (Anthony Thomas,

1988); *Haunted Summer* (Ivan Passer, 1988); *Sleepwalkers* (Mick Garris, 1992); *Institute Benjamenta* (Stephen and Timothy Quay, 1995); *Star Trek: First Contact* (1996); *The Commissioner* (George Sluizer, 1998); *Molokai* (Paul Cox, 1999); *The Little Vampire* (2000); *The Calling* (2000); *Superstition* (Kenneth Hope, 2001); and *Reign of Fire* (Rob Bowman, 2002). She has had better luck on British television: in the BBC serial of Stendhal's *Scarlet and Black* (Ben Bolt, 1993), as La Marquesa in *Sharpe's Honour* (Tom Clegg, ITV, 1994), and as an Italian lawyer in *Devil's Advocate* (Adrian Shergold, BBC, 1995).

In 1995 she made an isolated return to the stage to play Belvidera in Thomas Otway's *Venice Preserv'd* (Ian McDiarmid, Almeida).

L

Jane Lapotaire (b. Ipswich, 1944). An astute and graceful performer, Jane Lapotaire was the senior actress at the RSC in the 1990s. She played Gertrude in the Kenneth Branagh *Hamlet* (Adrian Noble, Barbican, 1992) as a despairing figure—she appeared to drink the poison knowingly—and was equally inspired as Mrs Alving in *Ghosts* (Katie Mitchell, TOP, 1993) and Katherine—emphasising the pain of exile by means of accent, gesture and expression—in *Henry VIII* (Gregory Doran, Swan, 1996).

Her earlier RSC roles were Viola in *Twelfth Night* (Peter Gill, RST, 1974); Lady Macduff/Weird Sister in the Nicol Williamson/Helen Mirren *Macbeth* (Trevor Nunn, RST, 1974); Sonya in *Uncle Vanya* (Nicol Williamson, TOP, 1974); Rosaline in *Love's Labour's Lost* (John Barton, RST, 1978); a remarkable interpretation of the great singer Piaf in Pam Gems's hit play (TOP, 1978); Lina in Shaw's *Misalliance* (John Caird, Barbican, 1986); and Maya in Miller's *The Archbishop's Ceiling* (Nick Hamm, Pit, 1986).

She is of French descent, the daughter of an orphan and an unknown father brought up by a foster mother in Norfolk (see her fine autobiography *Grace and Favour*, Macmillan, 1989). She trained in Bristol and was a member of the Bristol Old Vic Company, 1965-67, playing Ruth in *The Homecoming*, Vivie Warren in *Mrs Warren's Profession* and Natasha in *War and Peace*. She then joined Olivier's National Theatre Company at the Old Vic (1967), becoming a founder member of the National's satellite company at the Young Vic in 1970. At the Old Vic she played Judith in Strindberg's *The Dance of Death* (Glen Byam Shaw, 1967), Mrs Fainall in *The Way of the World* (Michael Langham, 1969), and Jessica to Olivier's Shylock in *The Merchant of Venice* (Jonathan Miller, 1970); at the Young Vic, Kate in *The Taming of the Shrew*, Jocasta in *Oedipus*, and Isabella in *Measure for Measure*. She returned to the National in 1983/84: Peter Gill's *Kick for Touch* (Cottesloe), Belvidera in Otway's *Venice Preserv'd* (Gill, Lyttelton), and the title role in *Antigone* (Gill/John Burgess, Cottesloe). Other appearances: Vera in *A Month in the Country* and Lucy in *A Room with a View* (Prospect, 1976); Rosalind in *As You Like It* (Gill, Nottingham Playhouse, 1976); the title role in *Saint Joan* (Compass, 1985); *L'Aide Memoire*, the inaugural production of Molière and Co. (1988); and Joy in *Shadowlands* (West End, 1989).

Her most prominent screen roles were Marie Curie (BBC, 1977); Lady Macbeth (Jack Gold, BBC, 1982); Helen in Nicholas Roeg's *Eureka* (1982); Princess Mary in *Lady Jane* (Trevor Nunn, 1986); and Olga in *Surviving Picasso* (James Ivory, 1996).

James Laurenson (b. Marton, New Zealand) trained at the London Academy of Dramatic Art and appeared with the Oxford Players before joining the RSC in 1964. Initially little more than a spear carrier, by the end of his second Stratford season, 1965, he had progressed to Longaville in *Love's Labour's Lost* (John Barton); First Basso in *The Jew of Malta* (Clifford Williams); Lucilius in *Timon of Athens* (John Schlesinger); and Guildenstern to Michael Williams's Rosencrantz in the David Warner *Hamlet* (Peter Hall). However, it was Prospect Theatre Company's acclaimed 1969 production of *Edward II* (Toby Richardson, Edinburgh Festival and Tour) that provided Laurenson with the best of his early opportunities—he played Gaveston to Ian McKellen's Edward.

Laurenson could have become one of the leading younger classical actors had not television, particularly the twenty-six episodes of the Australian series *Boney* in which he starred as the half-Aboriginal detective, taken up the relevant years. He re-established his reputation as a stage actor at the RSC, 1977-79, playing Charles the Dauphin/Jack Cade in the second and third parts of *Henry VI* (Terry Hands, RST); Duke Alessandro de Medici in *The Lorenzaccio Story* (Ron Daniels, TOP); Alsemero in *The Changeling* (Hands, Aldwych); Jack Benedict in *Saratoga* (Ronald Eyre, Aldwych); Cassio in *Othello* (Eyre, RST); and Cassius in *Julius Caesar* (Barry Kyle, RST). Laurenson has remained a respected and admired figure, the kind of actor who works constantly and who divides his time almost equally between stage and screen. He returned to Stratford to play Benedict Arnold in Richard Nelson's *The General from America* (Howard Davies, Swan, 1996); Friedrich in Heinrich Von Kleist's *The Prince of Homburg* (Neil Bartlett, Swan, 2002); and Danforth in Arthur Miller's *The Crucible* (Dominic Cooke, RST, 2006)—it was his fine achievement to suggest a small kernel of humanity within the character's severe fundamentalism.

At the National Theatre, he performed Fernando Gomez de Guzmanin in Declan Donnellan's production of Lope de Vega's *Fuente Ovejuna* (Cottesloe, 1989); Quentin in Arthur Miller's *After the Fall* (Michael Blakemore, Cottesloe, 1990); and Macduff in *Macbeth* (Richard Eyre, Olivier, 1993). He was Antony to Diana Rigg's Cleopatra in Dryden's *All for Love* and a formidable Claudius to Ralph Fiennes's *Hamlet*, both for Jonathan Kent at the Almeida (1991, 1995); Harry in Edward Albee's *A Delicate Balance* at the Theatre Royal Haymarket (Anthony Page, 1997); and James in Peter Nichols's *Passion Play* at the Donmar Warehouse (Michael Grandage, 2000). Most rewarding of all, during the summers of 2004 and 2006 he led Peter Hall's company at the Theatre Royal, Bath, in the most distinguished fashion— Ramsden in Shaw's *Man and Superman*; Don Luis in Molière's *Don Juan*; Pope Urban VIII in Timberlake Wertenbaker's *Galileo's Daughter*; and a chillingly unsympathetic Duke in *Measure for Measure*.

Laurenson created characters in the first Inspector Morse drama, *The Dead of Jericho* (ITV, 1987), *Prime Suspect 4* (ITV, 1995), *Sharpe* (ITV, 1996-97), Paul Abbott's *State of Play* (BBC, 2003), *Dalziel and Pascoe* (BBC, 2004), *Hustle* (BBC, 2004) and *Spooks* (BBC, 2007); and the films, *Women in Love* (Ken Russell, 1969), *Assault* (1971), *The Wall* (Alan Parker, 1982), *The Cat's Meow* (Peter Bogdanovich, 2001) and *Three Blind Mice* (Mathias Ledoux, 2003).

John Laurie (1897-1980, b. Dumfries, Scotland). A survivor of the Great War, John Laurie trained at the Central School in London and began his life as an actor in his hometown of Dumfries (*What Every Woman Knows*, 1921). He came to notice a year later playing Pistol in William Bridges-Adams's production of *The Merry Wives of Windsor* at the Lyric Hammersmith. Bridges-Adams included Laurie in his Stratford company of 1925, casting him as Autolycus in *The Winter's Tale*; Amiens in *As You Like It*; Feste in *Twelfth Night*; Speed in *The Two Gentlemen of Verona*; Don Pedro in *Much Ado About Nothing*; Ritornello in Sheridan's *The Critic*; Ross in *Macbeth*; Chatillon in *King John*; Ligarius in *Julius Caesar*; and Costard in *Love's Labour's Lost*. The beautiful and popular Florence Saunders, whom Laurie had married in 1924, played the leading female roles. Tragically, she died the following year at the age of thirty-five.

In the next decade Laurie became one of the master Shakespearean actors of his generation, a regular performer at Stratford and in the capital at the Old Vic, Regent's Park and elsewhere, renowned for his verse-speaking and his versatility—he played most of the tragic leads as well as the melancholy clowns, his speciality. In later years his forceful style perhaps dated him as an actor of that era (a friend of, and influence on, Laurence Olivier since the 1920s, Laurie might have expected to receive a call when Olivier started the National, but the great star had moved on and had no place for old troopers).

His other pre-war Stratford seasons were 1927, 1934 and 1939. He played Biondello in *The Taming of the Shrew*; Ross in *Macbeth*; Feste in *Twelfth Night*; the title role in *Hamlet*; Fag in *The Rivals*; Eros in *Antony and Cleopatra*; Amiens in *As You Like It* (all Bridges-Adams, 1927); Prokesch in Madge Pemberton's *The Son of Man* (Robert Atkins, 1934); Jaques in *As You Like It* (Baliol Holloway); the title role in *Richard III* (B. Iden Payne); the title role in *Othello* (Robert Atkins, Alec Clunes as Iago); Malvolio in *Twelfth Night* (Irene Hentschel); and Sicinius Velutus in *Coriolanus* (B. Iden Payne, all 1939).

At the Old Vic in 1928/29, directed by Andrew Leigh, he played Armando in *Love's Labour's Lost*; Sigurd in *The Vikings at Helgeland*; Touchstone in *As You Like It*; Feste in *Twelfth Night*; the title role in *Macbeth*; the title role in *Hamlet*; Buckingham in *Henry VIII*; Sir Hugh Evans in *The Merry Wives of Windsor*; and Adam in *Adam's Opera*. He spent the summers of 1933, 1934 and 1935 at Robert Atkins's Open Air Theatre, Regent's Park, as Orsino in *Twelfth Night*; Oliver in *As You Like It*; Lysander in *A Midsummer Night's Dream*; Alonzo in *The Tempest*; Aguecheek in *Twelfth Night*; and Flute in *A Midsummer Night's Dream*.

Laurie's non-Shakespearean performances included Tristan in *Tristan and Isolde* (London, 1927); Joel in *Judith of Israel* (1928); Seymour in *The Tudor Wench* (London, 1933); Faulkland in *The Rivals* (London, 1934); Sparkish in *The Country Wife* (London, 1934); Ferdinand in *The Duchess of Malfi* (London, 1935); Flamineo in *The White Devil* (London, 1935); Rosmer in *Rosmersholm* (London, 1936); Lovborg in *Hedda Gabler* (London, 1936); Shotover in *Heartbreak House* (London, 1943); Colonel Branden in *Sense and Sensibility* (London, 1946); the title role in *John Knox* (Glasgow, 1947); Syme in *The Human Touch* (London, 1949); Peterbono in *Thieves' Carnival* (London, 1952); Demokos in *Tiger at the Gates* (London, 1955); Firs in *The Cherry Orchard* (Chichester, 1966); and McGonagall in *The Hero of a Hundred Fights* (Perth, 1968).

From 1930 onwards Laurie worked prolifically as a character actor in British films. The films that have lasted are Hitchcock's *The Thirty-Nine Steps* (1935); Michael Powell's *Edge of the World* (1938), *I Know Where I'm Going!* (1945), and *The Life and Death of Colonel Blimp* (1943); Zoltan Korda's *The Four Feathers* (1939)—he played Khalifa; Olivier's *Henry V* (1944), *Hamlet* (1948) and *Richard III* (1954)—he played Captain Jamie, Francisco and Lord Lovell; Carol Reed's *The Way Ahead* (1944); and David Lean's *Hobson's Choice* (1953).

It is fitting that his last act as a classical actor was to return to the Stratford company, only recently renamed the RSC, to play Gloucester in Peter Brook's production of *King Lear* (1964). Laurie succeeded Alan Webb and played Gloucester at the Aldwych and on tour in America. Four years later he achieved national popularity as Fraser in *Dad's Army* (BBC, until 1977).

Jude Law (b. London, 1972). The son of teachers, Jude Law grew up in Lewisham, south London. He went to the local comprehensive, Kidbrooke School in Eltham (a school with a reputation for racism and violence), and then, from the age of fourteen, to Alleyn's, an enlightened public school in Dulwich.

From his early teens he acted with the National Youth Music Theatre, along with Johnny Lee Miller. He left Alleyn's at sixteen to play a wayward teenager in the Mancunian soap *Families* (ITV, 1990-92). Also on television, he was in *The Casebook of Sherlock Holmes* (ITV, 1990) and *The Marshal* (Alan Clayton, ITV, 1993).

His first break in the cinema came with the much-hyped flop *Shopping* (Paul Anderson, 1994). He married his co-star, Sadie Frost, and returned to the stage. At the National he played Michael in Jean Cocteau's *Les parents terribles* (Sean Mathias,

Lyttelton, 1994); at the RSC, the title role in David Lan's version of Euripides's *Ion* (Nicholas Wright, Pit, 1994-95). He began rehearsals for the Broadway transfer of *Les parents terribles* (renamed *Indiscretions*) before the end of *Ion*'s run.

He has followed an interestingly diverse career in films: *I Love You, I Love You Not* (Billy Hopkins 1996); Lord Alfred Douglas in *Wilde* (Brian Gilbert 1997); *Gattaca* (Andrew Niccol, 1997); *Bent* (Sean Mathias, 1997); *Midnight in the Garden of Good and Evil* (Clint Eastwood, 1997); *Music From Another Room* (Charlie Peters, 1998); *The Wisdom of Crocodiles* (Po-Chih Leong, 1998); *Existenz* (David Cronenberg, 1999); *Final Cut* (Dominic Anciano/Ray Burdis, 1998); Dickie Greenleaf in *The Talented Mr Ripley* (Anthony Minghella, 1999); *AI* (Steven Spielberg, 2001); *Enemy at the Gates* (Jean-Jacques Annaud, 2001); the assassin in *The Road to Perdition* (Sam Mendes, 2002); Inman in *Cold Mountain* (Minghella, 2003); *I Heart Huckabees* (David O. Russell, 2004); *Sky Captain and the World of Tomorrow* (2004); the title role in *Alfie* (Charles Shyer, 2004); Dan in *Closer* (Mike Nichols, 2004); Errol Flynn in Martin Scorsese's *The Aviator* (2004); *Breaking and Entering* (Minghella, 2006); and *Sleuth* (Kenneth Branagh, 2007).

Law's rare stage appearances have been for David Lan at the Young Vic: Giovanni in *'Tis Pity She's a Whore* (1999), and the title role in *Doctor Faustus* (2002).

Barbara Leigh-Hunt (b. Bath, 1935). Barbara Leigh-Hunt's career began at the Old Vic in 1960 with the roles of Helena in *A Midsummer Night's Dream* (Michael Langham), and Portia in *The Merchant of Venice* (Peter Potter). She next appeared in repertory at Nottingham, Guildford and Lowestoft. At the Bristol Old Vic, where she played opposite her future husband Richard Pasco, she was Rosemary in *A Severed Head* (1962); Rosaline in *Love's Labour's Lost* and Alice in *Henry V* (1964); the title role in *Saint Joan*, the title role in *Hedda Gabler* and Victoria in *Portrait of Queen* (1965-66); Lady Macbeth (1969); and Amanda in *Private*

Lies (1973). In 1967 she toured the US as Isabella in *Measure for Measure* and Ophelia in *Hamlet*.

At the RSC with Pasco from 1974 to 91, she played Madge Larrabee in *Sherlock Holmes* (Frank Dunlop, Aldwych, 1974); Nadya in Tom Stoppard's *Travesties* (Peter Wood, Aldwych, 1974); Mistress Ford in *The Merry Wives of Windsor* (Terry Hands, RST, 1975); Queen Elizabeth in the Ian Richardson *Richard III* (Barry Kyle, TOP, 1975); Paulina in *The Winter's Tale* (John Barton, RST, 1976); Helen in *Troilus and Cressida* (Barton/Kyle, RST, 1976); Goneril in the Donald Sinden *King Lear* (Nunn, RST, 1976); the Teacher in Stoppard's *Every Good Boy Deserves Favour* (Nunn, Festival Hall, 1977); Orbison in Howard Barker's *That Good Between Us* (Kyle, Warehouse, 1977); Gertrude in *Hamlet* (Barton, RST, 1980); Queen Margaret in the Alan Howard *Richard III* (Hands, RST, 1980); Lumina in *The Swan Down Gloves* (Ian Judge, RST, 1981); Raissa Pavlovna in *The Forest* (Adrian Noble, TOP, 1981); the Actress in *La Ronde* (Barton, Aldwych, 1982); and Lady Hunstanton in *A Woman of No Importance* (Philip Prowse, Barbican, 1991).

She was magnificently mean as the scheming Raissa in *The Forest* and has since cornered the market in fearsome matriarchs, most notably Big Mama in *Cat on a Hot Tin Roof* (Howard Davies, NT Lyttelton, 1988), Lady Bracknell in *The Importance of Being Earnest* (Hands, Birmingham Rep, 1995), and, on television, Lady Catherine de Bourgh in *Pride and Prejudice* (BBC, 1995). Her Lady Bracknell was formidable, of course, witheringly knowing and ironic, but there was a surprising undercurrent of tenderness. She found a brilliant solution to the 'A handbag!' challenge—she silently mouthed the words.

Anton Lesser (b. 1952) joined the RSC straight from RADA and was surprisingly cast as Richard of Gloucester in the three parts of *Henry VI* (Terry Hands, RST, 1977). His boyish Richard was an electrifying creation, the propitious beginning of a fine

313

classical career (he would return to the role ten years later in Adrian Noble's *The Plantagenets*).

Lesser has brought his own individuality to some of Shakespeare's greatest roles. There aren't many actors who could claim some, let alone all, of the following: Romeo (Daniels, RST, 1980); Troilus (Howard Davies, RST, 1985); Richard III (Noble, RST, 1988); Bolingbroke in *Richard II* (Daniels, RST, 1990); Petruchio in *The Taming of the Shrew* (Bill Alexander, RST, 1992); Ford in *The Merry Wives of Windsor* (David Thacker, RST, 1992); Iachimo in *Cymbeline* (Dominic Cooke, Swan, 2003); Leontes in *The Winter's Tale* (Cooke, Swan, 2006-07)—and, for other companies, Hamlet (Jonathan Miller, Warehouse, 1982); Feste in *Twelfth Night* (Kenneth Branagh, Renaissance, Riverside Studios, 1987); and Brutus in *Julius Caesar* (Deborah Warner, Barbican, 2005).

Alongside the Shakespeares, Lesser played Michael in David Rudkin's *The Sons of Light* (Ron Daniels, TOP, 1977); Allan in Strindberg's *The Dance of Death* (John Caird, Aldwych, 1978); and Darkie in Edward Bond's *The Fool* (Howard Davies, TOP, 1980). He starred in Richard Nelson's *Principia Scriptoriae* (David Jones, Pit, 1986), *Some Americans Abroad* (Roger Michell, Pit, 1989) and *Two Shakespearean Actors* (Michell, Swan, 1990).

Other theatre: Konstantin in *The Seagull* (Max Stafford-Clark, Royal Court, 1981), alongside Alan Rickman and Harriet Walter; Harry in Phil Young's *The Kissing God* (Hampstead Theatre, 1984); Yasmin Reza's *Art* (Matthew Warchus, Wyndham's, 1997); Shakespeare in Frank McGuinness's *Mutabilitie* (Trevor Nunn, NT Cottesloe, 1997); Elyot in *Private Lives* (Philip Franks, NT Lyttelton, 1999); and Charlotte Eilenberg's *The Lucky Ones* (Matthew Lloyd, Hampstead Theatre, 2002).

Television: *The Politician's Wife* (Graham Theakston, Channel Four, 1995); Pitt Crawley in *Vanity Fair* (BBC, 1998); Stephen Poliakoff's *Perfect Strangers* (BBC, 2001); *The Project* (BBC, 2002); *Foyle's War* (ITV, 2002); *Danielle Cable: Eyewitness* (ITV, 2003); Nick Dear's *Eroica* (BBC, 2003); Dickens in Peter Ackroyd's *London* (BBC, 2004).

Films: *The Assam Garden* (1985); *Fairytale: a True Story* (Charles Sturridge, 1997); *Esther Kahn* (Arnaud Desplechin, 2000); *Charlotte Gray* (Gillian Armstrong, 2001); *Imagining Argentina* (Christopher Hampton, 2003); *Miss Potter* (2006).

David Leveaux (b. London, 1957). The son of a cardiologist, educated at Rugby and Manchester University, David Leveaux had an early success with a production of Eugene O'Neill's *Moon for the Misbegotten* at the Riverside Studios (1983)—the American Repertory Theatre invited him to revive the production and when it played in New York he received a Tony nomination. For many years he has been a travelling director, working in Turkey, Germany, Finland and, most significantly, Japan: in 1989 he staged Christopher Hampton's *Les liaisons dangereuses* in Tokyo, and since 1993 he has spent part of each year as Artistic Director of Theatre Project Tokyo, a new company based in a converted dye works (he has directed western classics in Japanese via an interpreter).

At home he has worked for the major theatres without forming any lasting associations. He was at the RSC during Adrian Noble's first season, directing *'Tis Pity She's a Whore* with Saskia Reeves in the Swan, and *Romeo and Juliet* with Michael Maloney and Clare Holman in the main house. *'Tis Pity* was set in a mid-20th century Italy of gangsters and priests, of grey-black suits, high-heeled shoes, shadows and incense: it was as sultry and suspenseful as a Moravia novel. *Romeo and Juliet*, staged handsomely in candlelight before a screen of Renaissance paintings, was tragic in tone from scene one.

He often strips things down to essentials. During the 1990s, themes of desire and betrayal reoccurred in his choice of plays, and a ghostly sense of twilight in his presentation of them. At Chichester he staged an adaptation of Zola's *Thérèse Raquin* with Joanne Pearce and Neil Pearson (1990) and a renowned *Electra* with Zoë Wanamaker (1997); at the Almeida, three Harold Pinter plays—*Betrayal* (1991), *No Man's Land* (1992) and *Moonlight*

315

(1993); and at the Donmar, the musical *Nine* (1996) and Tom Stoppard's *The Real Thing* with Stephen Dillane and Jennifer Ehle (1999). His opera productions were similarly sombre: Britten's *The Turn of the Screw* (Scottish Opera); Mozart's *Le nozze di Figaro* (Scottish Opera, 1995); and Richard Strauss's *Salome* (ENO, 1995).

Work since 2000: Juliette Binoche in *Betrayal* (New York, 2000); Neil LaBute's *The Distance From Here* (Almeida at King's Cross, 2002); Antonio Banderas in *Nine* (New York, 2003); Stoppard's *Jumpers* (NT Olivier, 2003); *Fiddler on the Roof* (New York, 2004); *Sinatra* (Palladium, 2006); Kevin Kline in *Cyrano de Bergerac* (New York, 2007).

Damian Lewis (b. London, 1971) was educated at Eton and the Guildhall School of Music and Drama. His early theatre work included Romeo in *Romeo and Juliet* (Gwenda Hughes, Birmingham Rep, 1993); the title role in *Hamlet* (Regent's Park, 1994); Horace in *The School for Wives* (Jonathan Kent, Almeida, 1994); and Laertes in the Ralph Fiennes *Hamlet* (Kent, Almeida at the Hackney Empire, 1995).

He joined the RSC in London in 1996, taking over the role of Wittipol in Matthew Warchus's production of *The Devil is an Ass* (Pit). He then played the villainous Don John in *Much Ado About Nothing* (Michael Boyd, RST, 1996) with brooding vindictiveness, and, in contrast, the road builder Borghejm, calm and good-natured amid the wreckage of the Allmers (Robert Glenister, Joanne Pearce and Derbhle Crotty), in Adrian Noble's production of Ibsen's *Little Eyolf* (Swan, 1996-97). Posthumus in Noble's *Cymbeline* (RST, 1997) followed.

Lewis's early television work included *Mickey Love* (1993), *Poirot* (ITV, 1995), and *Warriors* (BBC, 1999). His performance as the American battalion leader in the Steven Spielberg/Tom Hanks production *Band of Brothers* brought him to prominence in 2001. He has since starred in *The Forsyte Saga* (BBC, 2002); *Jeffrey Archer: the Truth* (BBC, 2002); *Dreamcatcher* (Lawrence

Kasdan, 2003); *Colditz* (ITV, 2005); *An Unfinished Life* (Lasse Hallström, 2005); *Chromophobia* (Martha Fiennes, 2005); Stephen Poliakoff's *Friends and Crocodiles* (BBC, 2005); *Much Ado About Nothing* (BBC, 2005); *The Baker* (2007); *Confessions of a Diary Secretary* (ITV, 2007); and *The Escapist* (2007).

Returning to the stage, he played Daniel in Joanna Laurens's *Five Gold Rings* at the Almeida (Michael Attenborough, 2003); and Bernick in Ibsen's *Pillars of the Community* at the National (Marianne Elliott, Lyttelton, 2005).

John Light (b. Birmingham) started his theatre career at the RSC in 1995 playing Siczynski in Peter Gill's production of *A Patriot for Me* (Barbican). His work in Charles Wood's *The Tower* (Howard Davies, Almeida, 1995-96) earned him an Ian Charleson Award nomination. He was next in Edward Bond's *In the Company of Men* (Bond, RSC Pit, 1996); Samuel Adamson's *Clocks and Whistles* (Dominic Dromgoole, Bush, 1996); *The Cenci* (Almeida, 1997); David Haig's *My Boy Jack* (Hampstead Theatre, 1998); and Gill's *Certain Young Men* (Gill, Almeida, 1999).

In Adrian Noble's RSC production of Gill's version of *The Seagull* (Swan, 2000) he created a tense, needy Konstantin—the character's emotional volatility and pain were apparent in every look and gesture. In 2004 he played Stefan in a revival of Peter Flannery's *Singer* (Sean Holmes, Oxford Stage Company, Tricycle, 2004). For the RSC's Complete Works season (2006) he was cast in the major roles of Brutus in *Julius Caesar* (Holmes, RST) and Caliban in *The Tempest* (Rupert Gould, RST).

On the screen, he starred in the German television production *Dresden* (TV, 2006). Also: *Holding On* (Adrian Shergold, BBC, 1997); *The Unknown Soldier* (David Drury, ITV, 1998); *Cider With Rosie* (ITV, 1998); *Aristocrats* (BBC, 1999); *Love in a Cold Climate* (BBC, 2001); *Cambridge Spies* (BBC, 2003); *North and South* (BBC, 2004); and *Scoop* (Woody Allen, 2006).

Lighting. RSC productions have often been lit by the Company's in house lighting technicians.

John Bradley was the RSC's chief electrician/lighting engineer in Stratford from 1958 to 75. He lit most main house productions during these years. From 1975 to 93 he worked as the Company's Technical Manager.

Michael Calf (b. Hampshire) was the RSC's resident lighting designer in the London studios from 1980 to 84. He built the Pit's lighting rig and lit Howard Davies's *Good* (1981) and Adrian Noble's *The Winter's Tale* (Small-scale Tour, 1984).

Wayne Dowdeswell trained at the Bristol Old Vic Theatre School. He joined the RSC in 1978 and worked initially as an assistant electrician. He became The Other Place's chief electrician in 1984 and the Swan Theatre's lighting supervisor in 1986. He lit the Swan's opening season (1986), Gregory Doran's two seasons of rarities ('Jacobethans', 2002; 'Gunpowder', 2005), and, of particular note, Deborah Warner's *Titus Andronicus* (1987), Terry Hands's *The Seagull* (1990), and Adrian Noble's *The Cherry Orchard* (1995).

Brian Harris worked as a lighting assistant in the RST from 1972 to 73, and quickly emerged as a topflight designer. His RSC work included Buzz Goodbody's *King Lear* (TOP, 1974), Trevor Nunn's *Three Sisters* (Small-scale Tour, 1978) and Adrian Noble's *King Lear* (RST, 1982).

Vince Herbert has been the RSC's head of lighting since 2000. He lit Michael Boyd's *Hamlet* (RST, 2004) and *Twelfth Night* (RST, 2005).

Simon Kemp was The Other Place's Chief Electrician from 1996 to 01. He lit Steven Pimlott's *Richard II* (2000).

Leo Leibovici was the original Other Place's resident electrician and lighting designer, appointed by Buzz Goodbody. He lit most of the shows, from Goodbody's *Hamlet* (1975) to Adrian Noble's *Antony and Cleopatra* (1982). His work in the main house included Bill Alexander's *Richard III* (RST, 1984).

Stewart Leviton was the RSC's chief lighting engineer in London (at the Aldwych and then the Barbican) from 1969 to 84, designing regularly for Terry Hands and David Jones.

Ian Loffhagen succeeded Leo Leibovici at The Other Place. He lit Adrian Noble's *The Art of Success* (1986) and Nick Hamm's *Fashion* (1987).

Clive Morris joined the RSC in 1973 and headed the Stratford lighting department from 1975 to 98. From 1980 Terry Hands lit most of his own productions, in collaboration with Morris.

Chris Parry (1952-2007, b. Manchester) trained as a telephone engineer in his home town of Welshpool and joined the RSC as an electrician in 1976. He went on to make an outstanding contribution to the work of the RSC, both as a lighting supervisor (RST, 1976-89) and as a designer of noted artistry. After nearly ten years of waiting for an opportunity, he made his name with his first production—Howard Davies's *Les liaisons dangereuses* (TOP, 1985). His most striking RSC designs were conceived for productions by Adrian Noble in the main house, including *The Plantagenets* (1988) and *The Winter's Tale* (1992). He also lit Trevor Nunn's *Othello* (TOP, 1989). Parry moved to the United States at the end of the 1980s.

Geraint Pughe was one of the RSC's resident lighting supervisors at the Barbican from 1983 to 02, responsible for productions in the Pit. If most of his time was spent at the Barbican, he lit two outstanding productions during the 1990 Stratford season—Danny Boyle's *The Last Days of Don Juan* and Mendes's *Troilus and Cressida* (Swan).

Phyllida Lloyd (b. Bristol, 1957) studied English and drama at Birmingham University (1976-79). On graduating she worked briefly at BBC Pebble Mill as an assistant floor manager. She was an Arts Council trainee director at the Wolsey Theatre, Ipswich (1985), and came to notice as an associate director at the Everyman Theatre, Cheltenham (1986), staging *What the Butler Saw*, *A Midsummer Night's Dream*, *Much Ado About Nothing*,

Terry Johnson's *Insignificance*, Alan Ayckbourn's *Just Between Ourselves*, Dario Fo's *Accidental Death of an Anarchist*, Don Hale's *Every Black Day*, Emile Zola's *Earth* (also Edinburgh Festival), and Georg Büchner's *Woyzeck*.

She was an associate director at the Bristol Old Vic in 1989 (*The Comedy of Errors*, *A Streetcar Named Desire*, García Lorca's *Dona Rosita, the Spinster*) and at the Manchester Royal Exchange in 1990/91 (Wole Soyinka's *Death and the King's Horseman*, *Medea*, *The Winter's Tale*, *The School for Scandal*).

At the RSC, 1991-92, she introduced contemporary references into the obscure Restoration comedy *The Virtuoso*, conceiving one character as a Chelsea pensioner and another as a Soho 'madam'. Like so many of her productions it was fresh, colourful and visually ingenious. She is more versatile and eclectic than her contemporaries Deborah Warner and Katie Mitchell, working in different genres and all types of theatre space: Brecht's *The Threepenny Opera* (Donmar Warehouse, 1991); Chabrier's *L'Étoile* (Opera North, 1991); John Guare's *Six Degrees of Separation* (Royal Court, 1992); Terry Johnson's *Hysteria* (Royal Court, 1993); *Pericles* (NT Olivier, 1994); Britten's *Gloriana* (Opera North, 1994); *What the Butler Saw* (NT Lyttelton, 1995); *The Way of the World* (NT Lyttelton, 1995); *La Bohème* (Opera North, 1996); Luigi Cherubini's *Medée* (Opera North, 1996); *Dona Rosita, the Spinster* (Almeida, 1997); *The Prime of Miss Jean Brodie* (NT Lyttelton, 1998); *Carmen* (Opera North, 1998); *Macbeth* (Bastille, Paris, 1999); *Dialogues of the Carmelites* (ENO, 1999); the Abba musical *Mamma Mia!* (Prince Edward, 1999); Poul Ruders's *The Handmaid's Tale* (Kobenhavn, 2000); David Mamet's *Boston Marriage* (Donmar Warehouse, 2001); Britten's *Albert Herring* (Opera North, 2002); Verdi's *Macbeth* (ROH, 2002); *The Duchess of Malfi* (NT Lyttelton, 2003); *The Taming of the Shrew* (Globe, 2003); and Wagner's *The Rhinegold* (ENO, 2004).

Opera productions have dominated. *Gloriana* was a triumph of scene-setting and psychological drama, both grand and intimate; the tension of the death warrant scene (the agonised

320

scream of Essex's wife) matched the genius of Britten's dramatic scoring.

Mark Lockyer trained at RADA. His early opportunities came at the Derby Playhouse (*Carmen*), the Watford Palace (*Talk of the Devil*, 1985), the Birmingham Rep (Brocklehurst in *Jane Eyre, Julius Caesar, Peter Pan*, 1986-87), the Young Vic (*Outbreak of God in Area 9*, 1987), and the Liverpool Playhouse (*The Ragged Trousered Philanthropist*, 1988). From 1988 to 91 he was at the National, appearing in *The Changeling* (Howard Davies, Lyttelton); *Bartholomew Fair* (Richard Eyre, Olivier, 1989); *Ghetto* (Nicholas Hytner, Olivier, 1989); *The Madness of George III* (Nicholas Hytner, Lyttelton, 1991); and *Fuente Ovejuna* (Declan Donnellan, Cottesloe, 1991). Between and after his NT engagements he was Lucius in Stephen Jeffreys's *The Clink* (Anna Furze, Paines Plough, Riverside Studios, 1990), and Rupert in *The Prisoner of Zenda* (Matthew Francis, Greenwich Theatre, 1993).

At the RSC, 1993-97, his undeniable brilliance made him seem, at times, like the classical theatre's answer to Freddie Mercury. Undaunted by the distinguished senior players surrounding him in *King Lear* (Adrian Noble, RST, 1993) he gave Oswald an unusually strong presence, playing his pomposity and cowardice to the limit. This was followed by Gratiano in *The Merchant of Venice* (David Thacker, RST, 1993) and a hilarious, repulsive Stephano alongside David Bradley's Trinculo, two refugees from second-rate Music Hall, in *The Tempest* (Sam Mendes, RST, 1993). In 1995 he played a melancholy, highly-strung Mercutio in *Romeo and Juliet* (Noble, RST), and a vindictive Yasha in *The Cherry Orchard* (Noble, Swan).

After a few silent years he re-emerged in 2000 at Shakespeare's Globe: Laertes to Mark Rylance's *Hamlet* and Byplay in Richard Brome's *The Antipodes* (Gerald Freedman). He has since played Hermes in *Ion* (Gate, 2002); the lieutenant in Lope de Vega's *Peribanez* (Young Vic, 2003); Roderigo in *Othello* at the RSC (Gregory Doran, Swan, 2004); Malvolio in *Twelfth Night*

(David Farr, Bristol Old Vic, 2004); Peter Delvin in *Theatre of Blood* (Phelim McDermott, NT Lyttelton, 2005); Tibetan Grand Abbot in David Greig's adaptation of *Tintin* (Rufus Norris, Barbican, 2005-06); *Faustus* (Rupert Goold, Headlong, Hampstead Theatre, 2006); the reporter in *Vernon God Little* (Norris, Young Vic, 2007); and the surgeon in Marius von Mayenburg's *The Ugly One* (Ramin Gray, Royal Court, 2007).

Cherie Lunghi (b. London, 1953). Brought up by her mother and aunts in west London following the departure of her Italian father (the family ran a Kensington boarding house), Cherie Lunghi played Hedvig in *The Wild Duck* and Alice in *Alice in Wonderland* on BBC radio while still a pupil at the Arts Educational School in Hyde Park. After drama school (Central) she played Kitty in *The Thark*, Lisa in *Owners* and Irina in *Three Sisters* at the University Theatre, Newcastle (1973-74), and Kate in *She Stoops to Conquer* at the Nottingham Playhouse (1974). She was a switchboard operator and a programme-seller at the Royal Court before being cast in the role of Laura in *Teeth 'n' Smiles* (1975).

She was one of the leading young actresses at the RSC at the end of the 1970s: Hero in the Donald Sinden/Judi Dench *Much Ado About Nothing* (John Barton, RST, 1976); Perdita in *The Winter's Tale* (Barton, RST, 1976); Cordelia in the Sinden *King Lear* (Nunn, Aldwych, 1977); Rhoda in Howard Barker's *That Good Between Us* (Barry Kyle, Warehouse, 1977); Pat in C.P. Taylor's *Bandits* (Howard Davies, Warehouse, 1977); Genevieve in Brecht's *Days of the Commune* (Davies, Aldwych, 1977); Celia, succeeding Judith Paris, in *As You Like It* (Nunn, Aldwych, 1978); Lucy in *Saratoga, or, Pistols for Seven* (Ronald Eyre, Aldwych, 1978-79); and a fine Viola in *Twelfth Night* (Terry Hands, RST, 1979). A natural verse-speaker, she captured the role's allusive alchemy of sorrow and joy.

At the moment of her biggest success she left the RSC to play Guenevere in John Boorman's *Excalibur* (1981). This was followed by roles in *Letters to an Unknown Lover* (1985); *King David* (Bruce Beresford, 1985); *The Mission* (Roland Joffé, 1986); *To Kill a Priest* (1988); *Ransom* (1990); *Silent Cries* (1993); *Frankenstein* (Kenneth Branagh, 1994); *Jack and Sarah* (Tim Sullivan, 1995); and *Burn Hollywood Burn* (1997).

In 1993 she succeeded Felicity Kendal as Hannah in Tom Stoppard's *Arcadia* (Nunn, NT Lyttelton); and in 2000 she played Eleanor in Peter Nichols's *Passion Play* (Michael Grandage, Donmar Warehouse). These were rare stage appearances.

Christopher Luscombe. An alumnus of the very talented Cambridge Footlights team of the early 1980s, Christopher Luscombe is a wise interpreter of the eccentricities and obsessions of British comedy (how little, in essence, these have changed since the 16th century).

His first job was as a pantomime dame, understudying Terry Scott. He joined the RSC in 1991, the same year as his Cambridge contemporaries Hugh Bonneville and Sam Mendes. He effortlessly brought to life Valentine in *Twelfth Night* (Griff Rhys Jones, RST); Francis, the reluctant drawer ('Anon, anon, sir'), along with three other minor roles—Davy/Feeble/Travers—in the two parts of *Henry IV* (Adrian Noble, RST); and Dapper in Mendes's *The Alchemist* (Swan). On the transfer to London (1992) he added Pedro de Terreros in Richard Nelson's *Columbus and the Discovery of Japan* (John Caird, Barbican), and Vasya in Ostrovsky's *Artists and Admirers* (Phyllida Lloyd, Pit). The next six years belonged to the difficult art of Shakespearean comedy: Launcelot Gobbo in David Thacker's modern dress *The Merchant of Venice* (RST, 1993); Moth in Ian Judge's Edwardian, Oxbridge *Love's Labour's Lost* (RST, 1993); Dogberry in *Much Ado About Nothing* (Michael Boyd, RST, 1996-97); and Abraham Slender in *The Merry Wives of Windsor* (Judge, RST, 1996-97). Luscombe's achievement was to make these fools accessible. His Gobbo had the right tone of satirical cruelty, but was tenderly loyal to Kate Duchêne's Jessica. He transformed the boy Moth into an insufferably intelligent college chorister.

For the RSC's fringe festival Luscombe co-wrote with Bonne-ville, who also directed, the one-man show *Half-Time*, a satire on both theatrical and Cambridge life, in which Luscombe played all the characters, from the Master's wife to the decrepit porter (Buzz Goodbody Studio, 1992, Swan, 1997), and co-devised/directed, with Malcolm McKee, *The Shakespeare Revue*, an evening of sketches and songs (Swan, 1994). *The Shakespeare Revue* was revived in the Pit and later transferred to the Vaude-ville in the West End (1995).

In the years since Luscombe has followed a second career as a skilled director of comedies: the premiere staging of Noël Coward's final play, *Star Quality*, in his own adaptation (Apollo, 2001); Somerset Maugham's *Home and Beauty* (Lyric, 2002); the musical *Little Shop of Horrors* (West Yorkshire Playhouse, 2002-03); *The Importance of Being Earnest* (Theatre Royal, Bath, 2004); Alan Ayckbourn's *Things We Do For Love* (Harrogate Theatre, 2004); Bernard Shaw's *Candida* (Oxford Stage Company, Tour, 2004); Alan Bennett's *The Lady in the Van* (UK Tour, 2004); and Oscar Wilde's *Lord Arthur Savile's Crime* (Richmond Theatre, 2005).

Finbar Lynch (b. Dublin, 1959) used the stage name Barrie Lynch until 1997. His progress can be divided into Irish and English phases. The link was Adrian Noble's production of *Three Sisters*, which transferred from the Gate Theatre, Dublin, to the Royal Court, London, in 1990. Lynch's subtle playing of Tusenbach (not so much a soldier as a bookish academic—beard, long thinning hair, round spectacles) revealed this char-acter to be the truly tragic figure of the play: his doomed love for Niamh Cusack's Irina was poignantly expressed (they be-came a couple in real life).

His work in his native Ireland was, by all accounts, equally impressive (in 1988 he received the Irish Theatre Award for Best

Actor). At the Gate Theatre he played Jack Absolute in *The Rivals*, Charles Surface in *School for Scandal*, Bazarov in *Fathers and Sons*, Danceny in *Les liaisons dangereuses*, the title role in *Peer Gynt*, Sebastian in *Twelfth Night*, and Sydney in *Absurd Person Singular*; at the Abbey, Christy Mahon in *Playboy of the Western World*; and at the Gaiety Theatre, Gar Public in *Philadelphia Here I Come*, and Garry in *Noises Off*. Largely a Dublin secret, then, during the 1980s, although he did have one major British television role as an academic pursuing Leonie Mellinger in David Lodge's *Small World*.

After *Three Sisters* Lynch appeared at the Greenwich Theatre as Jean in *Miss Julie* (1990). In his first RSC season (1991-92) he played Bruce in Thomas Shadwell's *The Virtuoso* (Phyllida Lloyd, Swan); Proteus in *The Two Gentlemen of Verona* (David Thacker, Swan); Surly in Sam Mendes's production of *The Alchemist* (Swan); and, coming into his own, the predatory Wendoll, seducing Saskia Reeves at the meal table, in Thomas Heywood's *A Woman Killed With Kindness* (Katie Mitchell, TOP). He next played a dangerous Mark Antony in David Thacker's modern-dress production of *Julius Caesar* (TOP and Small-scale Tour, 1993); Tullus Aufidius in *Coriolanus* (Thacker, Swan, 1994); Lucio in *Measure for Measure* (Steven Pimlott, RST, 1994); and Puck in Adrian Noble's production of *A Midsummer Night's Dream* (RST, 1994). His original Puck was sly, sarcastic and not a little sadistic.

Subsequent work: Eddie in Sam Shepherd's *Fool for Love* (Ian Brown, Donmar Warehouse, 1996); Edmund in the Ian Holm *King Lear* (Richard Eyre, NT Cottesloe, 1997); Jim in the Tennessee Williams discovery *Not About Nightingales* (Trevor Nunn, NT Cottesloe, 1998); Enobarbus in the Helen Mirren/Alan Rickman *Antony and Cleopatra* (Sean Mathias, NT Olivier, 1998); Venus in Nick Whitby's *To the Green Fields Beyond* (Mendes, Donmar Warehouse, 2000); Tyrone in Eugene O'Neill's *A Moon for the Misbegotten* (Matthew Lloyd, Royal Exchange Manchester, 2001); Jesus in Steven Berkoff's *Messiah: Scenes from a Crucifixion* (Riverside Studios, 2001); the title role in *Macbeth* (James Phillips, Sheffield Crucible, 2003); Iago in *Othello* (Rupert Gould, Royal Theatre, Northampton, 2003); Polymestor in *Hecuba* (Jonathan Kent, Donmar Warehouse, 2004); McCann to Henry Goodman's Goldberg in Harold Pinter's *The Birthday Party* (Lindsay Posner, Birmingham Rep, 2005); Manders in Ibsen's *Ghosts* (Anna Mackmin, Gate, 2007); and Gibbs in Pinter's *The Hothouse* (Ian Rickson, NT Lyttelton, 2007). Returning to Stratford for the Complete Works festival (2006), he played Cassius in *Julius Caesar* (Holmes, RST) and Alonso in *The Tempest* (Gould, RST).

On the screen: *The Scold's Bridle* (Thacker, BBC, 1998); *Second Sight 2: Hide and Seek* (BBC, 2000); *Mind Games* (ITV, 2000); *To Kill a King* (2003); *Proof* (RTE, 2004); *Dalziel and Pascoe* (BBC, 2005).

David Lyon. David Lyon's RSC career began with small, often comedic, roles, but in middle age he has played authority figures with distinctive subtlety, notably Warwick in *The Plantagenets* (Adrian Noble, RST, 1988), Capulet in *Romeo and Juliet* (Michael Attenborough, Pit, 1997), and, for the 2000 'This England' cycle, Westmoreland in *Henry IV* (Attenborough, Swan) and *Henry V* (Edward Hall, RST).

His other RSC work: Archidamus in *The Winter's Tale* (John Barton, RST, 1976); Chandler in David Edgar's *Destiny* (Ron Daniels, TOP, 1976); a Gentleman in *King Lear* (Trevor Nunn, RST, 1976); Sexton in *Much Ado About Nothing* (Barton, Aldwych, 1977); Snug in *A Midsummer Night's Dream* (Barton, Aldwych, 1977); Bleech in Howard Barker's *That Good Between Us* (Barry Kyle, Warehouse, 1977); Wilcox in C.P. Taylor's *Bandits* (Howard Davies, Warehouse, 1977); Waitwell in *The Way of the World* (Barton, Aldwych, 1978); Hersch in *A Miserable and Lonely Death* (Walter Donohue, Warehouse, 1978); Hortensio in *The Taming of the Shrew* (Michael Bogdanov, RST, 1978); Tublin in Peter Whelan's *Captain Swing* (Bill Alexander, TOP, 1978); Dull in *Love's Labour's Lost* (Barton, RST, 1978); Maecenas/Demetrius in Peter Brook's *Antony and Cleopatra* (RST, 1978); Rick in Tom McGrath's *The Innocent* (Davies, Warehouse, 1979); Don Pedro in *Much Ado About Nothing* (Di Trevis, RST, 1988); and King Philip of France in *King John* (Deborah Warner, TOP, 1988).

At the National, Lyon has played Mowbray in Deborah Warner's production of *Richard II* (Cottesloe, 1995) and Albany in the Ian Holm *King Lear* (Cottesloe, 1997). Work elsewhere: *After Aida* (Old Vic); *Becket* (Elijah Moshinsky, Theatre Royal Haymarket, 1991); and Talbot in *Mary Stuart* (Patrick Sandford, Nuffield Theatre, Southampton, 2004).

M

Aidan McArdle (b. Dublin, 1970), a graduate of University College, Dublin, trained at RADA (1995-96) having already appeared at the Abbey Theatre, Dublin, as Osric in *Hamlet*, Don Parritt in *The Iceman Cometh* and Dromio in *The Comedy of Errors* (1993). On leaving the Academy he built a reputation on the London stage: Ya'acov in Julian Garner's *The Flight into Egypt* (John Dove, Hampstead Theatre, 1996); Martin in *When Brains Don't Count*, Paul in *In the Family*, Joe in *The Future is Betamax* (Young Playwrights Festival, Royal Court, 1996); Robbie in *Shopping and Fucking* (Max Stafford-Clark, Out of Joint, Tour, 1997); and Kaite O'Reilly's *Yard* (Julie-Anne Robinson, Bush, 1998).

He joined the RSC in 1999. In Michael Boyd's production of *A Midsummer Night's Dream* (RST, 1999) McArdle's singular Puck, cool and satirical, administered the potion by tossing soil from a wheelbarrow onto the lovers and watering it from a tin watering can. Also in the season at the RST and Barbican he played Roderigo in *Othello* (Michael Attenborough), and Alexas/Thidas in *Antony and Cleopatra* (Steven Pimlott). During the fringe festival he performed Conor McPherson's *Rum and Vodka* (Helen

Raynor, Buzz Goodbody Studio). He next became only the third actor in the RSC's history to play Richard of Gloucester in both *Henry VI Part 3* and *Richard III* ('This England: the Histories', Boyd, Swan, 2000-01, he was also Charles in *Henry VI Part 1*).

Subsequent theatre work: Murphy in Tennessee Williams's *Stairs to the Roof* (Lucy Bailey, Minerva, Chichester, 2001); the title role in *A Prayer for Owen Meany* (Mick Gordon, NT Lyttelton, 2002); Pip in David Farr's adaptation of *Great Expectations* (Gordon Anderson, Bristol Old Vic, 2003); Orestes to Catherine McCormack's Iphigenia in Goethe's *Under the Curse* (Joe Hill-Gibbins, Gate, 2003); Simon in Frank McGuinness's *There Came a Gypsy Riding* (Attenborough, Almeida, 2007).

On the screen, McArdle has played Dudley Moore in Terry Johnson's *Not Only But Always* (Channel Four, 2004), Einstein in *E=mc²* (Channel Four, 2005), Stravinsky in *Riot at the Rite* (BBC, 2005) and Richard Brinsley Sheridan in *The Duchess* (2008).

Richard McCabe (b. Glasgow). No actor of the last twenty-five years has a stronger stage personality than Richard McCabe. Constantly unpredictable, he has made a virtue out of nonchalance. His RSC 'Just William' Puck — school blazer and shorts, wings sticking out the back — was a remarkable re-invention of a familiar role: insolent, cocky, finding new verbal jokes in the text.

After RADA, McCabe worked at the Sheffield Crucible (*The Alchemist*; *The Changeling*), the Bolton Octagon (*Should Auld Acquaintance*; Mozart in *Amadeus*), the Plymouth Theatre Royal and the Leeds Playhouse (Mercutio in *Romeo and Juliet*). At the Manchester Royal Exchange in 1985/86 he played Simon in *Hay Fever* (James Maxwell) and Touchstone in *As You Like It* (Nicholas Hytner).

He joined the RSC in London in 1986 to play Bentley Summerhays in Shaw's *Misalliance* (John Caird, Barbican). Moving to Stratford (Swan, 1987), he was Sir Glorious Tiptoe in *The New Inn* (Caird), Lacy in *Hyde Park* (Barry Kyle), and Chiron in Deborah Warner's production of *Titus Andronicus*. On the transfer to London he added Umpleby in Howard Brenton's *The Churchill Play* (Kyle, Barbican, 1988). The RSC now cast him in leading roles. As well as Puck in John Caird's production of *A Midsummer Night's Dream* (RST, 1989), he played Truewit in Jonson's *The Silent Woman* (Danny Boyle, Swan, 1989); Wagner in *Dr Faustus* (Barry Kyle, Swan, 1989); Tranio in *The Taming of the Shrew* (Bill Alexander, RST, 1992); a wickedly charming Autolycus—he picked all of the Young Shepherd's pockets, rode off on the Young Shepherd's bicycle, then seduced the village girls with his accordion-playing and predatory hands—in *The Winter's Tale* (Adrian Noble, RST, 1992); Marlowe in Peter Whelan's *The School of Night* (Alexander, TOP, 1992); Flamineo, as if practising for Iago, in *The White Devil* (Gale Edwards, Swan, 1996); Plotwell in *Three Hours After Marriage* (Richard Cottrell, Swan, 1996); a prowling, intelligent Thersites in *Troilus and Cressida* (Ian Judge, RST, 1996); Iago in *Othello* (Michael Attenborough, RST, 1999); and the title role in *King John* (Joise Rourke, Swan, 2006).

Other theatre work: *The Tempest* (Bill Alexander, Birmingham Rep, 1994); Ford in *The Merry Wives of Windsor* (Terry Hands, NT Olivier, 1995); *Absolute Hell* (Anthony Page, NT Lyttelton, 1995); Fainall in *The Way of the World* (Phyllida Lloyd, NT Lyttelton, 1996); the title role in *Hamlet* (Alexander, Birmingham Rep, 1998); Austin in Ron Hutchinson's *The Beau* (Theatre Royal Haymarket, 2001); Mephostophiles to Jude Law's *Doctor Faustus* (David Lan, Young Vic, 2002); Salieri in *Amadeus* (Jonathan Best, City of London Sinfonia, Barbican, 2003); and the title role in Molière's *Scapino, or, The Trickster* (Silvin Purcarete, Chichester, 2005).

Colin McCormack (1941-2004, b. Cardiff) attended his local art college in Cardiff before winning a place at the Central School of Speech and Drama in London. His career began at the Bristol Old Vic (early 1960s), and is best summed up by a long association with the RSC. As a name, McCormack was little known to the public, but as a character actor he was part of the high-quality fabric that binds the elements of a production (and a company) together. Beginning in 1967 as a Stratford bit part player—Citizen in *Coriolanus* (John Barton); Courtier in *The Revenger's Tragedy* (Trevor Nunn); First Suitor in *All's Well That Ends Well* (Barton); Donalbain in *Macbeth* (Peter Hall); Third Musician in *Romeo and Juliet* (Karolos Koun)—, he returned to the RSC at some point during every subsequent decade of his life: Angus in *Macbeth* (Trevor Nunn, RST, 1974); Udy in Howard Barker's *The Hang of the Gaol* (Bill Alexander, Warehouse, 1978); Florence in *The Adventures of Awful Knawful* (John Caird/Howard Davies, Warehouse, 1978); Chachava in *The Caucasian Chalk Circle* and Borachio in *Much Ado About Nothing* (Caird/Davies, Small-scale Tour, 1979); Costall in Barker's *The Loud Boy's Life* (Davies, Warehouse, 1980); Macduff in *Macbeth* (Adrian Noble, RST, 1988); Mr Hardacre in Edward Bond's *Restoration* (Roger Michell, Swan, 1988); Sebastian in *The Tempest* (Nicholas Hytner, RST, 1988); Kent in *King Lear* (Cicely Berry, Almeida, 1989); Dolin in *A Clockwork Orange* (Ron Daniels, Barbican, 1990); Mike in Richard Nelson's *Goodnight Children Everywhere* (Ian Brown, TOP, 1997-98); Duke of Milan in *The Two Gentlemen of Verona* (Edward Hall, Swan, 1998); Baptista in *The Taming of the Shrew* (Lindsay Posner, Pit, 1999); Earl of Salisbury in *King John* (Gregory Doran, Swan 2001); Casca in *Julius Caesar* (Hall, RST, 2001); and three roles in Gregory Doran's season of rarities (Swan and Gielgud, 2002-03)—Lord Audley in *Edward III* (Anthony Clarke), Bramble in *Eastward Ho!* (Lucy Pitman-Wallace) and Pietro in *The Malcontent* (Dominic Cooke).

At the Royal Court he was in the original production of Jim Cartwright's seminal *Road* (Simon Curtis, Theatre Upstairs, 1986), as well as G.F. Newman's *Operation Bad Apple* (Max Stafford-Clark, 1982); Andrea Dunbar's *Shirley* (Carole Hayman, Theatre Upstairs, 1986); Griselda Gambaro's *Putting Two and Two Together* (Theatre Upstairs, 1991); and Timberlake Wertenbaker's *Three Birds Alighting in a Field* (Stafford-Clark, 1992).

Other notable appearances: *The Mother* (Di Trevis, NT Cottesloe, 1986); Islayev in *A Month in the Country* (Bill Pryde, Cambridge Theatre Company, Tour, 1987); Pinchwife in *The Country Wife* (Mike Alfreds, Cambridge Theatre Company, 1991); Chandebise/Poche in Feydeau's *A Flea in Her Ear* (Alfreds, Theatr Clwyd, 1993); Wangel in Ibsen's *The Lady from the Sea* (Sue Lefton, The Bridewell, Blackfriars, 1996); Kent in *King Lear* (Haymarket Theatre, Leicester, 1997); Estragon in *Waiting for Godot* (Matthew Smith, Mercury Theatre, Colchester, 2000); and Nicholas in Harold Pinter's *One for the Road* (Battersea Arts Centre 2003).

McCormack performed cameos in many popular television productions, including *Dixon of Dock Green* (BBC, 1974); *The Sweeney* (ITV, 1978); *Yes, Minister* (BBC, 1981); *Martin Chuzzlewit* (BBC, 1994); *Pie in the Sky* (BBC, 1996); *Inspector Morse* (ITV, 1997); and *Longitude* (Charles Strurridge, 2000).

Alec McCowen (b. Tunbridge Wells, 1925). Alec McCowen's career began during the war—he toured with ENSA (Entertainments National Service Association) from 1942. He next appeared in provincial repertory (York; Birmingham). Throughout the 1950s he worked in London in modern plays: *Escapade* (St James's, 1952); *The Matchmaker* (Theatre Royal Haymarket, 1954); *The Count of Clérambard* (Garrick, 1955); *The Caine Mutiny Court Martial* (Hippodrome, 1956); Jimmy Porter in *Look Back in Anger* (Royal Court, 1957, fourth cast); and Claverton-Ferry in T.S. Eliot's *The Elder Statesman* (Cambridge Theatre, 1958). At the Old Vic, 1959-61, he established his reputation as a classical actor playing Brisk in *The Double Dealer* (Michael Benthall, 1959); Touchstone in *As You Like It* (Wendy Toye, 1959); Algy to Judi Dench's Cecily in *The Importance of Being Earnest* (1959); Ford in *The Merry Wives of Windsor* (John Hale, 1959); the title role in *Richard II* (Val May, 1959); the Dauphin in *Saint Joan* (Douglas Seale, 1959); Mercutio in the Judi Dench/John Stride *Romeo and Juliet* (Franco Zeffirelli, 1960); Oberon in *A Midsum-*

mer *Night's Dream* (Michael Langham, 1960); and Malvolio in *Twelfth Night* (Colin Graham, 1961).

He was then at the RSC for four landmark years, acclaimed for his interpretations of Antipholus of Syracuse in *The Comedy of Errors* (Clifford Williams, RST, 1962), a famous Fool in the Paul Scofield *King Lear* (Peter Brook, RST, 1962), and Father Fontana in *The Representative* (Williams, Aldwych, 1963). He seemed on the brink of a long RSC career, but as things turned out he did not return to Stratford until the 1990s.

His choices during the years 1965 to 1992 were often surprising and usually memorable. They included Rolfe/Hadrian in Peter Luke's hit play *Hadrian VII* (Birmingham Rep, 1967); the title role in *Hamlet* (Birmingham Rep, 1970); Philip in Christopher Hampton's *The Philanthropist* (Robert Kidd, Royal Court, 1970); the title role in Simon Gray's *Butley* (Criterion, 1972); Alceste in *The Misanthrope* (John Dexter, NT Old Vic, 1973); Dysart in Peter Shaffer's *Equus* (Dexter, NT Old Vic, 1973); Higgins opposite Diana Rigg in *Pygmalion* (Albery, 1974); Antony in *Antony and Cleopatra* (Prospect, Edinburgh Festival and Old Vic, 1977); the acclaimed one-man show *St Mark's Gospel*, which he devised (Riverside Studios, 1978); Hitler in Hampton's *The Portage to San Cristobal of A.H.* (Mermaid, 1982); the one-man show *Kipling* (Mermaid, 1984); the one-man show *Shakespeare, Cole and Co.* (UK Tour, 1988); Father Jack in Brian Friel's *Dancing at Lughnasa* (Patrick Mason, Abbey Theatre, Dublin, 1990); and Michael in Frank McGuinness's *Someone Who'll Watch Over Me* (Robin Lefevre, Hampstead Theatre, 1992).

Back with the RSC after thirty years he played Prospero in *The Tempest* (Sam Mendes, RST, 1993), Edward Elgar in *Elgar's Rondo* (Swan, 1993), and Gaev in *The Cherry Orchard* (Adrian Noble, Swan, 1995). His scholarly, irascible Prospero surveyed the action from a high ladder. His dapper, unworldly Gaev was bucolic but vulnerable—he sucked sweets for comfort and at the moment of eviction broke down like a child. In 1997 he played the narrator in the National's production of *Peter Pan* (John

Caird, Olivier); in 1999, Reg in Ronald Harwood's *Quartet* (Christopher Morahan, Tour and Albery).

McCowen has worked steadily throughout his career as a character actor in British and American films. Seemingly unassuming and yet a true original, his talent has enriched many movies, including Charles Frend's *The Cruel Sea* (1953); Charles Crichton's *The Divided Heart* (1954); John Guillermin's *Town on Trial* (1956); Joseph Losey's *Time Without Pity* (1956); Roy Baker's *A Night to Remember* (1958); Tony Richardson's *The Loneliness of the Long Distance Runner* (1962); George Cukor's *Travels With My Aunt* (1972); Alfred Hitchcock's *Frenzy* (1972); and Martin Scorsese's *The Age of Innocence* (1993) and *Gangs of New York* (2002).

Ian McDiarmid (b. Carnoustie, Scotland, 1947) is a fastidious exponent of character roles, able to turn the blandest subject into a caricature. As a character actor in films he has made an impression disproportionate to the screen time allotted to his many doctors and scientists. But in the 1990s there was something else: with Jonathan Kent he transformed the Almeida into the most prestigious theatre in London.

He was educated at St Andrews University and the Royal Scottish Academy of Music and Drama. In the first phase of his career, he played Claudius in *Hamlet* at the Library Theatre, Manchester (1972); the title roles in *Galileo* and *Timon of Athens* and St Juste in *Danton's Death* at the Glasgow Citizens' (1971); Hitler in *Schweyk in the Second World War* at the Edinburgh Lyceum (1973); and the title role in *Peer Gynt* at the Oxford Playhouse. In 1974 he spent six months at the Théâtre National Populaire in Paris, and throughout his career he has been especially interested in the drama of continental Europe.

He was at the RSC from 1973 to 1986: the Judge in *Toad of Toad Hall* (Euan Smith, RST, 1973); Elbow in *Measure for Measure* (Keith Hack, RST, 1974); Trinculo in *The Tempest* (Hack, TOP, 1974); Roche in *Afore Night Come* (Ron Daniels, TOP, 1974);

Goebbels/Brettschneider in *Schweyk in the Second World War* (Howard Davies, TOP, 1976); Don John in *Much Ado About Nothing* (John Barton, RST, 1976); Comic in Charles Wood's *Dingo* (Barry Kyle, TOP, 1976); the Porter in Trevor Nunn's *Macbeth* (TOP, 1976); Turner in David Edgar's *Destiny* (Daniels, TOP, 1976); Billy in Howard Barker's *That Good Between Us* (Kyle, Warehouse, 1977); *The Days of the Commune* (Davies, Aldwych, 1977); Lang in *A Miserable and Lonely Death* (Walter Donohue, Warehouse, 1978); an ever-present Chorus, wry and sarcastic, in the Branagh/Noble *Henry V* (RST, 1984); Shylock, played with unusual levels of complexity as a repellent but hounded alien, in *The Merchant of Venice* (Kyle, RST, 1984); the broodingly intense Glaswegian John Tagg, a performance of mesmerising silences, in Trevor Griffiths's *The Party* (Davies, TOP, 1984); Edward Bond's trilogy *War Plays* (*Red Black and Ignorant*, *The Tin Cat People*, *Great Peace*, Nick Hamm, Pit, 1985); 'The Barker Plays' (*Crimes in Hot Countries*, *The Castle*, *Downchild*, Bill Alexander/Hamm, Pit, 1985); and Robespierre in Pam Gems's *The Danton Affair* (Daniels, Barbican, 1986).

Although he became identified with the RSC during this period he had some notable successes elsewhere: his performances as 'Einstein' in Terry Johnson's *Insignificance* at the Royal Court (Les Waters, 1982) and Brecht in *Tales from Hollywood* at the National (Peter Gill, Olivier, 1983) were particularly memorable. From 1986 to 1988 he was an associate director at the Manchester Royal Exchange, directing productions of Molière's *Don Juan* and Marivaux's *Slave Island* and playing the title role in *Edward II* and Phillip II in Schiller's *Don Carlos* (both Nicholas Hytner). His association with Howard Barker was continued at the Almeida where he directed *The Possibilities* (1988). In 1989 he starred in a West End production of Iris Murdoch's *The Black Prince* (Stuart Burge, Aldwych).

As co-Artistic Director of the Almeida (1989-02) he played leading roles in *The School for Wives* (Jonathan Kent, 1993), Giorgio Battistelli's *Experimentum Mundi* (1995), *Tartuffe* (Kent, 1996), *Ivanov* (Kent, 1997), *The Government Inspector* (Kent, 1997), *Doc-*

tor's Dilemma (Michael Grandage, 1998), *The Tempest* (Kent, 2000), and Battistelli's *The Embalmer* (2002), and he directed productions of *The Rehearsal* (1990), *Hippolytus* (1991), *A Hard Heart* (1992), *Siren Song* (1994) and *Venice Preserv'd* (1995). In 2004 at the Donmar Warehouse he starred in Pirandello's *Henry IV* (Grandage).

John McEnery (b. Birmingham, 1943). As a member of Laurence Olivier's National Theatre company at the Old Vic, John McEnery played Hamlet in the premiere production of Tom Stoppard's *Rosencrantz and Guildenstern are Dead* (Derek Goldby, 1967); Silvius in the all-male *As You Like It* (Clifford Williams, 1967); Costard in *Love's Labour's Lost* (Olivier, 1968); and Harry Havelock in Charles Wood's *H* (Geoffrey Reeves, 1969). Franco Zeffirelli cast him as Mercutio in his screen version of *Romeo and Juliet* (1968), the first in a series of films that are difficult to categorise: *The Lady in the Car with Glasses and a Gun* (Anatole Litvak, 1970); *Le bateau sur l'herbe* (Gérard Brach, 1970); *Bartleby* (Anthony Friedman, 1970); *Nicholas and Alexandra* (1971); *Days of Fury* (1973); *Little Malcolm* (1974); *Alle origini della mafia* (1974); *The Land That Time Forgot* (1975); *Galileo* (Joseph Losey, 1975); *Schizo* (1977); and *The Duellists* (Ridley Scott, 1977).

He first joined the RSC in 1975 to play Private Meek in *Too True to be Good* (Clifford Williams, Aldwych). His one prolonged phase of work with the Company was dominated by Shakespearean comedy: Antonio in *The Changeling* (Terry Hands, Aldwych, 1978); Pistol in *The Merry Wives of Windsor* (Trevor Nunn/John Caird, RST, 1979); Sir Andrew in *Twelfth Night* (Hands, RST, 1979); Roderigo in *Othello* (Ronald Eyre, RST, 1979); and Mr Snevellicci in *Nicholas Nickleby* (Nunn/Caird, Aldwych, 1980). He has returned twice: in 1991 to play Weston in Sam Shepard's *The Curse of the Starving Class* (Robin Lefevre, Pit), and in 2001 to create one of the leading roles in Nick Stafford's *Luminosity* (Gemma Bodinetz, Pit).

In 1995, at the National, he played Lord Castlereagh in Ernst Toller's *The Machine Wreckers* (Katie Mitchell), and Lord Willoughby in *Richard II* (Deborah Warner, both Cottesloe). Since 1997 he has been one of the regular senior players at Shakespeare's Globe. His fine character work has helped to give artistic credibility to a popular tourist attraction: Pistol in *Henry V* (Richard Olivier, 1997); a 'decrepit knight' in Thomas Middleton's *A Chaste Maid in Cheapside* (Malcolm McKay, 1997); Jaques in *As You Like It* (Lucy Bailey, 1998); Shortrod Harebrain in Middleton's *A Mad World, My Masters* (Sue Lefton, 1998); Enobarbus in *Antony and Cleopatra* (1999); the Fool in *King Lear* (Barry Kyle, 2001); John of Gaunt in *Richard II* (Tim Carroll, 2003); and the assassin in Marlowe's *Edward II* (Timothy Walker, 2003).

Other screen work: John Rokesmith in *Our Mutual Friend* (BBC, 1977); *Life of Shakespeare* (ITV, 1978); Lucio in *Measure for Measure* (BBC, 1979); Caligula in *A.D.* (1985); *Little Dorrit* (1988); *Precious Bane* (BBC, 1989); *The Krays* (1990); *The Fool* (1990); Osric in *Hamlet* (Zeffirelli, 1990); Uncle Ted in Hanif Kureishi's *The Buddha of Suburbia* (Roger Michell, BBC, 1993); *Black Beauty* (1994); and Jack Durbeyfield in *Tess of the D'Urbervilles* (ITV, 1998).

Peter McEnery (b. Walsall, 1940) made his stage debut, aged sixteen, at the Palace Pier Theatre in Brighton (1956). A year later he was working alongside Ralph Richardson in Robert Bolt's *Flowering Cherry* (Theatre Royal Haymarket). His boyish, pop star good looks were right for the time and he was cast in three major films released in 1960/61 — *Tunes of Glory* (Ronald Neame), *Beat Girl* and *Victim* (Basil Dearden). Cinema came to dominate his career, but first he made his mark at the RSC in both classical and modern roles, among them Laertes in *Hamlet* (Peter Wood, RST, 1961); Silvius in the Vanessa Redgrave *As You Like It* (Michael Elliott, RST, 1961); Tybalt in *Romeo and Juliet* (Peter Hall, RST, 1961); Johnny Hobnails in David Rudkin's

Afore Night Come (Clifford Williams, Arts Theatre, 1962); Patroclus in *Troilus and Cressida* (Hall, Aldwych, 1962); De Laubardemont in John Whiting's *The Devils* (Wood, Aldwych, 1962); and Bassanio in *The Merchant of Venice* (Williams, RST, 1965). Between RSC seasons he played Konstantin to Vanessa Redgrave's Nina in *The Seagull* (Tony Richardson, Queen's, 1964).

Among the films he made as a leading actor are *The Moon Spinners* (James Neilson, 1964); the Jane Fonda vehicle *La Curée* (*The Game is Over*, Roger Vadim, 1966); *J'ai tué Raspoutine* (1967); *Negatives* (Peter Medak, 1968); *Le mur de l'Atlantique* (1970); *Entertaining Mr Sloane* (1970); and *The Adventures of Gerard* (Jerzy Skolimowski, 1970).

Back at the RSC, 1977-90, he sought diversity, creating a decadent Lorenzo in *The Lorenzaccio Story* (Ron Daniels, TOP, 1977); Orlando in *As You Like It* (Trevor Nunn, RST, 1977); the imprisoned South Africa journalist in David Edgar's *The Jail Diary of Albie Sachs* (Howard Davies, Warehouse, 1978); the title role in *Pericles* (Daniels, TOP, 1979); Jerry in *Once in a Lifetime* (Nunn, Aldwych, 1979); Antipholus of Ephesus in *The Comedy of Errors* (Adrian Noble, RST, 1983); a fatalistic Brutus in *Julius Caesar* (Daniels, RST, 1983); Urbain Grandier in *The Devils* (John Barton, Pit, 1984); and Godber in Michael Hastings's *A Dream of People* (Janet Suzman, Pit, 1990). More recently, he played Hector in *Heartbreak House* at the Almeida (David Hare, 1997), and Claudius in the Simon Russell Beale *Hamlet* at the National (John Caird, Lyttelton, 2000-01).

Jo McInnes. One of the discoveries of the 1996/97 season, Jo (or Jay as she was then credited) McInnes gave memorable performances as the servant girl Hester in *The Herbal Bed* (Michael Attenborough, TOP) and Peggy in *The General from America* (Howard Davies, Swan). She has continued to win acclaim for her sensitive character playing: Nell Gwyn in April de Angelis's *Playhouse Creatures* (Peter Hall Company, Old Vic, 1997); a tender but unsentimental Sonya in the RSC's Young Vic production of *Uncle Vanya* (Katie Mitchell, 1998); a girl footballer in the television series *Playing the Field* (Catherine Morshead, BBC, 1998); Queen Isabella in *Edward II* (Richard Grandage, Sheffield Crucible, 2001); Sarah Kane's *4.48 Psychosis* (James Macdonald, Royal Court, 2001); Keith Allen's assistant in the Charlotte Gainsbourg movie *Ma femme est une actrice* (Yvan Attal, 2001); Hesp in Naomi Wallace's *The Inland Sea* (Dominic Dromgoole, Oxford Stage Company, 2002); Shona in Glyn Cannon's *On Blindness* (Vicky Featherstone, Paines Plough, Soho Theatre, 2004); and Martirio in García Lorca's *The House of Bernarda Alba* (Davies, NT Lyttelton, 2005).

She trained at the Mountview School and gained her early experience at the Haymarket Theatre, Basingstoke, the Salisbury Playhouse and the Angles Theatre, Wisbech. Work on the London fringe included *Medea* (Duke's Head), *Tales of Christmas Past* (Polka Children's Theatre), *Dora* (Hen and Chickens), *The Last of the Just* (Arts Theatre), and *The Mayflies* (Attic Theatre). Her first high-profile production was Howard Davies's NT revival of *The Children's Hour* (Lyttelton, 1994).

Ian McKellen (b. Burnley, Lancashire, 1939). Ian McKellen's progress to the top of the league of classical actors began at Bolton School, where, at the age of thirteen, he played Malvolio in *Twelfth Night*. At Cambridge (St Catharine's College) his precocious talent and vociferous appetite for challenging roles (including Justice Shallow in John Barton's *Henry IV*) made him a star actor of the Marlowe Society and provoked the interest of the London press. His contemporaries included Derek Jacobi (Hal in *Henry IV*), David Frost and, most significantly, Trevor Nunn. McKellen and Nunn acted together in the Marlowe Society's productions of *Doctor Faustus* (1960) and *Henry VI* (1961).

On graduating McKellen began four years of hard work on regional stages. Among the forty-odd roles he performed at the Belgrade Theatre, Coventry, the Arts Theatre, Ipswich, and the

Playhouse, Nottingham, were William Roper in Robert Bolt's *A Man for all Seasons* (his debut, 1961); Stan Dyson in Keith Waterhouse's *Celebration* (1961); Chief Weasel in *Toad of Toad Hall* (1961); Konstantin in *The Seagull* (1962); Claudio in *Much Ado About Nothing* (1962); Tom Midway in David Turner's *Semi-Detached* (1962); the title role in *David Copperfield* (1962); Tee Vee in the pantomime *Aladdin* (1962); the title role in *Henry V* (Robert Chetwyn, 1963); the title role in John Osborne's *Luther* (Chetwyn, 1963); Edmund Tyrone in Eugene O'Neill's *Long Day's Journey into Night* (Chetwyn, 1963); Julian in Peter Shaffer's *The Public Eye* (1963); John Bogle in Peter Ustinov's *The Life in My Hands* (1963); Tullus Aufidius in *Coriolanus* (Tyrone Guthrie, 1963); Winifred Hutchinson to John Neville's George Bernard Shaw in Harold Callen's *The Bashful Genius* (Frank Dunlop, 1964); Don Alvaro in Calderón's *The Mayor of Zalamea* (John Neville, 1964); and Arthur Seaton in *Saturday Night and Sunday Morning* (Dunlop, 1964). Later that year he made his London debut at the Duke of York's as Godfrey in James Saunders's *A Scent of Flowers*, a notable success.

In 1965 he was briefly a member of Laurence Olivier's National Theatre, playing Claudio in the Robert Stephens/Maggie Smith *Much Ado About Nothing* (Franco Zeffirelli, Old Vic), a Protestant Evangelist in John Arden's *Armstrong's Last Goodnight* (Chichester), and de Foenix in *Trelawney of the Wells* (Chichester). For some years, moving from theatre to theatre, he seemed creatively restless: Hanker in Donald Howarth's *A Lily in Little India* (Hampstead Theatre, 1965); Cobham in Arnold Wesker's *Their Very Own and Golden City* (John Dexter/William Gaskill, Royal Court, 1966); Napoleon in Shaw's *Man of Destiny* (Robert Kidd, Mermaid, 1966); Leonidik alongside Judi Dench and Ian McShane in Arbuzov's *The Promise* (Frank Hauser, Oxford Playhouse, 1966); Tom/Harold Gorringe in Peter Shaffer's *White Liars/Black Comedy* (Lyric, 1968); Pentheus in *The Bacchae* (Antony Tuckey, Liverpool Playhouse, 1969); Darkly in Barry Hines's *Billy's Last Stand* (Michael Wearing, Royal Court Upstairs, 1970); and Captain Plume in George Farquhar's *The*

Recruiting Officer (Richard Cottrell, Cambridge Theatre Company, Tour, 1970). Between 1968 and 71 McKellen appeared regularly with the touring company Prospect: his performances as Shakespeare's Richard II (Cottrell) and Hamlet (Chetwyn) and Marlowe's Edward II (Toby Robertson) established his reputation as a young classical actor who owed more to the high theatrical style of Laurence Olivier and John Gielgud than to the more realistic approach of immediate predecessors such as Ian Holm, Albert Finney, Alan Bates and Robert Stephens.

In 1971 he opened the Sheffield Crucible as Svetlovidov in Chekhov's *Swan Song* (David William). He devoted much of the early 1970s to the Actors' Company, which he co-founded. McKellen received the same pay as the other actors and took on minor as well as leading roles—the Page-boy in Feydeau's *Ruling the Roast* (Cottrell) and Giovanni in John Ford's *'Tis Pity She's a Whore* (David Giles, Tour and Edinburgh Festival, 1972); Prince Yoremitsu in Iris Murdoch's *The Three Arrows* (Noel Willman, Arts Theatre, Cambridge, 1972); Kruschov in Chekhov's *The Wood-Demon* (Giles) and Lady Wishfort's Footman in Congreve's *The Way of the World* (William, Tour and Edinburgh Festival, 1973). In 1974 the Actors' Company performed *The Wood-Demon*, *The Way of the World* and *King Lear* at the Brooklyn Academy of Music in New York: McKellen's performance as Edgar received the New York Drama Desk Award. The Actors' Company was not sustainable.

Given McKellen's Cambridge connection with John Barton and Trevor Nunn it is a little surprising that he did not join the RSC until 1974. His RSC career began at the Aldwych with the title roles in Marlowe's *Doctor Faustus* (Barton) and Wedekind's *The Marquis of Keith* (Ronald Eyre), Philip the Bastard in *King John* (Barton/Barry Kyle), and Aubrey Bagot in Shaw's *Too True to Be Good* (Clifford Williams). It was a typically diverse and challenging programme but immediately eclipsed by the 1976 Stratford season. McKellen played Romeo and Leontes in the main house and Macbeth at The Other Place, directed by Trevor Nunn. *Macbeth* was one of those rare occasions when a play, type of theatre, actor and director combine to create something out of the ordinary. The Other Place was the crucial factor. McKellen, in general a master technician specialising in intellectually gripping concepts rather than emotional reality, seemed dangerously possessed on this occasion. The thought-processes of Macbeth's criminal psychology hummed around the tiny theatre like an electric current. The sleeked back hair, pallid complexion and leather coat were almost unnecessary. The following year, in London, he added Face in *The Alchemist* (Nunn, Aldwych); Alex in Tom Stoppard and André Previn's *Every Good Boy Deserves Favour* (Nunn, Royal Festival Hall); Bernick in Ibsen's *Pillars of the Community* (Barton, Aldwych); Langevin in Brecht's *The Days of the Commune* (Howard Davies, Aldwych); and Kentridge in Norman Fenton and Jon Blair's *A Miserable and Lonely Death* (Walter Donohue, Warehouse). For the RSC's first small-scale tour, which he led, he played Sir Toby Belch in *Twelfth Night* (John Amiel) and Andrei in *Three Sisters* (Nunn, 1978).

If the scale of McKellen's RSC achievement has kept him linked to the Company, he has, since 1984, appeared more often at the National on the South Bank. Following a suburb opening treble of Pierre in Thomas Otway's *Venice Preserv'd* (Peter Gill, Lyttelton), Platonov in Chekhov's *Wild Honey* (Christopher Morahan, Lyttelton) and the title role in *Coriolanus* (Peter Hall, Olivier), McKellen accepted Hall's invitation to form and direct, with Edward Petherbridge, one of the National's companies. As leader of the McKellen/Petherbridge group he played Bosola in Webster's *The Duchess of Malfi* (Philip Prowse, Lyttelton, 1985), Inspector Hound/Mr Puff in the double-bill of Tom Stoppard's *The Real Inspector Hound* and Sheridan's *The Critic* (Stoppard/Sheila Hancock, Olivier, 1985) and Lopakhin in *The Cherry Orchard* (Mike Alfreds, Cottesloe, 1985). During the Richard Eyre era he played Max in *Bent* (Sean Mathias, Lyttelton, 1990); the title role—a uniformed fascist amid the English aristocracy, modelled on Oswald Mosley—in *Richard III* and Kent in the Brian Cox *King Lear* (Eyre and Deborah Warner respectively,

Lyttelton, 1990); Gennaro in Eduardo De Filippo's *Napoli Milionaria* (Eyre, Lyttelton, 1991); and the title role in *Uncle Vanya* (Mathias, Cottesloe, 1992). McKellen's Richard was deliberately revisionist in that the opportunities for black comedy were completely ignored. He returned to the National in 1997 for Nunn's first season, playing Stockmann in Ibsen's *An Enemy of the People* (Nunn, Olivier) and Mr Darling/Captain Hook in *Peter Pan* (John Caird, Olivier).

Elsewhere, his work has included Colin in David Rudkin's *Ashes* (Ron Daniels, Young Vic, 1975); Max in *Bent* (Chetwyn, Royal Court, 1979); Salieri in *Amadeus* (Hall, Broadhurst, New York, 1980); the extraordinary one-man show *Acting Shakespeare*, an evening of speeches with commentary, anecdotes and impersonations, performed throughout the world (1980-88); Boy in Sean Mathias's *Cowardice* (Anthony Page, Ambassadors, 1983); Jerome in Alan Ayckbourn's *Henceforward* (Vaudeville, 1988); the recital show *A Knight Out* (Lyceum, London, and Tour, 1994, Los Angeles, 1997, performed to raise funds for various theatrical and community causes, particularly AIDS research); leading Jude Kelly's 1998/99 repertory season at the West Yorkshire Playhouse—Dorn in *The Seagull*, Essendine in Ayckbourn's *Present Laughter* and Prospero in *The Tempest*; and Edgar in August Strindberg's *Dance of Death* (Mathias, Broadhurst, New York, 2001).

McKellen has only returned to the RSC to star in productions directed by Nunn (an Adrian Noble *Coriolanus* was discussed in 1983 but McKellen finally chose to play the role for Peter Hall at the National). In *Othello* (TOP, 1989) McKellen's Iago—a womanish NCO whose psychotic nature was convincingly hidden from the other characters while, paradoxically, being apparent in the most ordinary of gestures (for instance, the obsessive way he tidied the bunks in the barracks)—was among his most original creations. *King Lear* (Courtyard, 2007) was first-rate but both the performance and the production lacked the essential strangeness that Robert Stephens and Adrian Noble brought to the tragedy in 1993. In Nunn's haunting *The Seagull* (Courtyard,

2007) McKellen played Sorin with a veteran's command of every trick of the trade, and yet with true feeling. It was the latest stop in a long Chekhovian journey that had started forty-five years before with the role of Konstantin in the same play.

As a screen actor McKellen was for many years restricted to supporting roles, but he found success in Hollywood in the late 1990s: D.H. Lawrence in *Priest of Love* (Christopher Miles, 1981); Dr Theodore Cuza in *The Keep* (Michael Mann, 1983); Sir Andrew Charleson in *Plenty* (Fred Schepisi, 1985); Walter in *Walter and June* (1986); John Profumo in *Scandal* (Michael Caton-Jones, 1989); Geoffrey in *Six Degrees of Separation* (Fred Schepisi, 1993); Archibald Anson Gidde in *Tales of the City* (TV, 1993); Percy Corcoran in *The Ballad of Little Jo* (Maggie Greenwald, 1993); Death in *Last Action Hero* (1993); Bill Kraus in *And the Band Played On* (Roger Spottiswoode, 1993); Will Gates in *Restoration* (Michael Hoffman, 1995); *Jack and Sarah* (Tim Sullivan, 1995); *Cold Comfort Farm* (John Schlesinger, 1995); the title role in *Richard III* (Richard Loncraine, 1995); Nicholas II in *Rasputin* (TV, 1996); James Kennedy in *Amy Foster* (1997); Uncle Freddie in *Bent* (Mathias, 1997); James Whale in *Gods and Monsters* (Bill Condon, 1998); *Apt Pupil* (Bryan Singer, 1998); Magneto in *X-Men* (2000-06); Gandalf in *The Lord of the Rings* (Peter Jackson, 2001-03); *Asylum* (2005); *Neverwas* (2005); *Coronation Street* (ITV, 2005); Teabing in *The Da Vinci Code* (2006).

Hilton McRae (b. Dundee, 1949). When Hilton McRae joined the RSC in 1977 he looked like a typical, long-haired juvenile lead of the time, but was in fact a much more interesting figure, an Edinburgh law graduate who had started out in the theatre as a member of John McGrath's politically radical troupe 7:84 (contemporaries included Robbie Coltrane and Bill Paterson).

His ten years at the RSC were the most challenging and impressive of his career. In the main house, he was Eros/Boy Singer in Peter Brook's *Antony and Cleopatra* (RST, 1978); Orlando to Juliet Stevenson's Rosalind in Adrian Noble's *As You*

Like It (RST, 1985); Patroclus in Howard Davies's *Troilus and Cressida* (RST, 1985, his future wife, Lindsay Duncan, played Helen); and Antoine Saint-Just in Pam Gems's *The Danton Affair* (Daniels, Barbican, 1986). In the studio spaces, his credits included Jonson, Brecht, Shakespeare and new work—Kastril in *The Alchemist* (Trevor Nunn, TOP, 1977); Young Prochazska in *Schweyk in the Second World War* (Davies, Warehouse); Stephens in C.P. Taylor's *Bandits* (Davies, Warehouse, 1977); Mick in James Robson's *Factory Birds* (Bill Alexander, Warehouse, 1977); Launcelot Gobbo in *The Merchant of Venice* (John Barton, TOP, 1978); Daniel in Peter Whelan's *Captain Swing* (Alexander, TOP, 1978); McCulloch in Howard Brenton's *The Churchill Play* (Barry Kyle, TOP, 1978); Third Shepherd in *The Shepherds' Play* (Tucker, TOP, 1978-79); Heggie in Tom McGrath's *The Innocent* (Davies, Warehouse, 1979); Man at Rehearsal in Pam Gems's *Piaf* (Davies, Aldwych, 1980); and Danceny, succeeding Sean Baker, in Christopher Hampton's *Les liaisons dangereuses* (Davies, Ambassadors, 1986-87).

Other theatre: Steven Berkoff's *The Trial* (Roundhouse, 1973), *Agamemnon* (Greenwich, 1976), and *Acapulco* (King's Head, 1992); the title role in *Hamlet* (Christopher Fettes, New Shakespeare Company, Tour, 1983); the title role in *Macbeth* (Cliff Burnett, Dundee Rep, 1989); the Engineer in *Miss Saigon* (1990); Iago in *Othello* (Bill Alexander, Birmingham Rep, 1993); Lovborg to Geraldine James's Hedda in *Hedda Gabler* (Joseph Blatchley, Manchester Royal Exchange, 1993); Torvald in *A Doll's House* (Irina Brown, Birmingham Rep, 1996); Schwartz in *The Front Page* (Sam Mendes, Donmar Warehouse, 1997-98); Sam Carmichael in *Mamma Mia!* (Phyllida Lloyd, Prince Edward, 1999); Prince Nikki in *My One and Only* (Loveday Ingram, Chichester, 2001); and the title role in *Peer Gynt* (David Levin, Arcola, 2003).

Anna Madeley (b. London, 1977) trained at the Central School of Speech and Drama. Her early work included Norma in Amanda Whittington's *Be My Baby* (Abigail Morris, Soho Theatre Company, 1998); the first series of *Cold Feet* (ITV, 1998); *Sense and Sensibility* (Northcott Theatre, Exeter, 2000); Neil Monaghan's *Eye Contact* (Izzy Mant, Riverside Studios, 2000); and Catherine Cookson's *A Dinner of Herbs* (ITV, 2000).

She first appeared with the RSC as a child (Bill Alexander's *Merry Wives of Windsor*, Barbican, 1986). She rejoined the Company in 2001 to play Ilse in Peter Whelan's *A Russian in the Woods* (Robert Delamere, TOP); Martha in Wycherley's *Love in a Wood* (Tim Supple, Swan); and Erifila in Lope de Vega's *Madness in Valencia* (Jonathan Munby, TOP). As Whelan's war-damaged Berliner, caught between desperation and longing, anger and tenderness, she was both moving and alluring. Staying with the Company for Gregory Doran's season of rarities in the Swan, she was cast as Domitia in *The Roman Actor* (Sean Holmes) and Maria in *The Malcontent* (Dominic Cooke).

She has continued to impress: Yulka in Vassily Sigarev's *Ladybird* at the Royal Court (Ramin Gray, Theatre Upstairs, 2004); Lydia Languish in Sheridan's *The Rivals* at the Bristol Old Vic (Rachel Kavanaugh, 2004); Jenna in Laura Wade's *Colder Than Here* at the Soho Theatre (Abigail Morris, 2005); fatally attractive as the young Russian pole dancer in David Greig's *The Cosmonaut's Last Message to the Woman He Once Loved in the Former Soviet Union* at the Donmar Warehouse (Supple, 2005); Celia in Christopher Hampton's *The Philanthropist* at the Donmar (David Grindley, 2005); the boy hero of *Coram Boy* at the National (Melly Still, Olivier, 2005-06); and, on television, a nurse in *The Royal* (ITV, 2003-05), Mrs Beeton in *The Secret Life of Mrs Beeton* (BBC, 2006), a rape victim in *Consent* (Channel Four, 2007), and Lucy Steele in *Sense and Sensibility* (BBC, 2008).

Michael Maloney (b. Bury St Edmunds, Suffolk, 1957) played the Hamlet-obsessed actor in Kenneth Branagh's *In the Bleak Midwinter* (1995) and Leartes in Branagh's Hollywood *Hamlet* (1996). His distinctive vocal delivery, fast and emphatic, found its most suitable outlet in his own acclaimed performance of the role—a Hamlet showing the effects of extreme mental disquiet in every word and gesture (Philip Franks, Greenwich Theatre, 1996).

This was Michael Maloney's second classical triumph, following his watchful, enigmatic Hal in Adrian Noble's RSC production of *Henry IV* (RST, 1991). He first appeared with the RSC in 1982-83, as Donalbain in *Macbeth* (Howard Davies, RST); Ben in Edward Bond's *Lear* (Barry Kyle, TOP); Ferdinand to Alice Krige's Miranda in *The Tempest* (Ron Daniels, RST); Eros in the Helen Mirren/Michael Gambon *Antony and Cleopatra* (Noble, TOP); and Master Greenwit in *The Roaring Girl* (Kyle, Barbican). In 1991-92, along with Hal, he played Romeo opposite Clare Holman in *Romeo and Juliet* (David Leveaux, RST), and Frankford in *A Woman Killed with Kindness* (Katie Mitchell, TOP).

Elsewhere, he starred in Alan Ayckbourn's *Taking Steps* (Lyric Hammersmith, 1980); Anthony Minghella's *Two Planks and a Passion* (Greenwich Theatre, 1984); Daniel Mornin's *Built on Sand* (Royal Court, 1987); Jack Shepherd's *In Lambeth* (Donmar Warehouse, 1989), as William Blake; Peter Gill's *In the Blue* (NT Cottesloe, 1985); Paul Godfrey's in *Once in a While the Odd Thing Happens* (NT Cottesloe, 1990), as Benjamin Britten; and Christopher Hampton's *Alice's Adventures Underground* (Martha Clarke, NT Cottesloe, 1994), as Dodgson.

Maloney is saturnine in appearance, but projects melancholia rather that menace—hence the hapless innocents and depressives that feature among his television roles: the betrayed husband in Minghella's *What if it's Raining* (Channel Four, 1986); William Boot in *Scoop* (Gavin Millar, 1987); Lee opposite Juliet Stevenson in Minghella's *Living with Dinosaurs* (Paul Weiland, 1989); and Jaspar Pye in *Love on a Branch Line* (Martyn Friend, 1993).

His best film roles have come through Kenneth Branagh and Anthony Minghella: the Dauphin in *Henry V* (Branagh, 1989); Roderigo, a suburb cameo, in the Branagh/Fishburne *Othello* (Oliver Parker, 1995); and Mark in *Truly Madly Deeply* (Minghella, 1991).

Maloney returned to the RSC in 1999 to play Edgar in Yukio Ninagawa's production of *King Lear* (Tokyo, Barbican and RST). In 2001, at the Royal Court, he gave a powerful performance in Kevin Elyot's *Mouth to Mouth* (Ian Rickson). In 2004, reunited with Ninagawa, he played his second Hamlet (Barbican).

Tom Mannion (b. Glasgow). The son of a Glasgow shop-keeper, Tom Mannion trained for the stage at the Royal Scottish Academy of Music and Drama. He was first at the RSC from 1982 to 86. The presence he gave to small roles during the 1982/83 season—Murderer/Lennox in *Macbeth* (Howard Davies, RST); Servant/Knight in *King Lear* (Adrian Noble, RST); Soldier in Edward Bond's *Lear* (Barry Kyle, TOP); Mariner in *The Tempest* (Ron Daniels, RST); Decretas/Menecrates/Eros in *Antony and Cleopatra* (Noble, TOP)—led quickly to the title role in Nick Darke's *The Body* (Nick Hamm, Pit, 1983); Willem Van Es in Nicholas Wright's *The Custom of the Country* (David Jones, Pit, 1983); Christian de Neuvillette in the Derek Jacobi *Cyrano de Bergerac* (Terry Hands, Barbican, 1983); Lafayette in Caryl Churchill's *Softcops* (Davies, Pit, 1984); the Young Man in *Mary, After the Queen* (Kyle, The Warehouse, Stratford, 1985); Nil in Gorky's *Philistines* (John Caird, TOP, 1985); Cassio in *Othello* (Hands, RST, 1985); First Geologist in *Melons* (Alison Sutcliffe, Pit, 1986); Alex in *Mephisto* (Noble, Barbican, 1986); and Desmoulins in Pam Gems's *The Danton Affair* (Daniels, Barbican, 1986).

Mannion has continued to base his career in the theatre: Demetrius in *A Midsummer Night's Dream*, Littlewit in *Bartholomew Fair* (Peter Barnes), and Proteus in *The Two Gentlemen of Verona* (Ian Talbot) at the Open Air Theatre, Regent's Park (1987); Patrick in Ian Heggie's *American Bagpipes* (Caspar Wrede, Manchester Royal Exchange, 1988); the newspaper editor in *An Enemy of the People* (David Thacker, Young Vic, 1988); Rooney in Ted Moore's *The Marshalling Yard* (Bush, 1989); Sammy in Chris Hannan's *The Evil Doers* (Bush, 1990); James Doherty's *The Rising of the Moon* (Old Red Lion, Islington, 1991); James Stock's

Blue Night in the Heart of the West (Bush, 1991); Lussurioso in *The Revenger's Tragedy* (Jude Kelly, West Yorkshire Playhouse, 1992); outstanding as a Glaswegian Cyrano de Bergerac (Gerry Mulgrew, Communicado Theatre Company, Edinburgh Festival, 1992); Mitya in *The Brothers Karamazov* (Braham Murray, Manchester Royal Exchange, 1993); Wocky in Chris Hannan's *The Baby* (Bush, 1993); *The Trick is to Keep Breathing* (Michael Boyd, Tron, Glasgow, 1993); the title role in *Oedipus Tyrannos* (Kenny Ireland, Royal Lyceum, Edinburgh, 1994); the foreman in *Rutherford and Son* (Katie Mitchell, NT Cottesloe, 1994); Peachum in *The Threepenny Opera* (Phyllida Lloyd, Donmar Warehouse, 1994-95); Pintilje in David Lan's *The Ends of the Earth* (Andrei Serban, NT Cottesloe, 1996); Philip Barry's *Philadelphia Story* (Manchester Royal Exchange, Upper Campfield Market, 1996); Bill in David Farr's *Elton John's Glasses* (Terry Johnson, Palace Theatre, Watford, 1997); Billy in Chris Hannan's *Shining Souls* (Peter Hall Company, Old Vic, 1997); Shelagh Stephenson's *An Experiment With An Air Pump* (Manchester Royal Exchange, 1998); Larry in Patrick Marber's *Closer* (Marber, NT Lyric, 1998); Kuligin in Alexander Ostrovsky's *The Storm* (Hettie Macdonald, Almeida, 1998); *Art* (Matthew Warchus, West End, 1999); Archie in Tennessee Williams's *Baby Doll* (Lucy Bailey, Birmingham Rep, 1999); and Benedick in *Much Ado About Nothing* (Rachel Kavanaugh, Regent's Park, 2000).

From 2000 to 03 he was back at the RSC: Bosola in *The Duchess of Malfi* (Gale Edwards, Barbican, 2000); Mark Antony in *Julius Caesar* (Edward Hall, RST, 2001); Francis in David Farr's *Night of the Soul* (Farr, Pit, 2002); Frank Ford in *The Merry Wives of Windsor* (Rachel Kavanaugh) and Sicinius Velutus in *Coriolanus* (Farr, Swan and Small-scale Tour, 2002-03). In 2004 he played Claudius in Trevor Nunn's *Hamlet* at the Old Vic.

Lesley Manville (b. Brighton, 1956) emerged as one of her generation's most distinctive actresses in the theatre of the late 1970s and early 80s. Appearing, most notably, in new plays by

Peter Flannery, Hanif Kureishi, Andrea Dunbar and Caryl Churchill at the RSC's Warehouse and the Royal Court, she was a petite but forceful performer, able to humanise the most contrived character types.

She grew up in Brighton, the daughter of a taxi driver. Early in her career she appeared in the daytime soap *Emmerdale Farm* (1974-76). At the RSC in 1978 she worked exclusively in the Warehouse: Sister Croy in David Rudkin's *The Sons of Light* (Ron Daniels); Ali in Peter Flannery's *Savage Amusement* (John Caird); Isabel in Kate Collingwood's *Trust Us* (Walter Donohue, reading); the title role in Louise Page's *Lucy* (Mark Dornford-May, reading); and Second Student in John Hale's *Who Needs Enemies?* (Donohue, reading). In 1980 she played Jen in a fringe production of Doug Lucie's *Fear of the Dark* (Walter Donohue).

During the 1980s she moved between Sloane Square (where she met and married Gary Oldman), Stratford and the Barbican: Hanif Kureishi's *Borderline* (Stafford-Clark, Joint Stock, Royal Court, 1981); Sue in Andrea Dunbar's *Rita, Sue and Bob Too* (Royal Court, 1981); Marlene in Caryl Churchill's *Top Girls* (Royal Court, 1982); *Falkland Sound* (Royal Court, 1983); Pat in Edward Bond's *The Pope's Wedding* (Stafford-Clark, Royal Court, 1984); Liz in Bond's *Saved* (Danny Boyle, Royal Court, 1984); Polya in Gorky's *Philistines* (Caird, TOP, 1985); Phebe in *As You Like It* (Adrian Noble, RST, 1985); Cécile in *Les liaisons dangereuses* (Howard Davies, TOP, 1985); Dolores in *The Dead Monkey* (Roger Michell, RSC fringe production, TOP, 1985); Scilla in Churchill's *Serious Money* (Stafford-Clark, Royal Court, 1987); Sandra in Iain Heggie's *American Bagpipes* (Lindsay Posner, Royal Court, 1989); and Natasha in *Three Sisters* (Noble, Royal Court, 1990).

Away from the RSC and the Court she played Varya in *The Cherry Orchard* (Sam Mendes, Aldwych, 1989), and the title role opposite Finbar Lynch in *Miss Julie* (Greenwich Theatre, 1990). On screen, she appeared opposite Kenneth Branagh in *High Season* (Clare Peploe, 1987) and Gary Oldman in *The Price* (Alan Clarke, BBC, 1988). Her most significant work has been for Mike

Leigh—the films *High Hopes* (1988), *Secrets and Lies* (1996), *Topsy-Turvy* (1999), and *All or Nothing* (2002).

She returned to the RSC in 1994/95 to play Mrs Wittwoud in *The Wives' Excuse* (Stafford-Clark, Swan).

Trevor Martin first worked at the RSC in 1962, playing Hippolito in *Women Beware Women* (Anthony Page) at the Arts Theatre, and Captain in *Curtmantle* (Stuart Burge), Menelaus in *Troilus and Cressida* (Peter Hall), and Richelieu in *The Devils* (Peter Wood) at the Aldwych. From 1963 to 66 he was a member of the National Theatre company at the Old Vic (Rodas in *The Royal Hunt of the Sun*). From 1969 to 1980 he appeared regularly with Prospect, on tour and at the Old Vic (Lancaster in the Ian McKellen *Edward II*, Kent in the Timothy West *King Lear*).

In 1984 he joined the RSC's small-scale touring troupe to play Corey in *The Crucible* (Barry Kyle) and Old Shepherd in *The Winter's Tale* (Adrian Noble). He has since become a mainstay of the Company: Host of the Garter in *The Merry Wives of Windsor* (Bill Alexander, RST, 1985); Harry Caine in *The Dillen* (Kyle, TOP, 1985); Jack Timms in *Mary, After the Queen* (Kyle, The Warehouse, Stratford, 1985); Duke of Venice in *Othello* (Terry Hands, RST, 1985); Dr Neuwirth in Vaclav Havel's *Temptation* (Roger Michell, TOP, 1987); Samuel in Heidi Thomas's *Indigo* (Sarah Pia Anderson, TOP, 1987); Gremio in *The Taming of the Shrew* (Jonathan Miller, RST, 1987); Trundle in Ben Jonson's *The New Inn* (John Caird, Swan, 1987); Caius Lucius, succeeding Geoffrey Freshwater, in *Cymbeline* (Alexander, Pit, 1988); Tiresias in *Oedipus* (Donald Sumpter, Almeida, 1988); Antonio in *Much Ado About Nothing* (Alexander, RST, 1990); Mr Scott in Richard Nelson's *Two Shakespearean Actors* (Michell, Swan, 1990); Shamrayev in *The Seagull* (Hands, Swan, 1990); Baptista in *The Taming of the Shrew* (Alexander, RST, 1992); Eumaeus in Derek Walcott's *The Odyssey* (Gregory Doran, TOP, 1992); Soldan of Egypt in *Tamburlaine the Great* (Hands, Swan, 1992); Bennett in Tom Stoppard's *Travesties* (Noble, Barbican, 1993); Duncan, succeeding Joseph O'Conor, in the Antony Sher *Macbeth* (Doran, Swan, 1999-00); Duke of Austria/Peter of Pomfret in *King John* (Doran, Swan, 2001); Jago in Peter Barnes's *Jubilee* (Doran, Swan, 2001); Soothsayer in *Antony and Cleopatra* (Michael Attenborough, RST, 2002); and Antonio in *Much Ado About Nothing* (Doran, RST, 2002).

Other theatre: James in *Long Day's Journey into Night* (Arts, 1984); Martin in *The Royal Hunt of the Sun* (Tim Pigott-Smith, Compass, Tour, 1989); Mr Zaretsky in Herb Gardner's *Conversations with My Father* (Alan Ayckbourn, Scarborough, 1994); and Paul in Simon Bent's *Goldhawk Road* (Paul Miller, Bush, 1996).

Brewster Mason (1922-1987, b. Kidsgrove). By any measure Brewster Mason was an intimidating figure. (During a performance of the 1967 *Coriolanus* he lifted Helen Mirren off the ground by the neck for corpsing—see the BBC programme *Ruby Wax Meets Helen Mirren*, 1996.) One of the last of the old-style Shakespearean actors, he had the presence and vocal-power to make even the grandest of theatres seem intimate.

The war claimed his youth—he served in the Royal Navy (promoted from petty officer to lieutenant, he landed troops in north Africa and Italy)—so when he resumed his long interrupted course at RADA he was far more experienced in life than his peers. He made his debut in 1948 at the Lyric Hammersmith and came to notice playing Polixenes to John Gielgud's Leontes in Peter Brook's 1951 production of *The Winter's Tale* at the Phoenix. Gielgud became an important early influence, directing Mason in the West End—Borachio in *Much Ado About Nothing* (Phoenix, 1952), Sir Wilful Witwoud in *The Way of the World* (Lyric, 1953); and at Stratford—Northumberland in the Paul Scofield/Eric Porter *Richard II* (1952).

A senior player at the RSC from 1963 to 76, Mason gave richly detailed if classically orthodox performances in all genres—Kent in the Peter Brook/Paul Scofield *King Lear* (Aldwych, 1963); Warwick in *The Wars of the Roses* (Peter Hall, RST, 1963);

Goldberg—a rare contemporary role—in Harold Pinter's *The Birthday Party* (Aldwych, 1964); Boyet in *Love's Labour's Lost* (John Barton, RST, 1965); Alcibiades in *Timon of Athens* (John Schlesinger, RST, 1965); Claudius in the David Warner *Hamlet* (Hall, 1965); Sir Toby Belch in *Twelfth Night* (Clifford Williams, RST, 1966); Lafeu in *All's Well That Ends Well* (Barton, RST, 1967); the title role in *Julius Caesar* (Barton, RST, 1968); Sir Tunbelly Clumsey in *The Relapse* (Trevor Nunn, Aldwych, 1968); Wolsey in *Henry VIII* (Nunn, RST, 1969); Andrew Undershaft in *Major Barbara* (Williams, Aldwych, 1970); the title role in *Othello* (Barton, RST, 1971); and Falstaff to Alan Howard's Hal in *Henry IV* and *The Merry Wives of Windsor* (Terry Hands, 1975).

For ten years he worked outside of the RSC, partly in America (where he was a guest lecturer at the University of California, Irvine) but most notably at the National in *Major Barbara* (Peter Gill, Lyttelton, 1982), Giraudoux's *The Trojan War Will Not Take Place* (Harold Pinter, Lyttelton, 1983), Kaufman and Hart's *You Can't Take It With You* (Michael Bogdanov, Lyttelton, 1983), *Venice Preserv'd* (Peter Gill, Lyttelton, 1984) and Chekhov's *Wild Honey* (Christopher Morahan, Lyttelton, 1984). He returned to the RSC in 1986 to play John of Gaunt in the Jeremy Irons *Richard II* (Barry Kyle, RST). He died soon after the final London performance of *Richard II* in August 1987.

Daniel Massey (1933-1998, b. London) was born into the high society of the British theatre during the era of Noël Coward (his godfather). But beneath the surface of his stylish acting—he was the Scarlet Pimpernel of the English stage—one sensed an undertone of gravitas, even melancholy.

The son of distinguished actors (Raymond Massey and Adrianne Allen), Massey's career was set in motion by Coward, who cast his nine-year old godson as Bobby Kinross in *In Which We Serve* (1942). Following his education at Eton and King's College, Cambridge, Massey glided—by way of the Footlights (1956) and Agatha Christie's *Peril at End House* (Connaught

Theatre, Worthing, 1956)—into West End comedies and musicals. It was to be his milieu for the next twenty years: *The Happiest Millionaire* (1957); *Living for Pleasure* (Garrick, 1958); the Monty Norman musical *Make Me an Offer* (Stratford East, 1959); Charles Surface in John Gielgud's *The School for Scandal* (Haymarket, 1962); *The Three Musketeers* (Nottingham Playhouse, 1962); the Jerry Bock musical *She Loves Me* (New York, 1963); *Julius Caesar* (Royal Court, 1964); the tutor in Michael Redgrave's *A Month in the Country* (Yvonne Arnaud Theatre, Guildford, 1965); *Barefoot in the Park* (Piccadilly, 1965); Jack Absolute in *The Rivals* and John Worthing in *The Importance of Being Earnest* (Haymarket, 1966-67); *Abelard and Heloise* (Wyndham's, 1970); *Becket* (Yvonne Arnaud Theatre, Guildford, 1972); the musical *Popkiss* (Globe, 1972); Gaston in *Gigi* (New York, 1973); Lytton Strachey in Peter Luke's *Bloomsbury* (Phoenix, 1974); and *The Gay Lord Quex* (Albery, 1975). On the screen, he played Graham in John Osborne's *The Entertainer* (Tony Richardson, 1960), and starred alongside Robert Stephens in Michael Powell's *The Queen's Guards* (1961) and opposite Maggie Smith in *Go to Blazes* (1962). It is apposite that he enjoyed his biggest success portraying Noël Coward in *Star!* (Robert Wise, 1968).

Massey's priorities changed in the mid-1970s. He began a period of compelling classical and modern work that would take him from Shakespeare to Poliakoff by way of Calderón, Molière, Shaw, Granville-Barker, Horváth and Pinter. During four outstanding years at the National he seemed to be pursuing an actress (his wife Penelope Wilton) and a theme (the battle of the sexes): Don Juan in Horváth's *Don Juan Comes Back from the War* (Stewart Trotter, Cottesloe, 1978); Macduff in *Macbeth* (Peter Hall, Olivier, 1978); Shaw's *The Philanderer* (Christopher Morahan, Lyttelton, 1978); Robert alongside Michael Gambon and Penelope Wilton in Pinter's *Betrayal* (Hall, Lyttelton, 1978); John Tanner opposite Wilton in Shaw's *Man and Superman* (Morahan, Olivier, 1981); the Captain in Calderón's *The Mayor of Zalamea* (Michael Bogdanov, Cottesloe, 1981); Benedict opposite Wilton in *Much Ado About Nothing* (Peter Gill, Olivier, 1981); and Argan in *The Hypochondriac* (Bogdanov, Olivier, 1981). Then, at the RSC, 1983-85, he was Joe in William Saroyan's *The Time of Your Life* (Howard Davies, TOP); Aguecheek in *Twelfth Night* (John Caird, RST); an enigmatic and charismatic Duke, seducing Juliet Stevenson's Isabella by stealth, in *Measure for Measure* (Adrian Noble, RST); Nikolai Pesiakoff in Stephen Poliakoff's *Breaking the Silence* (Pit); and Henry Trebell in Granville-Barker's *Waste* (John Barton, Pit).

Massey's mellifluous voice was far less important than his Shavian wit and originality. He did return to the musical theatre to star in Sondheim's *Follies* (Shaftesbury Theatre, 1987), but serious drama remained at the centre of his work: Torvald in *A Doll's House* (Nick Dear, Haymarket, Leicester, 1989); Hector in Shaw's *Heartbreak House* (Trevor Nunn, Theatre Royal Haymarket, 1992); Don Armado—the last in his collection of semi-crazed fantasists—in the RSC's *Love's Labour's Lost* (Ian Judge, RST, 1993); General Burgoyne in Shaw's *The Devil's Disciple* (Morahan, NT Olivier, 1994); and Furtwangler in Ronald Harwood's *Taking Sides* (Harold Pinter, Minerva, Chichester, 1996).

Forbes Masson (b. Falkirk, 1963). At the Royal Scottish Academy of Music and Drama in the 1980s Forbes Masson teamed up with fellow student Alan Cumming to write and perform a cabaret double-act called *Victor and Barry* (they would later collaborate on the camp BBC situation comedy *The High Life*). Michael Boyd saw *Victor and Barry* and booked the show for the Tron Theatre in Glasgow. While Cumming went on to become an improbable star in America, Masson took routine TV work, trod the boards in Scotland and wrote comedy musicals (including *Mince* at the Dundee Rep, 2001). His re-working of pantomimes at the Tron have brightened Glasgow winters since 2001 (*Aladdie* in 2004 is probably the highlight).

Boyd brought Masson to the RSC in 2004. He has played three clowns (filtering the Elizabethan mayhem through his sharply sarcastic Scottish comedy style, post-modern irreverence and fine singing)—the Porter in *Macbeth* (Dominic Cooke, RST, 2004), Feste in *Twelfth Night* (Boyd, RST, 2005) and Dromio of Ephesus in *The Comedy of Errors* (Nancy Meckler, RST, 2005)—but also Horatio to Toby Stephens's Hamlet (Boyd, RST, 2004), Seneca in *The Pilate Workshop* (Boyd, TOP, 2004), and supporting roles in Boyd's complete Histories project (Courtyard, 2006-08)—Alençon, Edward and Holland in *Henry VI*, Bagot and Lord Marshal in *Richard II*, and Rumour in *Henry IV*. The multi-talented Forbes will surely be creating an RSC Christmas show before too long.

Joe Melia (b. London). An unconventional performer, Joe Melia worked regularly at the RSC between 1974 and 1990. In particular, he played Shakespeare's clowns with the cockney style of classic English screen comedy: Attendant in Philip Magdalany's *Section Nine* (Charles Marowitz, Aldwych, 1974); Father Froylan in Peter Barnes's *The Bewitched* (Terry Hands, Aldwych, 1974); Bill alongside Roy Kinnear in Victor Lanoux's *Can Opener* (Rory Dempster, The Place, 1974); Sergeant Fielding in *Too True to Be Good* (Clifford Williams, Aldwych, 1975); John Dory in *Wild Oats* (Williams, Aldwych, 1976); Corporal Len Bonny in *Privates on Parade* (Michael Blakemore, Aldwych, 1977); Touchstone in *As You Like It* (Hands, RST, 1980); Second Murderer in *Richard III* (Hands, RST, 1980); Rodney Gmawdrot in *The Swan Down Gloves* (Hands, RST, 1981); Thersites in *Troilus and Cressida* (Hands, Aldwych, 1981); Maurice in C.P. Taylor's *Good* (Howard Davies, Warehouse, 1981); Isaac Levine in *Flight* (Davies, TOP, 1986); the trickster Autolycus, a part which could have been written for him, in *The Winter's Tale* (Hands, RST, 1986); Sir Robert Walpole in *The Art of Success* (Adrian Noble, TOP, 1986); Mayor/Mullisheg in *The Fair Maid of the West* (Trevor Nunn, Swan, 1986); Chief of Police in *The Balcony* (Hands, Barbican, 1987); Alderman Smuggler in *The Constant Couple* (Roger Michell, Swan, 1988); Old Bellair in *The Man of Mode* (Gary Hynes, Swan, 1988); Parson in *Restoration* (Michell,

Swan, 1988); an American in Richard Nelson's *Some Americans Abroad* (Michell, Pit, 1989); Chorus in Peter Flannery's *Singer* (Hands, Swan, 1989); and Junius Brutus in *Coriolanus* (Hands/John Barton, RST, 1989).

Sam Mendes (b. Reading, 1965). Sam Mendes's grandfather was the Portuguese-born Trinidadian novelist Alfred H. Mendes, a key figure in the cultural and political opposition to British rule in the Caribbean before the war. His father taught English at Reading University; his mother writes children's stories.

Adrian Noble's RSC production of *Antony and Cleopatra* with Helen Mirren (1982) was an important early influence. Mendes started to direct plays at Cambridge. His professional breakthrough came when he was elevated from an assistant at Chichester to run the new studio space there, the Minerva Theatre (1989). He directed *Heartlands*, *Summerfolk* and *Love's Labour's Lost*, and was rewarded with an opportunity in the main house—Boucicault's *London Assurance*—when an established director withdrew. *London Assurance*, starring Paul Eddington, transferred to the Theatre Royal Haymarket. He next directed Judi Dench in *The Cherry Orchard* at the Aldwych.

Terry Hands brought Mendes into the RSC in 1990. He began in the Swan with *Troilus and Cressida*, a production of extraordinary theatrical lucidity, brilliantly cast. Biting, darkly comic productions of *The Alchemist* (Swan, 1991) and *Richard III* (TOP, 1992), starring Simon Russell Beale, followed. *The Tempest* (RST, 1993) was a first-rate main house production.

From 1992 to 2002 he was director of the Donmar Warehouse in Covent Garden. He persuaded the leaseholders to let him run the theatre as a producing house, and Equity to let him employ actors at provincial rates. His choices at the Donmar revealed a fondness for Stephen Sondheim (*Assassins*, 1992; *Company*, 1996) and were almost all Anglo-American: *Glengarry Glen Ross* (1994); *The Glass Menagerie* (1995); *Habeas Corpus* (1996); *The*

Front Page (1997); *The Fix* (1997); *To the Green Fields Beyond* (2000); *Uncle Vanya* (2002); and *Twelfth Night* (2002). The programming looked conservative when compared to that of the Almeida.

Other productions: *Kean* (Old Vic, also Toronto, 1990) with Derek Jacobi; *The Plough and the Stars* (Young Vic, 1991); *Oliver!* (London Palladium, 1994); and, at the National, Edward Bond's *The Sea* (Lyttelton, 1991); *The Rise and Fall of Little Voice* (Cottesloe, 1992) with Jane Horrocks; *The Birthday Party* (Lyttelton, 1994); and a fine *Othello* (Cottesloe, 1997) with Simon Russell Beale. In 1998 he directed Natasha Richardson in *Cabaret* on Broadway and Nicole Kidman and Iain Glen in *The Blue Room* at the Donmar. Soon after he shot *American Beauty* for Steven Spielberg's studio in Hollywood. The screenplay was risible but Mendes made an acclaimed film (and won five Oscars).

Mendes's direction of plays is almost faultless in its good taste, flair and sensitivity to the source material. However, as the critics' darling, some of his work has been overrated. The Mendes phenomenon is better explained by his self-confidence and personal charisma (in the wake of *American Beauty* Spielberg poured hundreds of thousands of dollars into the Donmar). One sees American traits and an American outlook, not only in his decision to make Hollywood rather than British films, but also in all those Sondheim and other American musicals at the Donmar.

The revelation of *American Beauty* was Mendes's command of the visual medium. *Road to Perdition* (2002) was even more striking, a succession of thematically linked images. The climatic scene in a beach house filled with white light, using reflections to give two points of view and achieving the ghostly effect of a developing photograph, shows the extent to which Mendes combines a gift for image making with skills learnt in the theatre: so often his frames are composed to suggest depth, giving a 3-D illusion of space.

Roger Michell (b. South Africa, 1956). The son of a diplomat, Roger Michell was born in South Africa and brought up in Damascus, Beirut and Prague. While at Queen's College, Cambridge, he received the RSC's Buzz Goodbody Award for his production of Edward Bond's *Bingo* (National Student Drama Festival, 1977). After Cambridge he worked at the Royal Court, assisting Samuel Beckett and John Osborne and directing Mike McGrath's *The Key Tag* and Nick Darke's *The Catch* in the Theatre Upstairs.

In the early 1980s his productions included David Mamet's *Sexual Perversity in Chicago* at the Hampstead Theatre and *Romeo and Juliet* at the Young Vic. He also co-wrote (with Richard Maher) and directed *The White Glove* and *Private Dick* at the Lyric Hammersmith.

He joined the RSC in 1985 as an assistant director. He worked on Bill Alexander's *The Merry Wives of Windsor* (RST), Terry Hands's *Othello* (RST) and Adrian Noble's *Mephisto* (Barbican). He was promoted to the directorial team and over the next four years staged small-scale productions of *The Taming of the Shrew*, *Hamlet* and *The Constant Couple*. Of more significance were his productions of new plays by Václav Havel, Nick Darke and Richard Nelson.

A freelance director since 1991, Michell has directed *Under Milk Wood* (NT Olivier, 1995); Martin Sherman's *Some Sunny Day* (Hampstead Theatre, 1996); Harold Pinter's *The Homecoming* (NT Lyttelton, 1997); Joe Penhall's *Blue/Orange* (NT Cottesloe, 2000); and Joanna Murray-Smith's *Honour* (NT Cottesloe, 2003). His first screen piece, Hanif Kureishi's *The Buddha of Suburbia* (BBC, 1993), was as accomplished as his stage work. He has since directed Nick Dear's adaptation of *Persuasion* (BBC, 1995); *Titanic Town* (1998); *My Night With Reg* (BBC, 1998); Richard Curtis's *Notting Hill* (1999); *Changing Lanes* (2002); Kureishi's *The Mother* (2003); and *Enduring Love* (2004).

Poppy Miller (b. Norwich) was educated at Cambridge University and the Webber Douglas Academy. She came to notice playing Hermione in Laurence Boswell's Euripides trilogy *Agamemnon's Children* at the Gate (1995), and Mary in *Mansfield Park* at Chichester (Michael Rudman, 1996). At the RSC, 1997-99, she was Win-the-Fight Littlewit in Ben Jonson's *Bartholomew Fair* (Laurence Boswell, Swan) and Silvia in *The Two Gentlemen of Verona* (Edward Hall, Swan).

Since leaving the RSC she has played Dona Elvira in Molière's *Don Juan* (Stephen Unwin, English Touring Theatre, 1999); Amy in *Amy's View* (Natalie Wilson, Salisbury Playhouse, 2003); Hope in Adrian Osmond's *Switchback* (Tron, Glasgow, 2004); Ophelia in *Hamlet* (Rupert Goold, Royal and Derngate Theatre, Northampton, 2005); Mrs Fainall in William Congreve's *The Way of the World* (Selina Cadell, Royal and Derngate Theatre, Northampton, 2007); and a beguiling Viola in *Twelfth Night* (Sean Holmes, Filter, 2007). She co-starred in the BBC's *Attachments* (2000-02), *Red Cap* (2004), *Derailed* (2005) and *New Tricks* (2006).

Joseph Millson (b. Berkshire, 1974). For an actor of obvious star-quality, Joseph Millson was a slow starter, treading water in the popular television soap *Peak Practice* and appearing on the fringe and in touring productions—Matt in Harvey Schmidt and Tom Jones's musical *The Fantasticks* (Dan Crawford, King's Head, 1996); Dickie Greenleaf in Phyllis Nagy's adaptation of *The Talented Mr Ripley* (Giles Croft, Watford, 1998); opposite his wife Caroline Fitzgerald in Craig Baxter's two-hander *Monogamy* (Stuart Mullins, Pursued by a Bear, Grace Theatre, 1999); Richard in Kate Miller's *Shipton Blank* (Amanda Hill, Riverside Studios, 2000); Stephen in George Eliot's *Mill on the Floss* (Polly Teale/Nancy Meckler, Shared Experience, 2001); Morville in Paul Webb's *Four Nights in Knaresborough* (Paul Miller, Tour, 2001); and Robert in Helen Edmundson's *The Clearing* (Teale, Shared Experience, 2002).

Things started to change in 2003/04. He followed a fine Orlando in Peter Hall's *As You Like It* at Bath with a successful move to the RSC: the Spanish Golden Age season (Swan, 2004)—Teodoro in *The Dog in the Manger* (Laurence Boswell) and Don Carlos in *House of Desires* (Nancy Meckler), crowd-pleasing examples of bravura comedy; and the Complete Works festival (Swan, 2006)—Benedick in *Much Ado About Nothing* (Marianne Elliott), and The Bastard in *King John* (Josie Rourke).

Helen Mirren (b. London, 1945) was born into a humble London family, but her father's lineage was Russian and aristocratic. Her grandfather was in London securing arms for the tsar when the Revolution struck. In exile with a young family, he struggled to earn a living, finally becoming a taxi driver. Her father married an English girl called Kitty Rogers and, ironically, became a Communist in the 1930s. He was an atheist but he sent his daughter to a convent school. The daughter, perhaps in rebellion against an upbringing that was rather puritanical, knew from an early age that she wanted to be an actress. To appease her parents she went to a teacher training college in Hampstead, but she followed her ambition with the National Youth Theatre and made a great impression, aged eighteen, as Cleopatra in *Antony and Cleopatra* (Old Vic, 1965).

She joined the RSC in 1967, making her debut as a citizen in *Coriolanus* (John Barton, RST). The tabloids, responding to her nude scenes in Michael Powell's *Age of Consent* (1969) and Ken Russell's *Savage Messiah* (1971), quickly labelled her 'Sex Queen of the RSC', but even in her twenties she refused to be predictable. For more than a decade she concentrated on classical roles at Stratford, bringing sensuality, vitality and vulnerability to Castiza in *The Revenger's Tragedy* (Trevor Nunn, RST, 1967); Diana in *All's Well That Ends Well* (John Barton, RST, 1967); Phebe in *As You Like It* (David Jones, RST, 1968); Cressida in *Troilus and Cressida* (John Barton, RST, 1968); Hero in *Much Ado About Nothing* (Nunn, RST, 1968); Win-the-Fight Littlewit in *Bar-*

tholomew Fair (Terry Hands, Aldwych, 1969); Susie Monican in O'Casey's *The Silver Tassie* (Jones, Aldwych, 1969); Ophelia to Alan Howard's prince in Trevor Nunn's production of *Hamlet* (RST, 1970); Lady Anne in *Richard III* (Terry Hands, RST, 1970); Julia in *The Two Gentlemen of Verona* (Robin Phillips, RST, 1970); Tatyana in Gorky's *Enemies* (Jones, Aldwych, 1971); Harriet in Etherege's *The Man of Mode* (Hands, Aldwych, 1971); a stunning Miss Julie (Phillips, The Place, 1971); Elyane in *The Balcony* (Hands, Aldwych, 1971); a predatory Lady Macbeth to Nicol Williamson's *Macbeth* (Nunn, RST, 1974); Queen Margaret in the three parts of *Henry VI* (Hands, RST, 1977); a mercurial Cleopatra opposite Michael Gambon in *Antony and Cleopatra* (Noble, TOP, 1982); and Moll Cutpurse in Middleton and Dekker's *The Roaring Girl* (Barry Kyle, Barbican, 1983).

Between RSC seasons, Mirren travelled to North Africa with Peter Brook's Centre Internationale de Recherches Théâtrales (1972); played the alcoholic rock singer in David Hare's *Teeth 'n' Smiles* (Royal Court, 1975); a remarkable, highly-sexed Nina in *The Seagull* and Ella in Ben Travers's *The Bed Before Yesterday* (both Lindsay Anderson, Lyric Theatre Company, 1975); Isabella in *Measure for Measure* (Peter Gill, Riverside Studios, 1979); Grace in Brian Friel's *Faith Healer* (Christopher Fettes, Royal Court, 1981); and the title role in *The Duchess of Malfi* (Adrian Noble, Royal Exchange, Manchester, 1980). She also appeared in films of varying quality: Hermia in an RSC movie of *A Midsummer Night's Dream* (Peter Hall, 1968); almost playing herself in Lindsay Anderson's dark fable *O Lucky Man!* (1973); Gertrude and Ophelia in *Hamlet* (Celestino Corondao, 1976); Pinter's *The Collection* (Michael Apted, 1976); the European soft-porn of *Caligula* (Tinto Brass, 1979); one of the children in Dennis Potter's *Blue Remembered Hills* (BBC, 1979); Bob Hopkins's mistress in *The Long Good Friday* (1979); *The Fiendish Plot of Dr Fu Manchu* (Piers Haggard, 1980); and Morgana in John Boorman's *Excalibur* (1981).

Since the mid-1980s films have dominated: *Cal* (Pat O'Connor, 1984); *The Mosquito Coast* (Peter Weir, 1986)—as Harrison Ford's wife, River Phoenix's mother; Peter Greenaway's *The Cook, the Thief, His Wife and Her Lover* (1989)—betraying her RSC Antony with her RSC Hamlet; *The Madness of King George* (Nicholas Hytner, 1994); *The Pledge* (Sean Penn, 2001); *Gosford Park* (Robert Altman, 2001); *Calendar Girls* (2003); and *The Queen* (Stephen Frears, 2006). In the *Prime Suspect* dramas (ITV, 1991-96, 2003, 2006) she brought to the role of a senior police detective an emotional and professional realism that went way beyond the expectations of the genre.

She has continued to work on the stage: the prostitute opposite Bob Peck's detective in Arthur Miller's *Two-Way Mirror* (David Thacker, Young Vic, 1989); Natalya in *A Month in the Country* (Bill Bryden, Albery, 1994); her third Cleopatra (Sean Mathias, NT Olivier, 1998); Alice opposite Ian McKellen in August Strindberg's *Dance of Death* (Mathias, New York, 2001); and Christine Mannon in Eugene O'Neill's *Mourning Becomes Electra* (Howard Davies, NT Lyttelton, 2003-04).

Richard Moore (b. Burnley) worked as a photographer for a local paper in his native Lancashire before winning a place at the Bristol Old Vic Theatre School (1961). His early opportunities included a leading role in Troy Kennedy Martin and John McGrath's six-part BBC series *Diary of a Young Man*, directed by Ken Loach (1964).

A fine character actor, particularly of Shakespearean comedy, Moore has been a member of the RSC since 1965, when he played minor roles in Brecht's *Puntila* (Michel Saint-Denis) and Robert Bolt's *The Thwarting of Baron Bolligrew* (Trevor Nunn) at the Aldwych. The following year, in Stratford, he was cast as Guildenstern in the David Warner *Hamlet* (Peter Hall) and Pistol in *Henry IV Part 2* and *Henry V* (John Barton). Moore's Pistol cast a long shadow. Nine years later he returned to the part for Terry Hands (the *Henries* and *The Merry Wives of Windsor*). In-between, he was Peter in the Ian Holm/Estelle Kohler *Romeo and Juliet* (Karolos Koun, RST, 1967); the Narrator in *Under Milk Wood*

(Hands, Theatregoround, 1968); Corin in *As You Like It* (David Jones, RST, 1968); Wagner in *Doctor Faustus* (Clifford Williams, RST, 1968); Ajax in the Michael Williams/Helen Mirren *Troilus and Cressida* (John Barton, RST, 1968); Estragon in *Waiting for Godot* (Gareth Morgan, Theatregoround, 1968); Harry in Sean O'Casey's *The Silver Tassie* (David Jones, Aldwych, 1969); Jordan Knockem in *Bartholomew Fair* (Hands, Aldwych, 1969); and Starveling in Peter Brook's *A Midsummer Night's Dream* (International Tour, 1972).

Long intervals have separated Moore's subsequent appearances with the Company: Capulet in the Sean Bean/Niamh Cusack *Romeo and Juliet* (Michael Bogdanov, RST, 1986); Doctor in *The Two Noble Kinsmen* (Barry Kyle, Swan, 1986); Mowbray in the Jeremy Irons *Richard II* (Kyle, RST, 1986); Bishop in *The Balcony* (Hands, Barbican, 1987); Captain Dan in *The Great White Hope* (Nicholas Kent, Mermaid, 1987); Launce in *The Two Gentlemen of Verona* (David Thacker, Swan, 1991); Herdsman in *The Thebans* (Adrian Noble, Swan, 1991); First Gravedigger in the Kenneth Branagh *Hamlet* (Noble, Barbican, 1992); and, for the Complete Works festival, Simonides in *Pericles* and the Old Shepherd in *The Winter's Tale* (Dominic Cooke, Swan, 2006-07).

Elsewhere, he has continued his collaboration with Terry Hands: Page in *The Merry Wives of Windsor* (NT Olivier, 1995); the schoolmaster in Friedrich Dürrenmatt's *The Visit* (Chichester, 1995); Gloucester in *King Lear* (Clwyd Theatr Cymru, 2001); and the Player in *Rosencrantz and Guildenstern Are Dead* (Clwyd Theatr Cymru, 2002).

Hattie Morahan (b. London, 1979) made an impressive debut at the age of seventeen in *The Peacock Spring*, a two-part BBC film set in post-colonial India (1996). Directed by her father, Christopher Morahan, she played the leading role, a diplomat's daughter who elopes with an Indian gardener (Naveen Andrews).

While an undergraduate at Cambridge, reading English, she made her name as one of the best university actresses. At the RSC, 2001-02, her first professional work in the theatre, she played Gentlewoman/Player in the Samuel West *Hamlet* (Steven Pimlott, RST); Lucy in William Wycherley's *Love in a Wood* (Tim Supple, Swan); Emela in David Edgar's *The Prisoner's Dilemma* (Michael Attenborough, TOP); and the hotel receptionist in David Farr's *Night of the Soul* (Farr, Pit). She presented a delectable paradox as Wycherley's Lucy, outwardly demure but sold willingly to an old miser (masquerading as a music teacher) by her mother and a bawd. Her suggestive delivery of the line 'I don't see your fiddle, sir, where is your little kit?' was a highlight of the show.

On leaving the RSC she was cast as Elaine in *Arsenic and Old Lace* (Matthew Francis, Strand, 2003); Louise de Vallière in Nick Dear's *Power* (Lindsay Posner, NT Cottesloe, 2003); and Ruby in Peter Flannery's *Singer* (Sean Holmes, Oxford Stage Company, Tricycle, 2004). She joined the front rank of young actresses playing the title role in Katie Mitchell's production of *Iphigenia at Aulis* (NT Lyttelton, 2004). She has since played Viola in *Twelfth Night* (Ian Brown, West Yorkshire Playhouse, 2005); Penelope in Philip King's *See How They Run* (Douglas Hodge, UK Tour, 2006); and, for Mitchell, Nina in *The Seagull* (NT Lyttelton, 2006), Clair in Martin Crimp's *The City* (Royal Court, 2008) and the woman in *...Some Trace of Her* (NT Cottesloe, 2008). Hattie Morahan's work on screen has included the BBC productions *Bodies* (2005) and *Sense and Sensibility* (2008); and the films *The Golden Compass* (2007) and *The Bank Job* (2008).

Christopher Morley (b. Newcastle) studied painting under Carl Cheek and began his career in the regional theatre of the late 1950s. He was based at the Belgrade Theatre, Coventry, from 1960 to 1963, and at the New Phoenix Theatre, Leicester, from 1964 to 1965. At the Royal Court in 1966 he designed William Gaskill's productions of Arnold Wesker's *Their Very Own and Golden City* and *Macbeth*.

Later that year he went to the RSC to resume a partnership with Trevor Nunn that had been formed at the Belgrade Theatre. Their overtly theatrical production of *The Revenger's Tragedy* challenged the prevailing RSC house style and established Nunn as a major new talent. When Nunn succeeded Peter Hall as artistic director Morley succeeded John Bury as Head of Design. He was responsible for the 1969 white box stage configuration and his spare, often monochrome, settings were highly influential. As well as collaborating with Nunn on *The Taming of the Shrew* (RST, 1967), *The Relapse* (Aldwych, 1967), *King Lear* (RST, 1968), *Much Ado About Nothing* (RST, 1968), *The Winter's Tale* (RST, 1969), *Hamlet* (RST, 1970) and 'The Romans' (RST, 1972), he designed John Barton's stylish *Twelfth Night* (RST, 1969) and Buzz Goodbody's *As You Like It* (RST, 1973). He stepped down as Head of Design in 1974 but remained an associate artist, designing Barton's studio productions of *The Merchant of Venice* (1978), *Life's a Dream* (1983), *The Devils* (1984), *Waste* (1985) and *Dreamplay* (1985); Barry Kyle's *Measure for Measure* (RST, 1978), *The White Guard* (Aldwych, 1979) and *Julius Caesar* (RST, 1979); David Jones's *Cymbeline* (RST, 1979); and Terry Hands's *Coriolanus* (RST, 1989).

Cherry Morris (b. London). A member of the RSC in the early years, 1961-63, Cherry Morris played Lady Capulet in *Romeo and Juliet* (Peter Hall, RST); Jura/Aniko in *The Caucasian Chalk Circle* (William Gaskill, Aldwych); Refugee in *Curtmantle* (Stuart Burge, Aldwych); Andromache in *Troilus and Cressida* (Hall, Aldwych); Sister Claire in *The Devils* (Peter Wood, Aldwych); Ceres in *The Tempest* (Clifford Williams, RST); Portia in *Julius Caesar* (John Blatchley, RST); and Eleanor, Duchess of Gloucester/Lady Bona in *The Wars of the Roses* (Hall, RST).

Remarkably, the character of Eleanor took her back to the RSC twenty-five years later—Adrian Noble's *The Plantagenets*

(RST, 1988). Now the right age for the senior character parts, she saw out the millennium with the RSC, working as hard as any young girl in the Company. As well as playing Queen Margaret in successive productions of *Richard III* (Sam Mendes, TOP, 1992; Steven Pimlott, RST, 1995), she was Queen Elinor in *King John* (Deborah Warner, TOP, 1988); Harriet Stanley in *The Man Who Came to Dinner* (Gene Saks, Barbican, 1989); Autie Rezi in Julius Hay's *Have* (Janice Honeyman, Pit, 1990); Aemilia in *The Comedy of Errors* (Ian Judge, RST, 1990); Polina in *The Seagull* (Terry Hands, Swan, 1990); Caroline Pontefract in *A Woman of No Importance* (Philip Prowse, Barbican, 1991); Chorus in *Murder in the Cathedral* (Pimlott, Swan, 1993); Old Lady Squeamish in *The Country Wife* (Max Stafford-Clark Swan, 1993); Madame Sylvie in Maureen Hunter's *Transit of Venus* (Alison Sutcliffe, TOP, 1993); Mrs Fezziwig in *A Christmas Carol* (Judge, Barbican, 1994); Boyette in *Love's Labour's Lost* (Judge, Barbican, 1995); Duchess of Vaubricourt in Eric Emmanuel Schmitt's *La nuit de Valognes* (Paul Garrington, TOP, 1996); Old Lady in *Henry VIII* (Gregory Doran, Swan 1996); Mistress Quickly in *The Merry Wives of Windsor* (Judge, RST, 1996); Lady Mulligan in *Camino Real* (Pimlott, Swan, 1997); Mariya in *Uncle Vanya* (Katie Mitchell, Young Vic, 1998); Agave in *Tales from Ovid* (Tim Supple, Swan, 1999); Ivy in *The Family Reunion* (Noble, Swan, 1999); and Old Edie in *A Warwickshire Testimony* (Alison Sutcliffe, TOP, 1999).

David Morrissey (b. Liverpool, 1964) started out in the youth company of the Liverpool Everyman. He left school at sixteen and won the lead role in Willy Russell's *One Summer* (Channel Four). After his training at RADA he toured with Cheek By Jowl as Sebastian in *Twelfth Night* (Declan Donnellan, 1986), and appeared at the Manchester Royal Exchange as Valentine White in *The Cabinet Minister* (Braham Murray, 1987). He was a member of the RSC for one two-year cycle (1988-89)—Philip the Bastard in *King John* (Deborah Warner, TOP), and Vernon/Duke of Clarence in *The Plantagenets* (Adrian Noble, RST). He next played the title role in *Peer Gynt* at the National (Donnellan, Olivier, 1990).

A leading actor ever since, Morrissey has worked most prominently in front of the camera, starring in such diverse works as *Framed* (ITV, 1993); *Being Human* (Bill Forsyth, 1993); Tony Marchant's *Holding On* (BBC, 1997); *Our Mutual Friend* (BBC, 1998); *Pure Wickedness* (BBC, 1999); *Born Romantic* (David Kane, 2000); Paul Abbott's *State of Play* (BBC, 2003); *The Deal* (Stephen Frears, Channel Four, 2003); *Blackpool* (BBC, 2004); and *Cape Wrath* (Channel Four, 2007). In 1999 he made a rare return to the stage to play Pip and Theo in Richard Greenberg's *Three Days of Rain* (Robin Lefevre, Donmar Warehouse).

Vicki Mortimer studied at the Slade School of Fine Art. Her long association with Katie Mitchell has produced a body of stylish and innovative work, at the RSC—*A Woman Killed With Kindness* (TOP, 1991), *The Dybbuk* (Pit, 1992), *Ghosts* (TOP, 1993), *The Phoenician Women* (TOP, 1995), *The Mysteries* (TOP, 1996), *Beckett Shorts* (TOP, 1997) and *Uncle Vanya* (Young Vic, 1998); the National—*Rutherford and Son* (Cottesloe, 1994), *The Machine Wreckers* (Cottesloe, 1995), Ted Hughes's version of *The Oresteia* (Cottesloe, 1999), *Ivanov* (Cottesloe, 2002), *Three Sisters* (Lyttelton, 2003), *The Seagull* (Lyttelton, 2006), *Waves* (Cottesloe, 2006), Martin Crimp's *Attempts On Her Life* (Lyttelton, 2007), and *...Some Trace of Her* (Lyttelton, 2008); and the Royal Court—Crimp's *The Country* (2000) and *The City* (2008).

But Vicki Mortimer does take breaks from the claustrophobic atmosphere of a Katie Mitchell project. She designed David Leveaux's *The Real Thing* (Donmar, 1999) and *Jumpers* (NT Lyttelton, 2003); Adrian Noble's *The Seagull* (RSC Swan, 2000); Matthew Warchus's *The Winter's Tale* (RSC Roundhouse, 2002); Michael Grandage's *The Wild Duck* (Donmar, 2005); Howard Davies's *The House of Bernarda Alba* (NT Lyttelton, 2005) and *Never So Good* (NT Cottesloe, 2008); and Nicholas Hytner's *Cosi fan tutte* (Glyndebourne, 2006), *The Man Of Mode* (NT Olivier, 2007), *Much Ado About Nothing* (NT Olivier, 2007-08) and *Major Barbara* (costumes only, NT Olivier, 2008).

She creates atmospheric settings with an elegant economy of means, and beautifully designed and tailored costumes, particularly for women.

Gerard Murphy (b. Newry, Northern Ireland, 1955) first appeared with the RSC in 1973, playing minor roles in Trevor Nunn's 'The Romans' (Aldwych) and David Rudkin's *Cries from the Casement* (Terry Hands, The Place). He came to notice at the Glasgow Citizens' in the years that followed: the title roles in *Chinchilla, Macbeth, Woyzeck* and *Coriolanus*; Mercutio in *Romeo and Juliet*; Pinchwife in *The Country Wife*; Miss Prism in *The Importance of Being Earnest*; and Ezra/Orin in *Mourning Becomes Electra*.

Revealed as a visceral performer of some originality, he rejoined the RSC in 1980 to play Johnny Boyle in *Juno and the Paycock* (Trevor Nunn, Aldwych). Then, in his first full season, 1981-82, he was cast as the Young Shepherd in *The Winter's Tale* (Ronald Eyre, RST), Frank opposite Harriet Walter and Juliet Stevenson in *The Witch of Edmonton* (Barry Kyle, TOP), and Hal in Nunn's production of the two parts of *Henry IV* (Barbican). Murphy, fair-haired and thickset, held his own against the svelte Timothy Dalton and later Hugh Quarshie (playing Hotspur). His strikingly original Hal was a rough and bitter creation.

Murphy and Quarshie were reunited for *The Two Noble Kinsmen* (Kyle, Swan, 1986), their characters' rivalry culminating (London run, Mermaid, 1987) in one of the most dangerously realistic sword fights seen on the English stage. In the 1986-87 cycle he was also Oberon in *A Midsummer Night's Dream* (Bill Alexander, RST); Sam Mowbray in *Country Dancing* (Alexander, TOP); Roger in *The Balcony* (Terry Hands, Barbican); Green Eyes and Solange in the Genet double-bill of *Deathwatch* and *The*

Maids (Pit), which he also co-directed; and Graham in Tony Marchant's *Speculators* (Kyle, Pit). He brought a Presbyterian preacher's intensity to the title role in *Doctor Faustus* (Kyle, Swan, 1989), played Petruchio in *The Taming of the Shrew* (Alexander, Small-scale Tour, 1990) without any notion of political correctness, and gave a masterly performance as Oedipus in Adrian Noble's *The Thebans* (Swan, 1991). As the blinded Oedipus, a hunched, mud-caked figure led by Joanne Pearce's Antigone, Murphy presented an unforgettable image of misery and stoicism. During the 1990 season he directed a graphic production of Marlowe's *Edward II* (Swan) featuring Simon Russell Beale.

Since 1993 he has appeared at the major regional theatres: Mosca in *Volpone* (Bill Alexander, Birmingham Rep, 1993); D'Amville in *The Atheist's Tragedy* (Anthony Clark, Rep, 1994); the title role in *Macbeth* (Glasgow Citizens', 1998); a brutish Claudius in the Richard McCabe *Hamlet* (Alexander, Rep, 1998); Mallory in Peter Barnes's *Dreaming* (Matthew Lloyd, Manchester Royal Exchange, 1999); the father in Eugene O'Neill's *A Moon for the Misbegotten* (Lloyd, Royal Exchange, 2001); George to Clare Higgins's Martha in *Who's Afraid of Virginia Woolf?* (Gareth Machin, Bristol Old Vic, 2002); Falstaff in the two parts of *Henry IV* (Bristol Old Vic, 2002); Pozzo in *Waiting for Godot* and Jack in *The Weir* (Rupert Goold, Royal Theatre, Northampton, 2003); Jack in Alan Ayckbourn's *A Small Family Business* (Ian Brown, West Yorkshire Playhouse, 2003); Eichmann in Donald Freed's *The White Crow* (Michael Vale, Mercury, Colchester, 2003); Sir David Ochterlony in *A Taste for Mangoes* (Jatinder Verma, Tara Arts, Wilton's Music Hall, 2003); the title role in *Volpone* (Greg Hersov, Royal Exchange, 2004); Samuel Byck in *Assassins* (Nikolai Foster, Sheffield Crucible, 2006); the Chorus in *Henry V* (Jonathan Munby, Royal Exchange, 2007). In 2008 he returned to the RSC to play Sergeant Browne in Leo Butler's *I'll Be the Devil* (Ramin Gray, Tricycle).

Music. Most RSC productions feature original music performed live (usually off-stage) by the Company's resident band. The RSC's music department has been run by three outstanding musicians.

Guy Woolfenden (b. 1937) was educated at Christ's College, Cambridge, and the Guildhall School of Music and Drama. He ran the RSC's music department from 1965 to 98, and composed the majority of RSC music during this period.

Stephen Warbeck (b. Southampton) read drama and French at Bristol University. One of the contemporary cinema's most accomplished composers of romantic music, he won an Oscar for *Shakespeare in Love* (1998) and has since scored *Billy Elliot* (2000), *Captain Corelli's Mandolin* (2001), *Birthday Girl* (2001), *Charlotte Gray* (2001), and *Proof* (2004). During the early part of his career, in the 1970s and 80s, he was a moderately successful actor as well as a theatre composer/music director. By the early 1990s he was in demand as a composer, scoring all of the *Prime Suspect* dramas (ITV, 1991-96) and Stephen Daldry's celebrated production of *An Inspector Calls* (NT Lyttelton, 1992). Warbeck first worked at the RSC in 1995, and ran the Company's music department from 1999 to 2003. His shows included Adrian Noble's *The Cherry Orchard* (Swan, 1995), *Cymbeline* (RST, 1997) and *The Tempest* (RST, 1998); Michael Boyd's *Romeo and Juliet* (RST, 2000); and Rachel Kavanaugh's *Alice in Wonderland* (RST, 2001).

John Woolf read music at St John's College, Cambridge, and studied the oboe at the Royal Academy of Music. He has been a member of both the City of Birmingham Symphony Orchestra and the Bournemouth Symphony Orchestra. He joined the RSC's house band in 1977; became music director, Stratford, in 1987; and Head of Music in 2003. He scored Michael Boyd's productions of *Hamlet* (2004) and the *Histories* (2007).

N

John Napier (b. 1944) studied theatre design under Ralph Koltai at the Central School of Art and Design (he had previously studied sculpture). After an impressive early career at Nottingham, Birmingham, the Royal Court and Sadler's Wells, he joined Koltai at the RSC. He was particularly prominent in 1976—he transformed, with Chris Dyer, the Royal Shakespeare Theatre (creating a platform stage with wooden galleries, the 'Wooden O'), and designed John Barton's 'Raj' *Much Ado About Nothing*, Trevor Nunn's musical *Comedy of Errors* and his studio *Macbeth*. In 1980 he worked on Barton's *The Greeks* and Nunn's *Nicholas Nickleby* (Aldwych). By this time he was specialising in mobile frame-based structures of impressive adaptability. When Nunn began the process of converting the Conference Room into the Swan Theatre it was Napier who drew up the first plans.

As one of the RSC's associate artists, John Napier also designed Barton's *King John* (RST, 1974), *Richard II* (RST, 1974) and *A Midsummer Night's Dream* (RST, 1977); Nunn's *Hedda Gabler* (Aldwych, 1975), *As You Like It* (RST, 1977), *Three Sisters* (Small-scale Tour, 1978), *The Merry Wives of Windsor* (RST, 1979), *Once in a Lifetime* (Aldwych, 1979), *Henry IV* (Barbican, 1982), *Peter Pan* (Barbican, 1982), *Les Misérables* (Barbican, 1985) and *The Fair Maid of the West* (Swan, 1986); Barry Kyle's *Richard III* (TOP, 1975); Terry Hands's *Twelfth Night* (RST, 1979); and Howard Davies's *Mother Courage* (Barbican, 1984).

Richard Nelson (b. Chicago, 1950). One of the RSC's few resident playwrights, Richard Nelson has written for the Swan and the Barbican's main stage. It is interesting that, during the 1980s and 90s, the RSC championed an American writer of well-made, deceptively lightweight plays and largely ignored the young talents of the Anglo-Irish theatrical revival; but Nelson's virtues include a fascination with different cultures and periods, subtlety of characterisation, and the ability to allow intensity of feeling to evolve beneath the humorous surface of the writing.

It was through David Jones that Nelson came to the RSC. Formerly colleagues at the Brooklyn Academy of Music in New York, Jones directed the British premiere of *Principia Scriptoriae* at the Pit in 1986. Nelson had struggled to achieve recognition in America, where his style and themes were perhaps not brash enough. In contrast, he felt immediately at home in the English theatre. His plays for the RSC have been, at turns, cleverly appropriate (*Two Shakespearean Actors*), ambitious (*Misha's Party*, co-written with the Russian dramatist Alexander Gelman), and unexpected (*Goodnight Children Everywhere*). *Madame Melville*, a tender rites of passage piece set in the Paris of the 1960s (an American boy has an affair with his French teacher), was written for the West End and performed by Macaulay Culkin and Irène Jacob in 2000.

John Nettles (b. St Austell, 1943). The popular star of *Bergerac* (BBC, 1981-91) made his name at the RSC in Shakespearean roles as diverse as Thersites in *Troilus and Cressida* (John Barton, RST, 1976); Albany in *King Lear* (Trevor Nunn, RST, 1976); Lucio in *Measure for Measure* (Kyle, RST, 1978); Bassanio in *The Merchant of Venice* (Barton, TOP, 1978); and Ventidius/Dolabella in Peter Brook's *Antony and Cleopatra* (RST, 1978). Overall, his contribution, ranging from new plays by Edward Bond, Howard Barker and David Edgar in the studios to bravura lightweight entertainments in the main house, was impressively eclectic: Maxwell in Edgar's *Destiny* (Ron Daniels, TOP, 1976); Godber in Barker's *That Good Between Us* (Kyle, Warehouse, 1977); Hoy in James Robson's *Factory Birds* (Bill Alexander, Warehouse, 1977); Peter in Barrie Keeffe's *Frozen Assets* (Kyle, Warehouse, 1977); Kung-tu in Bond's *The Bundle* (Howard Davies, Warehouse, 1977); Von Lieres in *A Miserable and Lonely Death* (Walter Donohue, Aldwych, 1978); Captain Thompson in Howard Brenton's *The Churchill Play* (Kyle, TOP, 1978); Alexei Turbin in

Bulgakov's *The White Guard* (Kyle, Aldwych, 1979); Harry Thunder in John O'Keeffe's *Wild Oats* (Clifford Williams, Aldwych, 1979); Ernest in Hart and Kaufman's *Once in a Lifetime* (Nunn, Aldwych, 1979); and the Count in Schnitzler's *La Ronde* (Barton, Aldwych, 1982).

After *Bergerac*, Nettles returned to Stratford to play a fine Leontes, exhausted by remorse, in *The Winter's Tale* (Adrian Noble, RST, 1992); Page in *The Merry Wives of Windsor* (David Thacker, RST, 1992); Octavius Caesar in *Antony and Cleopatra* (John Caird, RST, 1992); Merecraft, enjoyably devious and greedy, in *The Devil is an Ass* (Matthew Warchus, Swan, 1995); Brutus in *Julius Caesar* (Peter Hall, RST, 1995); and Buckingham in *Richard III* (Steven Pimlott, RST, 1995). Since 1997 he has starred in *Midsomer Murders* (ITV).

John Normington (1937-2007, b. Dukinfield, Cheshire) was a member of Peter Hall's RSC, a supporting player who most notably appeared in *The Wars of the Roses*, *Henry IV* and Harold Pinter's *The Homecoming*. Gravity, erudition, and a lovely way of playing comedy as if it was the least funny thing in the world typified Normington's style. The RSC had to compete with the National, the Royal Court and other theatres for the services of this formidable and splendidly adaptable master.

Normington trained as an opera singer at the Northern School of Music in Manchester. Following his National Service in the army, he worked in repertory at the Library Theatre, Manchester, and the Oxford Playhouse. He joined the RSC to play Jerry in William Gaskill's production of Fred Watson's *Infanticide in the House of Fred Ginger* at the Arts (1962), and was offered one of the new three-year contracts: Lucilius in *Julius Caesar* (John Blatchley, RST, 1963); Young Clifford in *The Wars of the Roses* (Peter Hall, RST, 1963); Bardolph in *Henry IV* and *Henry V* (Hall, RST, 1964); Antipholus of Ephesus in *The Comedy of Errors* (Williams, Aldwych, 1965); Sam in *The Homecoming* (Hall, Aldwych, 1965—he returned to the part for Hall's 1990

373

revival at the Comedy); the Dean in *Puntila* (Michel Saint-Denis, Aldwych, 1965); Witness 7 in *The Investigation* (Peter Brook, Aldwych, 1965); Sir Oblong in *The Thwarting of Baron Bolligrew* (Trevor Nunn, Aldwych, 1965); Glendower/Shallow in *Henry IV* (Barton, RST, 1966); Player Queen/Osric in *Hamlet* (Hall, RST, 1966); and Flute in Hall's RSC film of *A Midsummer Night's Dream* (1968).

His subsequent theatre work, a crowded parade of dissimilar characters, included, at the Royal Court, Feste in *Twelfth Night* (Jane Howell, 1968) and the Parson in Edward Bond's *The Fool* (Peter Gill, 1975); at the Bush, the schoolmaster in Robert Holman's *German Skerries* (Chris Parr, 1977); at the National, Dzershinsky in Robert Bolt's *State of Revolution* (Christopher Morahan, Lyttelton, 1977), Touchstone in *As You Like It* (John Dexter, Olivier, 1979), Clarence in *Richard III* (Morahan, Olivier, 1979), Joseph II in Peter Shaffer's *Amadeus* (Hall, Olivier, 1979), Conlag in Howard Brenton's *The Romans in Britain* (Michael Bogdanov, Olivier, 1980), *The Shoemakers' Holiday* (Dexter, Olivier, 1981), *The Oresteia* (Hall, Olivier, 1981), the Salvation Army colonel in *Guys and Dolls* (Richard Eyre, Olivier, 1982), Robespierre in *Danton's Death* (Peter Gill, Olivier, 1982), *Animal Farm* (Hall, Cottesloe, 1984), Arthur Miller's *The American Clock* (Peter Wood, Cottesloe, 1986), *The School for Scandal* (Wood, Olivier, 1990), the Old Shepherd in *The Winter's Tale* (Nicholas Hytner, Olivier, 2001), Lee Hall's version of Herman Heijermans's *The Good Hope* (Bill Bryden, Cottesloe, 2001), Watson in Simon Bent's *The Associate* (Paul Miller, Loft, 2002), and Sammy Lennon in Owen McCafferty's *Scenes from the Big Picture* (Peter Gill, Cottesloe, 2003); at the Almeida, Filippo in Pirandello's *The Rules of the Game* (Jonathan Kent, 1992).

Rejoining the RSC after a gap of twenty-five years, he was outstanding as Albany in the Robert Stephens *King Lear* (Adrian Noble, RST, 1993); Engstrand in Ibsen's *Ghosts* (Katie Mitchell, TOP, 1993); Holofernes in *Love's Labour's Lost* (Ian Judge, RST, 1993); Grove in Stephen Poliakoff's *Talk of the City* (Poliakoff, Swan, 1998); and as a member of Michael Boyd's first company

(2004)—Friar Laurence in *Romeo and Juliet* (Peter Gill), and the Fool, a sad-faced relic of vaudeville, in *King Lear* (Bill Alexander, RST). Illness meant that he was unable to accompany these productions to London. He returned to the stage in the final year of his life, as compelling as ever playing Peacey in Granville-Barker's *The Voysey Inheritance* at the National (Peter Gill, 2006), and Archie's father in John Osborne's *The Entertainer* at the Old Vic (Sean Holmes, 2007).

Jeremy Northam (b. Cambridge, 1961) came to prominence playing immoral characters with a sulky arrogance: in particular, he was suburb in a classy BBC adaptation of Barbara Vine's *A Fatal Inversion* (Tim Fywell, 1991), as the villain in the Sandra Bullock vehicle *The Net* (Irwin Winkler, 1995), and at the RSC as Horner in *The Country Wife* (Max Stafford-Clark, Swan, 1993).

The son of an academic and a teacher, he was born in Cambridge and brought up in that city and in Bristol. Oliver Neville, the actor and former head of RADA, was a neighbour and friend of the Northams in Bristol. Northam studied English at Bedford College, London, and then trained for the stage back in Bristol. Pantomimes in Salisbury led to his entry into the National as a bit player. His career was set up by a difficult beginning. As Daniel Day-Lewis's understudy in *Hamlet* (Richard Eyre, NT Olivier, 1989) it was Northam (playing Osric) who had to take over mid-performance on the day of Day-Lewis's collapse. He was rewarded with the lead in Harley Granville-Barker's *The Voysey Inheritance* (Eyre, Cottesloe, 1990).

Northam joined the RSC at the end of 1992 to play Philip alongside Judi Dench and Michael Pennington in the premiere production of Peter Schaffer's *The Gift of the Gordon* (Peter Hall, Pit). Then, as a member of the 1993-94 company, as well as his stylish Horner in *The Country Wife*, he gave a tellingly sombre account of Berowne in *Love's Labour's Lost* (Ian Judge, RST) and played the lead in Maureen Hunter's *Transit of Venus* (Alison Sutcliffe, TOP).

He has since concentrated on the movies: *Carrington* (Christopher Hampton, 1995); Knightley opposite Gwyneth Paltrow in *Emma* (Douglas McGrath, 1996); *Mimic* (Guillermo Del Toro, 1997); the judge in *Amistad* (Steven Spielberg, 1997); the property developer seduced by Anna Friel and Joely Richardson in Stephen Poliakoff's television film *The Tribe* (BBC, 1998); *The Ideal Husband* (1998); *Gloria* (1999); Sir Robert Morton in David Mamet's version of *The Winslow Boy* (1999); an escaped convict, a rare comedy role, in *Happy Texas* (1999); *The Golden Bowl* (James Ivory, 2000); the spymaster in *Enigma* (2001); Ivor Novello in *Gosford Park* (Robert Altman, 2001); *Possession* (2002); and the director in *A Cock and Bull Story* (Michael Winterbottom, 2005).

O

Timothy O'Brien (b. Shillong Assam, India, 1929). An influential designer at the RSC from 1966 to 1993, Timothy O'Brien worked regularly with John Barton, Terry Hands and David Jones. He first collaborated with Barton on student productions at Cambridge. On graduating he chose television over the stage: he was head of design at ABC Television for ten years from 1956.

O'Brien designed Trevor Nunn's *Tango* (Aldwych, 1966); John Schlesinger's *Days in the Trees* (Aldwych, 1966); Peter Hall's *Staircase* (Aldwych, 1966); John Barton's *All's Well That Ends Well* (RST, 1967), *Troilus and Cressida* (RST, 1968), *Measure for Measure* (RST, 1970), *Richard II* (RST, 1973), *La Ronde* (Aldwych, 1982) and *Three Sisters* (Barbican, 1988); David Jones's *As You Like It* (RST, 1967), *Enemies* (Aldwych, 1971), *The Lower Depths* (Aldwych, 1972), *The Island of the Mighty* (Aldwych, 1972), *Love's Labour's Lost* (RST, 1973), *Summerfolk* (Aldwych, 1974), *The Marrying of Ann Leete* (Aldwych, 1975), *The Zykovs* (Aldwych, 1976) and *Misha's Party* (Pit, 1993); Karolos Koun's

Romeo and Juliet (RST, 1967); Terry Hands's *The Merry Wives of Windsor* (RST, 1968), *The Latent Heterosexual* (Aldwych, 1968), *Pericles* (RST, 1969), *Women Beware Women* (RST, 1969), *Bartholomew Fair* (RST, 1969), *The Merchant of Venice* (RST, 1971), *The Man of Mode* (Aldwych, 1971) and *Love's Labour's Lost* (RST, 1990); Bill Alexander's *Cymbeline* (RST, 1989); and John Caird's *Columbus and the Discovery of Japan* (Barbican, 1992).

Joseph O'Conor (1916-2001, b. Dublin). In 1949 Joseph O'Conor alternated the roles of Othello and Iago with Donald Wolfit and played Hamlet under Wolfit's direction (Bedford Theatre, Camden Town). The season made his name as a leading Shakespearean, a position he was to keep (without seeking fame or glamour) for the next fifty years.

The son of Irish parents, O'Conor grew up in London and was educated at London University and RADA. His first appearance was as Flavius in *Julius Caesar* at the Embassy Theatre in 1939. After the war he started again with the role of Conrade in *Much Ado About Nothing* (Aldwych, 1946). While he continued to work in London, notably at the Open Air Theatre and the Arts, many of his most important performances were given on provincial stages—Christ in *The Mystery Plays* at York (1951, 1954); Benedick in *Much Ado About Nothing* at the Citizens' Theatre, Glasgow; and Kent in *King Lear*, Danton in *The Empty Chair*, Higgins in *Pygmalion*, Bottom in *A Midsummer Night's Dream*, Undershaft in *Major Barbara*, the title role in *Othello*, and Michael in his own play *The Iron Heart*, at the Bristol Old Vic (1956-58). The company he led at Bristol included Eric Porter, Peter O'Toole and Richard Harris. In 1958/59 he toured America with the Old Vic company (Chorus in *Henry V*; Polonius in *Hamlet*).

His appearances of the 1960s and 70s included Old Jolyon in *The Forsyte Saga* (BBC, 1966), Mr Brownlow in the film version of *Oliver!* (1968), and the Duke in *Measure for Measure* at the National (Jonathan Miller, Old Vic, 1974). Having worked for many years with increasing irregularity, and without forming an allegiance to any theatre, it was a great pleasure to see O'Conor based so visibly and with such quiet authority at the RSC: the title role in *Julius Caesar* (Ron Daniels, RST, 1983); Aegeon in *The Comedy of Errors* (Adrian Noble, RST, 1983); Escalus in *Measure for Measure* (Noble, RST, 1983); De Laubardemont in *The Devils* (John Barton, Pit, 1984); Swedish Commander in *Mother Courage* (Howard Davies, Barbican, 1984); Duke Frederick and Duke Senior in *As You Like It* (Noble, RST, 1985); Agamemnon in *Troilus and Cressida* (Davies, RST, 1985); Brabantio in *Othello* (Terry Hands, RST, 1985); Magnus in *Mephisto* (Noble, Barbican, 1986); Lord Summerhays in Bernard Shaw's *Misalliance* (John Caird, Barbican, 1986); Goodstock in Ben Jonson's *The New Inn* (Caird, Swan, 1987); the title role, succeeding David Waller, in *Julius Caesar* (Hands, Barbican, 1988); Chebutykin in *Three Sisters* (Barton, Barbican, 1988); Menenius in *Coriolanus* (Hands/Barton, RST, 1989); Lord Earner in Peter Flannery's *Singer* (Hands, Swan, 1989); and Gregor in *Moscow Gold* (Barry Kyle, Barbican, 1990). During the 1990s he played a polar survivor in the one-man play *The Forbidden Quest* (Peter Delpuit, 1993), and delivered fine cameo performances in the films *Elizabeth* (1998) and *Joan of Arc* (Luc Besson, 1999). His final role, a return to the RSC, was Duncan in the Antony Sher *Macbeth* (Gregory Doran, Swan, 1999-00).

Anthony O'Donnell received the Critics' Circle Best Newcomer Award for his work at the RSC in 1983. He had been acting for a decade, but the roles of Pompey in *Measure for Measure* (Adrian Noble, RST), Marall in *A New Way to Pay Old Debts* (Noble, TOP) and Clarion in *Life's a Dream* (John Barton, TOP) suited so well his short physique and pugnacious style of playing (revealing a natural clown) that they brought him to sudden notice. As Marall he wore a coat of black feathers and looked like a plump bird.

He first worked with the RSC in 1974: *Twelfth Night* (Peter Gill, RST); David Holman's *The World Turned Upside Down* (Buzz Goodbody, Tour of Schools); Taffy in David Rudkin's *Afore Night Come* (Ron Daniels, TOP); and Farm-hand in *Uncle Vanya* (Nicol Williamson, TOP). He took part in two readings at the Warehouse in 1978, playing Irish Man in *Landscape of Exile* (Howard Davies) and Jack in *Harry Mixture* (Mark Dornford-May), and found his RSC voice at the beginning of the 1980s: Snug in *A Midsummer Night's Dream* (Daniels, RST, 1981); Cuddy Banks in *The Witch of Edmonton* (Barry Kyle, TOP, 1981); Stout in *Money* (Bill Alexander, TOP, 1981); Benny in Peter Flannery's *Our Friends in the North* (John Caird, TOP, 1982); the Young Shepherd, succeeding Gerard Murphy, in *The Winter's Tale* (Ronald Eyre, Barbican, 1982); Tootles in *Peter Pan* (Trevor Nunn/Caird, Barbican, 1982-83); and Garage Mechanic in Max Frisch's *Triptych* (Terry Johnson, Pit, 1983). Following the 1983 season, he continued as Solinus in *The Comedy of Errors* (Noble, Barbican, 1984); Yuri in Charles Wood's *Red Star* (Caird, Pit, 1984); Sanguino in *Il Candelaio* (Clifford Williams, Pit, 1986); and Vet in Nick Darke's *The Dead Monkey* (Roger Michell, Pit, 1986). He returned in 1992/93 to play Lockit in *The Beggar's Opera* (Caird, Swan); Touchstone in *As You Like It* (David Thacker, RST); Lavatch in *All's Well That Ends Well* (Peter Hall, Swan); and Valeriy in *Misha's Party* (David Jones, Pit).

O'Donnell has also appeared at the National, the Almeida and the Donmar Warehouse: Harvey Duff in *The Shaughraun* (Howard Davies, NT Olivier, 1988); *Bartholomew Fair* (Richard Eyre, NT Olivier, 1988); *Ghetto* (Nicholas Hytner, NT Olivier, 1989); *The Miser* (Steven Pimlott, NT Olivier, 1991); *The Resistible Rise of Arturo Ui* (Di Trevis, NT Olivier, 1991); Wilful Witwoud in *The Way of the World* (Phyllida Lloyd, NT Lyttelton, 1995-96); Catherine Czercawska's *Wormwood* (Philip Howard, Traverse, 1997); the Ralph Fiennes *Ivanov* (Jonathan Kent, Almeida, 1997); *The London Cuckolds* (Terry Johnson, NT Lyttelton, 1998); the psychiatrist in *The Seven Year Itch* (Queen's, 2000); Sganarelle in *Don Juan* (Michael Grandage, Sheffield Crucible, 2001); the Fool in *King Lear* (Kent, Almeida at King's Cross, 2002); Sam Mendes's swansong at the Donmar—acting and singing beautifully as Waffles in *Uncle Vanya*, and Feste, here more than ever a world-weary, middle-aged troubadour of futility, in *Twelfth Night* (2002); Ragueneau in *Cyrano de Bergerac* (Davies, NT Olivier, 2004); Wolsey in *Henry VIII* (Gregory Thompson, AandBC Company, Holy Trinity Church, Stratford, 2006); and the policeman in Alistair Beaton's *King of Hearts* (Ramin Gray/Max Stafford-Clark, Hampstead Theatre, 2007).

One of Mike Leigh's regularly actors, O'Donnell created characters in *Nuts in May* (BBC, 1976), *Secrets and Lies* (1996) and *Vera Drake* (2004). Other notable work: Moth in Kenneth Branagh's *Love's Labour's Lost* (2000); *Two Men Went to War* (2002); *Charles II: the Power and the Passion* (Joe Wright, BBC, 2003); *Twenty Thousand Streets Under the Sky* (BBC, 2005); *Much Ado About Nothing* (BBC, 2005); and *Sweeney Todd* (BBC, 2006).

Gary Oldman (b. London, 1958) had a troubled childhood and adolescence in working-class New Cross, south London, from which acting and the theatre (he won a scholarship to Rose Bruford) offered a means of escape. His upbringing provided the material for his remarkable first feature as a writer/director, *Nil By Mouth* (1997), and can be detected in many of his screen performances. Throughout his career he has played highly-strung and brutal characters with a weary authenticity. His brilliance was evident in the early television piece *The Firm*, in which he played the leader of a gang of football hooligans (Alan Clarke, BBC, 1988). One sensed that this kind of urban monster was someone he knew well. His ability to threaten, along with an ear for accents, has brought him strong roles in American films, but of a limited kind—gangsters, corrupt cops, psychopaths. Able to conjure the damaged and the dead, he was remarkable as Sid Vicious, Joe Orton and Lee Harvey Oswald.

He emerged as one of his generation's most exciting actors in the theatre of the 1980s, a performer of pent-up energy and verbal precocity. Following work with the Greenwich Young People's Theatre he joined the Glasgow Citizens' and appeared in *The Massacre at Paris* (Philip Prowse, 1980), *Chinchilla* (Prowse, 1980), *A Waste of Time* (Prowse, 1980), and *Desperado Corner* (Di Trevis, 1981). In Prowse's production of Robert David MacDonald's *Summit Conference* (Lyric Hammersmith, 1982) he was the soldier seduced and humiliated by Glenda Jackson's Eva Braun and Georgina Hale's Clara Petacci. At the Royal Court in 1984 he met Leslie Manville, his future wife, and played the cockney PC in Ron Hutchinson's *Rat in the Skull* (Max Stafford-Clark), Scopey in Edward Bond's *The Pope's Wedding* (Stafford-Clark), and Mike in Bond's *Saved* (Danny Boyle). His first films were Mike Leigh's *Meantime* (1981), and *Remembrance* (1982).

Oldman was a member of the RSC in 1985-86: Edward Bond's *War Plays* (Nick Hamm, Pit); Major Carp/Petko, succeeding Andy Readman, in Nicholas Wright's *The Desert Air* (Adrian Noble, Pit); *Abel and Cain* ('Not the RSC' fringe festival, Almeida); Jack, the revolutionary leader, his first American, in Trevor Griffiths's *Real Dreams* (Ron Daniels, Pit); and Harold Pinter's *The Dumb Waiter* (Adrian Dunbar, 'Not the RSC Again' fringe festival, Almeida, 1986).

He was ferocious as Sordido, servant to Ward (Simon Russell Beale), in Howard Barker's updating of *Women Beware Women* (William Gaskill, Royal Court, 1986), and cruelly eloquent as Horner in *The Country Wife* (Nicholas Hytner, Manchester Royal Exchange, 1986). His stature was confirmed by the films *Sid and Nancy* (Alex Cox, 1986) and *Prick Up Your Ears* (Stephen Frears, 1987), and by Caryl Churchill's hit play *Serious Money*, in which he created the lead, a wide boy city dealer (Stafford-Clark, Royal Court, 1987).

After *Serious Money* Oldman went to America to make *Track 29* (Nicholas Roeg, 1988). An international film career followed: *Criminal Law* (Martin Campbell, 1988); a New York Irish gangster in *State of Grace* (Phil Joanou, 1990); Rosencrantz to Tim Roth's Guildenstern in *Rosencrantz and Guildenstern Are Dead* (Tom Stoppard, 1990); Lee Harvey Oswald in *JFK* (Oliver Stone,

1991); the title role in *Dracula* (Francis Coppola, 1992); a corrupt New York cop in *Romeo is Bleeding* (Peter Medak, 1993); Beethoven in *Immortal Beloved* (Bernard Rose, 1994); a corrupt New York cop in *Leon* (Luc Besson, 1994); the priest in *The Scarlet Letter* (Roland Joffé, 1995); Albert Milo in *Basquiat* (1996); the villain in *The Fifth Element* (Luc Besson, 1997); the Russian hijacker in *Air Force One* (Wolfgang Petersen, 1997); Dr Smith in *Lost in Space* (1998); Mason Verger in *Hannibal* (Ridley Scott, 2001); *Harry Potter and the Prisoner of Azkaban* (Alfonso Cuarón, 2004); *Batman Begins* (Christopher Nolan, 2005); and *Backwoods* (2006).

Peter O'Toole (b. 1932) grew up in Leeds, spent hours at the races helping his father, a bookmaker known as Spats because of his choice of shoes, and started his adult life as an apprentice photographer on the *Yorkshire Evening Post*. It was during his national service in the Navy—he served on a corvette, patrolling British fishing rights in the Atlantic—that he decided to become an actor. He applied to RADA and won a scholarship.

O'Toole's strong, flamboyant personality conquered RADA, then the Bristol Old Vic, 1955-58. His Bristol roles included Cornwall in the Eric Porter *King Lear* (1956); Bullock in *The Recruiting Officer* (1956); Alfred Doolittle in *Pygmalion* (1957); Lysander in *A Midsummer Night's Dream* (1957); Jimmy Porter in *Look Back in Anger* (1957); Tanner in *Man and Superman* (1958); the title role in *Hamlet* (1958); and Jupiter in Jean Giraudoux's *Amphitryon '38* (1958). In 1959, the year of his marriage to the actress Siân Phillips, he played Bamforth in Willis Hall's *The Long and the Short and the Tall* (Lindsay Anderson, Royal Court), a great success. He had presence, photogenic looks and a voice of range and expressiveness—but it was his rebelliousness, both on and off the stage, that struck a theatrical establishment only just getting used to working-class actors becoming stars.

Peter Hall had asked Paul Scofield to lead his first RSC ensemble. When Scofield withdrew at short notice Hall took a calculated risk and offered the roles of Petruchio in *The Taming of the Shrew*, Shylock in *The Merchant of Venice* and Thersites in *Troilus and Cressida* to the up-and-coming O'Toole. At first the risk paid off—O'Toole gave acclaimed performances. If we believe the legend, he also charmed Peggy Ashcroft, Kate to his Petruchio, argued publicly with John Barton and engineered his removal from the production, failed to turn up for sonnet classes, and won speed drinking competitions in the Dirty Duck pub. Hall wanted O'Toole to play Henry in Jean Anouilh's *Becket*, the title role in *Richard III* and Iago to John Gielgud's Othello, but the actor left the RSC without fulfilling his contract. He had been offered the role of Lawrence in *Lawrence of Arabia*. (Christopher Plummer was called in to play Henry and Richard III; Ian Bannen played Iago.)

Screen stardom had been O'Toole's goal since RADA. For a decade he went from film to film but struggled to repeat the great achievement of *Lawrence*. *Becket* (Peter Glenville, 1964) was performed with flare; *Lord Jim* (Richard Brooks, 1965) was an interesting failure; and the comedies *What's New, Pussycat* (Clive Donner, 1965) and *How to Steal a Million* (William Wyler, 1966) were typical entertainments of the period. With the exception of two high-profile failures at the Old Vic—*Hamlet* (opening Laurence Olivier's National Theatre) in 1963 and *Macbeth* in 1980—O'Toole appears to have chosen his infrequent stage appearances largely on personal grounds. They included seasons in Dublin and his old stamping ground of Bristol: Brecht's *Baal* (Phoenix, 1963); David Mercer's *Ride a Cock Horse* (Piccadilly, 1965); Jack Boyle in *Juno and the Paycock* and Tanner in *Man and Superman* (Gaiety, Dublin, 1966); Vladimir in *Waiting for Godot* (Abbey, Dublin, 1969); the title role in *Uncle Vanya*, Ben Travers's *Plunder*, King Magnus in *The Apple Cart* and Barry Collins's dramatic monologue *Judgement* (Bristol Old Vic, 1973-74); *Uncle Vanya* and *Present Laughter* (Chicago, 1978); *Man and Superman* (Theatre Royal Haymarket, 1982); *Pygmalion* (Shaftesbury, 1984); *The Apple Cart* (Theatre Royal Haymarket, 1986); and *Our Song* (Apollo, 1992).

Macbeth aside, during the 1980s O'Toole delivered his best work in years—the films *The Stunt Man* (Richard Rush, 1980), *My Favorite Year* (Richard Benjamin, 1982), and *The Last Emperor* (Bernardo Bertolucci, 1987), and the stage play *Jeffrey Bernard is Unwell* (Apollo, 1989), which allowed him to personate Jeffrey Bernard while seeming to be himself. He returned to the role in 1991 and 1999.

P

Cécile Paoli (b. France) was educated at the École Nationale Supérieure des Arts et Techniques du Théâtre, Paris, and at the Conservatoire de Marseilles. She made her debut in a 1980 BBC adaptation of H.E. Bates's *Fair Stood the Wind for France*, playing the girl who courageously helps an English airman shot down in wartime France. A beautiful beginning, it initiated a career that has seen her work on both sides of the Channel. At the RSC (1984-85) she was an irresistible Katharine in the Kenneth Branagh *Henry V* (Adrian Noble, RST), and was equally beguiling in the darker part of Mila, a Polish refugee, in Nicholas Wright's *The Desert Air* (Noble, TOP). On the transfer to London she added Kara in Trevor Griffiths's *The Party* (Howard Davies, Pit), and the Chorus Girl, the Wife, the Blind Woman, and the Dean of Medicine in Strindberg's *Dreamplay* (John Barton, Pit).

On British television, following *Fair Stood the Wind for France*, she played John Nettles's girlfriend in the first series of *Bergerac* (BBC, 1981); Isabelle de Chamonpierre in *The Ginger Tree* (BBC, 1989); a *femme fatale* in Malcolm Bradbury's EEC satire *The Gravy Train Goes East* (1991); sexy again in the Jilly Cooper nonsense *Riders* (ITV, 1993); Lucille in *Sharpe's Revenge* and *Sharpe's Waterloo* (Tom Clegg, ITV, 1997); and *Holby City* (BBC, 2004). Her films are: *Voyage to Rome* (Michel Lengliney, 1992); *Near Misses* (Baz Taylor, 1992); and *Kaspar Hauser* (Peter Sehr, 1994).

Cécile Paoli's theatre appearances in France have included: Gabriella in *Les Libertins* (Roger Planchon, Théâtre national populaire, Villeurbanne, 1994); Lumîr in Paul Claudel's trilogy *Les Coûfontaine* (Marcel Maréchal, Théâtre de Gironde, Saint-Médard-en-Jalles, 1996); Milady in *Les trois mousquetaires* (Maréchal, Théâtre du Rond-Point, Paris, 1999); Pauline in Corneille's *Polyeucte* (Thierry Harcourt, Théâtre Mouffetard, Paris, 2001); and Anne in Jean-Pierre About's *Le manège du pouvoir* (Thomas Le Douarec, Théâtre 14 Jean-Marie Serreau, Paris, 2002-03).

Richard Pasco (b. London, 1926). Before the age of twenty Richard Pasco worked as an apprentice assistant stage manager at the Q Theatre in London and made his first professional appearances in *She Stoops to Conquer* (1943) and *Zero Hour* (Lyric, 1944). Active service (1944-48) interrupted his career, but after the war he received an ex-serviceman's state grant to study at the Central School of Speech and Drama. He made his first visit to Stratford in 1950 and saw Anthony Quayle in *Henry VIII* (Tyrone Guthrie). Membership of the Stratford theatre became his goal.

After Central, Pasco worked at the Old Vic and the Birmingham Rep. In 1955 he played Fortinbras in the Peter Brook/Paul Scofield *Hamlet* (Phoenix). He emerged as a leading actor in the newly formed ESC at the Royal Court (1957): *The Member of the Wedding* (Tony Richardson); the second Jimmy Porter in *Look Back in Anger* (Richardson); Frank to Olivier's Archie Rice in *The Entertainer* (Richardson); the double-bill of Giraudoux's *The Apollo of Bellac* and Ionesco's *The Chairs* (Richardson); and Oliver Marlow Wilkinson's *How Can We Save Father?* (Peter Wood).

His West End appearances during the 1960s included Lyngstrand in Ibsen's *The Lady from the Sea* (Queen's, 1961); *The New Men* (Strand, 1962); Julian in Peter Shaffer's *The Public Eye* (Globe, 1963); and Konstantinovitch in Chekhov's *Ivanov* (Phoenix, 1965). At the Bristol Old Vic he played the title role in *Henry V*; Berowne in *Love's Labour's Lost* (1964); the title role in *Peer*

Gynt; Angelo in *Measure for Measure*; and the title role in *Hamlet* (1966).

He failed an audition with Peter Hall in 1964 but was successful in 1969, the beginning of a long RSC career of strong, beautifully spoken performances. As well as the leading roles of Becket in T.S. Eliot's *Murder in the Cathedral* (Terry Hands, Aldwych, 1972), both Richard and Bolingbroke (alternated with Ian Richardson) in *Richard II* (John Barton, RST, 1973) and Timon of Athens (Ron Daniels, TOP, 1980), Pasco played Polixenes in *The Winter's Tale* (Trevor Nunn, RST, 1969); Leantio in Middleton's *Women Beware Women* (Hands, RST, 1969); Proteus in *The Two Gentlemen of Verona* (Gareth Morgan, Theatregoround, 1969); Orsino in *Twelfth Night* (Barton, Aldwych, 1970—he took on the part at short notice following the sudden death of Charles Thomas); Buckingham in *Henry VIII* (Nunn, RST, 1969); Adolphus Cusins in *Major Barbara* (Clifford Williams, Aldwych, 1970); Richard in *Richard II* (Barton, RST, 1971); Don John in *Much Ado About Nothing* (Ronald Eyre, RST, 1971); Bologna in *The Duchess of Malfi* (Williams, RST, 1971); the Baron in Gorky's *The Lower Depths* (David Jones, Aldwych, 1972); Medraut in *The Island of the Mighty* (Jones, Aldwych, 1972); Jaques in *As You Like It* (Buzz Goodbody, RST, 1973); Philip the Bastard in *King John* (Barton, RST, 1974); Aleister Crowley in Snoo Wilson's *The Beast* (Howard Davies, The Place, 1974); Lord John Carp in Granville-Barker's *The Marrying of Ann Leete* (Jones, Aldwych, 1975); Jack Tanner in *Man and Superman* (Clifford Williams, Malvern Festival, 1977); Clarence in *Richard III* (Hands, RST, 1980); Arkady Schatslivtses, alongside his wife Barbara Leigh-Hunt, in *The Forest* (Adrian Noble, TOP, 1981); Sir Sackville Lump in *The Swan Down Gloves* (Hands, Aldwych, 1981); and the Poet in *La Ronde* (Barton, Aldwych, 1982).

From 1987 to 1994 Pasco worked at the National, performing such roles as the Father in *Six Characters in Search of an Author* (Michael Rudman, Olivier, 1987); Charlie Allen in *Racing Demon* (Richard Eyre, Cottesloe, 1990); Sir Peter Edgecombe in *Murmuring Judges* (Eyre, Olivier, 1991); Birling in Stephen Daldry's production of *An Inspector Calls* (Lyttelton, 1992); Malcolm Pryce in *Absence of War* (Eyre, Olivier, 1993); and Boss Findley in *Sweet Bird of Youth* (Eyre, Lyttelton, 1994). Pasco was contemplating his retirement when a chance meeting with Adrian Noble on the train to Warwick brought him back to the RSC to play Sorin in *The Seagull* (Swan, 2000).

Joanne Pearce (b. Cornwall). In productions directed by her husband, Adrian Noble, Joanne Pearce gave some of the most striking and unusual RSC performances of the 1980s and 90s. As Antigone in *The Thebans* (Swan, 1991) she guarded Gerard Murphy's Oedipus with the mute loyalty of a dog. As Doll in *Henry IV Part Two* (RST, 1991), wearing a red dress, high heels and a long hair pin she used as a weapon, she was both rough and vulnerable, and her duet with Robert Stephens's Falstaff, funny and sad ('I am old, I am old' 'I love thee better than I love e'er a scurvy young boy of them all'), was unforgettable. As Ophelia in the Kenneth Branagh *Hamlet* (Barbican, 1992) her madness— intimations of which were given early on in the performance— was free of cliché and extravagance.

She trained at the Guildhall School and worked extensively in provincial repertory (Manchester, Bristol, Leicester) in the early 1980s: roles included Dorinda in *The Beaux' Stratagem*; Cordelia in *King Lear*; Miranda in *The Tempest*; Asta in *Little Eyolf*; Alithea in *The Country Wife*; Lady Windermere in *Lady Windermere's Fan*; and Isabella in *Ring Around the Moon*. On television she appeared in the BBC's *The Two Gentlemen of Verona* and *The Comedy of Errors*, and gave a sensitive performance as the young wife in Ayckbourn's *Way Upstream* (BBC, 1987).

She joined the RSC in London in 1984, taking over the role of Olivia from Sarah Berger in John Caird's production of *Twelfth Night* (Barbican). Then, in the 1988-89 cycle, she played Olivia in *The Plain Dealer* (Ron Daniels, Swan) and Queen Elizabeth (plus La Pucelle in London) in *The Plantagenets* (Noble, RST, Barbican). She ended this period of work as Hilde Wangel in *The*

Master Builder (Noble, Barbican, 1989). Dressed in a white sailor suit, relentlessly probing John Wood's Solness, flirting then withdrawing, Pearce's Hilde was especially dangerous: at the climax she faced the audience transfixed like a groupie and revelling in the moment of catastrophe.

She then appeared in two forgettable films, Griff Rhys Jones and Mel Smith's unfunny comedy *Morons from Outer Space* and a cold war thriller called *Murder East Murder West*. She also had parts in the television serials *Reilly Ace of Spies* and *Lovejoy*. Returning to the RSC for the 1991/92 season, as well as Doll Tearsheet and Antigone, she played Doll Common in *The Alchemist* (Sam Mendes, Swan). In London she gave a typically intense performance as Leye in *The Dybbuk* (Katie Mitchell, Pit).

In 1994 she succeeded Felicity Kendall as Hanna in Stoppard's *Arcadia* (Trevor Nunn, West End) before heading back to Stratford to play Rita in *Little Eyolf* (Noble, Swan, 1996-97) and Imogen in *Cymbeline* (Noble, RST, 1997). One example of Pearce's imaginative playing: near the end of *Little Eyolf* Rita removed large pebbles from the pockets of her overcoat: this suggestion of a rejection of suicide, along with the closing image of Rita tentatively holding out her hand to Alfred, made Ibsen's difficult ending—their future devoted to impoverished children—moving and uncertain. In 2002/03 she played the White Witch in *The Lion, the Witch and the Wardrobe* (Noble, RST).

Other theatre since 1998: Catherine Johnson's *Shang-a-Lang* (Mike Bradwell, Bush, 1998-99); Simon Block's *A Place at the Table* (Julie-Anne Robinson, Bush, 2000); Bea in Shelagh Stephenson's *Ancient Lights* (Ian Brown, Hampstead, 2000); Hannie Rayson's *Life After George* (Michael Blakemore, Duchess, 2002); and Mrs Allonby in *A Woman of No Importance* (Noble, Theatre Royal Haymarket, 2003).

Bob Peck (1945-1999, b. Yorkshire). The son of an insurance man, a Methodist, Bob Peck grew up in Leeds and attended the Leeds Modern School. His performances in school productions led to membership of the National Youth Theatre, but he initially stepped back from pursuing a career as an actor. Instead, he studied art in his hometown and joined the local amateur dramatics society. Fate intervened when Alan Ayckbourn came to direct one of his plays. Impressed by Peck, he invited him to join the company of the Library Theatre, Scarborough.

For over five years Peck worked in provincial repertory. Among the parts he played were Sir Epicure Mammon in *The Alchemist*, Inspector Truscott in *Loot*, Pat in Brendan Behan's *The Hostage* (1972), Old Alan in Edward Bond's *The Pope's Wedding*, and Shakespeare in Bond's *Bingo* (1973). His breakthrough came in 1974 at the Royal Court, where he played Abercrombie in David Storey's *Life Class* (Lindsay Anderson).

The following year he joined the RSC. Beginning with supporting roles, he quickly became a prominent performer, the Company's resident brooder (nicknamed 'Pause Peck'). Tall and bearded with, at moments of intensity, bulging eyes, he was particularly persuasive as dark and dangerous characters, notably Soliony in *Three Sisters* (Trevor Nunn, Small-scale Tour, 1978), Iago in *Othello* (Ronald Eyre, RST, 1979), Sir Mulberry Hawk in *Nicholas Nickleby* (Nunn/John Caird, Aldwych, 1980), Macbeth (Davies, RST, 1982), and Caliban in *The Tempest* (Ron Daniels, RST, 1982). Also: First Player/First Gravedigger in the Ben Kingsley *Hamlet* (Buzz Goodbody, TOP, 1975); Mowbray in *Henry IV Part 2* (Terry Hands, RST, 1975); Surrey in John Ford's *Perkin Warbeck* (Barry Kyle, TOP, 1975); Uria Shelley in Brecht's *Man is Man* (Davies, TOP, 1975); Lord Hastings in *Richard III* (Kyle, TOP, 1975); Himmler in Brecht's *Schweyk in the Second World War* (Davies, TOP, 1976); Borachio in *Much Ado About Nothing* (John Barton, RST, 1976); Camillo in *The Winter's Tale* (Barton, RST, 1976); Macduff in the Ian McKellen *Macbeth* (Nunn, TOP, 1976); Richard Cleaver in David Edgar's *Destiny* (Ron Daniels, TOP, 1976); Kent in *King Lear* (Nunn, RST, 1976); Purvis in C.P. Taylor's *Bandits* (Davies, Warehouse, 1977); Papa in Brecht's *Days of the Commune* (Davies, Aldwych, 1977); Ferryman in Edward Bond's *The Bundle* (Davies, Warehouse, 1977);

Sir Wilfull Witwoud in *The Way of the World* (Barton, Aldwych, 1978); Proctor in *A Miserable and Lonely Death* (Walter Donohue, Warehouse, 1978); Malvolio in *Twelfth Night* (Jon Amiel, Small-scale Tour, 1978); George Page in *The Merry Wives of Windsor* (Nunn, RST, 1979); Cloten in *Cymbeline* (David Jones, RST, 1979); Edward in David Mercer's *No Limits to Love* (Howard Davies, Warehouse, 1980); Rivers in Peter Whelan's *The Accrington Pals* (Bill Alexander, Warehouse, 1981); the title role in Edward Bond's *Lear* (Barry Kyle, TOP, 1982); and Enobarbus in the Michael Gambon/Helen Mirren *Antony and Cleopatra* (Adrian Noble, TOP, 1982).

Peck's occasional early screen appearances included *Sunset Across the Bay* (1975), and the film *Royal Flash* (1975). After the success of the thriller *Edge of Darkness* (BBC, 1986), he worked constantly on television: *After Pilkington* (1987); *Children Crossing* (Angela Pope, BBC, 1990); *Who Bombed Birmingham?* (1990); Nigel Williams's *Centrepoint* (Piers Haggard, 1990); Nicias in *The War That Never Ends* (Jack Gold, BBC, 1991); *An Ungentlemanly Act* (1992); *Natural Lies* (1992); Gradgrind in Peter Barnes's adaptation of *Hard Times* (BBC, 1994); Shylock in *The Merchant of Venice* (1996); *Deadly Summer* (1997); *Hospital!* (1997); and *The Scold's Bridle* (David Thacker, 1998). He played supporting roles in the films *On the Black Hill* (Andrew Grieve, 1987); *The Kitchen Toto* (1987); *Slipstream* (Steven Lisberger, 1989); *The Lord of the Flies* (1990); *Jurassic Park* (Steven Spielberg, 1993); *Surviving Picasso* (James Ivory, 1996); and *Smilla's Sense of Snow* (Bille August, 1997).

Peck's final stage appearances were typically compelling: Athol Fugard's *The Road to Mecca* (Fugard, NT Lyttelton, 1985); Guy Jones in Ayckbourn's *A Chorus of Disapproval* (Ayckbourn, NT Olivier, 1985); Tom Paine in *In Lambeth* (Jack Shepherd, Donmar Warehouse, 1989); Arthur Miller's *Two-Way Mirror* and *The Price* (David Thacker, Young Vic, 1989-90); Goldberg in Pinter's *The Birthday Party* (Sam Mendes, NT Lyttelton, 1994); and John Rutherford in Githa Sowerby's *Rutherford and Son* (Katie Mitchell, NT Cottesloe, 1994).

Michael Pennington (b. Cambridge, 1943) read English at Trinity College, Cambridge, and began his career at the Arts Theatre. He first appeared with the RSC in 1965/66, playing Dumaine in *Love's Labour's Lost* (John Barton); Mathias in *The Jew of Malta* (Clifford Williams); Titus in *Timon of Athens* (John Schlesinger); Fortinbras in the David Warner *Hamlet* (Peter Hall); and Stark in Peter Weiss's *The Investigation* (Peter Brook, Aldwych). Following work in London, including Laertes in the Nicol Williamson *Hamlet* (Tony Richardson, Roundhouse, 1969), *Captain Jack's Revenge* (Nicholas Wright, Royal Court, 1971) and the anthropologist in Christopher Hampton's *Savages* (Robert Kidd, Royal Court, 1973), he returned to the RSC as a leading actor. A key figure of the years 1974 to 1981, he was Angelo in *Measure for Measure* (Keith Hack, RST, 1974); Ferdinand in *The Tempest* (Hack, TOP, 1974); Johnnie in David Rudkin's *Afore Night Come* (Ron Daniels, TOP, 1974); Mercutio in the Ian McKellen/Francesca Annis *Romeo and Juliet* (Trevor Nunn, RST, 1976); Hector in *Troilus and Cressida* (Barton/Barry Kyle, RST, 1976); Major Rolfe in David Edgar's *Destiny* (Daniels, TOP, 1976); Edgar in the Donald Sinden *King Lear* (Nunn, RST, 1976); Mirabell in *The Way of the World* (Barton, Aldwych, 1978); the Duke in *Measure for Measure* (Kyle, RST, 1978); an intellectually arrogant Berowne in *Love's Labour's Lost* (Barton, RST, 1978); the title role in *Hippolytus* (Daniels, TOP, 1978); Shervinsky in Bulgakov's *The White Guard* (Kyle, Aldwych, 1979); Donal Davoren in *The Shadow of a Gunman* (Michael Bogdanov, TOP, 1980); a noble if flawed Hamlet (Barton, RST, 1980)—the immaculate verse-speaking and gimmick-free characterisation made the interpretation seem old-fashioned when it was anything but; and Jack Beaty in Howard Brenton's *Thirteenth Night* (Kyle, Warehouse, 1981). If a scholarly, carefully considered approach to the craft of acting defines Pennington's elegant style, he has never been dryly cerebral—after all, in roles such as Mercutio, Hector and Hamlet he performed with anger and impetuosity.

From 1986 to 1993 Pennington directed, with Michael Bogdanov, the touring English Shakespeare Company and played Hal, Henry V, Richard II, Coriolanus, Leontes and Macbeth. His most prominent theatre work since the ESC folded has been for Peter Hall: Claudius in *Hamlet* at the Gielgud Theatre (1994); Trebell in Granville-Barker's *Waste*, a splendidly seedy Brute in Vanbrugh's *The Provok'd Wife* and Trigorin in *The Seagull* at the Old Vic (1997); Alceste in Molière's *The Misanthrope* at the Piccadilly (1998); and Dickens in Simon Gray's *Little Nell* at the Theatre Royal, Bath (2007). Elsewhere, his collection of characters has been richly diverse: Jaffeir in Thomas Otway's *Venice Preserv'd* (Peter Gill, NT Lyttelton, 1984); Henry in Tom Stoppard's *The Real Thing* (Peter Wood, Strand, 1985); Vershinin in *Three Sisters* (Adrian Noble, Gate Theatre, Dublin, 1990); the American army interrogator in Ronald Harwood's *Taking Sides* (Harold Pinter, Minerva, Chichester, 1995); Archie Rice in John Osborne's *The Entertainer* (Stephen Rayne, Watermill, Newbury, 1996); Prentice in Joe Orton's *What the Butler Saw* (Jeremy Sams, Theatre Royal, Bath, 2001); the clairvoyant in David Mamet's *The Shawl* (Angus Jackson, Sheffield Crucible, 2001); Walter Burns in *The Front Page* (Douglas Wager, Chichester, 2002); the title role in *John Gabriel Borkman* (Stephen Unwin, English Touring Theatre, Greenwich Theatre, 2003); Dorn in *The Seagull* (Peter Stein, Edinburgh Festival, 2003); the title role in Alan Bennett's *The Madness of George III* (Rachel Kavanaugh, West Yorkshire Playhouse, 2003); Cecil opposite Catherine McCormack in Hanif Kureishi's *When the Night Begins* (Anthony Clark, Hampstead Theatre, 2004); and Keith/Bernard in David Greig's *The Cosmonaut's Last Message to the Woman He Once Loved in the Former Soviet Union* (Tim Supple, Donmar Warehouse, 2005).

Pennington has maintained his association with the RSC, but only at intervals. He created roles in two new plays—Bill in Stephen Poliakoff's *Playing With Trains* (Daniels, Pit, 1989) and Edward opposite Judi Dench in Peter Shaffer's *The Gift of the Gorgon* (Hall, Pit, 1992); replaced Alan Bates at short notice to play the title role in *Timon of Athens* (Gregory Doran, RST, 1999);

and narrated Shakespeare's epic poem *Venus and Adonis: a Masque for Puppets* (Doran, TOP, 2004).

Edward Petherbridge (b. Bradford, 1936) trained at the Northern Theatre School and made his name as a member of Laurence Olivier's National Theatre company at the Old Vic. Most notably he created the role of Guildenstern in Tom Stoppard's *Rosencrantz and Guildenstern are Dead* (1967), and appeared opposite Maggie Smith as Ferdinand Gadd in *Trelawny of the Wells* (1965). On leaving the National in 1970 he played Alceste in *The Misanthrope* at the Nottingham Playhouse. His work for the Actors' Company, the troupe he co-founded with Ian McKellen and others, included the title role in *Tartuffe* and the Fool in *King Lear* (1972-75).

In 1978 he joined McKellen's RSC touring company to play Orsino in *Twelfth Night* (John Amiel) and Vershinin in *Three Sisters* (Trevor Nunn). He remained with the Company until 1984: Newman Noggs in *Nicholas Nickleby* (Nunn/John Caird, Aldwych, 1980); Golashchapov, succeeding Nigel Terry, in *The Suicide* (Ron Daniels, Warehouse, 1980); Otto in David Mercer's *No Limits to Love* (Howard Davies, Warehouse, 1980); the storyteller in *Peter Pan* (Caird, Barbican, 1983-84); and Armado in *Love's Labour's Lost* (Barry Kyle, RST, 1984).

In 1984 Petherbridge won an Olivier award for his performance in Eugene O'Neill's *Strange Interlude* (Duke of York's). From 1984-86, again with McKellen, he led a company of actors at the National and appeared in *The Duchess of Malfi*, *The Cherry Orchard*, *The Real Inspector Hound*, and *The Critic*. When this ended he began a period of freelance work: *Busman's Honeymoon* (Lyric, Hammersmith, 1988); the one-man show *Eight O'Clock Muse* (Riverside Studios, 1989); Alceste in *The Misanthrope* (Bristol Old Vic, 1989); *The Power and the Glory* (Chichester, 1990); *Cyrano de Bergerac* (Greenwich, 1990); *Point Valaine* and *Valentine's Day* (Chichester, 1991); and Noël Coward in *Noël and Gertie*

(Duke of York's, 1991). Most prominently, he starred in the BBC's *Lord Peter Wimsey* (1987).

In 1996 he returned to the RSC: Malvolio in *Twelfth Night* (Ian Judge, Barbican, 1996); Ford in *The Merry Wives of Windsor* (Judge, RST, 1996-97); the title role in *Cymbeline* (Adrian Noble, RST, 1997); Ghost/Player King in *Hamlet* (Matthew Warchus, RST, 1997); and *Krapp's Last Tape* (Edward Petherbridge and David Hunt, Pit, 1998).

Leslie Phillips (b. London, 1924) made his professional debut at the age of ten, playing a wolf in *Peter Pan* at the London Palladium (1935). Mrs Phillips, recently widowed, put her talented son on the stage to supplement the family's meagre income. The next eight years saw him appear with such figures as Rex Harrison, John Gielgud and Laurence Olivier. Called up at eighteen, his acquired upper-class voice (regional accents had yet to become acceptable in the theatre) secured him a commission in the Durham Light Infantry.

On returning to the stage after the war, he played Jimmy McBride in *Daddy Long-Legs* (Comedy, 1948); Jerry Winterton in *On Monday Next* (Embassy, 1949); Lord Fancourt Babberley in *Charley's Aunt* (Saville, 1950); Tony in *For Better, For Worse* (Comedy, 1952-53); Lupin Pooter in *The Diary of a Nobody* (Arts, 1954); Scruffy Pembridge in *The Lost Generation* (Garrick, 1955); Carliss in *The Whole Truth* (Aldwych, 1955); and Peter Croone in *Three-Way Stretch* (Aldwych, 1958). He became best known as a light comedian in British films, particularly associated with the upper-class skirt-chaser he played in the 'Carry On' and 'Doctor' comedies. His voice is instantly recognisable; it is the perfect instrument for adding a hint of sarcasm or a double meaning to innocent phrases. It explains why his public image is still that of a lecher in cravat and blazer. However, he also appeared in David Lean's *The Sound Barrier* (1952), George Cukor's *Les Girls* (1957), John Guillermin's *I Was Monty's Double* (1958), Robert Aldrich's *The Angry Hills* (1959), and *The Longest Day* (1962).

In middle age he reinvented his career by concentrating on dramatic roles. He was in Peter Nichols's *Passion Play* (Wyndham's), and the films *Out of Africa* (Sydney Pollack, 1985), *Empire of the Sun* (Steven Spielberg, 1987), and *Scandal* (Michael Caton-Jones, 1989). His rich but subtle characterisations enlivened many films and television dramas during the next two decades, among them *Chancer* (ITV, 1990); *Mountains of the Moon* (Bob Rafelson, 1990); *King Ralph* (1991); *The Changeling* (Simon Curtis, BBC, 1994); *August* (1996); Evelyn Waugh's *Sword of Honour* (Channel Four, 2001); Kingsley Amis's *Take a Girl Like You* (BBC, 2001); *Lara Croft: Tomb Raider* (2001); *Harry Potter and the Sorcerer's Stone* (Chris Columbus, 2001); and *Venus* (Roger Michell, 2006).

He was at the RSC for one two-year cycle, 1996-98, playing Falstaff in *The Merry Wives of Windsor* (Ian Judge, RST) and Gutman in Tennessee Williams's *Camino Real* (Steven Pimlott, Swan). He played Falstaff as a melancholy old roué. As the ring master of *Camino Real*, a hotel proprietor in a rumpled linen suit, he was menacingly enigmatic: greeting the beginning of each scene with its number proceeded by the word 'block' (as in 'Block one on the Camino Real'), his delivery of the words, like the whole performance, contained all kinds of bitter meaning and implied threat. His spot-on performance as Sir Plympton Makepeace, MP, in Peter Tinniswood's one-man play *On the Whole Life's Been Jolly Good* was a hit at the 1999 Edinburgh Festival.

Tim Pigott-Smith (b. Rugby, 1946) was brought up in Leicester but spent the final two years of his schooling in Stratford (his father edited the local paper). During school holidays he worked in the RSC paint shop. From Shakespeare's old school he went to Bristol University to study drama (1964-67). He trained at the Bristol Old Vic Theatre School, entering the Old Vic company in 1969, his first professional work. During a year touring with Prospect (1970-71) he played Laertes in the Ian McKellen *Hamlet*.

He joined the RSC in 1972 to appear in Trevor Nunn's 'Romans' season at the RST: Tullus Lieutenant in *Coriolanus*; Metellus Cimber in *Julius Caesar*; Proculeius in *Antony and Cleopatra*; and Bassianus in *Titus Andronicus*. In 1974 he was promoted to play Posthumus in *Cymbeline* (John Barton, RST), and Dr Watson in the John Wood *Sherlock Holmes* (Aldwych).

The popularity of *Holmes* initiated Pigott-Smith's screen career. His authoritative acting was a memorable feature of BBC drama of the mid to late 1970s: *Glittering Prizes* (1975); *Eustace and Hilda* (1977); *The Lost Boys* (1978); Angelo in *Measure for Measure* (1978); Hotspur in *Henry IV Part One* (1979); and Vasques in *'Tis Pity She's a Whore* (Roland Joffé, 1979). After *The Jewel in the Crown* (Christopher Morahan and Jim O'Brien, ITV, 1984), in which he enjoyed his biggest success as the sadistic Captain Merrick, he returned to the London stage, creating the role of Colin in Michael Frayn's *Benefactors* (Michael Blakemore, Vaudeville, 1984), and organising a one-man show called *Bengal Lancer* (Lyric Hammersmith, 1985). Perhaps to avoid further Merricks he took bland jobs—Agatha Christie's *Dead Man's Folly* (1986); *The Challenge* (1986); *The Chief* (ITV, 1990)—and missed out on the kind of chance in Hollywood that momentarily lifted the careers of his *Jewel* co-stars Charles Dance and Art Malik. Instead, he continued in the theatre. For three outstanding years from 1986 he worked for Peter Hall at the National: Stephen Poliakoff's *Coming into Land* (Lyttelton, 1986); Octavius Caesar in the Anthony Hopkins/Judi Dench *Antony and Cleopatra* (Olivier, 1987); Henry in David Edgar's *Entertaining Strangers* (Cottesloe, 1987); and the 'Late Romances'—Leontes in *A Winter's Tale*, Iachimo in *Cymbeline*, and Trinculo in *The Tempest* (Cottesloe, 1987). In 1989 he succeeded Anthony Quayle as Artistic Director of Compass Theatre, a position he held until the Arts Council withdrew the company's grant in 1992. He directed *Royal Hunt of the Sun*, and performed Brutus in *Julius Caesar* and Salieri in *Amadeus*.

Subsequent theatre: Rochester in *Jane Eyre* (Playhouse, 1993); director of the Damian Lewis *Hamlet* (Regent's Park, 1994); the National's 1996 season—Leicester in *Mary Stuart* (Howard Davies, Lyttelton), Subtle in *The Alchemist* (Bill Alexander, Olivier); Larry Slade in the Kevin Spacey *Iceman Cometh* (Davies, Almeida, 1998); Scrooge in *A Christmas Carol* (Lyric, Hammersmith, 2002-03); Ezra Mannon in *Mourning Becomes Electra* (Davies, NT Lyttelton, 2003-04); Agamemnon in *Hecuba* (Jonathan Kent, Donmar Warehouse, 2004); the bishop in Philip King's farce *See How They Run* (Douglas Hodge, Duchess, 2006); and, back at the RSC, a fascinatingly complex Cassius in *Julius Caesar* (Edward Hall, RST, 2001-02), and the Duke of Florence in *Women Beware Women* (Laurence Boswell, Swan, 2006).

Since the early 2000s Pigott-Smith's ability as a character actor has once more started to find recognition on the screen: General Ford in *Bloody Sunday* (Paul Greengrass, 2002); Bertrand Tavernier's *Laissez-passer* (2002); Martin Scorsese's *Gangs of New York* (2002); *Spooks* (BBC, 2002); *The Vice* (ITV, 2002-03); *Johnny English* (2003); General Feversham in *The Four Feathers* (Shekhar Kapur, 2003); Nick Dear's *Eroica* (BBC, 2003); *The Private Life of Samuel Pepys* (BBC, 2003); *London* (BBC, 2004); *North and South* (BBC, 2004); *Alexander* (Oliver Stone, 2004); *V for Vendetta* (2005); *Flyboys* (2006); *L'Entente cordiale* (2006).

Harold Pinter (b. London, 1930) grew up in Hackney and trained at RADA. During the years he spent as a struggling actor, living in guest houses and working in drab provincial theatres, he published poetry and short stories and wrote his first one-act plays, *The Room* (performed by students at Bristol University in 1957) and *The Dumb Waiter* (eventually staged by the Royal Court in 1960). He sent *The Birthday Party*, his first full-length work, to Peter Hall at the Arts Theatre Club, but Hall wasn't free. The play, directed by Peter Wood at the Arts Theatre, Cambridge, and the Lyric Hammersmith in 1958, was largely misunderstood, although Harold Hobson wrote a glowing notice in *The Sunday Times*. Pinter had found his voice. The play's setting—a seaside boarding house—is deliberately mundane, seedy and metaphorical. Its language is spare and poetic (Pinter's assortment of losers and predators use words as a means of inflicting all kinds and degrees of damage). Its theme is the constant threat of other people. Pinter's next full-length work, *The Caretaker*, brought him critical recognition and fame.

Hall was keen to secure Pinter's work for the RSC. He staged a play originally written for television, *The Collection* (1962), and invited the author to direct Patrick Magee, Brewster Mason, Bryan Pringle and Janet Suzman in a revival of *The Birthday Party* at the Aldwych (1964). The production opened a repertory of challenging contemporary works that became known as 'the dirty plays' season after the phrase used by an outraged Emile Littler.

Pinter's next work, *The Homecoming*, was duly delivered. Hall's associates, including Peter Brook and John Barton, were not convinced that the play had enough quality to play on the main stage. Hall overruled them. His direction matched the poetic economy of the writing (as did John Bury's ash-grey set). *The Homecoming* is about the struggle for dominance within an all-male London family and the disruption caused by the trophy wife one of the sons brings home from America. Is the family Jewish, inspired by the Hackney of Pinter's childhood? The answer, properly Pinteresque, is 'yes and no'. Hackney may have been the inspiration, but the play is about human psychology, male and female, at its most basic level. The theme is elevated by Pinter's mastery of language, metaphors and ambiguity. Hall's cast included Paul Rogers as the father, Ian Holm as Lenny, the pimp, and Vivien Merchant, Pinter's wife, as Ruth. After a provincial tour beginning in Cardiff the production played at the Aldwych (1965).

Pinter stayed with the RSC until Hall left to run the National in 1973. Terry Hands staged a revival of *The Dumb Waiter* for Theatregoround in 1967; and Hall directed *Landscape* and *Silence* as a double-bill in 1969, and *Old Times*, Pinter's first full-length work since *The Homecoming*, in 1971. During the same season Pinter directed a production of James Joyce's *Exiles*.

Tom Piper (b. London, 1964) has been the most influential designer at the RSC since 2000. He became interested in theatre design while studying at Trinity College, Cambridge. His friend Sam Mendes (they'd both gone up to Cambridge from Magdalen College School, Oxford) was directing student shows and Piper was soon designing them. He switched degree courses from Natural Sciences to Art History, and went on to study theatre design at the Slade School. He spent six months with Peter Brook's company in Paris, assisting Chloë Obolensky, the designer of Brook's production of *La tempête* (1990), and established his reputation at the Soho Poly Theatre, the Tabard Theatre, Chiswick (*A Cat in the Ghetto*), and the Orange Tree Theatre, Richmond. His partnership with Michael Boyd was formed at the Tron, Glasgow, with the Iain Glen *Macbeth* (1993) and *Dumbstruck* (1994).

Piper creates settings from pale wood or rusting metal, and favours clean lines and limited decoration—his structures have sculptural elegance. He first worked at the RSC in 1994; since 2003 he has been an associate artist and Boyd's head of design. If Piper's main current task is to make the Courtyard work as a blank page for inspired design, he's been given an impossible brief. If the new RST is like the Courtyard his role will surely become redundant.

Piper has designed all of Boyd's RSC productions—*The Broken Heart* (Swan, 1994); *Much Ado About Nothing* (RST, 1996); *The Spanish Tragedy* (Swan, 1997); *Measure for Measure* (RST, 1998); *Troilus and Cressida* (Pit, 1998); *A Midsummer Night's Dream* (RST, 1999); *Romeo and Juliet* (RST, 2000); *Henry VI* (Swan, 2000); *Richard III* (Swan, 2001); *The Tempest* (Roundhouse, 2002); *Hamlet* (RST, 2004); *Twelfth Night* (RST, 2005); and the *Henries* (Courtyard, 2006-08). Other RSC shows: *Spring Awakening* (Tim Supple, Pit, 1995); *A Patriot for Me* (Peter Gill, Barbican, 1995);

Bartholomew Fair (Laurence Boswell, Swan, 1997); *A Month in the Country* (Michael Attenborough, Swan, 1998); *King Lear* (Bill Alexander, RST, 2004); and *Solstice* (Zinnie Harris, TOP, 2005).

Elsewhere, Piper has worked with Mendes (*Cardboard City*, Soho Poly Theatre, 1989, *The Birthday Party*, NT Lyttelton, 1994); Brian Cox (*Mrs Warren's Profession*, Orange Tree, 1989, *The Master Builder*, Royal Lyceum, Edinburgh, 1993); Philip Franks (*The Duchess of Malfi*, Greenwich Theatre, 1995); Ron Daniels (*Blinded by the Sun*, NT Cottesloe, 1996); and Stephen Poliakoff (*Sweet Panic*, Hampstead Theatre, 1996).

Christopher Plummer (b. Toronto, 1929) made his name on Broadway and at Stratford, Ontario, where he was the most important homegrown actor to take leading roles in the first years of the Shakespeare Festival under William Gaskill and Michael Langham (1956-60). Throughout his career he has seemed both American (he has the look of a stereotypical US president) and English (a fine verse-speaker, his classical work places him in the orthodox tradition of Shakespearean acting).

Educated in Montreal, he began his career at the Canadian Repertory Theatre in Ottawa (Faulkland in *The Rivals*, 1950). Within five years he was acting in New York: George Phillips in *The Starcross Story* (Royale Theatre, 1954); Mancester Monaghan in *Home is the Hero* (Booth, 1954); Count Zichy in *The Dark is Light Enough* (ANTA, 1955); the Earl of Warwick in *The Lark* (Longacre, 1955); Lewis in *Night of the Auk* (Playhouse, 1956); and Nickles in *J.B.* (ANTA, 1958). His Stratford, Ontario, career began in 1956 with the title role in *Henry V*: the production travelled to the Edinburgh Festival. He subsequently played Hamlet, opening the festival's first permanent theatre (1957); Aguecheek in *Twelfth Night* (1957); Benedick in *Much Ado About Nothing* (1958); Leontes in *The Winter's Tale* (1958); Bardolph in *Henry IV Part One* (1958); and the Bastard in *King John* (1960).

His reputation crossed the Atlantic. Peter Hall brought him to the RSC in 1961 to play roles originally designated for Peter

O'Toole, directed by his Ontario colleagues: Benedick to Geraldine McEwan's Beatrice in *Much Ado About Nothing* (Michael Langham, RST); the title role in *Richard III* (William Gaskill, RST); and King Henry to Eric Porter's *Becket* (Peter Hall, Aldwych).

A BBC *Hamlet*, filmed in Elsinore, extended his popularity in Britain (1964), while *The Sound of Music* (1965) made him an international star. His stature as a Shakespearean has meant that, in features, he has often played famous men from history and literature, but his long list of credits also contains light comedies and musicals. Movies that contain essential Plummer performances: *The Night of the Generals* (1967); *The Battle of Britain* (1968); *The Royal Hunt of the Sun* (1969); *Waterloo* (1970); *The Man Who Would Be King* (John Huston, 1975); *Wolf* (Mike Nichols, 1994); *Dolores Claiborne* (Taylor Hackford, 1995); *Twelve Monkeys* (Terry Gilliam, 1996); *The Insider* (Michael Mann, 1999); and *Ararat* (Atom Egoyan, 2002).

In 1971/72 he joined Olivier's National Theatre at the Old Vic to appear in Jean Giraudoux's *Amphytrion 38* (Olivier) and Büchner's *Danton's Death* (Jonathan Miller). He has returned to the New York stage at intervals: the title role in *Cyrano* (1973); *The Good Doctor* (1974); Iago in *Othello* (1982); the title role in *Macbeth* (1988); Harold Pinter's *No Man's Land* (1994); *Barrymore* (1997); and the title role in *King Lear* (Miller, Lincoln Center, 2004).

Eric Porter (1928-1995, b. London). The son of a London bus conductor, Eric Porter studied electrical engineering at Wimbledon Technical College and started work at sixteen for the Marconi Company. At the same time he sought admission to RADA but was rejected. A district schools drama organiser, who had seen Porter's school performances, provided an introduction to Robert Atkins, director of the Shakespeare Memorial Theatre: this led to a non-speaking part in the SMT's production of *Twelfth Night*, visiting Cambridge (Arts Theatre, 1945), and bit parts at Stratford, including Mat Muggins in *She Stoops to Conquer* (1945). He made his London debut as Dunois' Page in *Saint Joan* (Travelling Repertory Company, Lyric Hammersmith, 1946).

After national service in the RAF (1946-47) he spent ten years building his reputation, at the Birmingham Rep (1948-50), the Bristol Old Vic (Becket in *Murder in the Cathedral*, the title roles in *King Lear, Uncle Vanya, Volpone*, 1954-56), the Old Vic (Jacques in *As You Like It*, Bolingbroke in *Richard II*, the title role in *Henry IV*, 1954-55), the Lyric Hammersmith (Bolingbroke to Paul Scofield's *Richard II*, Fainall in *The Way of the World*, Reynault in Peter Brook's *Venice Preserv'd*, for Gielgud's Company, 1953), and elsewhere (Peter Ustinov's *Romanoff and Juliet*, Piccadilly, 1956; Brook's *Time and Again*, Theatre Royal, Brighton, 1957). *Time and Again*, renamed *The Visit*, took him to New York in 1958. His performance as Rosmer in George Devine's production of Ibsen's *Rosmersholm* (Royal Court, 1959) brought him the Evening Standard Award for Best Actor.

He was a central member of Peter Hall's first Stratford ensemble in 1960, and, as an associate artist, spent the rest of that decade with the RSC. He was only in his thirties but he had an older man's authority, capable of a stern and forbidding demeanour that leant itself to rulers and churchmen—Ulysses in *Troilus and Cressida* (Hall, RST, 1960), the title role in Jean Anouilh's *Becket* (Hall, Aldwych, 1961), Macbeth (Donald McWhinnie, RST, 1962) and Bolingbroke in *Richard II* (Hall et al, RST, 1964) were formidably presented. He also played strong men in decline or crisis—Leontes in *The Winter's Tale* (Peter Wood, RST, 1960), Henry IV (the continuation of Bolingbroke, played in the same season), the title role in *Doctor Faustus* (Clifford Williams, RST, 1968)—and the deluded Malvolio in *Twelfth Night* (Hall, RST, 1960).

Between Stratford seasons Porter found television fame as Soames in *The Forsyte Saga* (BBC, 1967), and for the next two decades he worked as a screen actor. Then suddenly, at the end of the 1980s, he returned, as powerful as ever: Big Daddy in *Cat on a Hot Tin Roof* (Howard Davies, NT Lyttelton, 1988); the title role in *King Lear* (Jonathan Miller, Old Vic, 1989); Malvolio in *Twelfth Night* (Hall, Playhouse, 1991); and Serebriakov in Uncle Vanya (Sean Mathias, NT Studio, Cottesloe, 1992).

After Soames, his most memorable television roles were Karenin in *Anna Karenina* (BBC, 1977); Alanbrooke in *Churchill and the Generals* (BBC, 1979); Danforth in *The Crucible* (BBC, 1980); Polonius in *Hamlet* (BBC, 1980); Neville Chamberlain in *Winston Churchill: the Wilderness Years* (1981); Dimitri Bronowsky in *The Jewel in the Crown* (1984); Moriarty in *The Adventures of Sherlock Holmes* (1984, 1985); and Fagin in *Oliver Twist* (BBC, 1985).

Pete Postlethwaite (b. Warrington, 1945). Pete Postlethwaite's roots are in Lancashire, in teaching and in the English theatre. Seasons at the Bristol Old Vic and the Liverpool Everyman were followed by roles in new plays in London. At the Royal Court he appeared in Howard Brenton's *Magnificence* (Max Stafford-Clark, 1973), David Storey's *Cromwell* (Anthony Page, 1973) and Bill Morrison's *Flying Blind* (Alan Dossor, 1978). At the Lyric Hammersmith, in Alan Bleasdale's *Having a Ball* (1981) and Stephen Poliakoff's *Favourite Nights* (1981). Other early work in London included Willy Russell's *Breezeblock Park* (1975) and Mike Stott's *Funny Peculiar* (Mermaid, 1976), while on television he appeared in two pieces by Alan Bennett directed by Stephen Frears, *Doris and Doreen* (1978) and *Afternoon Off* (1979). In 1980, at the Manchester Royal Exchange, he blacked up to play Jones in Eugene O'Neill's *The Emperor Jones* (Richard Negri), and gave a memorable performance as Antonio alongside Helen Mirren, Bob Hoskins and Mike Gwilym in Adrian Noble's production of *The Duchess of Malfi*.

The success of the latter took Postlethwaite to the RSC, where he was cast as Macduff in the Bob Peck *Macbeth* (Howard Davies, RST, 1982); Cornwall in the Michael Gambon *King Lear* (Noble, RST, 1982); Soldier in Edward Bond's *Lear* (Barry Kyle,

TOP, 1982); Grumio in *The Taming of the Shrew* (Kyle, RST, 1982); Ragueneau in *Cyrano de Bergerac* (Terry Hands, Barbican, 1983); Hastings, succeeding Brian Blessed, in *Richard III* (Bill Alexander, Barbican, 1985); Exeter, succeeding Blessed, in the Kenneth Branagh *Henry V* (Noble, Barbican, 1985); Brodin in *Red Noses* (Hands, Barbican, 1985); the ruffian Bobadill, played as a self-deluding exhibitionist, in Ben Jonson's *Every Man in His Humour* (John Caird, Swan, 1986); Bottom, played with comic mastery as a dignified fantasist and serious mime artist, in *A Midsummer Night's Dream* (Bill Alexander, RST, 1986); and the sea-dog Roughman in Thomas Heywood's *The Fair Maid of the West* (Trevor Nunn, Swan, 1986).

Postlethwaite's film career took flight at the end of the 1980s. He is an exponent of both British angst and Hollywood fantasy: *A Private Function* (Malcolm Mowbray, 1985); the abusive father in *Distant Voices, Still Lives* (Terence Davies, 1988); *Alien 3* (David Fincher, 1992); *The Last of the Mohicans* (Michael Mann, 1992); Giuseppe Conlon in *In the Name of the Father* (James Sheridan, 1993); Kobayashi in *The Usual Suspects* (Bryan Singer, 1995); Father Laurence in *Romeo and Juliet* (Baz Luhrmann, 1996); *Brassed Off* (Mark Herman, 1996); *The Lost World: Jurassic Park* (Steven Spielberg, 1997); *Amistad* (Spielberg, 1997); *The Shipping News* (Lasse Hallström, 2001); *Dark Water* (Walter Salles, 2005); and *The Constant Gardener* (Fernando Meirelles, 2005). On television, he played Hakeswill in *Sharpe's Enemy* and *Sharpe's Company* (ITV, 1994).

Postlethwaite's rare theatre appearances since 1990: the bookie in Jim Cartwright's *The Rise and Fall of Little Voice* (Sam Mendes, NT Cottesloe, 1992); Max in *The Homecoming* (Gregory Hersov, Manchester Royal Exchange, 2002); *Scaramouche Jones* (Dublin Festival, 2001); a fine Prospero in *The Tempest* (Hersov, Manchester Royal Exchange, 2007); and the title role in *King Lear* (Rupert Goold, Liverpool Everyman, 2008).

Claire Price (b. Chesterfield, Derbyshire, 1972). 2002/03 was an outstanding year for Claire Price. She began the year at the Sheffield Crucible, playing Lady Anne opposite Kenneth Branagh in *Richard III* (Michael Grandage), and ended it at the RSC as Agnes opposite Ralph Fiennes in *Brand* (Adrian Noble, Swan). In-between she was Miranda in the Derek Jacobi *The Tempest* (Grandage), a Sheffield production that transferred to the Old Vic. It was back in 1999, at the RSC, that she first came to notice. Her success as Celia in *Volpone* (Lindsay Posner, Swan) and Princess Eboli in *Don Carlos* (Gale Edwards, TOP) led to the role of Berinthia in Trevor Nunn's *The Relapse* at the National (Olivier, 2001).

The daughter of the actor John Price, she read English at Queen Mary's College, London, before training at the Guildford School of Acting. Her early opportunities included Angela in David Williamson's *Dead White Males* (Nuffield Theatre, Southampton, 1996); Louisa in *Hard Times* (Sue Pomeroy, Good Company, Tour, 1997); and the title role in Howard Barker's *Ursula* (Wrestling School, Tour, 1998). Following her first season at the RSC she played Rosalind in *As You Like It* at the Manchester Royal Exchange (Marianne Elliott, 2000), and Olivia in *Twelfth Night* at the Liverpool Playhouse (James Kerr, 2001).

Since *Brand* Claire Price has played Roxane in the Stephen Rea *Cyrano de Bergerac* at the National (Howard Davies, Olivier, 2004); Queen Elizabeth in the Jacobi/Grandage *Don Carlos* at the Sheffield Crucible (2004); Beatrice in *Much Ado About Nothing* also at the Crucible (Josie Rourke, 2005); the title role in *Doctor Faustus* at the Bristol Old Vic (David Fielding, 2006); and, on television, DS Clarke in *Rebus* (2006-07).

Jonathan Pryce (b. Holywell, North Wales, 1947) made his name in the 1970s with four typically audacious and suspenseful theatre performances: Richard, a psychopath in a tracksuit, in *Richard III* (Alan Dossor, Liverpool Everyman, 1973); the shaven-headed comic in Trevor Griffiths's *Comedians* (Richard

Eyre, Nottingham Playhouse, 1975); Petruchio in *The Taming of the Shrew* (Michael Bogdanov, RST, 1978), the highlight of his first RSC season; and the title role in *Hamlet* (Eyre, Royal Court, 1980). At the beginning of Bogdanov's production of *The Shrew* an unruly drunk invaded the auditorium—he turned out to be Pryce.

Pryce trained at RADA. At the Liverpool Everyman during the early 1970s he led a troupe that included Antony Sher, Bernard Hill, Peter Postlethwaite and Julia Walters and directed productions of *The Taming of the Shrew, The Sea Anchor, Cantril Tales* and *A Taste of Honey.* At the RSC, 1978-79, as well as his chauvinistic Petruchio—gleefully bullying Paola Dionisotti's Kate—he played Angelo in *Measure for Measure* (Barry Kyle, RST) and Octavius in Peter Brook's *Antony and Cleopatra* (RST). He returned in 1986: his performance as *Macbeth* (Adrian Noble, RST) had typical originality and daring in its use of humour, vocal sounds and manic behaviour and was riveting in its externalisation of the agony of conscience. Elsewhere, his work included Mick in Howard Pinter's *The Caretaker* (Kenneth Ives, NT Lyttelton, 1980); Trigorin to Vanessa Redgrave's Arkadina in *The Seagull* (Lyric Hammersmith, 1985); and Astrov in *Uncle Vanya* (Michael Blakemore, Vaudeville, 1988).

Pryce's success as the Engineer in the musical *Miss Saigon* (Nicholas Hytner, Drury Lane, 1989) refashioned his career. He subsequently played Fagan in *Oliver!* (Sam Mendes, Palladium, 1994), Perón opposite Madonna in the movie of *Evita* (Alan Parker, 1996), and Higgins in *My Fair Lady* (Trevor Nunn, NT Lyttelton, 2001).

Pryce starred in two of the best British features of the 1980s, *The Ploughman's Lunch* (Ian McEwan/Richard Eyre, 1983) and Terry Gilliam's *Brazil* (1985). Since the beginning of the 1990s his versatile skill has been showcased in contrasting roles—James Lingk in *Glengarry Glen Ross* (James Foley, 1992); Rivière in Martin Scorsese's *The Age of Innocence* (1993); Lytton Strachey in *Carrington* (Christopher Hampton, 1995); the villain—a media mogul—in the Bond film *Tomorrow Never Dies* (1997); William

Rivers in *Regeneration* (Gillies MacKinnon, 1997); O'Rourke in *Ronin* (John Frankenheimer, 1998); Governor Swann in *Pirates of the Caribbean* (2003-07); King James in *The New World* (Terrence Malick, 2005); and Frazier in *Leatherheads* (George Clooney, 2008).

Q

Hugh Quarshie (b. Accra, Ghana, 1954). Hugh Quarshie's acting career began at Oxford University, where he was a co-director of the Oxford and Cambridge Shakespeare Company and played the title role in *Othello* for the University Dramatic Society (Playhouse, 1976). A charismatic actor whose interests extend beyond the theatre, he was President of the Oxford University African Society and on graduating (from Christ Church) worked for *West Africa Magazine*.

His early professional appearances, including *Charlie and the Chocolate Factory* (Round-a-Bout Theatre, Nottingham), *Black Ball Game* (Crucible, Sheffield), and *Whose Life is it Anyway?* (Savoy, 1979), were followed by a small role in the film *Dogs of War* (John Irvin, 1980).

He joined the RSC in 1981, cast as Aaron and Outlaw in John Barton's double-bill of *Titus Andronicus* and *The Two Gentlemen of Verona* (RST), and Cleomenes in *The Winter's Tale* (Ronald Eyre, RST). On the transfer to London (1982), he played Vernon/Hastings in *Henry IV* (Trevor Nunn, Barbican) before succeeding Timothy Dalton as Hotspur. In 1986/87 he was an arrogant, image-conscious Tybalt in *Romeo and Juliet* (Michael Bogdanov, RST), and brought considerable presence to the uncomplicated roles of Arcite in *The Two Noble Kinsmen* (Barry Kyle, Swan), Banquo in the Jonathan Pryce *Macbeth* (Adrian Noble, RST), and Belville in *The Rover* (John Barton, Swan). In 1995/96 he was a cool, stylish Mephistopheles in Michael Bogdanov's modern-dress production of *Faust* (Swan), Loveless in

The Relapse (Ian Judge, Swan), and Mark Antony in Peter Hall's *Julius Caesar* (RST).

Between RSC seasons, he played the title role in *The Admirable Crichton* (James Maxwell, Manchester Royal Exchange, 1984-85); Jack Jefferson in Howard Sackler's *The Great White Hope* (Nicolas Kent, Tricycle, 1985); Levee in August Wilson's *Ma Rainey's Black Bottom* (Howard Davies, NT Cottesloe, 1989); Sky Masterson in *Guys and Dolls* (Bogdanov, Deutsches Schauspielhaus, Hamburg, 1990); and the American doctor in Frank McGuinness's *Someone to Watch Over Me* (Robin Lefevre, Hampstead Theatre, 1992).

Quarshie has performed one of the leading roles in the BBC's *Holby City* since 2002. *The Murder of Stephen Lawrence* (Paul Greengrass, 1999) contains his best work on screen.

R

George Raistrick (1931-1995) trained at the London Academy of Music and Dramatic Art. He joined the RSC in 1978 to play Egeus in *A Midsummer Night's Dream* (John Barton) and Menecrates in *Antony and Cleopatra* (Peter Brook) and stayed for twelve years. He avoided the histories (so often the character actor's graveyard at Stratford), preferring the more idiosyncratic worlds of the comedies.

Alongside his classical work—Vincentio in *The Taming of the Shrew* (Michael Bogdanov, RST, 1978), Balderdash in George Farquhar's *The Twin Rivals* (John Caird, TOP, 1981), Carter in Dekker, Ford and Rowley's *The Witch of Edmonton* (Barry Kyle, TOP, 1981), Capulet in *Romeo and Juliet* (Caird, Small-scale Tour, 1983), Snout in *A Midsummer Night's Dream* (Sheila Hancock, Small-scale Tour, 1983), Dull in *Love's Labour's Lost* (Kyle, RST, 1984), Friar Bernardine in Marlowe's *The Jew of Malta* (Kyle, Swan, 1987), Baptista in *The Taming of the Shrew* (Jonathan Miller, RST, 1987), Elbow in *Measure for Measure* (Nicholas Hytner, RST, 1987), Dogberry in *Much Ado About Nothing* (Alexander, RST, 1990) and Old Spencer in Marlowe's *Edward II* (Gerard Murphy, Swan, 1990)—he created roles in Peter Whelan's *Captain Swing* (Alexander, TOP, 1978), Nigel Baldwin's *Men's Beano* (Alexander, Warehouse, 1979), Peter Flannery's *Our Friends in the North* (Caird, Pit, 1982), Louise Page's *Golden Girls* (Kyle, TOP, 1984), Robert Holman's *Today* (Alexander, TOP, 1984) and Richard Nelson's *Two Shakespearean Actors* (Roger Michell, Swan, 1990). He also brought his moody individuality to Gerald Morn in Howard Brenton's *The Churchill Play* (Barry Kyle, TOP, 1978); Hetman in Mikhail Bulgakov's *The White Guard* (Kyle, Aldwych, 1979); Lamp in John O'Keeffe's *Wild Oats* (Williams, Aldwych, 1979); Bishop in Hart and Kaufman's *Once in a Lifetime* (Trevor Nunn, Aldwych, 1979); Mr Graves in Edward Bulwer-Lytton's *Money* (Alexander, TOP, 1981); Smee in *Peter Pan* (Nunn/Caird, Barbican, 1982-83); the lawyer in Strindberg's *Dreamplay* (Barton, Pit, 1985); and Mr Kenwigs in *Nicholas Nickleby* (Nunn/Caird, RST, 1985-86).

On leaving the RSC Raistrick was cast by Sam Mendes in *The Rise and Fall of Little Voice* (NT Cottesloe, 1992), and *Cabaret* (Donmar Warehouse, 1993). At the time of his death in 1995 he was playing Arturo Taddei in *La grande magia* at the National (Richard Eyre, Lyttelton).

Emily Raymond (b. Los Angeles, 1967). The daughter of the British actors Gary Raymond and Delena Kidd, Emily Raymond studied at Manchester Polytechnic and made her professional debut as Nina in *The Seagull* at the Birmingham Rep (Anthony Clark, Studio, 1990). Her next engagements were Miranda in *The Tempest* at the Manchester Royal Exchange (Braham Murray, 1990); and Helena in *A Midsummer Night's Dream*, Lady Macduff in *Macbeth* and Fatima in *The Boys From Syracuse* at the Open Air Theatre, Regent's Park (1991).

She joined the RSC in 1992 and gave fine performances in the Swan as the spirited Meriel in Richard Brome's *A Jovial Crew*

(Max Stafford-Clark); Mrs Vixen in *The Beggar's Opera* (John Caird); Mariana in Peter Hall's *All's Well That Ends Well*; and Isabella in *The Changeling* (Michael Attenborough).

Leading roles at lower-profile theatres followed: Gloria in *You Never Can Tell* (Mercury Theatre, Colchester); Juliet in *Romeo and Juliet* (Gateway Theatre, Chester); Curly's Wife in *Of Mice and Men* (Dominic Cooke, Nottingham Playhouse, 1994). She then re-entered the national spotlight at Chichester, playing Julia in *The Rivals* and Olwyn in *Dangerous Corner* (1994).

In 1995 she was both funny and affecting as Helena in Adrian Noble's RSC production of *A Midsummer Night's Dream* (Barbican). In 2000/01 she played Lydia in *The Rivals* (Lindsay Posner, Swan) and Adriana in *The Comedy of Errors* (Lynne Parker, RST); in 2004/05, Lady Capulet in *Romeo and Juliet* (Peter Gill) and Goneril in *King Lear* (Bill Alexander, RST).

Corin Redgrave (b. London, 1939) was one of the best fencers of his generation, a British title holder at junior level. He graduated from King's College, Cambridge, with a first in English, and then, inevitably, joined the family firm—acting. From the start he seemed a dissatisfied actor: during the crucial years he became an active member of the Workers' Revolutionary Party, and, in partnership with his sister Vanessa, was lampooned by the tabloids as a champagne socialist and crank.

At Cambridge, as well as acting alongside Ian McKellen, Derek Jacobi, Trevor Nunn and others, he directed student productions, including a one-play adaptation of *Henry VI* with McKellen and Nunn. On graduating he took up an appointment as Tony Richardson's assistant at the Royal Court. Richardson persuaded him to continue as an actor and he played Lysander in *A Midsummer Night's Dream* (Richardson, 1962) and the pilot in Arnold Wesker's *Chips With Everything* (John Dexter, 1962). His subsequent early stage work included *The Right Honourable Gentleman* (West End, 1964, with Anthony Quayle and Anna Massey) and *Lady Windermere's Fan* (1966). His early films were

Crooks in Cloisters (1963); *A Man for All Seasons* (Fred Zinne-mann, 1966); *The Deadly Affair* (Sidney Lumet, 1967); Richardson's *The Charge of the Light Brigade* (1968); *The Magus* (Guy Green, 1968); *Oh! What a Lovely War* (Richard Attenbor-ough, 1969); *When Eight Bells Toll* (1971); and *Von Richtohofen and Brown* (Roger Corman, 1971). On television he played the lead, opposite Susan George and Judy Geeson, in the soap *The New-comers* (1966), and the villain in an adaptation of *The Tenant of Wildfell Hall* (BBC, 1967). He was in episodes of *The Avengers* (1964) and *Callan* (1971).

He joined the RSC for one two-year cycle, 1972-73, and played Octavius Caesar in *Julius Caesar* and *Antony and Cleopatra* (Trevor Nunn/Buzz Goodbody, RST) and Antipholus of Syra-cuse in *The Comedy of Errors* (Clifford Williams, RST). This was at the height of his activism with the Workers' Revolutionary Party, and members of the Arts Council expressed unease about his presence in the publicly-funded RSC. Redgrave believes that the BBC blacklisted him for over twenty years.

It was not until the 1980s that he re-emerged as an actor with roles in John Boorman's *Excalibur* (1981), Nicholas Roeg's *Eureka* (1982), and the mini-series *Wagner* (1983). Since the beginning of the 1990s he has been busier, and more powerful, than ever be-fore, both as a freelance actor and as the director of Moving Theatre, the company he co-founded with Vanessa Redgrave: the title role in *Coriolanus* (Jane Howell, Young Vic, 1989); Ros-mer to Francesca Annis's Rebekka in *Rosmersholm* (Annie Castledine, Young Vic, 1992); Moving Theatre's first two years—an adaptation of Robert Shaw's *The Flag* (Redgrave played the lead and directed) at the Bridge Lane Theatre (1994), the Bosnian *Silk Drums*, *Antony and Cleopatra* and Maureen Law-rence's *Real Writing* (Redgrave directed his wife Kika Markham as Anna Akhmatova) at the Riverside Studios (1995), Sara Salih's *Ousama* at the Brixton Shaw Theatre (1995), and *Julius Caesar* (Redgrave directed and played the title role) at the Abbey Theatre, Houston (1996); Frank Elgin, a role originally played by his father, in Clifford Odet's *The Country Girl* (Annie Castledine,

411

Greenwich Theatre, 1995); Horatio in Martin Sherman's *Some Sunny Day* (Roger Michell, Hampstead Theatre, 1996); Marat in *Marat/Sade* (Jeremy Sams, NT Olivier, 1997); the Duke of Windsor in Snoo Wilson's *HRH* (Playhouse, 1997); Sir Hugo in Noël Coward's *Song at Twilight* (Sheridan Morley, King's Head, 1999); the title role in *Macbeth* (Tom Morris, BAC, 2000); Hirst to John Wood's Spooner in Harold Pinter's *No Man's Land* (Pinter, NT Lyttelton, 2001-02); Crocker-Harris in Terence Rattigan's *The Browning Version* (Mark Clements, Derby Playhouse, 2002); Anthony Blunt in his own monologue *Blunt Speaking* (Clements, Minerva, Chichester, 2002); George in Joanna Murray-Smith's *Honour* (Michell, NT Cottesloe, 2003); opening the new Garrick Theatre in Lichfield — Captain Brazen in *The Recruiting Officer* (Redgrave/Castledine, complete with a new political epilogue by Tony Harrison), and Samuel Johnson in Maureen Lawrence's *Resurrection* (2003); Archie Rice in John Osborne's *The Entertainer* (John Tiffany, Liverpool Playhouse, 2004); and the title role in *Pericles* (Globe, 2005).

Redgrave returned to the RSC during the Adrian Noble era to play George Washington in Richard Nelson's *The General from America* (Howard Davies, Swan, 1996), and he led Michael Boyd's first full season of work (2004/05) — the title role in *King Lear* (Bill Alexander, RST), and the one-man show *Tynan* (Swan).

Contempt for the Establishment can be seen in his many depictions of politicians and officials: as Dixon in *In the Name of the Father* (Jim Sheridan, 1993) and the prison governor in Tennessee Williams's *Not About Nightingales* (Nunn, NT Cottesloe, 1998) his face had a pallor of corruption and callousness. He continued the prison injustice theme by performing Wilde's *De Profundis* (Moving Theatre, NT 'Platform', 1998).

He wrote much of his ailing father's autobiography, *In My Mind's Eye* (1983), and two years later published a fine memoir called *Michael Redgrave, My Father* (Richard Cohen Books). The book reveals the extent to which he is haunted by his father.

Vanessa Redgrave (b. London, 1937) emerged from the shadow of her father at Stratford, where in 1959 she followed small parts in *Othello* (Tony Richardson) and *All's Well That Ends Well* (Tyrone Guthrie) with Helena in *A Midsummer Night's Dream* (Peter Hall) and Valeria in the Laurence Olivier *Coriolanus* (Hall). Although golden-haired and beautiful, her strapping physique had earned her the nickname 'Big Van' at drama school. Blessed with natural ability, she progressed to Rosalind in *As You Like It* (Michael Elliott, RST, 1961) and Kate in *The Taming of the Shrew* (Maurice Daniels, Aldwych, 1961). She only played Rosalind because Dorothy Tutin fell ill, but her performance was received with rapture, an absolute rarity; she was suddenly the most fêted actress of a brilliant generation. She stayed with the RSC only for another year, playing Imogen in *Cymbeline* (William Gaskill, RST, 1962), before embarking on a film career. *Morgan, a Suitable Case for Treatment* (Karel Reisz, 1966), in which she is blonde and vivacious, and *Blow-Up* (Michelangelo Antonioni, 1967), in which she is dark and enigmatic, brought her to international prominence. Her reputation as a film actress rests on these and only a handful of other movies — *Isadora* (Reisz, 1968), *The Devils* (Ken Russell, 1971), *Julia* (Fred Zinnemann, 1976), *Wetherby* (David Hare, 1985), and *Howards End* (James Ivory, 1992).

She was her father's favourite and grew up wanting to be an actress. Following her training at Central she worked in repertory at the Frinton Summer Theatre (1957). Before her breakthrough in *As You Like It* she appeared in two productions with Sir Michael, *A Touch of the Sun* (Saville, 1958) and Robert Bolt's *The Tiger and the Horse* (Queen's, 1960), as well as *Look on Tempests* (1960) and *The Lady from the Sea* (Queen's, 1960).

The movies claimed her, but her status derives principally from the range and quality of her stage work. Notable performances have included Nina in *The Seagull* (Tony Richardson, Queen's, 1964); Jean Brodie in *The Prime of Miss Jean Brodie* (Wyndham's, 1966); Ellida in *The Lady from the Sea* (Elliott, Man-

413

chester Royal Exchange, 1978); Miss Tina in her father's adaptation of Henry James's *The Aspern Papers* (Theatre Royal Haymarket, 1984); Arkadina in *The Seagull* (Lyric Hammersmith, 1985); Mrs Alving in *Ghosts* (David Thacker, Young Vic, 1986); Mrs Hushabye in *Heartbreak House* (Trevor Nunn, Theatre Royal Haymarket, 1992); Ella in *John Gabriel Borkman* (Richard Eyre, NT Lyttelton, 1996); Ranevskaya in *The Cherry Orchard* (Nunn, NT Cottesloe, 2000); and Mary Tyrone in *Long Day's Journey into Night* (Robert Falls, New York, 2003).

Throughout her career she has worked with family members, friends and lovers, particularly her brother Corin, husband of 1962-67 Tony Richardson, Franco Nero, and Timothy Dalton. She appeared opposite Dalton in *The Taming of the Shrew* and *Antony and Cleopatra* (Toby Robertson, Theatr Clwyd, 1986), and *A Touch of the Poet* (Thacker, Young Vic, 1988). She and her daughter Joely Richardson portrayed the same character at different ages in *Wetherby* (1985). In 1990 she was joined by her sister Lynn and niece Jemma in *Three Sisters* (Queen's).

Roger Rees (b. Aberystwyth, 1944) was nine when his father, a policeman, moved the family from Wales to London (Balham). A talented artist, Rees studied painting at Camberwell Art School and the Slade. He was painting scenery at the Wimbledon Theatre when its manager offered him a part in a play (*Hindle Wakes*).

His emergence as a new RSC talent at the end of the 1970s followed ten years hard work as a young supporting player in the Company's ranks: unnamed parts in *The Taming of the Shrew* (Trevor Nunn, RST, 1967); Courtier in *The Revenger's Tragedy* (Nunn, RST, 1967); unnamed parts in *As You Like It* (David Jones, RST, 1967); Attendant in *The Relapse* (Nunn, Aldwych, 1967); Volumnius in *Julius Caesar* (John Barton, RST, 1968); Fenton in *The Merry Wives of Windsor* (Terry Hands, RST, 1968); Caddo in *Indians* (Jack Gelber, Aldwych, 1968); Patchbreech in *Pericles* (Hands, RST, 1969); First Servant in *The Winter's Tale*

(Nunn, RST, 1969); Curio in *Twelfth Night* (Barton, RST, 1969); Sir Henry Guildford in *Henry VIII* (Nunn, RST, 1969); Damashke in *The Plebeians Rehearse the Uprising* (David Jones, Aldwych, 1970); Stephen Undershaft in *Major Barbara* (Clifford Williams, Aldwych, 1970); Sir Pierce in *Richard II* (Barton, RST and Theatregoround, 1971); First Officer in Barton's *Twelfth Night* (RST, 1971); Claudio in *Much Ado About Nothing* (Ronald Eyre, RST, 1971); Roderigo in *Othello* (Barton, RST, 1971); Gratiano in *The Merchant of Venice* (Hands, Aldwych, 1972); Balin in *The Island of the Mighty* (Jones, Aldwych, 1972); and Young Courtly in *London Assurance* (Ronald Eyre, US Tour, 1974-75).

From 1976 his expressively energetic style was given full reign in both comedic and dramatic roles: Benvolio in *Romeo and Juliet* (Nunn, RST, 1976); Malcolm in *Macbeth* (Nunn, TOP, 1976); Young Shepherd in *The Winter's Tale* (Barton, RST, 1976); Antipholus of Syracuse in *The Comedy of Errors* (Nunn, RST, 1976); Ananias in *The Alchemist* (Nunn, TOP, 1977); Petulant in *The Way of the World* (Barton, Aldwych, 1978); Tusenbach in *Three Sisters* and Aguecheek in *Twelfth Night* for the first Small-scale Tour (Nunn and John Amiel, 1978); Posthumus to Judi Dench's Imogen in *Cymbeline* (Jones, RST, 1979); Podsekalnikov in Nikolai Erdman's *The Suicide* (Ron Daniels, TOP, 1979); Tusenbach in *Three Sisters* (Nunn, TOP, 1979); the title role in *Nicholas Nickleby* (Nunn, Aldwych, 1980); the title role in *Hamlet* (Ron Daniels, RST, 1984); and Berowne in *Love's Labour's Lost* (Barry Kyle, RST, 1984). These performances revealed an ability to shift mood line by line. He made Dickens's upright hero interesting through impetuosity. His Hamlet was surprisingly bitter.

Between RSC seasons, Rees played Young Marlow in *She Stoops to Conquer*, the brother in Brecht's *Fears and Miseries in the Third Reich*, Pierre in Ionesco's *Aunt Sally*, Kit in *French Without Tears*, Simple Simon in *Jack and the Beanstalk*, Algernon in *The Importance of Being Earnest* and Stanley in *The Birthday Party* (Cambridge Theatre Company, 1972-73, 1975); Vosco in *Paradise* (Theatre Upstairs, Royal Court, 1975); and Henry in Stoppard's *The Real Thing* (Strand, 1982). Since leaving the Company he has worked as a screen character actor in America, appearing in such diverse pieces as the films *Mountains of the Moon* (Bob Rafelson, 1990), *Robin Hood, Men in Tights* (Mel Brooks, 1993), *A Midsummer Night's Dream* (Michael Hoffman, 1999), *Frida* (Julie Taymor, 2002) and *The Tulse Luper Suitcases* (Peter Greenaway, 2003); and the television shows *Cheers* (1989-93) and *The West Wing* (2000-05).

Saskia Reeves (b. London, 1962). A Londoner, Saskia Reeves trained at the Guildhall School and worked for her Equity card in community and pub theatre (Covent Garden). She appeared in *Faust* at Clwyd, and first came to notice, a petite green-eyed girl with a beguiling manner, as a member of Cheek By Jowl, playing Hermia in *A Midsummer Night's Dream* and Harriet in Etherege's *Man of Mode* (both Declan Donnellan, Donmar Warehouse, 1985). At the Hampstead Theatre in 1986 she worked with Mike Leigh (*Smelling a Rat*) and starred opposite David Suchet as the disabled actress in Tom Kempinski's *Separation* (Michael Attenborough). She next played Greta in Steven Berkoff's *Metamorphosis* at the Mermaid (1986); Honey in *Who's Afraid of Virginia Woolf?* and Isabella in *Measure for Measure* at the Young Vic (David Thacker, 1987); Viola in *Twelfth Night* at the Manchester Royal Exchange (Braham Murray, 1988); and Jaq in Caryl Churchill's *Icecream* at the Royal Court (Max Stafford-Clark, 1989).

Her early film and television work, equally impressive, included the comedy *Antonia and Jane* (BBC, 1991), the powerful short *In My Defence* (BBC, 1990) and two Irish subjects directed by Thaddeus O'Sullivan and played out with the intensity of Greek tragedy, *December Bride* (1990) and *In the Border Country* (Channel Four, 1991). Her break in films came when she played the incestuous sister in Stephen Poliakoff's *Close My Eyes* (1991). In all of these she took a potentially melodramatic role and stripped it to the bone: intense but economical acting.

416

At the RSC in 1991/92 she performed in the smaller spaces. As Annabella in David Leveaux's modern-dress production of *'Tis Pity She's a Whore* (Swan) and Anne in Katie Mitchell's *A Woman Killed With Kindness* (TOP) she gave restrained, sensual performances. As Miranda in *The Virtuoso* (Phyllida Lloyd, Swan) she was acerbic in a pink party dress. Sylvia in *The Two Gentlemen of Verona* (David Thacker, Swan) was too dull a part to interest her much.

On leaving the Company, she played Regan in *King Lear* at the Royal Court (Max Stafford-Clark, 1993), and then starred in the films *Traps* (Pauline Chan, 1994), *I.D.* (Philip Davis, 1995), and, most notably, *Butterfly Kiss* (Michael Winterbottom, 1995), playing Amanda Plumber's mousy sidekick. In Malcolm McKay's BBC television film based on Zola's *La bête humaine*, *Cruel Train* (1996), she created a London *femme fatale*, a perform-ance of unglamorous pride and fatal hunger: working-class accent, red mouth used as a weapon. Her stage career continued with leading roles in Stephen Poliakoff's *Sweet Panic* (Hamp-stead Theatre, 1996); Cheek By Jowl's *Much Ado About Nothing* (Donnellan, International Tour, 1998); Rita Dove's *The Darker Face of the Earth* (NT Cottesloe, 1999); Tennessee Williams's *Orpheus Descending* (Nicholas Hytner, Donmar Warehouse, 2000); Roland Schimmelpfennig's *The Woman Before* (Richard Wilson, Royal Court, 2005); and Athol Fugard's *Hello and Goodbye* (Paul Robinson, English Touring Theatre, Trafalgar Studios, 2008).

Ian Richardson (1934-2007, b. Edinburgh) trained at the Col-lege of Dramatic Art in Glasgow and began his career at the Birmingham Rep (1958-59).

He was a major figure at the RSC from the Company's incep-tion in 1960/61 to 1975. Few actors have played as many classical roles; fewer still with such precision and style, for Richardson was easily the most imperious (and chilling) actor of his generation. The crystal clarity of his voice and the sheer in-ventiveness of his imagination linked all of the work: Sir

Andrew Aguecheek in *Twelfth Night* (Peter Hall, RST, 1960); Oberon to Judi Dench's Titania in *A Midsummer Night's Dream* (Hall, RST, 1962); Antipholus of Ephesus and Antipholus of Syracuse in *The Comedy of Errors* (Clifford Williams, RST, 1962, 1965); Edmund, succeeding James Booth, in the Paul Scofield *King Lear* (Peter Brook, Aldwych, 1964); Marat in *Marat/Sade* (Brook, Aldwych, 1964); Vendice in *The Revenger's Tragedy* (Trevor Nunn, RST, 1966); Ford in *The Merry Wives of Windsor* (Terry Hands, RST, 1968, 1975); the title role in *Pericles* (Hands, RST, 1969); Berowne to Estelle Kohler's Rosaline in *Love's Labour's Lost* (David Jones, RST, 1973); the title role in *Richard III* (Barry Kyle, TOP, 1975); and, for John Barton, the title role in *Coriolanus* (RST, 1967), Cassius in *Julius Caesar* (RST, 1968), Prospero in *The Tempest* (RST, 1970), Angelo to Estelle Kohler's Isabella in *Measure for Measure* (RST, 1970) and both Richard and Bolingbroke, alternated with Richard Pasco, in the renowned *Richard II* (RST, 1973).

Fifteen years of concentrated theatre. It was not surprising that television dominated the second phase of Richardson's career: he reached a large public as Bill Haydon, the mole, in *Tinker, Tailor, Soldier, Spy* (BBC, 1979) and, especially, as the sinister Urquhart in *House of Cards, To Play the King* and *The Final Cut* (BBC, 1990-95).

In 2002 he returned to the RSC to perform, with Donald Sinden, Derek Jacobi and Janet Suzman, John Barton's *The Hollow Crown* (Australian Tour and RST).

Alan Rickman (b. London, 1946). Brought up in Acton, west London, the son of working-class parents, Alan Rickman won a scholarship to a public school (Latymer Upper in Hammersmith) and went on to study art and design at the Chelsea College of Art and the Royal College of Art. He worked as a graphic designer until his mid-twenties, when he took up a place at RADA. He gained his early experience at some of the major provincial theatres: Dabble in *Lock Up Your Daughters*

(1974) and Andrew Hunter in *There's a Girl in my Soup* (1975) at the Library Theatre Manchester; Paris in *Romeo and Juliet* (Michael Bogdanov, 1975) at the Haymarket, Leicester; the title role in *Nijinsky* (1976), Daniel in *The Carnation Gang* (1976), Rubek in *When We Dead Awaken* (1976) and Jaques in *As You Like It* (Peter James, 1977) at the Sheffield Crucible; Laertes in *Hamlet* (1976), Uriah Shelly in *Man is Man* (1976) and Mar Ubu in *Ubu Rex* (1977), the last two directed by Adrian Noble, at the Bristol Old Vic; the title role in *Sherlock Holmes* (1976) and Wittipol in Peter Barnes's adaptation of *The Devil is an Ass* (1976) at the Birmingham Rep (1977). On television he played Tybalt in *Romeo and Juliet* (Alvin Rakoff, BBC, 1978) and Vidal in *Thérèse Raquin* (Simon Langton, BBC, 1979).

He joined the RSC in 1978, cast as Ferdinand in *The Tempest* (Clifford Williams, RST); Boyet in *Love's Labour's Lost* (John Barton, RST); Thidias/Alexas in *Antony and Cleopatra* (Peter Brook, RST); and Farquarson in Peter Whelan's *Captain Swing* (Bill Alexander, TOP). For six years he worked mostly in new plays, on the fringe and at the Royal Court: the title role in Peter Barnes's *Antonio* (Nottingham Playhouse, 1979); seven roles in Brecht's *Fears and Miseries of the Third Reich* (Giles Havergal, Glasgow Citizens', 1979); Nigel in Stephen Poliakoff's *The Summer Party* (Peter James, Sheffield Crucible, 1980); Barnes's version of Wedekind's *The Devil Himself* (Lyric Studio, Hammersmith, 1980); Hugh in Dusty Hughes's *Commitments* (Richard Wilson, Bush, 1980); Aston in an Irish *The Seagull* (Max Stafford-Clark, Royal Court, 1981); Stephen Davis's *The Last Elephant* (Bush, 1981); *The Brothers Karamazov* (Edinburgh Festival, 1981); Bob in Dusty Hughes's *Bad Language* (Hampstead, 1983); Dennis in Snoo Wilson's *Grass Widow* (Royal Court, 1983); and Gayman in a Women's Playhouse Trust production of Aphra Behn's *The Lucky Chance* (Royal Court, 1984).

Rickman's progress into the public's consciousness was decidedly slow. As an actor his identity—cerebral, dry and sardonic—is very strong, and for years this meant that he was left slightly on the outside of a conventional career. But from the start he was an admired figure in the profession, working constantly with the same people, among them Peter Barnes, Adrian Noble, Richard Wilson, Stephen Poliakoff and Dusty Hughes, and taking on the role of confidant to friends such as Juliet Stevenson (they met at the RSC in 1978), Harriet Walter and Ruby Wax. Rickman and Ruby Wax followed each other around in the late 1970s, working together at Sheffield, Bristol and the RSC, and Rickman later produced and directed her early efforts as a writer and comedienne: *Desperately Yours*, which started life as an RSC fringe show (1978-79) but ended up in New York (1980); *Live Wax* (Edinburgh Festival, 1986); and *Wax Acts* (West End, 1992). Not satisfied with the actor's role, he became a member of the board at the Bush.

Rickman's lugubrious, predatory Obadiah Slope in *The Barchester Chronicles* (David Giles, BBC, 1982) was a major success. In 1985 he returned to the RSC along with Juliet Stevenson to play leading parts: Jaques in *As You Like It* (Noble, RST); Achilles in *Troilus and Cressida* (Howard Davies, RST); Valmont in *Les liaisons dangereuses* (Davies, TOP); and Höfgen in *Mephisto* (Noble, Barbican). All showcased Rickman's talent for projecting disdain, duplicity and boredom. He missed out on the film version of *Les liaisons* but achieved international fame playing a classy villain in two Hollywood hits, Hans Gruber in *Die Hard* (John McTiernan, 1988) and the Sheriff of Nottingham in *Robin Hood: Prince of Thieves* (Kevin Reynolds, 1991).

His subsequent film roles have included Jamie opposite Juliet Stevenson in *Truly Madly Deeply* (Anthony Minghella, 1991); Sinclair, laid-back and enigmatic, in *Close My Eyes* (Stephen Poliakoff, 1991); Lukas Hart III in *Bob Roberts* (Tim Robbins, 1992); Colonel Brandon, so laid-back he seemed half asleep, in *Sense and Sensibility* (Ang Lee, 1995); O'Hara in *An Awfully Big Adventure* (Mike Newell, 1995); De Valera in *Michael Collins* (Neil Jordan, 1996); an angel in *Dogma* (1999); Snape in *Harry Potter* (since 2001); and Harry in *Love Actually* (2003).

Only occasionally seen on the stage since 1990, Rickman played Hamlet in a production directed by Robert Sturua at the

Riverside Studios (1992); a glum Antony opposite Helen Mirren in *Antony and Cleopatra* at the National (Sean Mathias, Olivier, 1998); and Elyot opposite Lindsay Duncan in *Private Lives* at the Albery (Davies, 2001). He directed both the stage production of Sharman Macdonald's *The Winter Guest* (West Yorkshire Playhouse, 1995) and the film version, released in 1997.

Richard Ridings (b. Henley, 1958). Richard Ridings's career as a character actor has been built on his imposing physical presence and his ability to portray dullards and hard men. He trained at the Bristol Old Vic Theatre School and his early theatre work included Hull Truck's productions of John Godber's *Bouncers* and *Up 'n' Under* (Tour, 1984); Mad Mick in *Putting on the Ritz* (Leicester Haymarket, 1987); and Bill Walker in *Major Barbara* (Chichester, 1988). On the big screen his first roles were of a limited kind—a German guard in *Lassiter* (1984), a policeman in *Clockwise* (1986), a skinhead in *The Fourth Protocol* (1987), a Viking in *Erik the Viking* (Terry Jones, 1989), and the appropriately named Hugh Primates in *Fierce Creatures* (Fred Schepisi/Robert Young, 1997).

But Ridings is a deceptively subtle actor. At the RSC, 1990-91, he gave stature to three supporting roles in Shakespeare: Ajax in *Troilus and Cressida* (Sam Mendes, Swan); Cornwall in *King Lear* (Nicholas Hytner, RST); and a comically slow-speaking Dull in *Love's Labour's Lost* (Terry Hands, RST). The song which closed Hands's production came to a surprising climax when Ridings's beaming blockhead produced a pitch-perfect falsetto note.

Notable screen work: Cotton in Malcolm McKay's *Cruel Train* (BBC, 1996); Bernard—a variation on Dull—in *Common as Muck* (Metin Huseyin, BBC, 1996-97); the Reverend Thwackum in *Tom Jones* (Huseyin, BBC, 1997); *The Messenger: the Story of Joan of Arc* (Luc Besson, 1999); *This is Personal: the Hunt for the Yorkshire Ripper* (ITV, 2000); *Fat Friends* (ITV, 2000); *The Pianist* (Roman Polanski, 2002); *Lara Croft Tomb Raider: the Cradle of Life* (Jan de Bont, 2003); and *The Brothers Grimm* (Terry Gilliam, 2004).

Diana Rigg (b. Doncaster, 1938) spent her early childhood in India where her father, an engineer, worked on the railways. She trained for the stage at RADA and made her first appearance as Natella in Brecht's *The Caucasian Chalk Circle,* a RADA production that visited the York Festival (1957). Following repertory at Chesterfield and York, she joined the Stratford Memorial Theatre Company (1959) and walked-on in the Paul Robeson/Sam Wanamaker *Othello* (Tony Richardson), *All's Well That Ends Well* (Tyrone Guthrie), *A Midsummer Night's Dream* (Peter Hall), the Laurence Olivier *Coriolanus* (Hall), and the Charles Laughton *King Lear* (Glen Byam Shaw). Staying on as a member of the new RSC, she progressed to leading roles: Andromache in *Troilus and Cressida* (Hall, RST, 1960); Phillipe Trincant in *The Devils* (Peter Wood, Aldwych, 1961); Gwendolen in *Becket* (Hall, Aldwych, 1961); Bianca to Vanessa Redgrave's Kate in *The Taming of the Shrew* (Maurice Daniels, Aldwych, 1961); the Presidente de Tourvel in *The Art of Seduction* (John Barton, Aldwych, 1962); Helena in *A Midsummer Night's Dream* (Hall, RST, 1962); Adriana to Ian Richardson's Antipholus of Ephesus in *The Comedy of Errors* (Clifford Williams, RST, 1962); Cordelia in the Paul Scofield *King Lear* (Peter Brook, RST, 1962); and Monika Stettler in *The Physicists* (Brook, Aldwych, 1963).

She was, then, by her middle twenties one of the RSC's brightest talents, and it was a stroke of inspiration by the makers of *The Avengers* to cast this young classical actress as Emma Peel (ITV, 1965-67). She returned to the RSC to play Viola in *Twelfth Night* (Williams, RST, 1966) and to repeat her Helena in Peter Hall's film of *A Midsummer Night's Dream* (1968). She then took up the opportunities in movies created by the success of *The Avengers*: James Bond's wife in *On Her Majesty's Secret Service* (1969); *The Assassination Bureau* (1969); Portia in *Julius Caesar* (1970); *The Hospital* (1971); and *Theatre of Blood* (1973).

Her career remained centred on the theatre. At the National (Old Vic, 1972-75, South Bank, 1978) she was Dorothy in Tom

Stoppard's *Jumpers* (Peter Wood, 1972); Annabella in *'Tis Pity She's a Whore* (Roland Joffé, 1972); Lady Macbeth, opposite Anthony Hopkins, in *Macbeth* (Michael Blakemore, 1972); the heartless *femme fatale* Célimène, opposite Alec McCowen, in Tony Harrison's updating of *The Misanthrope* (John Dexter, 1973); the Governor's Wife in *Phaedra Britannica* (Dexter, 1975); and Ilona in Molnár's *The Guardsman* (Wood, Lyttelton, 1978). Elsewhere, she starred as Heloise in *Abelard and Heloise* (Wyndham's, 1970); Eliza in *Pygmalion* (Albery, 1974); Ruth opposite John Thaw in Stoppard's *Night and Day* (Wood, Phoenix, 1978); Lady Ariadne Utterword in *Heartbreak House* (Theatre Royal Haymarket, 1983); Rita in *Little Eyolf* (Lyric Hammersmith, 1985); Cleopatra in *Antony and Cleopatra* (Robin Phillips, Chichester, 1985); and Phyllis in *Follies* (Mike Ockrent, Shaftesbury, 1987).

During the 1990s she created an outstanding body of work for Jonathan Kent at the Almeida, a theatre she helped put on the map: Cleopatra in Dryden's *All For Love* (1991); the title role in *Medea* (1992); Martha opposite David Suchet in *Who's Afraid of Viginia Woolf?* (Howard Davies, 1996); the title role in Ted Hughes's version of Racine's *Phèdre* (Almeida at Malvern and the Albery, 1998); and Agrippina in Racine's *Britannicus* (Albery, 1998). These performances were portrayed in some quarters as a comeback, but in fact were the continuation of a career dominated by the classics. Her recent stage appearances have included the mother in Charlotte Jones's *Humble Boy* (John Caird, NT Cottesloe, 2001); John Barton's *The Hollow Crown*, an isolated return to the RSC (Australian Tour, 2002); and Mrs Venable in Tennessee Williams's *Suddenly Last Summer* (Michael Grandage, Lyceum, Sheffield, 2004).

Linus Roache (b. Burnley, Lancashire, 1964) first acted as a child, appearing for a few weeks in *Coronation Street* alongside his father William Roache (Ken Barlow) and playing a plague victim in *The Onedian Line* (1976). Moving between the classical theatre and serious films, he came through in the late 1980s and early 90s as one of the most uncompromising actors of his generation, wary of both routine work and stardom.

His early years were spent in Lancashire but after the divorce of his parents (his mother is actress Anna Cropper) he moved to London and then to Sussex. Following his training at Central he worked at the Contact Theatre, Manchester (Pavel in *The Mother*) and the Royal Theatre, Northampton (Geoffrey in *A Taste of Honey*). He played Clive in *Five Finger Exercise* for the Cambridge Theatre Company on tour and made his London debut at the Royal Court as Billy in Karim Alrawi's *A Colder Climate* (1986).

He joined the RSC in 1987 and stayed until 1991, one of the exceptional group of actors produced by the Company during Terry Hands's final years as director (contemporaries included Ralph Fiennes, Simon Russell Beale and Richard McCabe). In his first season, 1987-88, he played Martius/Lucius in *Titus Andronicus* (Deborah Warner, Swan); William in *Indigo* (Sarah Pia Anderson, TOP); Sacha in John Berger's *A Question of Geography* (John Caird, TOP); Mark Antony, succeeding Nicholas Farrell, in *Julius Caesar* (Terry Hands, Barbican); Eric Blair in *Devine Gossip* (Barry Kyle, Pit); and the disabled Tom in Lucy Gannon's *Keeping Tom Nice* (Bill Buffery, Almeida). The promise of this work was fully realised during the next two-year cycle: Don Juan in *The Last Days of Don Juan* (Danny Boyle, Swan); Edgar in the John Wood *King Lear* (Nicholas Hytner, RST); and Aumerle in *Richard II* (Ron Daniels, RST). His lean face and arrogant gaze presented a young Don Juan who cared only for the chase.

In the most prominent of his subsequent stage and screen roles he has dared to make cold and feckless characters unsympathetic: Freddie opposite Penelope Wilton in Rattigan's *The Deep Blue Sea* (Karel Reisz, Almeida, 1992); the anti-hero of the wartime series *Seaforth* (BBC, 1994); Father Greg Pilkington in *Priest* (Antonia Bird, 1994); and Merton Densher opposite Helena Bonham Carter in *The Wings of the Dove* (Iain Softley, 1997). The latter re-started a career that he had deliberately stalled by refusing to make a second series of *Seaforth* and by taking a long sabbatical following the release of *Priest*.

In 1997 he appeared with Timothy Spall and Desmond Barrit in Caryl Churchill's short piece *This is a Chair* (Stephen Daldry, Royal Court at the Duke of York's). In 1998 he made a significant return to the RSC for Katie Mitchell's production of *Uncle Vanya* (Young Vic). Leaning towards the other characters with a penetrating stare, Roache's compelling Astrov was painfully self-aware and unusually hard ('If you had to shoot at something why didn't you choose your own head?' was delivered deadpan). In 2000 he joined the Almeida Company to play Bolingbroke in *Richard II* and Aufidius in *Coriolanus* opposite Ralph Fiennes (Gainsborough Studios). Films have dominated: *Shot Through the Heart* (1998); Denis Law in *Best* (2000); Samuel Coleridge in *Pandaemonium* (Julian Temple, 2000); *Hart's War* (2002); *The Gathering Storm* (Richard Loncraine, BBC, 2002); *Beyond Borders* (Martin Campbell, 2003); *The Chronicles of Riddick* (David Twohy, 2004); *The Forgotten* (Joseph Ruben, 2004); *Batman Begins* (Christopher Nolan, 2005); *Find Me Guilty* (Sidney Lumet, 2006); *The Namesake* (Mira Nair, 2006); *Broken Thread* (2007).

Norman Rodway (1929-2001), a Dubliner born in London, read Classics at Trinity College and worked as a schoolmaster, lecturer and accountant (for Guinness) before starting his acting career. He established his reputation at the Gate, Dublin, and scored an early success in London playing the title role in Hugh Leonard's *Stephen D*, an adaptation of James Joyce's *A Portrait of the Artist as a Young Man* (St Martin's, 1963). He appeared with Judi Dench in the British feature *Four in the Morning* (Anthony Simmons, 1966) and in Orson Welles's *Chimes at Midnight*, as Hotspur (1966). In his first, remarkable season with the RSC (1966) he played Witness 8 in *The Investigation* (Peter Brook, Aldwych); Hotspur to Ian Holm's Hal in the first part of *Henry IV* (John Barton/Trevor Nunn/Clifford Williams, RST); Feste in

Twelfth Night (Williams, RST); and Spurio in *The Revenger's Tragedy* (Nunn, RST). From flawed heroes to clowns, Rodway was in his element.

He remained with the RSC for much of the rest of his career. With his distinctive voice, strong physique and bird-like face, he played a wide spectrum of roles, English, Irish and Russian, in a style that was deft, imperturbable and often wittily ironic: Mercutio in *Romeo and Juliet* (Karolos Koun, RST, 1967); Edmund in the Eric Porter *King Lear* (Nunn, RST, 1968); Thersites in *Troilus and Cressida* (Barton, RST, 1968); Don Pedro in *Much Ado About Nothing* (Nunn, RST, 1968); Bates in Harold Pinter's *Silence* (Peter Hall, Aldwych, 1969); Tom Quar'lous in Ben Jonson's *Bartholomew Fair* (Terry Hands, Aldwych, 1969); the title role in *Richard III* (Hands, RST, 1970); Philip the Bastard in *King John* (Buzz Goodbody, RST, 1970); Snout in Brook's *A Midsummer Night's Dream* (RST, 1970); Trinculo in *The Tempest* (Barton, RST, 1970); Sergei in Gorky's *Summerfolk* (David Jones, Aldwych, 1974); Holofernes in *Love's Labour's Lost* (Jones, RST, 1975); Dazzle in Dion Boucicault's *London Assurance* (Ronald Eyre, Albery, 1975); Muratov in Gorky's *The Zykovs* (Jones, Aldwych, 1976); Harry Hope in Eugene O'Neill's *The Iceman Cometh* (Howard Davies, Aldwych, 1976); Lebedev in Chekhov's *Ivanov* (Jones, Aldwych, 1976); Sir George Thunder in John O'Keeffe's *Wild Oats* (Williams, Aldwych, 1976); Protassov in Gorky's *Children of the Sun* (Hands, Aldwych, 1979); Seamus in Sean O'Casey's *The Shadow of a Gunman* (Michael Bogdanov, TOP, 1980); Captain Boyle in O'Casey's *Juno and the Paycock* (Nunn, Aldwych, 1980); and Ovchukhov in Solzhenitsyn's *The Love-Girl and the Innocent* (Williams, Aldwych, 1981).

His first long break from the RSC was ended in 1990 when he gave fine performances as Pandarus—presented as an untrustworthy charmer in a striped blazer—in *Troilus and Cressida* (Sam Mendes, Swan) and Gloucester in *King Lear* (Nicholas Hytner, RST). In 1997 he took on the roles of the Chorus, the Archbishop of Canterbury, Sir Thomas Erpingham, the Governor of Harfleur and the Duke of Burgundy in *Henry V* (Ron Daniels, RST).

Elsewhere, his theatre work included Enobarbus in *Antony and Cleopatra* (Robin Phillips, Chichester, 1985); Hugh in Brian Friel's *Translations* (Mendes, Donmar Warehouse, 1993); Judge Brack in the Juliet Stevenson *Hedda Gabler* (Davies, NT Olivier, 1989); Sorin alongside Judi Dench in *The Seagull* (John Caird, NT Olivier, 1994); and Oberon in *A Midsummer Night's Dream* (Jonathan Miller, Almeida, 1996).

Rodway's performance as Hotspur in *Chimes at Midnight* remained the high point of his work on screen. Later roles included Cummings in *Reilly Ace of Spies* (ITV, 1983); the Marquis of Queensbury to Michael Gambon's Wilde in *Oscar* (Henry Herbert, BBC, 1986); Roland Marshall in *Inspector Morse, Deceived by Flight* (ITV, 1989); Hitler in *The Empty Mirror* (1996); and Werner Noth in *Mother Night* (Keith Gordon, 1996).

Paul Rogers (b. Plympton, Devon, 1917) trained at the Michael Chekhov Theatre Studio, Dartington Hall, and made his first appearance as Charles Dickens in *Bird's Eye of Valour* (Scala, 1938). He was a member of the 1939 Stratford company, playing, among other roles, Curtis in Theodore Komisarjevsky's *The Taming of the Shrew*. He served in the Royal Navy during the war, finally returning to the stage in 1946 and finding success at the Bristol Old Vic at the end of the decade.

He emerged as a fine Shakespearean at the Old Vic in London during the 1950s. The names of the leading parts he played during six crowded seasons, 1951-58, makes for astonishing reading, for no other actor has covered the canon so thoroughly: Malvolio in *Twelfth Night* (Hugh Hunt); Bottom in *A Midsummer Night's Dream* (Tyrone Guthrie); Iago in *Othello* (Michael Langham); Shylock in *The Merchant of Venice* (Hunt); Cassius in *Julius Caesar* (Hunt); the title role in *Henry VIII* (Guthrie); the title role in *Macbeth* (Richard Benthall); Don Armado in *Love's Labour's Lost* (Frith Banbury); Petruchio in *The Taming of the Shrew* (Denis Carey); Touchstone in *As You Like It* (Robert Helpmann); Falstaff in *Henry IV* (Douglas Seale); Brutus in *Julius Caesar* (Benthall); Leontes in *The Winter's Tale* (Benthall); Falstaff in *The Merry Wives of Windsor* (Seale); Pandarus in *Troilus and Cressida* (Guthrie); Mercutio in *Romeo and Juliet* (Helpmann); and the title role in *King Lear* (Seale). In 1960 he toured with the Old Vic company to Moscow, Leningrad and Warsaw.

During the 1950s he also fitted in two T.S. Eliot premieres, *The Confidential Clerk* (Edinburgh Festival and Lyric, 1953) and *The Elder Statesman* (Edinburgh Festival and Cambridge Theatre, 1958)—he created the roles of Sir Claude Mulhammer and Lord Claverton. On leaving the Old Vic he appeared in the West End as Mr Fox in *Mr Fox of Venice* (Piccadilly, 1959); Johnny Condell in *One More River* (Duke of York's, 1959); Nickles in Archibald MacLeish's *J.B.* (Phoenix, 1961); Reginald Kinsale in Peter Ustinov's *Photo Finish* (Saville, 1962); and Sorin in Tony Richardson's production of *The Seagull* (Queen's, 1964).

Rogers joined the RSC in 1965. His career with the Company was curiously muted, as if his great spell at the Old Vic had left him with nothing to prove. He played Falstaff in the two parts of *Henry IV* (John Barton/Trevor Nunn/Clifford Williams, RST, 1966); Apemantus in *Timon of Athens* (John Schlesinger, RST, 1965); the Mayor in *The Government Inspector* (Peter Hall, Aldwych, 1966); Bottom in Hall's film of *A Midsummer Night's Dream* (1968); Carnaby Leete in Granville-Barker's *The Marrying of Ann Leete* (David Jones, Aldwych, 1975); Mr Portland in Graham Greene's *The Return of A.J. Raffles* (Jones, Aldwych, 1975); and Antipa in Gorky's *The Zykovs* (Jones, Aldwych, 1976). His key role was Max in Harold Pinter's *The Homecoming* (Hall, Aldwych, 1965). Sitting in an armchair that was part throne, part cage, Rogers used his imposing physical presence and a growling delivery to convey the misery as well as the vindictiveness of Pinter's declining brute.

During the 1970s and 1980s he was at the National for three seasons. The first, 1974/75, took him back to the Old Vic: Peter Nichols's *The Freeway* (Jonathan Miller); A.E. Ellis's *Grand Manoeuvres* (Michael Blakemore); and Boss Mangan in *Heartbreak House* (Schlesinger). On the South Bank he played the

Zauberkönig in Ödön von Horváth's *Tales from the Vienna Woods* (Maximilian Schell, Olivier, 1977); Voltore in *Volpone* (Hall, Olivier, 1977); Henry Huxtable in Granville-Barker's *The Madras House* (William Gaskill, Olivier, 1977); Chasuble in *The Importance of Being Earnest* (Hall, Lyttelton, 1982); and Hornby in Harold Pinter's *A Kind of Alaska* (Hall, Cottesloe, 1982). In 1989, once again at the Old Vic, he played Gloucester in *King Lear* (Jonathan Miller).

Rogers's acting graced a long list of British movies, although there are no masterpieces among them. The most significant are *Beau Brummell* (1954); *The Beachcomber* (1954); *Svengali* (1954); *Our Man in Havana* (Carol Reed, 1960); *The Trials of Oscar Wilde* (Ken Hughes, 1960); *Billy Budd* (Peter Ustinov, 1962); *Decline and Fall of a Birdwatcher* (1968); *The Reckoning* (Jack Gold, 1969); *Three into Two Won't Go* (Hall, 1969); and *The Looking Glass War* (1970).

Amanda Root (b. Chelmsford, 1963) was a remarkably complete actress even in her early twenties, when physically she looked little more than a child. With her dark soulful eyes she could command a stage, and the RSC saw her talent very early on, casting her as Juliet opposite Daniel Day-Lewis in *Romeo and Juliet* and Hermia in *A Midsummer Night's Dream* (John Caird and Sheila Hancock respectively, Small-scale Tour and TOP, 1983-84).

She was an acclaimed Juliet, but the production was marred by Day-Lewis's withdrawal. Later in the 1984 season she played Jessica in *The Merchant of Venice* (Caird, RST), Moth in *Love's Labour's Lost* (Barry Kyle, RST), and Lucy in Robert Holman's *Today* (Bill Alexander, TOP). She did not stay with the RSC for the London performances of these productions, but returned in 1988/89 to play a young Lady Macbeth in *Macbeth* (Adrian Noble, RST), Harriet in *The Man of Mode* (Garry Hynes, Swan), Angelica in *The Constant Couple* (Roger Michell, Swan), and Betty McNeil in Richard Nelson's *Some Americans Abroad* (Michell, Pit). She achieved even more in 1990/91: Cressida opposite Ralph Fiennes in *Troilus and Cressida* (Sam Mendes, Swan); Rosaline in *Love's Labour's Lost* (Terry Hands, RST); and Nina in *The Seagull* (Hands, Swan).

Between RSC seasons she appeared at the Lyric Hammersmith in García Lorca's *The House of Bernarda Alba* (Núria Espert, 1986), and at the National in Paul Godfrey's *Once in a While the Odd Thing Happens* (Godfrey, Cottesloe, 1990). On leaving the Company she starred opposite Alec McCowen in *Caesar and Cleopatra* (Matthew Francis, Greenwich, 1992). Reunited with her RSC colleagues Susan Fleetwood, Ciaran Hinds and Simon Russell Beale, she delivered a beautiful performance as Anne in the Nick Dear's television adaptation of *Persuasion* (Michell, BBC, 1995); and was equally fine in *Breaking the Code* (Herbert Wise, BBC, 1996), *The Forsyte Saga* (ITV, 2002-03), *Daniel Deronda* (BBC, 2002), *Love Again* (BBC, 2003) and *Enduring Love* (Michell, 2004). She returned to the stage in 2000 to play Edith in Yasmina Reza's *Conversations After a Burial* (Howard Davies, Almeida).

Clifford Rose (b. Hamnish, Hertfordshire, 1929) was a founding member of the RSC and stayed with the Company until the end of the 1960s. Returning to Stratford as a white-haired senior player, he was one of the mainstays of Adrian Noble's Company.

In that first decade he played supporting roles in some of the RSC's most important productions—Priam in *Troilus and Cressida* (Hall, RST, 1960); Adam in *As You Like It* (Michael Elliott, RST, 1961); Starveling in *A Midsummer Night's Dream* (Hall, RST, 1962); Dromio of Ephesus in *The Comedy of Errors* (Clifford Williams, RST, 1963); Duke of Exeter in *The Wars of the Roses* (Hall, RST, 1963); Albany in *King Lear* (Peter Brook, American Tour, 1964); Coulmier in *Marat/Sade* (Brook, Aldwych, 1964); *US* (Brook, Aldwych, 1966); Simon Norton in *The Silver Tassie* (David Jones, Aldwych, 1969); Wasp in *Bartholomew Fair* (Terry Hands, Aldwych, 1969); and Antonio in *The Revenger's Tragedy* (Trevor Nunn, Aldwych, 1969). He was also Sir Eglamour in *The*

Two Gentlemen of Verona (Hall, RST, 1960); Stephano in *The Merchant of Venice* (Michael Langham, RST, 1960); Silvio in *The Duchess of Malfi* (Donald McWhinnie, Aldwych, 1960); Verges in *Much Ado About Nothing* (Langham, RST, 1961); Marcellus in *Hamlet* (Peter Wood, RST, 1961); Sir Robert Brakenbury in *Richard III* (William Gaskill, RST, 1961); Gratiano in *Othello* (Franco Zeffirelli, RST, 1961); Froth in *Measure for Measure* (John Blatchley, RST, 1962); Starveling in *A Midsummer Night's Dream* (Hall, RST, 1962); Christopher Sly in *The Taming of the Shrew* (Maurice Daniels, RST, 1962); Duncan in *Macbeth* (McWhinnie, RST, 1962); Cornelius in *Cymbeline* (Gaskill, RST, 1962); Soothsayer in *Julius Caesar* (Blatchley, RST, 1963); Shallow in *The Merry Wives of Windsor* (Blatchley, Aldwych, 1964); Mountjoy in *Henry V* (Barton/Trevor Nunn, Aldwych, 1965); Frederick in Brecht's *Puntila* (Michel Saint-Denis, Aldwych, 1965); Witness 6 in *The Investigation* (Brook/Jones, Aldwych, 1965); Emmanuel Lutz in *The Meteor* (Williams, Aldwych, 1966); Obadiah Bobblenob in *The Thwarting of Baron Bolligrew* (Nunn, Aldwych, 1966); Engstrand in *Ghosts* (Alan Bridges, Aldwych, 1967); Nestor in *Troilus and Cressida* (Barton, RST, 1968); and Don John in *Much Ado About Nothing* (Nunn, Aldwych, 1969).

Except for a provincial tour of Barton's *The Hollow Crown* (1975), Rose worked outside of the RSC for the next twenty years. He reached a large audience on television as Snell in *Callan* (1967-73); Kessler in *Secret Army* (BBC, 1977-79); Quintus Slide in *The Pallisers* (BBC, 1977); and Professor Gracey in *Fortunes of War* (James Cellan-Jones, BBC, 1987). The RSC missed his experience and fine verse-speaking. Since his return he has played Lafeu in *All's Well That Ends Well* (RST, 1989) and Andropov in *Moscow Gold* (Barbican, 1990) for Barry Kyle; Scroop in the two parts of *Henry IV* (RST, 1991), Tiresias in *The Thebans* (Swan, 1991) and the Ghost in the Kenneth Branagh *Hamlet* (Barbican, 1992) for Adrian Noble; Second Priest in *Murder in the Cathedral* (Swan, 1993) and Stanley in *Richard III* (RST, 1995) for Steven Pimlott; Gonzalo in *The Tempest* (RST, 1993) for Sam Mendes; the Lord Chief Justice in *Henry IV* (Swan, 2000) and

Lepidus/Proculeius in *Antony and Cleopatra* (RST, 2002) for Michael Attenborough; the Duke in *Othello* (Swan, 2004) for Gregory Doran; and Francis Nurse in *The Crucible* (RST, 2006) for Dominic Cooke.

Mary Rutherford (b. Toronto, 1945). A talented young leading actress at the RSC, 1969-75, Mary Rutherford initially played unnamed parts in two productions at the Aldwych—*Troilus and Cressida* (John Barton) and Sean O'Casey's *The Silver Tassie* (David Jones)—but she was quickly promoted: Punk Alice/Hero in Ben Jonson's *Bartholomew Fair* (Terry Hands, Aldwych, 1969); Juliet in *Measure for Measure* (Barton, RST, 1970); Elizabeth in *Richard III* (Hands, RST, 1970); a vivacious Hermia in Peter Brook's *A Midsummer Night's Dream* (RST, 1970); Nadya in Gorky's *Enemies* (Jones, Aldwych, 1971); Thief (Marlyse) in Jean Genet's *The Balcony* (Hands, Aldwych, 1971); Calpurnia in *Julius Caesar* (Trevor Nunn/Buzz Goodbody, Aldwych, 1973); Octavia in *Antony and Cleopatra* (Nunn/Goodbody, Aldwych, 1973); Alice Faulkner in *Sherlock Holmes* (Frank Dunlop, Aldwych, 1974); and Olivia in *Twelfth Night* (Peter Gill, RST, 1974).

Elsewhere: Fraulein Rabenjung in *The Tutor* (Royal Court, 1968); various parts in *The Hero Rises Up* (London, 1968); Glumdalclitch in *Gulliver's Travels* (London, 1969); Haze Cooke in *Yelapal* (London, 1969); Lika in *The Promise* (Welsh Theatre Company, 1972); Ingrid in *Peer Gynt* (Newcastle, 1973); Juliet opposite Jonathan Kent in *Romeo and Juliet* (Michael Bogdanov, Leicester Haymarket, 1974); Lady Percy/Joan of Arc/Lady Anne in *The Wars of the Roses* (Bogdanov, ESC, Tour, 1987-88); opposite Alan Bates in Thomas Bernard's *The Showman* (Jonathan Kent, Almeida, 1993); Jack Shepherd's *Chasing the Moment* (Pleasance, Edinburgh Festival, 1995); and the Mother in *Too Clever By Half* (Progress Theatre, Reading, 2004).

Barrie Rutter (b. Hull, 1946). The son of a Hull fishworker, Barrie Rutter trained at the National Youth Theatre and the

Royal Scottish Academy of Music and Drama and made his professional debut in 1968.

He was a powerfully authentic figure at the RSC from 1975 to 79, and again in 1987/88: Macmorris in *Henry V* (Terry Hands, RST, 1975); Peto in *Henry IV* (Hands, RST, 1975); *The Mouth Organ* (Cicely Berry, TOP, 1975); Heron in John Ford's *Perkin Warbeck* (John Barton, TOP, 1975); Dick the Butcher in *Henry VI* (Hands, RST, 1977); Gustavus Adolphus in Pam Gems's *Queen Christina* (Penny Cherns, TOP, 1977); First Roman Citizen in *Coriolanus* (Hands, RST, 1977); the devisor of *Old Tyme Music Hall* (RST, 1978); Will in Pete Atkin's *A & R* (Walter Donohue, Warehouse, 1978); Lollio in *The Changeling* (Hands, Aldwych, 1978); the Deputy Director in Václav Havel's *Temptation* (Roger Michell, TOP, 1987); Pilia-Borza in *The Jew of Malta* (Kyle, Swan, 1987); and Grumio in *The Taming of the Shrew* (Jonathan Miller, RST, 1987).

Inspired by his experience performing leading roles in Tony Harrison's *The Oresteia* (Peter Hall, 1981), *The Mysteries* (Bill Bryden, 1985), and *The Trackers of Oxyrhynchus* (Harrison, 1990) at the National Theatre, Rutter founded, in 1992, Northern Broadsides, a Halifax-based company dedicated to the performing of classic plays with northern voices. For Broadsides he has starred in and directed *Richard III* (1992); *Antony and Cleopatra* (1995); *Samson Agonistes* (1998); *King Lear* (1999); Ted Hughes's *Alcestis* (2000); *Antigone* (2003); and *The Merchant of Venice* (2004).

Daniel Ryan (b. 1968) gained his early experience at the Manchester Youth Theatre. He joined the RSC on leaving the London Academy of Music and Dramatic Art, and has returned at intervals to play single roles, each one a significant step up: Soldier in *All's Well That Ends Well* (Barry Kyle, Barbican, 1990); Citizen in *Pericles* (David Thacker, Pit, 1990); Citizen in *Coriolanus* (Terry Hands/John Barton, Barbican, 1990); Catesby in *Richard III* (Sam Mendes, TOP and Small-scale Tour, 1992); Jack Lane in Peter Whelan's *The Herbal Bed* (Michael Attenborough, Duchess, 1997); and Bottom in *A Midsummer Night's Dream* (Michael Boyd, RST, 1999). Ryan played Bottom as a neat, sharp, rather humourless young man, a wide boy with pretensions (goatee beard; dark grey suit). At the National he played Alan in *Life After Life* (Loft, 2002); at the Royal Court, Matt in Roy Williams's *Fallout* (Ian Rickson, 2003).

Ryan's work on screen has included Dennis Potter's *Lipstick on Your Collar* (Channel Four, 1993); *Men Only* (Peter Webber, Channel Four, 2001); Mike Leigh's *All or Nothing* (2002); Andrew Gilligan in *The Government Inspector* (Peter Kosminsky, Channel Four, 2005); *The Street* (BBC, 2006); *Bon Voyage* (ITV, 2006); *Consent* (Channel Four, 2007); and *Confessions of a Diary Secretary* (ITV, 2007).

Mark Rylance (b. Ashford, 1960) grew up in America (his parents, both teachers, emigrated to Milwaukee when he was two years old). He returned to England in his late teens to take up a place at RADA.

He was a founding member of the London Theatre of Imagination, playing Iago in *Othello* and Leonato in *Much Ado About Nothing*. From the start his theatre work was varied and interesting: Soldier Two in Carlo Goldoni's *The Battlefield* (Robert David MacDonald), Michael in *The Caucasian Chalk Circle* (Giles Havergal), Archivist in *Don Juan* (Philip Prowse), and Bazza in *Desperado Corner* (Di Trevis) at the Glasgow Citizens' (1980-81); Arturo in *The Resistible Rise of Arturo Ui* at the Contact Theatre Manchester; Madam in Genet's *The Maids* for Shared Experience at the Lyric Hammersmith (Mike Alfreds); Vincenzo Rocca alongside Greta Scacchi and Kevin McNally in Malcolm McKay's *Airbase* at the Oxford Playhouse (1985); Shelley in Brenton's *Bloody Poetry* at the Royal Court (1988); and Prince Djalma/Agricola in *The Wandering Jew* and Leonardo in *Countrymania* at the National (Alfreds, 1987-88).

He was at the RSC from 1982 to 1990, and remains an associate. During his first season, 1982/83, he was cast in roles that suited his slight physique: Michael in *Arden of Faversham* (Terry Hands, TOP); Gravedigger's Boy in Edward Bond's *Lear* (Barry Kyle, TOP); Lucentio in *The Taming of the Shrew* (Kyle, RST); Ariel in *The Tempest* (Ron Daniels, RST); Jack Dapper in *The Roaring Girl* (Kyle, Barbican); and the title role in *Peter Pan* (John Caird/Trevor Nunn, Barbican). It was on his return to the Company in 1988 that he joined the first division of classical actors. His disturbed, pyjama-clad Hamlet in Ron Daniels's production (RST, 1989) was arguably the most original of its time. In the same vein, he brought to the title role in *Romeo and Juliet* (Hands, Swan, 1989) a manic intensity, as if desire was drug-induced. He followed these performances with an anguished, non-heroic king in *Henry V* (Kyle, Theatre For a New Audience, New York, 1993), and a sharp, funny Benedick opposite Janet McTeer in *Much Ado About Nothing* (Matthew Warchus, Queen's Theatre, 1993).

Significant screen work followed these successes: John Healy in *The Grass Arena* (Gilles MacKinnon, 1991); Ferdinand in Peter Greenaway's *Prospero's Books* (1991); the butler Raunce in *Loving* (Diarmuid Lawrence, BBC, 1995); Jakob, alongside his RSC contemporary Alice Krige, in *Institute Benjamenta* (Stephen and Timothy Quay, 1995); William Adamson in Philip Haas's *Angels and Insects* (1995); and Kerry Fox's lover in Patrice Chéreau's *Intimacy* (2001).

Inspired by the example of Kenneth Branagh, Rylance formed his own company, Phoebus Cart, at the beginning of the 1990s, and directed a production of *The Tempest* (1991) which played outdoors at the Rollright Stones in Warwickshire and at the Globe construction site—through this he met Sam Wanamaker and was invited to join the Globe directorate. However, directing is not his strength: his 'Hare Krishna' *Macbeth* (1995) became legendary for all the wrong reasons.

He was Artistic Director of the Globe from 1996 to 2005. He believes that Francis Bacon wrote the plays, and links the Globe to Stonehenge as a circular space imbued with spiritual energy. This foolish way of thinking cannot be separated from the qualities that make him special as an actor—quirkiness, imagination and softly-spoken lyricism. Regrettably, though, a performance at Rylance's Globe could seem like an entertainment session in a holiday camp. He failed to attract topflight directors, and his preference for all-male productions limited the appeal of much of the work. Rylance played both leading and supporting roles: Henry V (Richard Olivier, 1997); Mr Allwit in *The Chaste Maid of Cheapside* (1997); Bassanio in *The Merchant of Venice* (1998); Hippolito in *The Honest Whore* (1998); Cleopatra in *Antony and Cleopatra* (1999); Hamlet (2000); Posthumus/Cloten in *Cymbeline* (2001); Olivia in *Twelfth Night* (2002); Richard II (2003); and Prospero in *The Tempest* (2005).

S

Rebecca Saire (b. London, 1963) was only fifteen when she played Juliet in the BBC's *Romeo and Juliet* (Alvin Rakoff, 1978). This is the kind of beginning that often comes to nothing, but Rebecca Saire has forged a successful adult career. Her early theatre appearances included May in Tom Taylor's *The Ticket-of-Leave-Man* at the National (Piers Haggard, Cottesloe, 1981), and seasons at the Mill, Sonning, and the Redgrave Theatre, Farnham—Polly in *The Gingerbread Lady*, Laura in *The Glass Menagerie*, Suzannah in *Bedroom Farce* and Mary Yellen in *Jamaica Inn*.

In 1985 (which saw the release of her first film, *The Shooting Party*) she joined the RSC to play Madeline Bray in the revival of *Nicholas Nickleby* (Trevor Nunn and John Caird, RST). Then in 1989/90 she was a slim, rather forbidding Ophelia to Mark Rylance's idiosyncratic prince in *Hamlet* (Ron Daniels, RST), Madame Centaur in Ben Jonson's *The Silent Woman* (Danny Boyle, Swan), and Szofi in Julius Hay's *Have* (Janice Honeyman, Pit). In 1991/92 she played Bianca in *The Taming of the Shrew* (Bill Alexander, RST), Rachel in Richard Brome's *A Jovial Crew* (Max

Stafford-Clark, Swan), Diana in Peter Hall's production of *All's Well That Ends Well* (Swan, Pit), and Audry in Peter Whelan's play about Marlowe (Richard McCabe), *The School of Night* (Alexander, TOP). On the transfer to London she was a brittle Gwendolen in Tom Stoppard's *Travesties* (Adrian Noble, Barbican, 1993).

Elsewhere: Louise in Strindberg's *Thunder in the Air* (Derek Martinus, Gate, 1989); Clea in Peter Shaffer's *Black Comedy* (Palace Theatre, Watford, 1995); *East Lynne* (Philip Franks, Greenwich Theatre, 1996); Isabella in *Northanger Abbey* (Greenwich Theatre, 1996); Eliante in Molière's *The Misanthrope* (Peter Hall, Piccadilly, 1998); Brenda in John Patrick Shanley's *Four Dogs and a Bone* (Crispin Bonham Carter, Etcetera, 1999); and Sybil in Noël Coward's *Private Lives* (Franks, NT Lyttelton, 1999).

Adrian Schiller (b. Oxford) came to notice at the RSC playing the Porter in *Macbeth* (Tim Albery, RST, 1996) and Trinculo in *The Tempest* (Adrian Noble, RST, 1998). Trinculo was a particular joy, a melancholy malcontent in jester's cap, so drunk that he spoke and moved in slow-motion.

But Schiller is not only an expert at clowns. In *Measure for Measure* (Michael Boyd, RST, 1998) his Lucio, wearing a red cravat and stained waistcoat, flaunting a silver cigarette case, was louche, dark and arrogant. The character dominated the play. And his other work has been equally distinctive: Dr Julio in *The White Devil* (Gayle Edwards, Swan, 1996); Paris's Servant in *Troilus and Cressida* (Ian Judge, RST, 1996); Police Officer/Prison Officer in Koltès's *Roberto Zucco* (James Macdonald, TOP, 1997); Touchstone in *As You Like It* (Gregory Doran, RST, 2000); Mercutio in *Romeo and Juliet* (Boyd, RST, 2000); Fluellen in *Henry V* (Edward Hall, RST, 2000); the title role in a fringe festival *Hamlet* (Samuel West, TOP, 2000); and Cassius in *Julius Caesar* (David Farr) paired with Panthino in *The Two Gentlemen of Verona* (Fiona Buffini, Swan and Small-scale Tour, 2004-05).

Schiller's work for other theatres has included Tailor's Apprentice in *Le bourgeois gentilhomme* (Richard Jones, NT Lyttelton, 1992); Berowne opposite Rebecca Johnson in *Love's Labour's Lost* (Rachel Kavanaugh, Regent's Park, 2001); Malcolm in *Macbeth* (Edward Hall, Albery, 2002); Jaggers in David Farr's version of *Great Expectations* (Gordon Anderson, Bristol Old Vic, 2003); Charles to Amanda Drew's *Madame Bovary* (Polly Teale, Shared Experience, Lyric Hammersmith, 2003); and Leicester in Schiller's *Mary Stuart* (Patrick Sandford, Nuffield Theatre, Southampton, 2004).

Paul Scofield (1922-2008, b. Hurstpierpoint, Sussex) emerged to a rare degree of critical and public adoration while still in his early twenties. If the sporadic work of his old age put in doubt the legitimacy of the purple prose of Kenneth Tynan and J.C. Trewin, there was no denying the scope of his talent. He caused as big a stir (and wounded as many hearts) playing the Young Shepherd in *The Winter's Tale* as the title role in *Hamlet*. Scofield's rise owed something to his partnership with Peter Brook under Barry Jackson at the Birmingham Rep and the RSC, his marriage to Joy Parker, and his refusal to compromise in movies. If Scofield's physical presence appealed to everyone, his mannered vocal style divided opinion. However, as much as anything, it was the range of his voice that allowed him to play older men and to alternate romantic leads with sardonic character parts.

He was brought up in the Sussex village of Hurstpierpoint, where his father was headmaster of the local school. He discovered Shakespeare early: as a schoolboy in Brighton he played Juliet in a school production of *Romeo and Juliet* and appeared as a crowd extra in *The Only Way* at the Theatre Royal (1935). Juliet was followed by Rosalind and Hal in *Henry IV* (1938). He trained at the Croydon Rep Theatre School (1939) and the London Mask Theatre School, Westminster Theatre, where he walked-on in *Under the Elms* and *Cornelius* and spoke a few lines as Third Clerk/First Soldier in Drinkwater's *Abraham Lincoln* (all Henry Cass, 1940). He played his first leading roles at the Bideford Repertory Theatre (1941), and then toured with ENSA as Vincentio/Tranio in *The Taming of the Shrew* (Robert Atkins, 1941).

In 1942 he appeared with Basil C. Langton's Travelling Repertory Theatre at the Birmingham Rep, playing Stephen Undershaft in *Major Barbara*, Horatio in *Hamlet* and meeting Joy Parker (Ophelia). He stayed with the TRT for the next two years, touring munitions factories. In 1945 he returned to the Birmingham Rep, this time as a member of Barry Jackson's resident company. It was here that he met the twenty-year-old Peter Brook. Some commentators perceived a new beginning for English theatre in the partnership of Brook and Scofield as acclaimed productions of *Man and Superman*, *King John* and *The Lady of the Sea* opened in quick succession.

When Jackson took charge of Stratford in 1946 he based his first seasons around Brook and Scofield. Scofield played with melancholy restraint as Don Armado in *Love's Labour's Lost* (1946) and Mercutio in *Romeo and Juliet* (1947). He was also Cloten in *Cymbeline* (Nugent Monck, 1946); Henry V (Dorothy Green, 1946); a menacing Lucio in *Measure for Measure* (Frank McMullan, 1946, 1947); Mephistophilis in *Doctor Faustus* (Walter Hudd, 1947); Aguecheek in *Twelfth Night* (Hudd, 1947); the title role in *Pericles* (Monck, 1947); a lyrical Hamlet in Michael Benthall's production (1948, the role alternated with Robert Helpmann); a loveable Young Shepherd in *The Winter's Tale* (Anthony Quayle, 1948); and Troilus in *Troilus and Cressida* (Quayle, 1948). In 1952 he played Don Pedro in John Gielgud's London revival of the 1950 Stratford *Much Ado About Nothing* (Phoenix).

During the next decade he worked in London, joining John Gielgud's company at the Lyric Hammersmith to play the title role in *Richard II* and Pierre in Brook's production of *Venice Preserv'd* (1952-53), and starring in such popular West End product as *A Question of Fact* (Piccadilly, 1953-54), *A Dead Secret* (Piccadilly, 1957), *Expresso Bongo* (Saville, 1958), Graham Greene's *The Complaisant Lover* (Globe, 1959), and Robert Bolt's *A Man For All Seasons* (Globe, 1960). His collaboration with Brook continued with a famous season at the Phoenix consisting of *Hamlet*, Graham Greene's *The Power and the Glory* and T.S. Eliot's *The Family Reunion* (1955-56). In each Scofield played a haunted anti-hero. The anguish and melancholy, power and subtlety, nobility and stoicism of his Hamlet moved and excited a generation of theatregoers. The production visited the Moscow Art Theatre for a two-week season.

In 1959 Peter Hall asked Scofield to return to Stratford to lead the re-named company, with an initial commitment of three years from 1960. He agreed to the roles of Shylock, Petruchio and Thersites in *Troilus and Cressida*, but withdrew on the eve of rehearsals. This caused a crisis, but such was Scofield's stature that two years later Hall tried again with an offer of *King Lear* directed by Brook. With contracts signed Scofield sent a doctor's note. Instead of cancelling Hall postponed *King Lear* to the autumn. As usual, Brook began his exploration of the play without preconceptions, discarding over a century of performance tradition. Consequently, Scofield's Lear was an implacable autocrat who wrecked lives, a bully with cropped hair, physically threatening, very much the author of his own fate. Famously, the phrase 'I shall go mad' was delivered not as a premonition but as a warning. After the storm Lear became a figure of desolation and of the grotesque (Shakespeare as a precursor of Samuel Beckett—this was a revelatory moment in the performance history of Shakespeare, although the idea had been explored by Jan Kott in *Shakespeare Our Contemporary*, published as Brook was working on the production). After playing in Stratford and London (1962-63), *King Lear* visited Paris (1963) and the United States (1964). Scofield stayed with the RSC until 1968, playing the title role in *Timon of Athens* (John Schlesinger, RST, 1965); Khlestakov in Gogol's *The Government Inspector* (Hall, Aldwych, 1966); Charles Dyer in *Staircase* (Hall, Aldwych, 1966); Dragon in *The Thwarting of Baron Bolligrew* (Trevor Nunn, Aldwych,

1966); and the title role in *Macbeth* (Hall, RST, 1967). In 1966 he joined Hall and Brook as a co-director of the Company. If *The Government Inspector* showcased his brilliant character work, the eagerly anticipated *Macbeth* (Scofield's first Shakespeare since *Lear*; Hall's first since the 1965 *Hamlet*) was a rare failure. Scofield, mercurial as ever, left the Company at the end of the run and refused to make the projected film of the production.

From the late 1960s to the end of the 70s his theatre work was dominated by new plays and included three productions at the Royal Court: Laurie in John Osborne's *The Hotel in Amsterdam* (Anthony Page, Royal Court, 1968); the title role in *Uncle Vanya* (Page, Royal Court, 1970); Voigt in Carl Zuckmayer's *The Captain of Köpenick* (Frank Dunlop, NT Old Vic, 1971); Pirandello's *The Rules of the Game* (Page, NT New, 1971); the kidnapped diplomat in Christopher Hampton's *Savages* (Robert Kidd, Royal Court, 1973); Prospero in *The Tempest* (Leeds Playhouse, 1975); the title role in Athol Fugard's *Dimetos* (Nottingham Playhouse, 1976); and Freddie in Ronald Harwood's *A Family* (Casper Wrede, Manchester Royal Exchange, 1978). He decided against returning to the RSC to star in Peter Brook's production of *Antony and Cleopatra*. At the National (Olivier, 1977-79), he accepted the roles of Volpone (Hall), Constantine Madras in Granville-Barker's *The Madras House* (William Gaskill), and Salieri in Peter Shaffer's *Amadeus* (Hall). Scofield's Salieri changed in an instant from youth to old age, from grace to tortured villainy. He stayed on at the National to play Othello (Hall, Olivier, 1980)—not a success: it effectively put an end to the notion that great white actors can black-up for the part—, Don Quixote (Bill Bryden, Olivier, 1982), and Oberon in *A Midsummer Night's Dream* (Bryden, Cottesloe, 1982).

From the early 1980s Scofield's appearances on the stage were few and far between. If *I am Not Rappaport* (Apollo, 1986-87) and Jeffery Archer's *Exclusive* (Strand, 1989) were bizarre choices, he was seen at his best in *Heartbreak House* (Nunn, Theatre Royal Haymarket, 1992) and *John Gabriel Borkman* (Richard Eyre, NT Lyttelton, 1996).

If Scofield never considered himself to be a film actor he still won the Best Actor Oscar for *A Man For All Seasons* (Fred Zinnemann, 1966). His other notable movies were John Frankenheimer's *The Train* (1964); Peter Brook's *King Lear* (1971); Kenneth Branagh's *Henry V* (1989); Robert Redford's *Quiz Show* (Robert Redford, 1995); and Nicholas Hytner's *The Crucible* (1996).

Fiona Shaw (b. County Cork, Ireland, 1958) read philosophy at University College, Cork, before training for the stage at RADA. Like her RSC contemporary Juliet Stevenson, she has increasingly based her interpretations on feminist readings. Following an unhappy experience playing Kate in *The Taming of the Shrew* for Jonathan Miller—Miller would not allow the inclusion of modern sexual politics—she has only occasionally worked with male directors. Her collaboration with Deborah Warner has produced a string of daring performances, but the work has sometimes been unsubtle in its denial of ambiguity. In performance she can come across as a militant visionary, and for this reason we might think of her as the Saint Joan of Stratford or the Virginia Woolf of the West End.

She won the Bancroft Gold Medal at RADA and made her professional debut as Rosaline in *Love's Labour's Lost* (Bolton, 1982). She next played Julia in *The Rivals* at the National (Peter Wood, Olivier, 1983) and Mary Shelley in Howard Brenton's *Bloody Poetry* at the Hampstead Theatre (1984).

At the RSC, 1985-89, she emerged as one of the best actresses of her generation, conspicuously intelligent but showing few hints of the absolute performer she was to become: Tatyana Vasilyevna in *Philistines* (John Caird, TOP, 1985); a wise Celia to Juliet Stevenson's Rosalind in *As You Like It* (Adrian Noble, RST, 1985); Madame de Volanges in *Les liaisons dangereuses* (Howard Davies, TOP, 1985); Erika Brückner to Alan Rickman's Brückner in *Mephisto* (Noble, Barbican, 1986); Beatrice opposite Nigel Terry in *Much Ado About Nothing* (Ron Daniels) and Portia in

The Merchant of Venice (Roger Michell, Small-scale Tour, 1986); Mistress Carol in *Hyde Park* (Barry Kyle, Swan, 1987); Katherine opposite Brian Cox in *The Taming of the Shrew* (Miller, RST, 1987); Lady Frampul in *The New Inn* (Caird, Swan, 1987); and the title role—shorn hair, black shift—in *Electra* (Pit, 1988), her first production with Deborah Warner and the first example of emotional extremism in her work.

Since leaving the RSC she has worked predominantly at the National: *Mary Stuart* (Greenwich, 1988); Rosalind in *As You Like It* (Old Vic, 1989); *The Good Person Of Sechuan* (Warner, NT Olivier, 1989); *Machinal* (Stephen Daldry, NT Lyttelton, 1993); the title role, manic from beginning to end, in *Hedda Gabler* (Warner, Abbey Theatre, Dublin, 1991); May in Beckett's *Footfalls* (Warner, Garrick, 1994); the title role in *Richard II* (Warner, NT Cottesloe, 1995); an effectively dramatic rendering of T.S. Eliot's *The Waste Land* in atmospheric settings (Warner, Wilton's Music Hall, Whitechapel, 1997, etc.)—with suburb mimicry she released the many London voices of Eliot's poem; Millamant opposite Roger Allam in *The Way of the World* (Phyllida Lloyd, NT Lyttelton, 1995); Joan in Honegger's cantata *Joan of Arc at the Stake* (Warner, Prom Concert, RAH, 1997); Jean Brodie in *The Prime of Miss Jean Brodie* (Lloyd, NT Lyttelton, 1998); the title role in *Medea* (Warner, Abbey Theatre, Dublin, 2000); *The PowerBook* (Warner, NT Lyttelton, 2002); Arkadina in Peter Stein's *The Seagull* (King's Theatre, Edinburgh Festival, 2003); and Portia in *Julius Caesar* (Warner, Barbican, 2005).

Sebastian Shaw (1905-1994, b. Holt, Norfolk). The long, distinguished career of Sebastian Shaw spanned seventy years and linked the pre-war Stratford of William Bridges-Adams with the modern company of Peter Hall, Trevor Nunn and Terry Hands. He joined the Stratford theatre at the age of twenty in 1926 and was still walking its stage in his eighties, a grandly charismatic elder statesman. He was a leading man in British movies of the

1930s and, his patrician features having become jowly with age, a fine character actor in the theatre of the 1960s, 70s and 80s.

He was a pupil at Gresham's School, Holt, where his father, the composer Geoffrey Shaw, taught music. (His was a well-to-do family dedicated to music—uncle Martin and grandfather James were also composers.) Theatre fascinated him from an early age. He appeared in a children's play at the Royal Court (1914), and played Petruchio to W.H. Auden's Kate in a school production of *The Taming of the Shrew*. For a career he originally chose the fine arts and did not change his mind until he had almost finished his studies at the Slade. He was briefly at RADA. Work in provincial repertory (Bristol, Liverpool and Hull) led to the leading juvenile roles at Stratford.

During the spring rehearsals for the 1926 Stratford season the theatre burned to the ground and the actors found themselves playing in a converted cinema in Greenhill Street. The company was led by Randle Ayrton, a famous Stratfordian who rarely performed in London. Shaw played Hal to Ayrton's Falstaff, and Romeo to his Mercutio. His other roles were Demetrius in *A Midsummer Night's Dream*; Green in *Richard II*; Bassanio in *The Merchant of Venice*; Fenton in *The Merry Wives of Windsor*; Citizen in *Coriolanus*; Ferdinand in *The Tempest*; and Metellus Cimber in *Julius Caesar*. All were directed by Bridges-Adams. In the West End he starred in Patrick Hamilton's *Rope* (1929); *Romeo and Juliet* (Embassy, Swiss Cottage, 1932); Ivor Novello's *Sunshine Sisters* (1933); *Double Door* (1934); J.M. Barrie's *A Kiss for Cinderella* (1937); and Robert Morley's *Goodness, How Sad!* (1938).

Shaw could play most of the staple character-types of the movies and worked prolifically for British studios during the 1930s. However, the films are largely forgotten. Shaw was not taken up by Alfred Hitchcock, and only once by Michael Powell (*The Spy in Black*, 1939). During the war he served in the RAF and appeared, alongside Richard Attenborough, in John Boulting's RAF film *Journey Together* (1944). In the 1950s he worked less than before, mostly on the stage: Heracles in *The Thracian Horses* (1946); Filmer Jesson in Pinero's *His House in Order* (New

Theatre, 1951); and Lucifer in *Brother Lucifer* (Shrewsbury Festival, 1957).

Shaw's years of relative decline came to an end when, in 1965, he joined the Royal Court to appear in new plays by John Osborne (*A Patriot for Me*, directed by Anthony Page), Arnold Wesker (*Their Very Own and Golden City*, directed by William Gaskill), Ann Jellicoe (*Shelley*), and N.F. Simpson (*The Cresta Run*). His performance as the union organiser in the Wesker was particularly admired.

In 1966 he returned to Stratford and began his long RSC career. He was Duncan to Paul Scofield's Macbeth (Peter Hall, RST, 1967); Friar Laurence in *Romeo and Juliet* (Karolos Koun, RST, 1967); Gloucester to Eric Porter's Lear (Trevor Nunn, RST, 1968); Ulysses in *Troilus and Cressida* (John Barton, RST, 1968); Leonato in *Much Ado About Nothing* (Nunn, RST, 1968); Justice Overdo in Ben Jonson's *Bartholomew Fair* (Terry Hands, Aldwych, 1969); Vincentio to Estelle Kohler's Isabella in *Measure for Measure* (Barton, RST, 1970); Polonius to Alan Howard's Hamlet (Nunn, RST, 1970); General Pechenegov in Gorky's *Enemies* (David Jones, Aldwych, 1971); the Duke of York in *Richard II* (Barton, RST, 1973); Boyet in *Love's Labour's Lost* (Jones, RST, 1973); Cymbeline (Barton/Barry Kyle, RST, 1974); Semyon in Gorky's *Summerfolk* (Jones, Aldwych, 1974); Shabelsky in Chekhov's *Ivanov* (Jones, Aldwych, 1976); Charles VI to Kenneth Branagh's Henry V (Adrian Noble, RST, 1985); Tubal in *The Merchant of Venice* (John Caird, RST, 1984); and the First Gravedigger in *Hamlet* (Ron Daniels, RST, 1984). Shaw's commitment to new writing was equally compelling—Sir Gerald Catesby in David Mercer's *Belcher's Luck* (Jones, Aldwych, 1966); Sir Oblong Fitz Oblong in Robert Bolt's *The Thwarting of Baron Bolligrew* (Nunn, Aldwych, 1966); Valletta in Trevor Griffiths's *Occupations* (Buzz Goodbody, The Place, 1971); Judge Michael Argyle in *The Oz Trial* (Goodbody, The Place, 1971); Best Friend in Edward Albee's *All Over* (Hall, Aldwych, 1972); and Professor Marvel/The Wizard in *The Wizard of Oz* (Ian Judge, Barbican, 1988-89).

Elsewhere, he played the Judge in *Whose Life Is It Anyway?* (Mermaid, 1978), and Jimmy in Brian Friel's *Translations* (Donald McWhinnie, Hampstead Theatre, 1981). His later screen work included the films *Return of the Jedi* (1983) and *High Season* (Clare Peploe, 1987), and the television dramas *Timon of Athens* (BBC, 1981), *Reilly, Ace of Spies* (1983), *Chimera* (1991), *Chernobyl: the Final Warning* (1991), *The Nation's Health* (Channel Four), and *Growing Rich* (ITV, 1991).

Shaw married the actress Margaret Delamere in 1929. She died in 1956. His play *The Cliff Walk* was produced at the Yvonne Arnaud Theatre, Guildford, in 1967; his novel *The Christening* was published in 1975. He wrote the lyrics to his father's opera *All at Sea*, performed at the Royal College of Music in 1956. Two of Shaw's plays—*The Glass Maze* and *Take a Life*—were performed by his RSC colleagues during the 1985 fringe festival at the Almeida.

Michael Sheen (b. Newport, Wales, 1969) was brought up in Port Talbot, the town that famously produced Richard Burton and Anthony Hopkins. He went to RADA and began his career at the highest level, appearing opposite Vanessa Redgrave in Martin Sherman's *When She Danced* (Globe, 1991). He next played Romeo in *Romeo and Juliet* (Gregory Hersov, Manchester Royal Exchange, 1992); Perdican in Alfred de Musset's *Don't Fool With Love* (Declan Donnellan, Cheek By Jowl, 1993); Fred in the premiere production of Harold Pinter's *Moonlight* (David Leveaux, Almeida, 1993); the title role in Ninagawa's 'virtual reality' *Peer Gynt* (Barbican, 1994); and Jimmy Porter to Claire Skinner's Alison in John Osborne's *Look Back in Anger* (Hersov, Manchester Royal Exchange, 1995). In 1997 he was outstanding as both Lenny in Pinter's *The Homecoming* at the National (Roger Michell, Lyttelton) and Henry V at the RSC (Ron Daniels, RST). Subsequent appearances: a second *Look Back in Anger* (Hersov, NT Lyttelton, 1999, opposite Emma Fielding); Mozart in *Amadeus* (Peter Hall, Old Vic, 1999); the title role in Albert Camus's

Caligula (Michael Grandage, Donmar Warehouse, 2003); the title role in David Farr's *The UN Inspector* (Farr, NT Olivier, 2005); and David Frost in Peter Morgan's *Frost/Nixon* (Grandage, Donmar, 2006).

Sheen has made moves to control his own destiny as an actor and director. In early 1997 Thin Language, the Welsh company he ran with Simon Harris, mounted a production (directed by Sheen) of Harris's play *Badfinger* at the Donmar. Also in 1997 he joined forces with Helen McCrory and Robert Delamere to set up a new writing production company called Foundry.

He gave an extraordinary performance as the mentally disturbed Joe, servant to Paul Rhys, in Barbara Vines's *Gallowglass* (BBC, 1995), and, directed by Stephen Frears, played Tony Blair in Peter Morgan's *The Deal* (Channel Four, 2003) and *The Queen* (2006).

Morgan Sheppard. Born in London but raised in Dublin, Morgan Sheppard served in the Norwegian Merchant Navy before gaining a scholarship to RADA (1956-58). His early theatre work included repertory at the Nottingham Playhouse (Keith Waterhouse's *Celebration*, 1961). An important character actor at the RSC from 1963 to 1974, he was a member of Peter Brook's group, appearing in the 'Theatre of Cruelty' seasons (1963-64), *Marat/Sade* (Aldwych, 1964), *The Investigation* (Aldwych, 1965) and *US* (Aldwych, 1966), but he was equally at home in such comedic classical roles as Bardolph in *The Merry Wives of Windsor* (John Blatchley, RST, 1964), Lory in *The Relapse* (Trevor Nunn, Aldwych, 1968) and Pistol in both *The Merry Wives of Windsor* (Terry Hands, RST, 1968) and *Henry V* (John Barton, Theatregoround and RST, 1971).

Also: Mr Hawkes in *Afore Night Come* (Clifford Williams, Aldwych, 1964); First Knight in *The Jew of Malta* (Williams, Aldwych, 1964); *Expeditions Two* (Aldwych, 1965); Williams in *Henry V* (Barton/Nunn, Aldwych, 1965); Surkkala-the-Red in Brecht's *Squire Puntila* (Michel Saint-Denis, Aldwych, 1965);

Glauser in Friedrich Dürrenmatt's *The Meteor* (Williams, Aldwych, 1966); Christopher Sly in *The Taming of the Shrew* (Nunn, RST, 1967); Duke Frederick in *As You Like It* (David Jones, RST, 1967); Marullus/Messala in *Julius Caesar* (Barton, RST, 1968); Wild Bill Hickok in *Indians* (Jack Gelber, Aldwych, 1968); ABC Round-up in Jules Feiffer's *God Bless* (Geoffrey Reeves, Aldwych, 1968); Antiochus/Boult in *Pericles* (Hands, RST, 1969); Antigonus in *The Winter's Tale* (Nunn, RST, 1969); Antonio in *Twelfth Night* (Barton, RST, 1969); Shakebag in *Arden of Faversham* (Buzz Goodbody, Roundhouse, 1970); Mason in Günter Grass's *The Plebeians Rehearse the Uprising* (Jones, Aldwych, 1970); Bolingbroke in *Richard II* (Barton, Theatregoround and RST, 1971); Borachio in *Much Ado About Nothing* (Ronald Eyre, RST, 1971); Duke of Venice in *Othello* (Barton, RST, 1971); Alfred in *Toad of Toad Hall* (Euan Smith, RST, 1972); Kleshch in Gorky's *The Lower Depths* (Jones, Aldwych, 1972); Third Priest in *Murder in the Cathedral* (Hands, Aldwych, 1972); Bedwy in *The Island of the Mighty* (Jones, Aldwych, 1972); *Cries from the Casement* (Hands, The Place, 1973); First Citizen in *Coriolanus* (Nunn/Goodbody, Aldwych, 1973); and Jim Craigin in *Sherlock Holmes* (Frank Dunlop, UK and US Tour, 1974).

Antony Sher (b. Cape Town, 1949) has been one of the defining members of the RSC since the early 1980s. An equally talented artist and writer, his book *The Year of the King* (Chatto, 1985) is the most valuable ever written about the RSC and among the best accounts of acting in the theatre. His background as an artist is perhaps the key to his method as an actor. He constructs characters from images, changing his appearance for each role and deliberately submerging his own personality. This approach looks back to Laurence Olivier, but Sher comes up with startlingly original, often revisionist, interpretations. He performs with the controlled aggression and fast reflexes of a lightweight boxer.

He left South Africa for England in 1968 in the hope of studying at a top drama school. Turned down by RADA and Central he finally won a place at the Webber Douglas Academy. His early experience included work at the Edinburgh Lyceum, the Nottingham Playhouse and the Liverpool Everyman, where he played Buckingham to Jonathan Pryce's *Richard III* (Alan Dossor, 1973) and Ringo in the musical *John, Paul, Ringo... and Bert* (1974). As Buckingham he appeared with sleeked back hair to provoke a laugh on the line 'My hair doth stand on end to hear her curses'. His career took flight in the latter half of the 1970s: he played the title role in *The Government Inspector* (William Gaskill, Edinburgh Festival), Anson in David Hare's *Teeth 'n' Smiles* (Hare, Royal Court, 1975), and Clive in Caryl Churchill's *Cloud Nine* (Max Stafford-Clark, Joint Stock, Royal Court, 1979). He reached a wide audience on television playing the lead in Malcolm Bradbury's *The History Man* (BBC), and transformed himself into a Saudi Arabian businessman for Mike Leigh's hit play *Goose-pimples* (Hampstead Theatre, 1981). Briefly at the National, he was Austin opposite Bob Hoskins in Sam Shepard's *True West* (John Schlesinger, Cottesloe, 1981).

At the RSC he has been drawn to outsiders and anti-heroes. He began with a famous Fool in Adrian Noble's production of *King Lear* (RST, 1982). Sher and Noble conceived the Fool as a small, crippled clown with red nose, bowler hat and child's violin. The Fool and Lear (Michael Gambon) performed some of their scenes as a Vaudeville double-act, a deliberately jarring image in the context of Shakespeare's play. In the same season he played the title role in Bulgakov's *Molière* (Bill Alexander, TOP), and in London, returning from injury (his Achilles tendon snapped during a performance of *Lear*, forcing him to miss the last few months of the Stratford year), the title role in *Tartuffe* (Alexander, Pit, 1983) and Martin Glass in David Edgar's *Maydays* (Ron Daniels, Barbican, 1983). He next gave his most audacious performance, as Richard III (Alexander, RST, 1984). In *The Year of the King* he describes how the physical appearance of his Richard grew from the image of a 'bottled spider' (hence the famous crutches) and a study of real deformities. It was a performance of relentless energy and the blackest humour.

Sher's RSC work continued with: Flote in *Red Noses* (Terry Hands, Barbican, 1985); an intense, unassimilated Shylock, deliberately unsympathetic, in *The Merchant of Venice* (Alexander, RST, 1987); Malvolio in *Twelfth Night* (Alexander, RST, 1987); Vindice in *The Revenger's Tragedy* (Di Trevis, Swan, 1987); Johnnie opposite Estelle Kohler in Athol Fugard's *Hello and Goodbye* (Janice Honeyman, Almeida, 1988); the title role in Peter Flannery's *Singer* (Hands, Swan, 1989); the title role in *Tamburlaine the Great* (Hands, Swan, 1992); Henry Carr in Tom Stoppard's *Travesties* (Noble, Barbican, 1993); the title role in *Cyrano de Bergerac* (Gregory Doran, Swan, 1997); Leontes in *The Winter's Tale* (Doran, RST, 1998); the title role in *Macbeth* (Doran, Swan, 1999-00); Domitian in *The Roman Actor* (Sean Holmes) and Malvole in *The Malcontent* (Dominic Cooke, Swan, 2002); and Iago in *Othello* (Doran, Swan, 2004). Sher was typically dynamic as Macbeth and Iago, but more original as Leontes: the interpretation suggested a profound psychosis (there was one Olivier moment—at breaking-point he fell backwards in a dead fall).

Other theatre: Arnold in *Torch Song Trilogy* (Albery, 1985); the title role in Sartre's *Kean* (Noble, Apollo, 2007); and, at the National, Arturo Ui in *The Resistible Rise of Arturo Ui* (Di Trevis, Olivier, 1991), Astrov in *Uncle Vanya* (Sean Mathias, Cottesloe, 1992), the title role in *Titus Andronicus* (Doran, NT Studio and Market Theatre Johannesburg co-production, Cottesloe, 1995), and Stanley Spenser in Pam Gems's *Stanley* (John Caird, Cottesloe, 1996).

Sher's first play, *ID*, was premiered at the Almeida in 2003 (Nancy Meckler). It was followed by *Primo*, a portrait of Primo Levi (Richard Wilson, NT Cottesloe, 2004); and *Giant*, about the rivalry of Michelangelo and Leonardo over an apprentice (Doran, Hampstead Theatre, 2007).

John Shrapnel (b. Birmingham, 1942). Son of the distinguished journalist Norman Shrapnel (parliamentary correspondent of *The Guardian* from the 1950s to the 1970s), John Shrapnel acted with the Marlowe Society while studying at St Catharine's College, Cambridge, and began his professional career in repertory at Birmingham, Leicester and Nottingham. His roles at Nottingham included Dunois in *Saint Joan*, Mick in Pinter's *The Caretaker*, Biff in Miller's *Death of a Salesman* and Claudio in *Measure for Measure*.

He first joined the RSC in Stratford in 1968, cast as Charles in *As You Like It* (David Jones), Patroclus in *Troilus and Cressida* (John Barton) and Balthasar in *Much Ado About Nothing* (Trevor Nunn).

On tour with Prospect during the early 1970s he played Edgar in *King Lear* and Berowne in *Love's Labour's Lost*. Then, at the National (Old Vic, 1972-73), he delivered a versatile quartet: Charles Surface in *The School for Scandal* (Jonathan Miller); Endicott in *The Front Page* (Michael Blakemore); Banquo in *Macbeth* (Blakemore); and Pentheus in Euripides's *The Bacchae* (Roland Joffé). He played supporting roles in the films *Nicholas and Alexandra* (Franklin Schaffner, 1971), *Pope Joan* (Michael Anderson, 1972) and *Hennessy* (Don Sharp, 1975). For the BBC, he was Sussex in *Elizabeth R* (1971), and McKendrick in Tom Stoppard's *Professional Foul* (Michael Lindsay-Hogg, 1977).

Shrapnel returned to the RSC in 1979. He has played figures of flawed authority from apparatchiks to kings with steely elegance: Vaguin in Gorky's *Children of the Sun* (Terry Hands, Aldwych, 1979); Agamemnon/Apollo in *The Greeks* (Barton, Aldwych, 1980); Hugh in David Mercer's *No Limits to Love* (Howard Davies, Warehouse, 1980); Jeremy in David Edgar's *Maydays* (Ron Daniels, Barbican, 1983); Sigmund in Arthur Miller's *The Archbishop's Ceiling* (Nick Hamm, Pit, 1986); George Selincourt in *A Penny for a Song* (Davies, Barbican, 1986); Foustka in Vaclav Havel's *Temptation* (Roger Michell, TOP, 1987); the title role in Ted Hughes's adaptation of *Oedipus* (Donald Sumpter, Almeida, 1988); Angelo, succeeding Sean Baker, in *Measure for Measure* (Nicholas Hytner, Barbican, 1988); Creon in *The Thebans* (Adrian Noble, Swan, 1991); Azriel in Solomon Anski's *The Dybbuk* (Katie Mitchell, Pit, 1992); and Claudius in the Kenneth Branagh *Hamlet* (Noble, Barbican, 1992).

Elsewhere: Verne in Mark Lee's *California Dog Fight* (Bush, 1985); Gibbs in Harold Pinter's *The Hothouse* (David Jones, Minerva, Chichester, 1995); the Captain in *South Pacific* (Nunn, NT Olivier, 2001-02); the title role in *Julius Caesar* (Deborah Warner, Barbican, 2005); and Gloucester in *King Lear* (Rupert Goold, Liverpool Everyman, 2008).

Josette Simon (b. Leicester, 1960) trained at the Central School of Speech and Drama. Her career changed course when she joined the RSC from the sci-fi television series *Blake's Seven* (BBC, 1980-81). Beginning quietly in 1982/83—Weird Sister in *Macbeth* (Howard Davies, RST); Josetta in *Much Ado About Nothing* (Terry Hands, RST); Anitra in *Peer Gynt* (Ron Daniels, TOP); Spirit in *The Tempest* (Daniels, RST); Iras in *Antony and Cleopatra* (Adrian Noble, TOP); Tendai in Nicholas Wright's *The Custom of the Country* (Pit, 1983)—she quickly progressed to leading roles: Nerissa in *The Merchant of Venice* (John Caird, RST, 1984); an ambitious young athlete in Louise Page's *Golden Girls* (Barry Kyle, TOP, 1984); Lindie Mann in Trevor Griffiths's *The Party* (Davies, TOP, 1984); an elegant, disdainful Rosaline to Roger Rees's Berowne in *Love's Labour's Lost* (Kyle, RST, 1984); Young Girl in Edward Bond's *War Plays* (Nick Hamm, Pit, 1985); and a coolly enigmatic Isabella, rejecting Roger Allam's Duke, in *Measure for Measure* (Nicholas Hytner, RST, 1987).

She was next in Arthur Miller's *After the Fall* (Michael Blakemore) and Webster's *The White Devil* (Philip Prowse) at the National (1990-91); Ibsen's *The Lady from the Sea* at the Lyric Hammersmith (1994); and *The Taming of the Shrew* at the Leicester Haymarket (1995). Her screen appearances during these years included the films *Cry Freedom* (Richard Attenborough,

1987) and *Milk and Honey* (1995), and the television dramas *Somewhere to Run* (ITV, 1989), *Nice Town* (BBC, 1992), *Dalziel and Pascoe* (BBC, 1998) and *Silent Witness* (BBC, 1998).

In 1999 she returned to the RSC to play Titania (doubled with Hippolyta) in *A Midsummer Night's Dream* (Michael Boyd, RST), and Queen Elisabeth in Schiller's *Don Carlos* (Gale Edwards, TOP).

Donald Sinden (b. Plymouth, 1923). The son of a chemist, Donald Sinden was brought up in the Sussex village of Ditchling where the family home doubled as a shop. His early academic progress was interrupted by serious illness (asthma) and he left school at fifteen. He found a position as an apprentice in joinery to T.B. Colman and Son, a firm of shopfitters in Hove (he hoped to become a draughtsman). He had no interest in the theatre, but fate intervened. A cousin who acted with an amateur group in Brighton persuaded Sinden to take his place in a play called *A Modern Aspasia*. Sinden took to acting, continued with the company, and was seen by Charles Smith, director of the Theatre Royal, Brighton, and founder of MESA (Mobile Entertainments Southern Area). For the duration of the war he worked out his apprenticeship with Colman's (now making ammunition boxes) while performing with MESA at night. Sinden had been pronounced unfit for active service; membership of MESA was classified as war work. He lived a double-life, never telling his Colman workmates about MESA and out of their presence carefully developing an actor's persona—he had the tall good looks of a leading man but the famous voice, strong and clipped, had to be acquired. MESA travelled to bases throughout Sussex, Hampshire, Kent and Surrey, and performed such plays as *George and Margaret*, *Private Lives* and *French Without Tears* in village halls and Nissen huts.

At the end of his apprenticeship he abandoned Colman's and enrolled at the Webber Douglas Academy, then temporarily based in Hampshire. He performed with MESA between terms.

A MESA production, *The Normandy Story*, was picked up by ENSA (Entertainments National Service Association) and Sinden spent the last year of the war entertaining troops and released prisoners in Europe and India.

On his return to England he began his Stratford career as a member of the 1946 and 1947 companies. In 1946, the first year of Peter Brook and Paul Scofield, his work included Adrian in *The Tempest* (Eric Crozier); Arviragus in *Cymbeline* (Nugent Monck); Dumain in Brook's production of *Love's Labour's Lost*; Grey in the Scofield *Henry V* (he was due to play the Dauphin but the director, Dorothy Green, demoted him when he arrived unshaven for the first rehearsal); and Le Beau/William in *As You Like It* (Herbert M. Prentice). In 1947 he met his future wife, Diana Mahony, and played Paris in *Romeo and Juliet* (Brook); Aumerle in *Richard II* (Walter Hudd); and Lorenzo in *The Merchant of Venice* (Michael Benthall). At the end of the Stratford season the company took Brook's *Romeo and Juliet* to London: because of the indisposition of Laurence Payne Sinden played Romeo for most of the engagement.

During the next few years he appeared with the Old Vic Company at the New Theatre, London; with Peggy Ashcroft and Ralph Richardson in *The Heiress* at the Theatre Royal Haymarket (John Gielgud, 1949-50); and at the Bristol Old Vic as Nicholas in *The Lady's Not For Burning*, Mr Honeywood in Goldsmith's *Good Natured Men* and Pistol in *The Merry Wives of Windsor* (1950).

At the beginning of the 1950s Sinden broke into movies with *The Cruel Sea* and accepted a contract with the Rank organisation. It was not until his return to the RSC and his performance as York to Peggy Ashcroft's Margaret in *The Wars of the Roses* (Peter Hall, RST, 1963) that his stature as a classical actor— deeply resonant characterisations, musical verse-speaking— became clear. Sinden remained with the RSC for the next seventeen years, entertaining and enlightening audiences in a wide spectrum of work, including Sir Novelty Fashion in *The Relapse* (Trevor Nunn, Aldwych, 1967); Malvolio—a masterpiece of physical invention and unforeseen vocal inflections—in *Twelfth Night* (John Barton, RST, 1969); the title role in *Henry VIII* (Nunn, RST, 1969); Sir William Harcourt Courtly in Boucicault's *London Assurance* (Ronald Eyre, Aldwych, 1970); Benedick to Judi Dench's Beatrice—a great autumnal duet—in *Much Ado About Nothing* (Barton, RST, 1976); a fine King Lear (Nunn, RST, 1976); and Othello (Ronald Eyre, RST, 1979).

Posterity, left with the films, may falsely view Donald Sinden as a minor star who specialised in looking urbane in uniforms and tropical suits. His work in the popular situation comedies *Two's Company* (1977-80) and *Never the Twain* (1981-83) established his latter-day public persona—that of a fruity-voiced thespian waiting, according to the satirical puppet show *Spitting Image*, for a knighthood.

Claire Skinner (b. Hemel Hempstead, Hertfordshire, 1965) trained at the London Academy of Music and Dramatic Art. Early in her career she was a member of Alan Ayckbourn's company at Scarborough, playing Norma and Tracey in *The Revenger's Comedies*, Blanche in *Wolf at the Door* (an adaptation of Henry Becque's *Les Corbeaux*), and Desdemona opposite Michael Gambon in *Othello* (1989-90).

She could have concentrated on ingénue roles into her thirties but instead sought diversity. She played the sensible daughter, a tomboy working as a plumber, in *Life is Sweet* (Mike Leigh, 1991); Lenny Henry's bossy sous-chef in the first series of *Chef* (BBC, 1993); an elegant girl in *Naked* (Leigh, 1993); a bespectacled Cecily in *The Importance of Being Earnest* (Nicholas Hytner, Aldwych, 1993); the ghostly Bridget in Harold Pinter's *Moonlight* (David Leveaux, Almeida, 1993); Alison to Michael Sheen's Jimmy in *Look Back in Anger* (Gregory Hersov, Manchester Royal Exchange, 1995); Laura in *The Glass Menagerie* (Sam Mendes, Donmar Warehouse, 1995); a fragile Desdemona in Mendes's production of *Othello* (NT Cottesloe, 1997); and Hermione in *The Winter's Tale* (Hytner, NT Olivier, 2001). At the

RSC she was a member of the ensemble formed by Trevor Nunn to open the new Other Place in 1991. She played Hermine in Pam Gems's *The Blue Angel* and conveyed both vulnerability and determination as Isabella in *Measure for Measure*.

Other notable screen work: *Clockwork Mice* (Vadim Jean, 1995); *Smilla's Feeling for Snow* (Bille August, 1997); *A Dance to the Music of Time* (Channel Four, 1997); *Sleepy Hollow* (Tim Burton, 1999); *Mauvaise passe* (Michel Blanc, 1999); *Second Sight* (BBC, 2000); Stephen Poliakoff's *Perfect Strangers* (BBC, 2001); Tony Marchant's *Swallow* (Channel Four, 2001); Andy Hamilton's *Bedtime* (BBC, 2001) and *Trevor's World of Sport* (BBC, 2003); Nick Dear's *Eroica* (Simon Cellan Jones, BBC, 2003); *Life Begins* (ITV, 2004); *The Trial of Tony Blair* (Cellan Jones, Channel Four, 2007); *Outnumbered* (BBC, 2007); *And When Did You Last See Your Father?* (Anand Tucker, 2007); Fanny Dashwood in *Sense and Sensibility* (BBC, 2008).

Jonathan Slinger performed with the Accrington Amateurs before taking up a place at RADA in 1991. He made his debut playing Yepikhodov in a Leicester Haymarket production of *The Cherry Orchard* (Misha Mokeiev, 1994). His breakthrough role was Harry Percy in the Deborah Warner/Fiona Shaw *Richard II* at the National (Cottesloe, 1995). Warner later cast him as Carstairs in her film *The Last September* (1999) and as the tutor in *Medea* (Queen's, 2001).

The young Slinger had the presence, inventiveness and technical skill to make a significant impression in supporting roles. At the Globe he was Florizel in *The Winter's Tale* (David Freeman) and Amintor in *The Maid's Tragedy* (Lucy Bailey, 1997); at the Manchester Royal Exchange, Touchstone in *As You Like It* (Marianne Elliott, 2000). He then returned to the National: Harry Trench in Bernard Shaw's *Widowers' Houses* (Fiona Shaw, Cottesloe, 2000); Nicholas Sazonov/Sleptsov in Tom Stoppard's *The Coast of Utopia* (Trevor Nunn, Olivier, 2002); Philippe in

Nick Dear's *Power* (Lindsay Posner, Cottesloe, 2002); and Delio in *The Duchess of Malfi* (Phyllida Lloyd, Lyttelton, 2003).

Since 2005 Slinger has been a member of the RSC. During his first season he was a very corporal, clumsily funny but casually vindictive red-headed Puck in *A Midsummer Night's Dream* (Gregory Doran, RST); the Trader in David Greig's *The American Pilot* (Ramin Gray, TOP); and Dromio of Syracuse in *The Comedy of Errors* (Nancy Meckler, RST). He stayed on to play both leading and supporting roles in Michael Boyd's Complete Works/Histories project at the Courtyard (2006-08) — the Bastard of Orleans/Richard in *Henry VI*, the title role in *Richard III*, the title role in *Richard II*, Fang/Francis Feeble in the second part of *Henry IV* and Captain Fluellen in *Henry V*. As Richard III, shaven-headed and black suited, he gave a dazzlingly virtuosic display in the familiar manner of sinister comedy adopted by most modern-day Crookbacks. (Will a director ever dare to make Richard a less entertaining psychopath?) His fanatical Fluellen was only a little less deranged.

Sound. The RSC's sound designers rarely achieve recognition, perhaps because soundtracks are designed to work subliminally.

Andrea J. Cox studied Physics and Philosophy at Liverpool University. She gained her early experience at the Liverpool Everyman and the Bristol Old Vic. She was a member of the Stratford sound department from 1987 to 2007, designing atmospheric soundtracks for Sam Mendes's *Troilus and Cressida* (Swan, 1990), Adrian Noble's *The Thebans* (Swan, 1991), Max Stafford-Clark's *A Jovial Crew* (Swan, 1992), Katie Mitchell's *Ghosts* (TOP, 1993), Michael Boyd's *Henry VI* (Swan, 2000), and Steven Pimlott's *Richard II* (TOP, 2000).

Jeremy Dunn trained at the Northcott Theatre, Exeter, and worked at the Bristol Old Vic and for West End and touring organisations before joining the RSC in 1990. He worked as a sound supervisor in the Pit and as a member of the RSC's touring unit until his appointment as head of sound in 2000.

John A. Leonard (b. 1951) trained at the Bristol Old Vic Theatre School and joined the staff of the Bristol Old Vic, initially as a stagehand, in 1971. He ran the sound department at a time when Bristol was home to a generation of outstanding young artists, including, in quick succession, the future RSC directors Howard Davies, Bill Alexander, John Caird and Adrian Noble. Leonard similarly moved to the RSC: beginning as a sound engineer at the Warehouse, he was promoted to head the sound department in 1984. During his time with the RSC Leonard created tapes for most productions in the London studios and, working with his colleagues Roland Morrow and Frank Bradley, many in the main house. He left the RSC in 1988.

Tim Oliver joined the RSC in 1988. He was previously the resident sound designer at the Chichester Festival Theatre. He has created soundtracks for Michael Attenborough's *The Herbal Bed* (TOP, 1996), Gregory Doran's *Cyrano de Bergerac* (Swan, 1997), Michael Boyd's *The Spanish Tragedy* (Swan, 1997), and Laurence Boswell's *The Dog in the Manger* (Swan, 2004).

Paul Slocombe joined the RSC in 1982 and headed the Stratford sound department from 1986 to 97. He designed tapes for many productions in the RST during these years.

Timothy Spall (b. London, 1957). The son of a Post Office worker and a hairdresser, Timothy Spall was raised on a council estate in Battersea, south London. He spent his spare time serving with the army cadets (Clapham Junction Third Royal Tank Regiment) and working at Battersea fun fair. Encouraged by his mother (an amateur singer) and by his ability to make people laugh as the Lion in a school production of *The Wizard of Oz*, he successfully auditioned for a place at the National Youth Theatre. His rare gifts were recognised early on, at RADA (where he played Macbeth and Othello and won the Bancroft Gold Medal), and at the RSC, his home from 1979 to 1981. From the start he was a master of dysfunctional characters, the flawed and the seedy, but also of the self-deluded, the good and the plain ordinary; there was, and is, humour and candour in his subtle rendering of the human condition.

After RADA, in 1978, he appeared at the Birmingham Rep, playing Graziano in Arnold Wesker's *The Merchant*, Baptista in *Kiss Me Kate* and Laurence in David Edgar's *Mary Barnes* (Peter Farago, 1979). He made his film debut in The Who's *Quadrophenia* (Franc Roddam, 1979). Then at the RSC he played Peter Simple in *The Merry Wives of Windsor* (Trevor Nunn/John Caird, RST, 1979); First Lord in *Cymbeline* (David Jones, RST, 1979); Waiter/Undertaker in Erdman's *The Suicide* (Ron Daniels, TOP, 1979); Mech/Bollebol in Brecht's *Baal* (Jones, TOP, 1979); Andrei in *Three Sisters* (Nunn, TOP, 1979); Young Wackford/Mr Folair in *Nicholas Nickleby* (Nunn/Caird, Aldwych, 1980); and Rafe in Beaumont's *The Knight of the Burning Pestle* (Michael Bogdanov, Aldwych, 1981).

On leaving the RSC he went into television. He was in Mike Leigh's *Home Sweet Home* (BBC, 1982) and became well-known as the obtuse Brummie electrician in *Auf Wiedersehen Pet* (1984-89). A few years later he was given his own drama series, *Frank Stubbs Promotes* (ITV, 1993-94), and a starring role, alongside Josie Lawrence (playing his wife) and Brenda Blethyn, in *Outside Edge* (1994). His collaboration with Mike Leigh continued with the award-winning features *Life is Short* (1990) and *Secrets and Lies* (1996). He also worked for Ken Russell (Dr Polidori in *Gothic*, 1986), Clint Eastwood (Hodkins in *White Hunter, Black Heart*, 1990), Bernardo Bertolucci (Jill Bennett's repugnant son in *The Sheltering Sky*, 1990), and Kenneth Branagh (Rosencrantz in *Hamlet*, 1996).

He joined John Sessions at the Almeida for Brecht's *Man Equals Man* (1986), and was at the National in 1992 playing Monsieur Jourdain in *Le bourgeois gentilhomme* (Richard Jones, Lyttelton) and Bottom in *A Midsummer Night's Dream* (Robert Lepage, Olivier).

Serious illness halted his career for a while, but he came back as strong as ever in Caryl Churchill's *This is a Chair* (Stephen Daldry, Royal Court at the Duke of York's, 1997); *The Wisdom of Crocodiles* (Po-Chih Leong, 1998); Tim Firth's *Neville's Island* (Terry Johnson, ITV, 1998); *Our Mutual Friend* (BBC, 1998), as Mr Venus; Dick Clement and Ian La Frenais's rock band movie *Still Crazy* (Brian Gibson, 1998), as the drummer; Stephen Poliakoff's *Shooting the Past* (BBC, 1999); Mike Leigh's *Topsy-Turvy* (1999); Kenneth Branagh's *Love's Labour's Lost* (1999), as Don Armado; *The Clandestine Marriage* (Christopher Miles, 1999); *Vatel* (Roland Joffé, 2000); *Intimacy* (Patrice Chéreau, 2001); Poliakoff's *Perfect Strangers* (BBC, 2001); *Vacuuming Completely Nude in Paradise* (Danny Boyle, 2001); *Lucky Break* (Peter Cattaneo, 2001); *Vanilla Sky* (Cameron Crowe, 2001); Leigh's *All or Nothing* (2002); *Nicholas Nickleby* (2002); the return of *Auf Wiedersehen, Pet* (BBC, 2002-04); *The Last Samurai* (Edward Zwick, 2003); *Harry Potter and the Prisoner of Azkaban* (Alfonso Cuarón, 2004); *The Street* (BBC, 2006-07); *A Room with a View* (ITV, 2007), as Mr Emerson; *Olivier Twist* (BBC, 2007), as Fagin; and *Sweeney Todd* (Tim Burton, 2007).

Elizabeth Spriggs (1929-2008, b. Buxton). Originally an opera singer, the redoubtable Elizabeth Spriggs began her acting career at the Bristol Old Vic in 1953. Within a few years she was starring as Cleopatra in *Antony and Cleopatra* and Madame Ranevsky in *The Cherry Orchard* (Birmingham Rep, 1958). At the RSC for fourteen years from 1962, she played the Shakespearean roles that could have been written for her—Gertrude in *Hamlet* (Peter Hall, RST, 1965), Mistress Quickly in the two parts of *Henry IV* (John Barton et al, RST, 1966), the Nurse in *Romeo and Juliet* (Karolos Koun, RST, 1967), Mistress Ford in *The Merry Wives of Windsor* (Terry Hands, RST, 1968), Paulina in *The Winter's Tale* (Trevor Nunn, Aldwych, 1970), Maria in *Twelfth Night* (Barton, Aldwych, 1970) and Beatrice in *Much Ado About Nothing* (Ronald Eyre, RST, 1971). Her interpretations were bravura in the best sense: grand, life-affirming and abundant with character detail. However, she was equally persuasive when playing less extravagantly in contemporary works—Rossignol in Peter Weiss's *Marat/Sade* (Peter Brook, Aldwych, 1964); Claire in Edward Albee's *A Delicate Balance* (Hall, Aldwych, 1969); Eleanor in David Mercer's *Duck Song* (David Jones, Aldwych, 1974); and Queen Mariana in Peter Barnes's *The Bewitched* (Hands, Aldwych, 1974).

On leaving Stratford Elizabeth Spriggs was seen at the National and increasingly on television. The drama serials *Shine On Harvey Moon* (1982-85), *Oranges Are Not the Only Fruit* (1990), *Middlemarch* (1994), *Martin Chuzzlewit* (1995) and *Playing the Field* (1998) brought her before a wide public. She was a memorable presence in the films *Sense and Sensibility* (Ang Lee, 1995) and *Paradise Road* (Bruce Beresford, 1997).

Max Stafford-Clark (b. Cambridge, 1941) was educated at Trinity College, Dublin. As a selector and director of new writing, he has been a constantly influential figure. At the Traverse Theatre, Edinburgh, in the late 1960s, with Joint Stock during the 1970s, at the Royal Court from 1979 to 93, and with Out of Joint since, he has worked tirelessly at the coalface of contemporary writing.

Writers who have benefited from his advocacy include: David Hare—*Fanshen* (1975); Caryl Churchill—*Light Shining in Buckinghamshire* (1976), *Cloud Nine* (1979), *Top Girls* (1982), *Serious Money* (1987); Timberlake Wertenbaker—*Our Country's Good* (1988), *Three Birds Alighting On a Field* (1991); Andrea Dunbar—*Rita, Sue and Bob Too* (1982); Michael Hastings—*Tom and Viv* (1984); Ron Hutchinson—*Rat in the Skull* (1984); Stephen Jeffreys—*The Libertine* (1994); Sebastian Barry—*The Steward of Christendom* (1995), *Our Lady of Sligo* (1998); April de Angelis—*The Positive Hour* (1997), *A Laughing Matter* (2002); and Mark Ravenhill—*Shopping and Fucking* (1996), *Some Explicit Polaroids* (1999).

In 1992 Stafford-Clark accepted an invitation from Adrian Noble to work at the RSC on 17th century texts. He directed outstanding productions in the Swan of the rarity *A Jovial Crew* (1992) and William Wycherley's *The Country Wife* (1993).

Barry Stanton joined Peter Brook's RSC experimental group in 1966 and appeared in the controversial protest piece *US* (Aldwych). Physically commanding and skilfully adaptable, he was subsequently cast in mainstream roles, including Arthur Landau in Paddy Chayefsky's *The Latent Heterosexual* (Terry Hands, Aldwych, 1968); the President in Jules Feiffer's *God Bless* (Geoffrey Reeves, Aldwych, 1968); Lord Hastings in *Richard III* (Hands, RST, 1970); Voltemand in the Alan Howard *Hamlet* (Trevor Nunn, RST, 1970); first Snug and then Bottom in Brook's *A Midsummer Night's Dream* (RST, 1970; International Tour, 1972-73); Caliban in *The Tempest* (John Barton, RST, 1970); Oswald in Brook's film of his 1962 *King Lear* (1970); Captain Boboyedovin in Gorky's *Enemies* (David Jones, Aldwych, 1971); George in Jean Genet's *The Balcony* (Hands, Aldwych, 1971); Dr Bravo in Peter Barnes's *The Bewitched* (Hands, Aldwych, 1974); Lucio in *Measure for Measure* (Keith Hack, RST, 1974); and Banquo in the Nicol Williamson/Helen Mirren *Macbeth* (Nunn, RST, 1974).

After the 1975 season he left the Company and pursued character parts in films and on television. Michael Bogdanov's English Shakespeare Company gave him a new lease of theatrical life at the end of the 1980s—he was masterly as Falstaff and York in *The Wars of the Roses* (Old Vic and International Tour, 1989). In the 1990s he appeared in *Johnny on the Spot* (Richard Eyre, NT Olivier, 1994), *The Woman in Black* (Fortune, 1996) and Stephen Daldry's *An Inspector Calls* (Garrick, 1997).

He rejoined the RSC briefly in 1990—Redozubov in Gorky's *Barbarians* (Jones, Barbican)—and has been back in earnest since 1998: Stephano in *The Tempest* (Adrian Noble, RST, 1998); Noel in Robert Holman's *Bad Weather* (Steven Pimlott, TOP, 1998); a temperamental and threatening Shamrayev in *The Seagull* (Noble, Swan, 2000); a repulsive Sir Toby Belch in *Twelfth Night* (Lindsay Posner, RST, 2001); Dr Johnson in Peter Barnes's *Jubilee* (Gregory Doran, Swan, 2001); and the 2002 Gunpowder season (Swan)—Leonides in Middleton and Rowley's *A New Way to Please You* (Sean Holmes), Berenthius in Massinger's *Believe What You Will* (Josie Rourke), and Tiberius in Jonson's *Sejanus: His Fall* (Doran).

Katy Stephens (b. Southampton) trained at the Royal Welsh College of Music and Drama and appeared in pantomimes and plays at the Belgrade, Coventry, and the Mercury, Colchester, for ten years from 1996, the jealously-guarded secret of patrons of these theatres. As well as entertaining audiences each Christmas as a glamorous villainess or principal boy, she played Viola in *Twelfth Night* (Bob Eaton, 1999); the Bride in García Lorca's *Blood Wedding* (Sue Lefton, 2001); Natasha in *Three Sisters* (2003); Lady Macbeth in *Macbeth* (2004); Creusa in Euripides's *Ion* (David Hunt, 2004); and Masha in *The Seagull* (David Hunt, 2005).

Michael Boyd must have been keeping his eye on the Belgrade, for in 2006 he brought Katy Stephens to the RSC to play Margaret of Anjou in the three parts of *Henry VI*. Margaret is an iconic role in the Company's history because of its size, rarity and pedigree (Peggy Ashcroft, Helen Mirren and Penny Downie). If that wasn't enough, Katy Stephens was also cast as Joan of Arc in the same production. Ashcroft had brought to her interpretation of Margaret decades of Shakespearean experience. It is legitimate to wonder why the RSC no longer attracts actresses of the stature of Ashcroft and Mirren, while acclaiming Katy Stephens's achievement in embodying Margaret's dangerous sexuality and ruthless ambition. During the history cycle (Courtyard and Roundhouse, 2007-08), she was also the Duchess of Gloucester in *Richard II* and Lady Northumberland in the second part of *Henry IV*.

463

Robert Stephens (1931-1995, b. Bristol). Robert Stephens's career divides into three acts. In act one he emerged as a leading actor at the Royal Court and the National. Already a performer of originality, daring and predatory charisma, he was one of the few to make headway within Olivier's regime. He married Maggie Smith and played Holmes in Billy Wilder's *The Private Life of Sherlock Holmes* (1970). Act two saw his departure from the National, the breakup of his marriage, and over a decade of routine television parts. In act three he re-emerged as a great classical actor, this time at the RSC.

He was born in Bristol, the first child of a building labourer and a factory worker. In his autobiography, *Knight Errant* (Hodder and Stoughton, 1995), he describes a childhood of little money, less love, and pervading violence (he was regularly beaten by his mother). He discovered his gift for acting at school and at the local youth club. He went on a National Association of Boys Clubs drama course, and won a scholarship to attend the Bradford Civic Theatre School, run by Esmé Church (1949-51). At Bradford he erased his Bristol accent, and married a fellow student after she became pregnant (his wife returned to Ireland and they never lived together). At the end of the course he toured with the Caryl Jenner Mobile Theatre Company, then began weekly rep in Morecambe (1951). In 1953 he played an Arab in the farce *Not a Clue* and met his second wife, the actress Tarn Bassett. It was at the Library Theatre, Manchester, that he started to find his voice: Iago, Biff in *Death of a Salesman*, Cassius in *Julius Caesar*, Voltore in *Volpone*, Horner in *The Country Wife*, and Dunois in *Saint Joan* (1955).

During his first year at the Royal Court he was cast in both supporting and leading roles: Judge Haythorne in *The Crucible* (George Devine, 1956); Ronald Duncan's *Don Juan* and *The Death of Satan* (Devine, 1956); Nigel Dennis's *Cards of Identity* (Tony Richardson, 1956); *The Good Woman of Setzuan* (Devine, 1956); Dorilant in *The Country Wife* (Devine, 1956); Jean Giradoux's

The Apollo de Bellac (Richardson); Jim in Michael Hastings's *Yes–and After* (John Dexter, 1957); Nigel Dennis's *The Making of Moo* (Richardson, 1957); Oliver Marlow Wilkinson's *How Can We Save Father?* (Peter Wood, 1957); Krank in John Arden's *The Waters of Babylon* (Graham Evans, 1957); and Graham (plus Olivier's understudy) in John Osborne's *The Entertainer* (Richardson, Palace, 1957). His performance as the failed writer in Osborne's *Epitaph for George Dillon* made his name in 1958. The production transferred to Broadway, where Stephens was fêted by the New York arts mafia. Returning to London he played opposite Vivien Leigh in Noël Coward's Feydeau adaptation *Look After Lulu* (Richardson, Royal Court, 1959), and Margaret Leighton in John Mortimer's *Wrong Side of the Park* (Peter Hall, Cambridge Theatre, 1960). He created the role of Peter in Wesker's *The Kitchen* (Royal Court, 1959).

Stephens almost joined the RSC in 1960 (he auditioned for the role of Iago in the John Gielgud *Othello*, but Franco Zeffirelli went with Ian Bannen), and again in 1962 when he reluctantly turned down Iachimo in William Gaskill's production of *Cymbeline*. Under contract to Twentieth Century Fox (the result of his success in *Dillon*), he was playing a minor part in *Cleopatra* and trapped by the film's protracted shoot.

In 1963 he was one of the first actors to join Laurence Olivier's National Theatre company. If Olivier made the National in his own image, Stephens's presence in the company constantly threatened to break the mould. His partnership with Maggie Smith gave the National of the 1960s much of its theatrical flair and glamour. Every time they appeared together the NT had a hit: Captain Plume/Silvia in *The Recruiting Officer* (William Gaskill, 1963); Sandy/Myra in Noël Coward's *Hay Fever* (Coward, 1964); Benedick/Beatrice in Franco Zeffirelli's *Much Ado About Nothing* (1965); Vershinin/Masha in *Three Sisters* (Olivier, 1967); Archer/Mrs Sullen in *The Beaux' Stratagem* (Gaskill, 1970); and Loevborg/Hedda in Ingmar Bergman's *Hedda Gabler* (1970). On screen, in *The Prime of Miss Jean Brodie* (Ronald Neame, 1969), he gave one of his many near self-portraits as the art teacher infatuated with Smith's Jean Brodie but unable to resist a nubile schoolgirl. It was a suburb performance, but second fiddle to Smith. As her career soared (she won the best actress Oscar for Brodie), this became a pattern. Stephens's biggest solo success came in 1964, when he played Atahuallpa in Peter Shaffer's *The Royal Hunt of the Sun* (Dexter). Other work at the National: Horatio in *Hamlet* (Olivier, 1963); the Dauphin in *Saint Joan* (John Dexter, 1963); Max Frisch's *Andorra* (Lindsay Anderson, 1964); Man in Beckett's *Play* (George Devine, 1964); Lindsay in John Arden's *Armstrong's Last Goodnight* (Gaskill/Dexter, 1965); *Trelawny of the Wells* (Desmond O'Donovan, 1965); Harold in Shaffer's *Black Comedy* (Dexter, 1966); John Osborne's Lope de Vega adaptation *A Bond Honoured* (Dexter, 1966); Kurt in Strindberg's *The Dance of Death* (Glen Byam Shaw, 1967); the title role in *Tartuffe* (Tyrone Guthrie, 1967); John Maddison Morton's *Most Unwarrantable Intrusion*, which he directed (1968); Somerset Maugham's *Home and Beauty* (Frank Dunlop, 1968); and John Spurling's *Macrune's Guevara*, which he co-directed with Frank Dunlop (1969).

Olivier never repaid the loyalty of star players like Stephens and Anthony Hopkins, holding back the major Shakespearean roles even though he was too old for them himself. He made Stephens an associate director in 1969, but their relationship declined rapidly: Stephens started to set up his own productions with Maggie Smith and Olivier shut the door on both of them. It was a time of growing turmoil. Billy Wilder cast Stephens as Holmes in what promised to be a major film. It was his big chance for stardom and the pressure was such that he took an overdose of sleeping pills during the shoot. He put his own individuality into the role, but *The Private Life of Sherlock Holmes* failed at the box office. At the same time his marriage to Maggie Smith was coming to an end. There was one final production and it was more than apposite, Coward's *Private Lives* (John Gielgud, Queen's, 1972). In 1975 he met his fourth wife, the actress Patricia Quinn (they played opposite each other in Anthony Shaffer's *Murderer*).

Stephens career went into relative decline after 1970. The low point was a production of *Othello* at the Open Air Theatre, Regent's Park (1976). There were successes. In 1974 he led a company for Jonathan Miller at the Greenwich Theatre, playing Trigorin in *The Seagull*, Claudius in *Hamlet* and Pastor Manders in *Ghosts*, and the following year he succeeded John Neville in the RSC's *Sherlock Holmes* on Broadway. He had two spells with Peter Hall's National on the South Bank: in 1978 he played Gaev in *The Cherry Orchard* (Hall, Olivier), the Mayor in *Brand* (Christopher Morahan, Olivier), and scored an Old Vic style hit as Maskwell in Congreve's *The Double Dealer* (Peter Wood, Olivier); in the mid-1980s, as a member of Bill Bryden's group, he succeeded Paul Scofield as Oberon in *A Midsummer Night's Dream* (Cottesloe, 1983), played opposite Ralph Richardson in Eduardo de Filippo's *Inner Voices* (Mike Ockrent, Lyttelton, 1983), and doubled the roles of Herod and Pontius Pilate in *The Mysteries* (Bryden, Cottesloe, 1985). In 1982 he decided against joining the RSC to play Falstaff in Trevor Nunn's production of *Henry IV*. He took many television and film roles during this period, his skill and instinct for character evident in even the least ambitious of them. His performance as the writer dying of drink and failure in *Fortunes of War* (BBC, 1987) was particularly memorable.

Adrian Noble wanted Stephens to lead his first RSC company (1991), and offered Falstaff in the two parts of *Henry IV* (Noble, RST) and the title role in *Julius Caesar* (Steven Pimlott, RST). Stephens had been away from the stage for five years; he was ready to return to a repertory company. His remarkable Falstaff was a charming, predatory, cagey and mean old operator — the performance seemed to encapsulate Dylan Thomas's 'rage, rage against the dying of the light'. Every performance was subtly different, an improvisation within the margins of the play. Stephens's distinctive, alliterative delivery of the lines highlighted key phrases ('I am old, old', 'If I had a thousand sons'). He spoke the speech on honour ('...honour is a mere scutcheon') leaning against the proscenium wall, spitting out the obscure final word to give it meaning. The title role in *King Lear* followed (Noble, RST, 1993). Stephens was seriously ill, but it was a masterly performance, a deeply moving elegy from Dover on (speaking the line 'When we are born we cry that we are come to this great stage of fools. This is a good block' he slapped the Stratford stage with the palm of his hand as though it represented all the theatres of his life). His premature death robbed the English stage of a flawed but fascinating actor, the most talented since Scofield.

Toby Stephens (b. London, 1969). The son of Robert Stephens and Maggie Smith, Toby Stephens trained at the London Academy of Music and Dramatic Art and immediately won an important role in Peter Hall's television adaptation of *The Camomile Lawn* (Channel Four, 1991). He then joined the RSC to play, in his first season (1992-93), an arrogant, aristocratic Bertram in *All's Well That Ends Well* (Peter Hall, Swan), King of Argier/Celebinus in *Tamburlaine the Great* (Terry Hands, Swan), and Pompey in *Antony and Cleopatra* (John Caird, RST). In London (Pit) he added Piccolomini in Schiller's *Wallenstein* (Tim Albery) and Beamish in Michael Hastings's *Unfinished Business* (Steven Pimlott).

He returned to Stratford as a leading actor, the youngest ever RSC Coriolanus (David Thacker, Swan, 1994). He also played Lysander in *A Midsummer Night's Dream* (Adrian Noble, RST), and Claudio in *Measure for Measure* (Pimlott, RST).

In the years since he has inevitably given preference to the cinema: *Photographing Fairies* (Nick Willing, 1996); Orsino in *Twelfth Night* (Trevor Nunn, 1996); Victorin Hulot in *Cousin Bette* (1998); Lensky in *Onegin* (Martha Fiennes, 1999); Clint Eastwood's younger self in *Space Cowboys* (2000); Gatsby in *The Great Gatsby* (Robert Markowitz, TV, 2001); the villain in the Bond film *Die Another Day* (2002); *Severance* (2006). And to television: Gilbert Markham in *The Tenant of Wildfell Hall* (BBC, 1996); Stephen Poliakoff's *Perfect Strangers* (BBC, 2001); Philby in *Cam-*

bridge Spies (Tim Fywell, BBC, 2003); *Poirot: Five Little Pigs* (Paul Unwin, ITV, 2003); *Waking the Dead* (BBC, 2005); Tony Armstrong Jones in *The Queen's Sister* (Channel Four, 2005); *Sharpe's Challenge* (ITV, 2006); Rochester in *Jane Eyre* (BBC, 2006); Custer in *The Wild West* (2007).

Stephens's theatre career continued with a season at the Almeida—Hippolytus in *Phèdre* and Nero in *Britannicus* (both Jonathan Kent, Albery, 1998)—and three roles for Peter Hall at the Haymarket—Stanley to Jessica Lange's Blanche in *A Streetcar Named Desire* (1997), the title role in Simon Gray's *Japes* (2001), and Anthony in *The Royal Family* (2001). In 2004 he returned to the RSC to play the title role in *Hamlet* (Michael Boyd, RST), and Jesus in *The Pilate Workshop* (Boyd, TOP).

Juliet Stevenson (b. Essex, 1956) won the Bancroft Gold Medal at RADA and first worked in children's theatre, touring with the Theatre Centre. She joined the RSC by chance, called up at the eleventh hour because an injured actress had to withdraw, and in that first season (1978-79) found herself playing a spirit in *The Tempest* (Clifford Williams, RST); Curtis in *The Taming of the Shrew* (Michael Bogdanov, RST); both nun and whore in *Measure for Measure* (Barry Kyle, RST); Iras in Peter Brook's production of *Antony and Cleopatra* (RST); Aphrodite/Artemis in *Hippolytus* (Ron Daniels, TOP); Caroline in Howard Brenton's *The Churchill Play* (Kyle, Warehouse); Yelena in Bulgakov's *The White Guard* (Kyle, Aldwych); Octavia as well as Iras during the London run of *Antony and Cleopatra* (Aldwych); and Miss Chasen in *Once in a Lifetime* (Trevor Nunn, Aldwych).

She quickly became the best young actress in the Company. Despite an intellectual feminism that led her to deny the sexual complexity of Cressida and Hedda, she is an actress of rare feeling and restrained sensuality: Lady Percy in *Henry IV* (Bill Alexander, Small-scale Tour, 1980); Hippolyta and Titania in Ron Daniels's 'Victorian' *Midsummer Night's Dream* (RST, 1981); Susan in *The Witch of Edmonton* (Kyle, TOP, 1981); Clara Douglas in Edward Bulwer-Lytton's *Money* (Alexander, TOP, 1981); striking in black as a young Isabella, intelligent and resourceful, in *Measure for Measure* (Adrian Noble, RST, 1983); tender as the loyal maid Polya in Stephen Poliakoff's *Breaking the Silence* (Daniels, Pit, 1984); ironically dyeing her hair blonde as feminism came to the fore for Cressida in *Troilus and Cressida* (Howard Davies, RST, 1985) and Rosalind in Noble's radical *As You Like It* (RST, 1985); exceptional as the destroyed Madame de Tourvel in *Les liaisons dangereuses* (Davies, TOP, 1985).

Theatre dominated her twenties, although early on she appeared in two television series, *Maybury* and *The Mallens*. Since leaving the RSC in 1986 she has concentrated on dramatic screen roles, most memorably producing inspired performances as Rosalind Franklin, the King's College London scientist who discovered DNA, in *Life Story* (Mick Jackson, BBC, 1987), and Nina in Anthony Minghella's *Truly Madly Deeply* (1991). Other work of note: *Drowning By Numbers* (Peter Greenaway, 1987); Nora in *A Doll's House* (David Thacker, BBC, 1991); *In the Border Country* (Thaddeus O'Sullivan, Channel Four, 1991); Fraulein Burstner in *The Trial* (David Jones, 1993); Isobel in *The Secret Rapture* (Howard Davies, 1993); Flora in Paula Milne's *The Politician's Wife* (Graham Theakston, Channel Four, 1995); Mrs Elton in *Emma* (1996); *Mona Lisa Smile* (Mike Newell, 2003); *Being Julia* (István Szabó, 2004); Annie Pierrepoint in *The Last Hangman* (Adrian Shergold, 2005); *Infamous* (2006); *And When Did You Last See Your Father?* (Anand Tucker, 2007).

Juliet Stevenson's theatre appearances since 1986 have included: the title role in García Lorca's *Yerma* (Di Trevis, NT Cottesloe, 1987); Hedda in *Hedda Gabler* (Howard Davies, NT Olivier, 1989); Lanford Wilson's *Burn This* (Robert Allan Ackerman, Lyric, 1990), opposite John Malkovich; *Death and the Maiden* (Lindsay Posner, Royal Court, 1992); the title role in *The Duchess of Malfi* (Philip Franks, Greenwich Theatre, 1995); Grusha in Brecht's *The Caucasian Chalk Circle* (Simon McBurney, NT Olivier, 1997); the six miniatures of *Beckett Shorts*, an isolated return to the RSC (Katie Mitchell, TOP, 1997); Amanda to Anton

Lesser's Elyot in *Private Lives* (Franks, NT Lyttelton, 1999); Corinna in Martin Crimp's *The Country* (Mitchell, Royal Court, 2000); Hetty in Imogen Stubbs's *We Happy Few* (Nunn, Gielgud, 2004); and Arkadina in *The Seagull* (Mitchell, NT Lyttelton, 2006).

Patrick Stewart (b. Mirfield, West Yorkshire, 1940) worked as a junior reporter on a local paper before gaining a place at the Bristol Old Vic Theatre School (1957). His early career included repertory at Lincoln, Manchester (Library Theatre), Sheffield, Liverpool and Bristol, and an international tour with the Old Vic Company.

He was a core member of the RSC from 1966 to 1982. Despite having the voice and presence to tackle the big leading roles, he continued to play supporting parts for much of his time with the Company—such luxury casting helped to establish the RSC in the 1960s and 70s. Stewart was classical and contemporary. He was both a comedian and a tragedian. As a young actor he may have lost out because of this versatility.

His RSC career began at the Aldwych in 1966 with the role of Witness 3 in Peter Brook's production of Peter Weiss's *The Investigation*. By that summer he was in Stratford playing Sir Walter Blunt/Lord Mowbray in *Henry IV* (John Barton/Trevor Nunn); the First Player in the David Warner *Hamlet* (Peter Hall); the Dauphin in the Ian Holm *Henry V* (Barton/Nunn); and Hippolito in *The Revenger's Tragedy* (Nunn). Stewart, like the other leading RSC members of the 1960s and 70s, rarely took a break: Grumio in *The Taming of the Shrew* (Nunn, RST, 1967); the Banished Duke in *As You Like It* (David Jones, RST, 1967); Worthy in *The Relapse* (Nunn, Aldwych, 1967); Cornwall in *King Lear* (Nunn, RST, 1968); Touchstone in *As You Like It* (Jones, RST, 1968); Hector in *Troilus and Cressida* (Barton, RST, 1968); Borachio in *Much Ado About Nothing* (Nunn, RST, 1968); Teddy Foran in Sean O'Casey's *The Silver Tassie* (Jones, Aldwych, 1969); Lantern Leatherhead in Ben Jonson's *Bartholomew Fair* (Terry Hands,

Aldwych, 1969); Edward IV in *Richard III* (Hands, RST, 1970); the title role in *King John* (Buzz Goodbody, RST and Theatregoround, 1970); Launce in *The Two Gentlemen of Verona* (Robin Phillips, RST, 1970); Stephano in *The Tempest* (Barton, RST, 1970); Snout in Brook's *A Midsummer Night's Dream* (Aldwych, 1971); Skrobotov in Gorky's *Enemies* (Jones, Aldwych, 1971); Kabak in Trevor Griffiths's *Occupations* (Goodbody, The Place, 1971); Roger in Jean Genet's *The Balcony* (Hands, Aldwych, 1971); Aufidius in *Coriolanus* (Nunn/Goodbody, RST, 1972); Cassius in *Julius Caesar* (Nunn/Goodbody, RST, 1972); Enobarbus in *Antony and Cleopatra* (Nunn/Goodbody, RST, 1972); Astrov in *Uncle Vanya* (Nicol Williamson, TOP, 1974); Luvborg opposite Glenda Jackson in *Hedda Gabler* (Nunn, Aldwych, 1975); Larry Slade in Eugene O'Neill's *The Iceman Cometh* (Howard Davies, Aldwych, 1976); Shakespeare in Edward Bond's *Bingo* (Davies, TOP, 1976); Oberon in *A Midsummer Night's Dream* (Barton, RST, 1977); Knatchbull in Howard Barker's *That Good Between Us* (Kyle, Warehouse, 1977); Basho in Bond's *The Bundle* (Davies, Warehouse, 1977); Colonel Goosen in Norman Fenton's *A Miserable and Lonely Death* (Walter Donohue, Aldwych, 1978); Engels in *Landscape of Exile* (Davies, Warehouse, 1978); Shylock in *The Merchant of Venice* (Barton, TOP, 1978); Enobarbus in *Antony and Cleopatra* (Brook, RST, 1978); the King in David Rudkin's *Hippolytus* (Daniels, TOP, 1978); Myshlaevsky in Bulgakov's *The White Guard* (Kyle, Aldwych, 1979); Leontes in *The Winter's Tale* (Ronald Eyre, RST, 1981); Sir Eglamour/Titus in Barton's double-bill of *The Two Gentlemen of Verona* and *Titus Andronicus* (RST, 1981); and the title role in *Henry IV* (Nunn, Barbican, 1982). In 1985/86 he moved briefly to the National to play King David and then the title role in Peter Shaffer's *Yonadab* (Peter Hall, Olivier).

During these years Stewart appeared in the films *Hennessy* (Don Sharp, 1975); *Excalibur* (John Boorman, 1981); *Dune* (David Lynch, 1984); *The Doctor and the Devils* (Freddie Francis, 1985); and *Lady Jane* (Nunn, 1986). On television, he was Claudius in *Hamlet* (Rodney Bennett, BBC, 1980), and Karla in *Tinker, Tailor,*

Soldier, Spy (John Irvin, BBC, 1980) and *Smiley's People* (Simon Langton, BBC, 1982).

The second, American, phase of his career began when he was cast as Jean-Luc Picard in *Star Trek: the Next Generation* (1987). *Star Trek* (of which he was also a producer and sometime director) dominated a dull Hollywood screen career: *L.A. Story* (1991); King Richard in *Robin Hood: Men in Tights* (Mel Brooks, 1993); four *Star Trek* movies (1994-02); *Dad Savage* (1997); Dr Jonas in the Mel Gibson thriller *Conspiracy Theory* (Richard Donner, 1997); and three *X-Men* movies (Bryan Singer, 2000-06).

Stewart resumed his theatre career in America in the mid-1990s: Prospero in *The Tempest* (Broadhurst Theater, New York, 1996); the title role in *Othello* (Jude Kelly, The Shakespeare Theater, Washington DC, 1997); and Lyman Felt in Arthur Miller's *The Ride Down Mount Morgan* (David Esbjornson, Public Theater, New York, 1998). Returning to England, he played the title role in J.B. Priestley's *Johnson Over Jordan* at the West Yorkshire Playhouse (Jude Kelly, 2001); Solness in *The Master Builder* at the Albery (Anthony Page, 2003); Robert in David Mamet's *A Life in the Theatre* at the Apollo (Lindsay Posner, 2005); the title role in *Macbeth* and Malvolio in *Twelfth Night* at Chichester (Rupert Goold/Philip Franks, 2007); and, back with the RSC, Antony in *Antony and Cleopatra* (Gregory Doran, Swan, 2006), Prospero in *The Tempest* (Goold, RST, 2006) and Claudius in *Hamlet* (Doran, Courtyard, 2008).

Malcolm Storry (b. Hull, 1948) studied at Bretton Hall College (Wakefield) and began his theatre career working as an Assistant Stage Manager at the Library Theatre, Manchester (1969). His early progress included membership of Charles Marowitz's Open Space Theatre and Richard Eyre's Nottingham Playhouse. For Marowitz, he played the Duke in *An Othello*, Hoss in Sam Shepard's *The Tooth of Crime* and the Drum Major in *Woyzeck* (1972-73); for Eyre, Yasha in *The Cherry Orchard* (1977).

He joined the RSC in 1978, and became an associate artist in 1994. There is something unassuming about Storry despite his commanding physical presence and gravitas. He took time to step forward as one of the leaders of the Company, eventually starring as Volpone (Lindsay Posner, Swan, 1999), Prospero in *The Tempest* (Michael Boyd, Roundhouse, 2002) and Bottom in *A Midsummer Night's Dream* (Gregory Doran, RST, 2005). His acting is honest and direct, free of rhetorical gestures. Kent in the Michael Gambon *King Lear* (Adrian Noble, RST, 1982), Stoman in Trevor Griffiths's *The Party* (Howard Davies, TOP, 1984), Williams in *Henry V* (Noble, RST, 1984) and the damaged giant Manik, henchman to Antony Sher, in Peter Flannery's *Singer* (Terry Hands, Swan, 1989) are good examples of his versatility, but any of the following would do as well: Jimmy Umpleby in Howard Brenton's *The Churchill Play* (Barry Kyle, TOP, 1978); Joseph in *The Shepherd's Play* (John Tucker, Aldwych, 1978); Galanba in Bulgakov's *The White Guard* (Kyle, Aldwych, 1979); Theo in Pam Gems's *Piaf* (Davies, Warehouse, 1979); John Dory in *Wild Oats* (Clifford Williams, Aldwych, 1979); Jack in Brenton's *Sore Throats* (Kyle, Warehouse, 1979); Yegor in Gorky's *The Children of the Sun* (Hands, Aldwych, 1979); Farquarson in Peter Whelan's *Captain Swing* (Bill Alexander, Warehouse, 1979); Clive Heap in Peter Prince's *Television Times* (Stephen Frears, Warehouse, 1980); Venturewell's Man in *The Knight of the Burning Pestle* (Michael Bogdanov, Aldwych, 1981); the Soldier in *La Ronde* (John Barton, Aldwych, 1982); Banquo in the Bob Peck *Macbeth* (Davies, RST, 1982); Foreman/Stranger in Edward Bond's *Lear* (Kyle, TOP, 1982); One Eye in Bulgakov's *Molière* (Alexander, TOP, 1982); Macduff in *Macbeth* (Davies, Barbican, 1983—Storry and Pete Postlethwaite exchanged the roles they had played in Stratford); James Grain in David Edgar's *Maydays* (Ron Daniels, Barbican, 1983); Lacenaire in Caryl Churchill's *Softcops* (Davies, Pit, 1984); Buckingham in the Antony Sher *Richard III* (Alexander, RST, 1984); Aufidius in *Coriolanus* (Hands, RST, 1989); Bajazeth in *Tamburlaine the Great* (Hands, Swan, 1992); De Flores in *The Changeling* (Michael Attenborough, Swan, 1992); and Enobarbus in *Antony and Cleopatra* (Steven Pimlott, RST, 1999).

Storry has occasionally appeared elsewhere: Yasmina Reza's *Art* (Matthew Warchus, Wyndham's, 1997-98); the Labour leader in *The Absence of War* (Birmingham Rep, 2003); Danforth in *The Crucible* (Hands, Clwyd Theatr Cymru, 2003); and De Guiche in *Cyrano de Bergerac* (Howard Davies, NT Olivier, 2004).

Geoffrey Streatfeild joined the RSC in 2000, his first work in the theatre, to play the minor roles of Young Clifford, Vernon and Lovell in Michael Boyd's productions of the three parts of *Henry VI* and *Richard III* (Swan). ('First work' is rather misleading—Streatfeild had undergone a long apprenticeship at the National Youth Theatre, Manchester University and RADA.)

The next few years saw him play the Officer in Harold Pinter's *Mountain Language* at the Royal Court (Katie Mitchell, 2001); Chorus in Euripides's *Bacchai* at the Olivier (Peter Hall, 2002); Graziano in *The Merchant of Venice* at Chichester (Gale Edwards, 2003); the tortured Stanhope, vividly presented, in *Journey's End* in the West End (David Grindley, Comedy Theatre, 2004); and Irwin in Alan Bennett's *The History Boys* at the Lyttelton (Nicholas Hytner, 2004). His success as Stanhope led to the role of Gent in *Twenty Thousand Streets Under the Sky* (BBC, 2005).

Streatfeild returned to Stratford as one of the leaders of the history cycle ensemble (Courtyard, 2006-08): Suffolk/Rivers in *Henry VI*, Rivers in *Richard III*, Hal in *Henry IV* and the title role in *Henry V*.

Imogen Stubbs (b. Newcastle, 1961) gave an unforgettable performance in *The Two Noble Kinsmen* (Barry Kyle, Swan, 1986). There was a subtle amalgam of humour and longing in her interpretation of the Gaoler's Daughter, a lovesick girl descending into madness. She played the 'mad scene' as though transported by the fantasy (the Gaoler's Daughter believes herself to be in the crow's nest of a ship) and the pity of the moment, tapping into real grief. She spoke the lines with a skill of spontaneity and emphasis, so that over two decades later they still belong to her voice ('they shall stand in fire up to the naval and in ice up to th' heart, and there th'offending part burns, and the deceiving part freezes...').

She came to the RSC from RADA, where her contemporaries included Ralph Fiennes, Iain Glen and Jane Horrocks. Before that she read English at Exeter College, Oxford, played Irina in *Three Sisters* and Cressida for the Oxford University Dramatic Society, and acted in a film with her Oxford contemporaries Hugh Grant and James Wilby (*Privileged*, Michael Hoffman, 1982). She was a schoolgirl at St Paul's and Westminster. Fifteen years after her first RSC season—she was also a spirited Helena in John Barton's Swan production of Aphra Behn's *The Rover* and Queen Isabel in *Richard II* (Kyle, RST), playing opposite Jeremy Irons—there is a feeling of unfulfilled promise about Imogen Stubbs. She has returned to the RSC only once, in 1989, to play a fine Desdemona in *Othello* (Trevor Nunn): in the intimate Other Place, where you could smell her perfume and the lemonade in her glass, her performance was beautifully modulated and touching, but curiously muted until the death scene when Desdemona fought for her life against Willard Whites's Othello—murder on the stage has rarely been as shocking. It is a cause of some regret that she did not follow the example of predecessors such as Judi Dench, Helen Mirren and Estelle Kohler and stay longer at the RSC.

Work outside of the RSC has included: Ellie in *Heartbreak House* (Nunn, Theatre Royal Haymarket, 1991); the title role in *Saint Joan* (Gale Edwards, Strand Theatre, 1993); Yelena in *Uncle Vanya* (Bill Bryden, Chichester, 1996); a graceful, hungry Stella in Peter Hall's *A Streetcar Named Desire* (Theatre Royal Haymarket, 1997); Polly in Ben Elton's two-hander *Blast from the Past* (Jude Kelly, West Yorkshire Playhouse, 1998); Anna in Patrick Marber's *Closer* (Lyric, 1998, succeeding Frances Barber); Emma in Harold Pinter's *Betrayal* (Nunn, NT Lyttelton, 1998); Amanda in *The Relapse* (Nunn, NT Olivier, 2001); Masha in *Three Sisters* (Patrick Sandford, Nuffield Theatre, Southampton, 2002); *Mum's the Word* (Albery, 2003); her own play *We Happy Few* (Stephen Rayne, Malvern, 2003); Gertrude in *Hamlet* (Nunn, Old Vic, 2004); Marianne opposite Iain Glen in Ingmar Bergman's *Scenes From a Marriage* (Nunn, Belgrade, Coventry, 2008). For the most part she has concentrated on television and film work, good performances in mostly forgettable pieces. Restricted to supporting roles, she played Lucy Steele in *Sense and Sensibility* (Ang Lee, 1995). She had a rare opportunity to shine as Viola in Trevor Nunn's film of *Twelfth Night* (1996).

David Suchet (b. London, 1946) trained at the London Academy of Music and Dramatic Art and worked extensively in provincial repertory before joining the RSC in 1973. By 1979 he had emerged as one of the Company's most powerful leading actors: Tybalt in *Romeo and Juliet* (Terry Hands, RST, 1973); Orlando opposite Eileen Atkins in *As You Like It* (Buzz Goodbody, RST, 1973)—he replaced the injured Bernard Lloyd; Tranio in the Susan Fleetwood/Alan Bates *The Taming of the Shrew* (Clifford Williams, RST, 1973); Mole in *Toad of Toad Hall* (Euan Smith, RST, 1973); Hubert in *King John* (Barry Kyle/Barton, RST 1974); the Fool in *King Lear* (Goodbody, TOP, 1974); Pisanio in *Cymbeline* (Kyle/Barton/Williams, RST, 1974); Nikolai Petrovich Zamislov in Gorky's *Summerfolk* (David Jones, Aldwych, 1974); Willmer in Strindberg's *Comrades* (Kyle, The Place, 1974); Ferdinand in *Love's Labour's Lost* (Jones, Aldwych, 1975); Caliban in *The Tempest* (Williams, RST, 1978); Grumio in the Jonathan Pryce/Paola Dionisotti *The Taming of the Shrew* (Michael Bogdanov, RST, 1978); Sir Nathaniel in *Love's Labour's Lost* (Barton, RST, 1978); Pompey in Peter Brook's *Antony and Cleopatra* (RST, 1978); Herman Glogauer in *Once in a Lifetime* (Trevor Nunn, Aldwych, 1979); Angelo, succeeding Jonathan Pryce, in *Measure for Measure* (Kyle, Aldwych, 1979); a calm Bolingbroke in the Alan Howard *Richard II* (Hands, RST, 1980); Edward IV in *Rich-*

ard III (Hands, RST, 1980); a sympathetic Shylock in *The Merchant of Venice* (Barton, RST, 1981); a thuggish, narcissistic Achilles in Terry Hands's production of *Troilus and Cressida* (Aldwych, 1981); Mazda in *The Swan Down Gloves* (Aldwych, 1981); Tom Stoppard's *Every Good Boy Deserves Favour* (1983); and Iago to Ben Kingsley's Moor in *Othello* (Hands, RST, 1985).

Since leaving the RSC his profile has been primarily that of a character actor on television (star of *Agatha Christie's Poirot* since 1989) and in mainstream movies, but between assignments he has returned to theatre: Tom Kempinski's *Separation* (Michael Attenborough, Hampstead Theatre, 1986); the title role in *Timon of Athens* (Trevor Nunn, Young Vic, 1991); the American professor opposite Lia Williams in David Mamet's *Oleanna* (Harold Pinter, Royal Court, 1993); George opposite Diana Rigg in *Who's Afraid of Virginia Woolf?* (Howard Davies, Almeida, 1996); *Saturday, Sunday, Monday* (Chichester, 1998); Salieri in *Amadeus* (Peter Hall, Old Vic, 1998); and Gregor Antonescu in Terence Rattigan's *Man and Boy* (Maria Aitken, Duchess, 2005).

Suchet's career in movies has included both British and American productions — *The Missionary* (Richard Loncraine, 1982); *Greystoke* (Hugh Hudson, 1984); *The Little Drummer Girl* (George Roy Hill, 1984); *The Falcon and the Snowman* (John Schlesinger, 1985); *A World Apart* (Chris Menges, 1988); *To Kill a Priest* (Agnieszka Holland, 1988); the terrorist leader in *Executive Decision* (Stuart Baird, 1996); the detective in *A Perfect Murder* (Andrew Davis, 1998); Napoleon in *Sabotage!* (2000); *Foolproof* (2003); *The Bank Job* (2008). He has reserved some of his best work for television: the title role in *Freud* (BBC, 1983); Blott in *Blott on the Landscape* (BBC, 1984); Bloom in the *Ulysses* episode of 'Great Writers' (Channel Four, 1988); Verloc in *The Secret Agent* (1992); *Cruel Train* (BBC, 1995); Augustus Melmotte in *The Way We Live Now* (BBC, 2002); Wolsey in *Henry VIII* (ITV, 2003); and the title role in *Maxwell* (BBC, 2007).

Tim Supple (b. Lewes) read English at Cambridge and started his career directing young actors at the Theatre Royal, York. In the 1980s and early 90s he followed a disparate career, dividing his time between workshop productions and the mainstream— *Guys and Dolls* (Haymarket, Leicester, 1988); David Holman's Christmas show for children, *Whale* (NT Lyttelton, 1989); *Accidental Death of an Anarchist* (NT Cottesloe, 1991); *Billy Budd* (Sheffield Crucible, 1991); John Sessions's *Travelling Tales* (Theatre Royal Haymarket, 1991); the Kenneth Branagh *Coriolanus* (Renaissance, Chichester, 1992); *Billy Liar* (NT Cottesloe, 1992); and a version of the epic of Gilgamesh, *He Who Saw Everything* (NT Cottesloe, 1993).

As artistic director of the Young Vic (1993-99), working with his partner Melly Still, he directed productions—often of classic stories aimed at the young—in a style that was both basic and chic: *Grimm's Tales* (1994); *The Jungle Book* (1995); Ted Hughes's version of García Lorca's *Blood Wedding* (1996); *More Grimm's Tales* (1997); *As I Lay Dying* (1998); and *Twelfth Night* (1998). He took this style to the National (Salman Rushdie's *Haroun and the Sea of Stories*, 1998) and to the RSC, where his productions of *The Comedy of Errors* (TOP, 1996) and *A Servant to Two Masters* (TOP, 1999) were particularly admired.

In 2000 he returned to large-scale work, not his forte, directing Nick Dear's *The Villain's Opera* and *Romeo and Juliet* at the National (Olivier).

Kit Surrey. Following his training at the Wimbledon School of Art, Kit Surrey worked as a design assistant at the Glasgow Citizens' (late 1960s). He was Head of Design at the Northcott Theatre, Exeter, from 1974 to 1976, the year he began his long association with the RSC. Working in particular with Bill Alexander, his best sets were conceived for The Other Place and The Warehouse: *Dingo* (Barry Kyle, TOP, 1976); *Captain Swing* (Bill Alexander, TOP, 1978); *The Churchill Play* (Kyle, TOP, 1978); *The Suicide* (Ron Daniels, TOP, 1979); *Sore Throats* (Kyle, Warehouse,

1979); *Men's Beano* (Alexander, Warehouse, 1979); *The Accrington Pals* (Alexander, Warehouse, 1981); *A Doll's House* (Adrian Noble, TOP, 1981); *Lear* (Kyle, TOP, 1982); *Golden Girls* (Kyle, TOP, 1984); *The Merchant of Venice* (Alexander, RST, 1987); *Twelfth Night* (Alexander, RST, 1987); *The Comedy of Errors* (Nick Hamm, Small-scale Tour, 1987); *Cymbeline* (Alexander, Pit, 1988); *Playing With Trains* (Ron Daniels, Pit, 1989); *Much Ado About Nothing* (Alexander, RST, 1990); and *The Bright and Bold Design* (Alexander, Pit, 1991).

Janet Suzman (b. Johannesburg, 1939) studied English and French at the multi-racial Witwatersrand University in the late 1950s. She was a member of the drama society but most of her energy went into the student protest against the Extension of University Education Bill. The bill was a means of introducing Apartheid into higher education, and when it was passed in 1959 Suzman decided to leave South Africa for England. As the niece of the opposition MP Helen Suzman she had been watched and even interviewed by the South African Special Branch.

In England she set out to become a professional actress. She trained at the London Academy of Music and Dramatic Art and made her first appearance as Liz in Keith Waterhouse's *Billy Liar* at the Tower Theatre, Ipswich (1962). She joined the RSC for the 1963 season, made an immediate impact as Joan of Arc in *The Wars of the Roses* (Peter Hall) and was rapidly promoted. Projecting a strong image of integrity and intelligence she claimed many of Shakespeare's heroines (making them more independent-minded than seductively feminine) in a ten-year journey that took her from the early comedies to the late tragedies: Luciana in *The Comedy of Errors* (Clifford Williams, RST, 1963); Lady Percy in the first part of *Henry IV* (Hall/John Barton, RST, 1964); Lady Anne in *Richard III* (Hall/Barton, RST, 1963); Rosaline in *Love's Labour's Lost* (Barton, RST, 1965); Portia in *The Merchant of Venice* (Williams, RST, 1965); Timandra in *Timon of Athens* (John

Schlesinger, RST, 1965); Ophelia, succeeding Glenda Jackson, in *Hamlet* (Hall, RST, 1965); Kate in *The Taming of the Shrew* (Trevor Nunn, RST, 1967); Celia to Dorothy Tutin's Rosalind in *As You Like It* (David Jones, RST, 1967); Beatrice opposite Alan Howard in *Much Ado About Nothing* (Nunn, RST, 1968); Rosalind in *As You Like It* (Jones, RST, 1968); Cleopatra opposite Richard Johnson in *Antony and Cleopatra* (Nunn/Buzz Goodbody, RST, 1972); and Lavinia in *Titus Andronicus* (Nunn/Goodbody, RST, 1972). Her non-Shakespearean roles were Lulu in Harold Pinter's *The Birthday Party* (Pinter, Aldwych, 1964); Berinthia in *The Relapse* (Nunn, Aldwych, 1967); and, re-emerging as a South African, Hester opposite Ben Kingsley in Athol Fugard's *Hello and Goodbye* (Peter Stevenson, The Place, 1973).

On the screen she gave a moving performance as Sheila in Peter Nichol's *A Day in the Death of Joe Egg* (Peter Madek, 1970) and brought unexpected complexity and grace to Hollywood's *Nicholas and Alexandra* (Franklin Schaffner, 1971). Although she continued to perform leading characters in classical drama—Masha in *Three Sisters* (Jonathan Miller, Cambridge, 1976); Brecht's Good Woman of Setzuan (Royal Court, 1977); Hedda Gabler (Duke of York's, 1977); the Duchess of Malfi (Birmingham Rep, 1979); Racine's Andromache (Miller, Old Vic, 1988); Phaidra in *Hippolytus* (Andrei Serban, Almeida, 1991); and both Clytemnestra and Helen of Troy in the RSC's *The Greeks* (Barton, Aldwych, 1980)—she increasingly looked for projects that allowed her to reconnect with her homeland and sought new challenges in teaching and directing. She starred in Fugard's *Boesman and Lena* at the Hampstead Theatre (1984), and the anti-Apartheid movie *A Dry White Season* (1990). Most notably she returned to Johannesburg (Market Theatre) to create South African versions of classic texts with multi-racial casts: *Othello* (1987); Brecht's *The Good Woman of Setzuan* renamed *The Good Woman of Sharksville* (1996); and, reunited with her RSC contemporary Estelle Kohler, a haunting *Cherry Orchard* (1997). Among her other productions as a director were Michael Hastings's *A Dream of People* at the RSC (Pit, 1990); *The Cruel Grasp* at the Edinburgh Festival (1991); Feydeau's *No Flies on Mr Hunter* at the Chelsea Centre (1992); Arthur Miller's *Death of a Salesman* at Theatr Clwyd (1993); and Pam Gems's *The Snow Palace* at the Tricycle Theatre (1998).

Janet Suzman returned to Stratford in 2002 to perform with Donald Sinden, Ian Richardson and Derek Jacobi a new version of John Barton's *The Hollow Crown*. During the Complete Works Festival of 2006/07 her Baxter Theatre (Cape Town) production of *Hamlet* visited the Swan and she played Volumnia in *Coriolanus*, the old RST's final show (Gregory Doran).

T

Owen Teale (b. Swansea, 1961). Owen Teale's significant early stage roles were O'Brien in Catherine Cookson's *The Fifteen Streets* (Rob Bettinson, Belgrade, Coventry, 1988); Sergei Esenin, the Russian poet, to Sheila Gish's Isadora Duncan in Martin Sherman's *When She Danced* (Tim Luscombe, King's Head, 1988); Antipholus of Syracuse in *The Comedy of Errors* (Phyllida Lloyd, Bristol Old Vic, 1989); and Titus in Racine's *Berenice* (Tim Albery, NT Cottesloe, 1990).

He was a member of the RSC during the Robert Stephens era, playing a powerful Hotspur in *Henry IV Part One* (Adrian Noble, RST, 1991); Mark Antony in *Julius Caesar* (Steven Pimlott, RST, 1991); Edmund in *King Lear* (Noble, RST, 1993); Bassanio in *The Merchant of Venice* (David Thacker, RST, 1993); and Navarre in *Love's Labour's Lost* (Ian Judge, RST, 1993).

He enjoyed a big success as Torvald opposite Janet McTeer in *A Doll's House* (Anthony Page, Playhouse and New York, 1996, Tony Award for Best Actor), and has continued to seek challenging work: the title role in *Macbeth* (Terry Hands, Clwyd Theatr Cymru, 1999); Richard in Martin Crimp's *The Country* (Katie Mitchell, Royal Court, 2000); the title role in *Ivanov* (Mitchell, NT Cottesloe, 2002); Adam opposite Rachel Sanders in Arnold Wesker's two-hander *The Four Seasons* (Hands, Clwyd Theatr Cymru, 2002); and Kurt in Strindberg's *Dance of Death* (Sean Mathias, Lyric, 2003).

David Tennant (b. Bathgate, Scotland, 1971) made a strong impression in his first RSC production, *As You Like It* (Steven Pimlott, RST), by transforming the often wearisome clown Touchstone into a sardonically bright, endearingly funny Scot. His other roles during the 1996/97 season were Jack Lane in Peter Whelan's *The Herbal Bed* (Michael Attenborough, TOP), and Hamilton in Richard Nelson's *The General from America* (Howard Davies, Swan). Wit and versatility have marked his subsequent progress as an actor, not least at the RSC where, in 2000, he played Jack Absolute in *The Rivals* (Lindsay Posner, Swan), Antipholus of Syracuse (as a 1930s matinee idol) in *The Comedy of Errors* (Lynne Parker, RST), and Romeo in *Romeo and Juliet* (Michael Boyd, RST); and, in 2008, directed by Gregory Doran, the title role in *Hamlet* and Berowne in *Love's Labour's Lost*.

David MacDonald was born in the West Lothian town of Bathgate, the son of a Church of Scotland minister. On graduating from the Royal Scottish Academy of Music and Drama he adopted the pseudonym David Tennant (Equity already had a member called David MacDonald), and quickly came to notice: a manic depressive in the television drama series *Takin' Over the Asylum* (BBC, 1994); Kenny in Iain Heggie's *An Experienced Woman Gives Advice* at the Manchester Royal Exchange (Matthew Lloyd, 1995); and Nick in Joe Orton's *What the Butler Saw* at the National (Phyllida Lloyd, Lyttelton, 1995). Between his first and second RSC seasons he was Mickey in David Rabe's *Hurlyburly* (Wilson Milam, Queen's Theatre, 1997); the critic in *The Real Inspector Hound/Black Comedy* (Gregory Doran, Comedy Theatre, 1998); Pavel opposite Anne-Marie Duff in *Vassa* (Howard Davies, Almeida, 1999); and Edgar in *King Lear* (Gregory Hersov, Manchester Royal Exchange, 1999). Since 2002 he has created roles in three new works, and starred in a revival of a

20th century classic: Robert opposite Jaqueline Defferary in Roland Schimmelpfennig's *Push Up* (Theatre Upstairs, Royal Court, 2002); Jeff, the security guard, in Kenneth Lonergan's *Lobby Hero* (Mark Brokaw, Donmar Warehouse, 2002); Katurian in Martin McDonagh's *The Pillowman* (John Crowley, NT Cottesloe, 2003); and Jimmy Porter opposite Kelly Reilly in John Osborne's *Look Back in Anger* (Richard Baron, Theatre Royal, Bath, 2005).

Among Tennant's films are *Jude* (Michael Winterbottom, 1996); *Bite* (1997); *LA Without a Map* (1998); *The Last September* (Deborah Warner, 1999); *Bright Young Things* (Stephen Fry, 2003); and *Harry Potter and the Goblet of Fire* (Mike Newell, 2005). On television he has starred in *He Knew He Was Right* (BBC, 2004); *Blackpool* (BBC, 2004); *Casanova* (BBC, 2005); *The Quatermass Experiment* (BBC, 2005); and *Doctor Who* (BBC, 2005-08).

Nigel Terry (b. Bristol, 1945). Although best known for his performances in the later films of Derek Jarman, Nigel Terry has created a significant body of work on the stage.

On graduating from the Central School of Speech and Drama, he won the role of John in the Hollywood movie *The Lion in Winter* (Anthony Harvey, 1968). His early plays included Harald Mueller's *Big Wolf* (William Gaskill, 1972) and Edward Bond's *The Fool* (Peter Gill, 1975) at the Royal Court.

In his first and longest spell with the RSC, he played Soranzo in *'Tis Pity She's a Whore* (Ron Daniels, TOP, 1977); Duke of Exeter in *Henry VI Part 3* (Terry Hands, RST, 1977); Duke Magnus in *Queen Christina* (Penny Cherns, TOP, 1977); John in David Rudkin's *The Sons of Light* (Daniels, TOP, 1977); Rackham in *The Women-Pirates* (Daniels, Aldwych, 1978); Lawson in Stephen Poliakoff's *Shout Across the River* (Bill Alexander, Warehouse, 1978); George in Mary O'Malley's *Look Out... Here Comes Trouble* (John Caird, Warehouse, 1978); Turk in Howard Barker's *The Hang of the Gaol* (Alexander, Warehouse, 1978); Madchat in *The Adventures of Awful Knawful* (Caird/Howard Davies, Warehouse,

1978-79); Cleon in *Pericles* (Daniels, TOP, 1979); Dominikovi in *The Suicide* (Daniels, TOP, 1979); Ekart in Brecht's *Baal* (David Jones, TOP, 1979); and Casca/Pindarus in *Julius Caesar* (Barry Kyle, RST, 1979). For the 1986 small-scale tour he was Benedick in *Much Ado About Nothing* (Daniels) and Shylock in *The Merchant of Venice* (Roger Michell). In 1988/89 he created the role of Savage in Howard Barker's *The Bite of the Night* (Danny Boyle, Pit), and played the title role in *Pericles* (David Thacker, Swan) and Bosola in *The Duchess of Malfi* (Alexander, Swan). In 2000 he starred as Trigorin in Adrian Noble's production of *The Seagull* (Swan).

Elsewhere: the title role in Molière's *Don Juan* (Gill, NT Cottesloe, 1981); Jack in Sebastian Barry's *Our Lady of Sligo* (Max Stafford-Clark, Out of Joint, 1998); Don Gutierre in *The Doctor of Honour* (Lindsay Posner, Cheek By Jowl, 1989); Vershinin in *Three Sisters* (Stafford-Clark, Out of Joint, 1995); Daniel Hill's *Cracked* (Terry Johnson, Hampstead, 1997); McCann in Harold Pinter's *The Birthday Party* (Joe Harmston, Piccadilly, 1999); and the tramp in Pinter's *The Caretaker* (Adrian Stokes, Mercury Theatre, Colchester, 2002).

Terry starred in John Boorman's *Excalibur* (1981), and in Derek Jarman's *Caravaggio* (1986), *The Last of England* (1987), *War Requiem* (1989), *Edward II* (1991), and *Blue* (1993).

David Thacker (b. 1950) studied at York University and worked for ten years in regional theatres before succeeding Frank Dunlop as artistic director of the Young Vic (1984). It was the beginning of a new era for the venue. Thacker sidelined the traditional youth policy, programmed the plays of a select group of classical and modern masters (Shakespeare, Ibsen, Eugene O'Neill, Arthur Miller, Edward Albee), and pursued prestige in casting. At a time when fringe venues either served a minority interest or staged left-wing new writing and little else, Thacker's Young Vic was commendably ambitious, the precursor of Jonathan Kent's Almeida and Sam Mendes's Donmar.

In listing Thacker's Young Vic work it is the names of the leading players that indicate the appeal of those years: Vanessa Redgrave and Tom Wilkinson in Ibsen's *Ghosts* (1986); Billie Whitelaw and Patrick Stewart in Albee's *Who's Afraid of Virginia Woolf?* (1987); Saskia Reeves in *Measure for Measure* (1987); Tom Wilkinson in Ibsen's *An Enemy of the People* (1988); Vanessa Redgrave and Timothy Dalton in O'Neill's *A Touch of the Poet* (1988); Helen Mirren and Bob Peck in Miller's *Two-Way Mirror* (1989); Susannah York in *The Glass Menagerie* (1989); Natasha Richardson in O'Neill's *Anna Christie* (1990); Trevor Eve and Rudi Davies in *The Winter's Tale* (1991); and Zoë Wanamaker in Miller's *The Last Yankee* (1993).

In 1993 Thacker left the Young Vic and accepted the position of resident director at the RSC (he had previously staged two enjoyably accessible productions in the Swan—*Pericles* in 1989 and *The Two Gentlemen of Verona* in 1991). The Stratford main stage exposed a fatal lack of inspired stagecraft in his direction: *As You Like It* (1992); *The Merry Wives of Windsor* (1992); *The Merchant of Venice* (1993).

His strength lies in interpreting the work of 20th century American playwrights, those great heavy plodders of world drama. His relationship with Arthur Miller, established at the Young Vic, was particularly rewarding—*A View from the Bridge* (Bristol Old Vic, 1994); *Broken Glass* (NT Lyttelton, 1994); *Death of a Salesman* (NT Lyttelton, 1996).

John Thaw (1942-2002, b. Manchester). One of Britain's most popular television stars, John Thaw played strong characters, often mavericks, but gave them a suggestion of vulnerability. The edgy impetuosity of Regan in *The Sweeney* (1974-78), the grumpy sensitivity of Morse (1987-01), and the earnest charm of Kavanagh in *Kavanagh QC* (1995-01), proved irresistible, perhaps because they seemed to fit Thaw so easily. It was hard to see through these roles to Thaw's other work, especially his stage appearances.

Born in Manchester, Thaw worked in a bakery before winning a place at RADA. At the beginning of his career he joined the RSC to play Sordido in *Women Beware Women* (Anthony Page, Arts, 1962). In the 1960s he appeared in popular programmes such as *Z Cars* and *Francis Durbridge Presents*, but it was not until *The Sweeney* that he became a household name. His sparse theatre roles included Dick Wagner opposite Diana Rigg in the premiere production of Tom Stoppard's *Night and Day* (Peter Wood, Phoenix, 1978), Musgrave in *Serjeant Musgrave's Dance* (John Burgess, NT Cottesloe, 1981), and Joe Keller in Arthur Miller's *All My Sons* (Gregory Hersov, Manchester Royal Exchange, 1988). In 1983, back with RSC after twenty years, Thaw played Nick, the barman, in William Saroyan's *The Time of Your Life* (Howard Davies, TOP), Sir Toby Belch in *Twelfth Night* (John Caird, RST), and Wolsey in *Henry VIII* (Davies, RST). He left the Company at the end of the Stratford year (Stephen More played Wolsey in London). His one theatre role of the 1990s was George Jones in David Hare's *The Absence of War* (Richard Eyre, NT Olivier, 1993).

Charles Thomas (1940-1970, b. Cardiff) trained at the Rose Bruford College of Speech and Drama. He joined the RSC in 1964 to play supporting parts in Peter Hall's History cycle— Aumerle in *Richard II*, Edmund Mortimer in *Henry IV* and *Henry VI*, and Catesby in *Richard III*. By 1970 he had made his name as one of the RSC's best young actors: Berowne to Janet Suzman's Rosaline in *Love's Labour's Lost* (John Barton, RST, 1965); Lorenzo in *The Merchant of Venice* (Clifford Williams, RST, 1965); Laertes in the David Warner *Hamlet* (Peter Hall, RST, 1965); Tranio in *The Taming of the Shrew* (Trevor Nunn, RST, 1967); Oliver in *As You Like It* (David Jones, RST, 1967); Loveless in Vanbrugh's *The Relapse* (Nunn, Aldwych, 1967); Mark Antony in *Julius Caesar* (Barton, RST, 1968); the anthology *Room for Company* (Gareth Morgan, Theatregoround, 1968); Hal/Henry V in *When Thou Art King* (Barton, Theatregoround, 1969); the ward in

Women Beware Women (Terry Hands, RST, 1969); and Orsino to Judi Dench's Viola in *Twelfth Night* (Barton, RST, 1969).

Touring Australia with the *Twelfth Night* company in February 1970, Thomas was found dead in his Melbourne hotel room. He had taken an overdose of sleeping pills and anti-depressants.

Mark Thompson (b. London, 1957). A designer who specialises in clean, vibrantly-coloured settings, Mark Thompson has formed partnerships with many of the most important directors of his generation, including Nicholas Hytner, Steven Pimlott, Phyllida Lloyd (his exact contemporary at Birmingham University), Sam Mendes and Matthew Warchus.

He studied drama at Birmingham and originally intended to act or direct, but soon sensed that his talent lay in design (architecture had been his main interest at school). He persistently applied for design jobs and was finally taken on as an assistant at the Swan Theatre, Worcester. He next went to Exeter's Northcott Theatre, where he met Nicholas Hytner.

At the RSC he has designed *Measure for Measure* (Nicholas Hytner, RST, 1987); *The Wizard of Oz* (Ian Judge, Barbican, 1987); *Much Ado About Nothing* (Di Trevis, RST, 1988); *The Comedy of Errors* (Judge, RST, 1990); *Hamlet* (Matthew Warchus, RST, 1997); and *The Unexpected Man* (Warchus, Pit, 1998).

Thompson's work elsewhere has included, for Nicholas Hytner, *The Scarlet Pimpernel* (Chichester, 1985), *The Country Wife* (Manchester Royal Exchange, 1986), *The Wind in the Willows* (NT Olivier, 1991), *The Madness of George III* (NT Lyttelton, 1991), *The Lady in the Van* (Queen's, 1999) and *Henry IV* (NT Olivier, 2005); for Steven Pimlott, *Joseph and the Amazing Technicolor Dreamcoat* (Palladium, 1991), *Butterfly Kiss* (Almeida, 1994), *Neverland* (Royal Court, 1998) and *Dr Dolittle* (Apollo Hammersmith, 1998); for Phyllida Lloyd, *Six Degrees of Separation* (Royal Court, 1992), *Hysteria* (Royal Court, 1993), *Pericles* (NT Olivier, 1994), *What the Butler Saw* (NT Lyttelton, 1995) and *Mamma Mia!* (Prince Edward, 1999); for Sam Mendes at the Donmar Warehouse, *Company* (1996), *The Front Page* (1997) and *The Blue Room* (1998); for Matthew Warchus, *Art* (Wyndham's, 1996); for David Leveaux, *Betrayal* (Almeida, 1991); for Stephen Daldry, *The Kitchen* (Royal Court, 1994); for Trevor Nunn, *Arcadia* (NT Lyttelton, 1993); and, for Adrian Noble, Verdi's *Macbeth* (The Met, New York, 2007).

David Threlfall (b. Manchester, 1953). The son of a builder, brought up in the Burnage area of Manchester, David Threlfall trained at Manchester Polytechnic and first came to notice alongside Ray Winstone in Alan Clarke's *Scum* (BBC, 1977). He then joined the RSC to appear in new plays in the Warehouse (1978)—Blackie in David Rudkin's *The Sons of Light* (Ron Daniels), Fitz in Peter Flannery's *Savage Amusement* (John Caird), Jake in Pete Atkin's *A and R* (Walter Donohue), and Mike in Stephen Poliakoff's *Shout Across the River* (Bill Alexander). The characters were dynamically presented—Threlfall had presence, energy and the gift of unpredictability. He moved to Stratford for the 1979 season, where his originality was apparent in a peculiar interpretation of Marc Antony in *Julius Caesar* (Barry Kyle, RST): he concentrated on private turmoil rather than public rhetoric. His other roles, 1979/80, were Abraham Slender in *The Merry Wives of Windsor* (Trevor Nunn/John Caird, RST); Second Lord/First British Captain in *Cymbeline* (David Jones, RST); Viktor in *The Suicide* (Daniels, TOP); and the crippled Smike in *Nicholas Nickleby* (Nunn/Caird, Aldwych). The latter performance was a *tour de force* of physical and vocal transformation, unsentimental but affecting. He returned to the Company in 1984 to play Joe Shawcross in Trevor Griffiths's *The Party* (Howard Davies, TOP).

In the years since his career has been quieter than expected. He defined the Tory 1980s as the reptilian politician Leslie Titmuss in John Mortimer's *Paradise Postponed* (1986) and *Titmuss Regained* (1991), and the New Labour 2000s as the despicable scrounger Frank Gallagher in Paul Abbott's *Shameless* (Channel

Four, 2004-08). He brought a brooding quality of unspoken threat to Gregers Werle in *The Wild Duck* (Peter Hall, Phoenix, 1990). He was memorable as Oedipus in *Oedipus Rex* (Manchester Royal Exchange, 1987); Ian in Stephen Bill's *Over a Barrel* (Michael Attenborough, Palace Theatre, Watford, 1990); Bolingbroke opposite Fiona Shaw in *Richard II* (Deborah Warner, NT Cottesloe, 1995); Loevborg opposite Harriet Walter in *Hedda Gabler* (Lindy Davies, Minerva, Chichester, 1996); Norman Nestor in Richard Hope's *Odysseus Thump* (Jude Kelly, West Yorkshire Playhouse, 1997); Essendine in *Present Laughter* (Matthew Lloyd, Manchester Royal Exchange, 1998); the title role in *Peer Gynt* (Braham Murray, Manchester Royal Exchange, 1999); the consultant in Joe Penhall's *Blue/Orange* (Roger Michell, NT Duchess, 2001); Orgon in *Tartuffe* (Lindsay Posner, NT Lyttelton, 2002); the title role in *Skellig* (Nunn, Young Vic, 2003-04); and Michael in Frank McGuinness's *Someone Who'll Watch Over Me* (Dominic Dromgoole, New Ambassadors, 2005).

David Troughton (b. London, 1950). An important member of the RSC since the early 1980s, David Troughton started with the Porter in *Macbeth* (Howard Davies, RST, 1982) and for some years comedic roles dominated, reflecting his ability as a true if idiosyncratic clown. He played Conrade in *Much Ado About Nothing* (Terry Hands, RST, 1982); Aslak in *Peer Gynt* (Ron Daniels, TOP, 1982); Bouton in *Molière* (Bill Alexander, TOP, 1982); Clown in the Michael Gambon/Helen Mirren *Antony and Cleopatra* (Adrian Noble, TOP, 1982); Sebastian in *The Roaring Girl* (Barry Kyle, Barbican, 1983); the Essex idiot Blunt, robbed and left naked by a whore, in *The Rover* (John Barton, Swan, 1986); and Cob in *Every Man in his Humour* (John Caird, Swan, 1986). The climax of this first phase came in 1989 with his performance as Bottom in John Caird's production of *A Midsummer Night's Dream* (RST), a masterpiece of pure comedy.

He now joined the first division of classical actors: the villainous Cloten in *Cymbeline* (Bill Alexander, RST, 1989); Hector in *Troilus and Cressida* (Sam Mendes, Swan, 1990); Kent in the John Wood *King Lear* (Nicholas Hytner, RST, 1990); Holofernes in *Love's Labour's Lost* (Ian Judge, RST, 1993); Zanetto/Tonino in Goldoni's *The Venetian Twins* (Michael Bogdanov, Swan, 1993); a wounded, beast-like Caliban in *The Tempest* (Mendes, RST, 1993); Fitzdottrel in *The Devil is an Ass* (Matthew Warchus, Swan, 1995); the title role, played as a sinister clown, in *Richard III* (Steven Pimlott, RST, 1995); Lopakhin in Adrian Noble's production of *The Cherry Orchard* (Swan, 1995); and Boling-broke—both political thug and tortured king—in *Richard II* (Pimlott, TOP, 2000) and the two parts of *Henry IV* (Michael Attenborough, Swan, 2000).

Troughton's work elsewhere has included: *Don Juan* (Peter Gill, NT Cottesloe, 1981); John Arden's *Serjeant Musgrave's Dance* (John Burgess, NT Cottesloe, 1981); *A Month in the Country* (Gill, NT Olivier, 1981); Martin in Sam Shepard's *Fool for Love* (Gill, NT Cottesloe, 1984); Mr Antrobus in Thornton Wilder's *The Skin of Our Teeth* (David Lan, Young Vic, 2004); the Duke in *Measure for Measure* (Simon McBurney, NT Olivier, 2004); and George Aldred in David Edgar's *Playing With Fire* (Attenborough, NT Olivier, 2005). On television, he played Tom in Alan Ayckbourn's *The Norman Conquests* (Herbert Wise, ITV, 1977), and Bob Buzzard in Andrew Davies's *A Very Peculiar Practice* (BBC, 1986-88).

Dorothy Tutin (1930-2001, b. London). At the age of nineteen Dorothy Tutin played Princess Margaret in *The Thistle and the Rose* (the Boltons, 1949). A year later she appeared at the Old Vic opposite Alec Clunes in *Henry V* (Glen Byam Shaw). She came to prominence in the mid-1950s with a string of acclaimed leading performances—Rose in Graham Greene's *The Living Room* (Wyndham's, 1953); Sally Bowles in *I Am a Camera* (New Theatre, 1954); Joan in Jean Anouilh's *The Lark* (1955); Hedwig in *The Wild Duck* (Saville, 1955); and Jean Rice in John Osborne's *The Entertainer* (Tony Richardson, Royal Court, 1957). In British movies, she played Cecily in *The Importance of Being Earnest* (Anthony Asquith, 1951), Polly in *The Beggar's Opera* (Peter Brook, 1954), and Lucie Manette in *A Tale of Two Cities* (Ralph Thomas, 1958).

She first joined the Stratford Memorial Company in 1952 to play Hero in the London performances of John Gielgud's production of *Much Ado About Nothing* (Phoenix). In 1958 she began her Stratford career with Juliet in *Romeo and Juliet* (Glen Byam Shaw), Viola in *Twelfth Night* (Peter Hall), and Ophelia in the Michael Redgrave *Hamlet* (Shaw). She toured with the Company to Leningrad and Moscow that December.

She remained with the RSC until the early 1970s: Portia in *The Merchant of Venice* (Michael Langham, RST, 1960); Viola in *Twelfth Night* (Hall, RST, 1960); Cressida opposite Denholm Elliott in *Troilus and Cressida* (Hall/Barton, RST, 1960); Sister Jeanne in *The Devils* (Peter Wood, Aldwych, 1961); *The Hollow Crown* (Barton, Aldwych, 1961); Juliet opposite Brian Murray in *Romeo and Juliet* (Hall, RST, 1961); Desdemona opposite John Gielgud in *Othello* (Franco Zeffirelli, RST, 1961); Varya in *The Cherry Orchard* (Michel Saint-Denis, RST, 1961); Cressida opposite Ian Holm in *Troilus and Cressida* (Hall, Aldwych, 1962); Polly Peachum in *The Beggar's Opera* (Wood, Aldwych, 1963); Rosalind in *As You Like It* (David Jones, RST, 1967); Alice in *Arden of Faversham* (Buzz Goodbody, Theatregoround, 1970); and Kate in Pinter's *Old Times* (Hall, Aldwych, 1971).

On leaving the RSC she gave an extraordinary performance as Sophie Brzeska in Ken Russell's *Savage Messiah* (1972). She played Natalya Petrovna in *A Month in the Country* at Chichester (1974), Cleopatra opposite Alec McCowen in *Antony and Cleopatra* for Prospect (Old Vic, 1977), and ended the decade with Peter Hall at the National—Madame Ranevsky in *The Cherry Orchard* (Hall, Olivier, 1978), Lady Macbeth to Albert Finney's *Macbeth* (Hall, Olivier, 1978), Lady Plyant in *The Double Dealer* (Peter Wood, Olivier, 1978), Stoppard's *Undiscovered Country* (Wood, Olivier, 1979), and Lady Fancyfull in *The Provok'd Wife* (Wood, Lyttelton, 1980).

From 1980 she worked mostly at Chichester and in the West End: *Reflections* (Theatre Royal Haymarket, 1980); Hester in Terence Rattigan's *The Deep Blue Sea* (Greenwich, 1981); *After the Lions* (Royal Exchange Manchester, 1982); Pinter's *A Kind of Alaska* (Duchess Theatre, 1985); *The Chalk Garden* (Chichester, 1986); *Are You Sitting Comfortably* (Watford, 1986); *Brighton Beach Memoirs* (Aldwych, 1987); *Thursday's Ladies* (Apollo, 1987); *Harlequinade* and *The Browning Version* (Royalty, 1988); *A Little Night Music* (Chichester, 1989); *Henry VIII* (Chichester, 1991); Pinter's *Party Time* (Almeida, 1991); Arkadina in *The Seagull* (Toby Robertson, Theatr Clwyd, 1992); *Getting Married* (Chichester, 1993); Rhoda in Rodney Ackland's *After October* (Keith Baxter, Minerva, Chichester, 1997); and Fonsia opposite Joss Ackland in *The Gin Game* (Frith Banbury, Savoy, 1999).

Margaret Tyzack (b. 1931) won the Gilbert Prize for Comedy at RADA and made her first professional appearance at the Civic Theatre, Chesterfield. In 1962 she joined the RSC to play Vassillissa in Gorky's *The Lower Depths* (Toby Robertson, Arts Theatre). This was the beginning of a sporadic but long-term association with the Company. In 1972/73 she played Volumnia in *Coriolanus*, Portia in *Julius Caesar* and Tamora in *Titus Andronicus* (Trevor Nunn/Buzz Goodbody, RST); in 1974/75, Maria Lvovna in *Summerfolk* (David Jones, Aldwych); in 1983, the Countess of Rossillion, succeeding Peggy Ashcroft, in *All's Well That Ends Well* (Nunn, Barbican); and in 1999, Amy in T.S. Eliot's *The Family Reunion* (Adrian Noble, Swan).

Theatre work elsewhere: Lady Macbeth (Nottingham, 1962); Miss Frost in *The Ginger Man* (Royal Court, 1964); Madame Ranevsky in *The Cherry Orchard* (Exeter, 1969); Jacqui in *Find Your Way Home* (Open Space Theatre, 1970); Queen Elizabeth in *Vivat! Vivat Regina!* (Piccadilly, 1971); *Richard III*, *All's Well That Ends Well*, *Ghosts* (Stratford, Ontario, 1977); *People Are Living There* (Manchester Royal Exchange, 1979); Martha in *Who's Afraid of Virginia Woolf?* (Nancy Meckler, NT Lyttelton, 1981);

An Inspector Calls (Greenwich, 1983); *Tom and Viv* (Max Stafford-Clark, Royal Court, 1984); *Mornings at Seven* (Westminster, 1984); *Night Must Fall* (Greenwich, 1986); Peter Shaffer's *Lettice and Lovage* (Michael Blakemore, Globe, 1987); Miss Prism in *The Importance of Being Earnest* (Nicholas Hytner, Aldwych, 1993); *An Inspector Calls* (Stephen Daldry, Aldwych, 1994); Tom Stoppard's *Indian Ink* (Aldwych, 1995); Muriel in Alan Bennett's *Talking Heads* ('Soldiering On', Minerva, Chichester, 1996); Brian Friel's *Give Me Your Answer, Do!* (Robin Lefevre, 1998); and Mrs Baldwin in *His Girl Friday* (Jack O'Brien, NT Olivier, 2003).

Among Margaret Tyzack's films are Stanley Kubrick's *2001: A Space Odyssey* (1968) and *A Clockwork Orange* (1971), and Stephen Frears's *Prick Up Your Ears* (1987). On television, she was memorable in *The Forsyte Saga* (BBC, 1967) and *I, Claudius* (BBC, 1976).

V

Hugh Vanstone came to notice lighting productions for Steven Pimlott at the English National Opera (including *La Bohème*, 1993) and Neil Bartlett at the Lyric, Hammersmith. Vanstone's magical use of light, both painterly and sculptural, created the moody, glamorous world of Bartlett's *Romeo and Juliet* (1995). He has since been in constant demand. At the RSC he has lit Adrian Noble's *Romeo and Juliet* (RST, 1995) and *Cymbeline* (RST, 1997); Steven Pimlott's *Richard III* (RST, 1995), *Bad Weather* (TOP, 1998) and *Antony and Cleopatra* (RST, 1999); Gale Edwards's *The Taming of the Shrew*, (RST, 1995); Ron Daniels's *Slaughter City* (Pit, 1996); Richard Cottrell's *Three Hours After Marriage* (Swan, 1996); and Matthew Warchus's *Hamlet* (RST, 1997), *The Unexpected Man* (Pit, 1988) and *The Winter's Tale* (Roundhouse, 2002). Vanstone often works with the designer Mark Thompson on productions by Warchus (*Art*, Wyndham's, 1996; the RSC work), and Sam Mendes (*The Front Page*, Donmar, 1997; *The Blue Room*, Donmar,

1998). Other productions: Phyllida Lloyd's *Dialogues des Carmé-lites* (ENO, 1999) and *Mary Stuart* (Donmar, 2005); Nicholas Hytner's *The Lady in the Van* (Queen's, 1999) and *Orpheus Descending* (Donmar, 2000); Trevor Nunn's *The Cherry Orchard* (NT Cottesloe, 2000) and *The Lady from the Sea* (Almeida, 2003); Mendes's *Uncle Vanya* and *Twelfth Night* (Donmar, 2002); John Crowley's *The Pillowman* (NT Cottesloe, 2003); and Michael Grandage's *Pacific Overtures* (Donmar, 2003) and *Grand Hotel* (Donmar, 2004).

Zubin Varla trained at the Guildhall School of Music and Drama and came to notice at Regent's Park playing Jack in *Lady Be Good* (Ian Talbot, 1992), Romeo opposite Rebecca Callard in *Romeo and Juliet* (Judi Dench, 1993), and Sir Galahad in *A Connecticut Yankee at the Court of King Arthur* (Talbot, 1993). At the Bush he played Rezmi in *In the Heart of America* (1994); in the West End, Jamie in Jonathan Harvey's *Beautiful Thing* (Hettie MacDonald, Duke of York's, 1994).

He joined the RSC for the 1995/96 season and played a petulant, doom-laden Romeo opposite Lucy Whybrow in *Romeo and Juliet* (Adrian Noble, RST), Celio in *The Painter of Dishonour* (Laurence Boswell, TOP), and Euphorion in *Faust* (Michael Bogdanov, Swan). He won acclaim as Judas in the West End revival of *Jesus Christ Superstar* (Gale Edwards, Lyceum, 1996), then returned to the RSC: the title role in Bernard-Marie Koltès's *Roberto Zucco* (James Macdonald, TOP, 1997-98); Winwife in *Bartholomew Fair* (Laurence Boswell, Swan, 1997-98); Caliban in *The Tempest* (Macdonald, Pit, 2000); Saleem Sinai in *Midnight's Children* (Tim Supple, Barbican, 2003); and Brutus in *Julius Caesar* (David Farr) paired with the clown Thurio in *The Two Gentlemen of Verona* (Fiona Buffini, Small-scale Tour, 2004-05).

Other theatre: the Client in Koltès's *In the Solitude of Cotton Fields* (Actors Touring Company, Aldwych Tube Station, 2001); *Teeth 'n' Smiles* (Sheffield Crucible, 2002); Johnny in Athol Fugard's *Hello and Goodbye* (Paul Robinson, Southwark Playhouse,

2003); Mozart to Richard McCabe's Salieri in a concert staging of Peter Shaffer's *Amadeus* (City of London Sinfonia, Barbican, 2003); and, at the National, Christian in *Cyrano de Bergerac* (Howard Davies, Olivier, 2004), Fulganzio in Brecht's *The Life of Galileo* (Davies, NT Olivier, 2006), Martin Crimp's *Attempts on Her Life* (Katie Mitchell, Lyttelton, 2007), and Gustave in Victoria Benedictsson's *The Enchantment* (Paul Miller, Cottesloe, 2007).

Philip Voss (b. Leicester, 1936) was at the beginning of his career as an actor when he went to Stratford in 1960 to walk-on in Peter Wood's *The Winter's Tale*, Peter Hall's *Twelfth Night* and *Troilus and Cressida*, and Donald McWhinnie's *The Duchess of Malfi*. The following year, at the Aldwych, he was promoted to play Louis XIII in John Whiting's *The Devils* (Wood) and the Provost Marshal in Jean Anouilh's *Becket* (Hall).

Voss's career evolved slowly. It was not until the 1980s that he achieved significant recognition, first with Shared Experience—Juster in the British premiere of Maria Irene Fornes's *Abingdon Square* (Nancy Meckler, Soho Theatre, 1989)—and then at the National (1987-90)—Rodin in *The Wandering Jew* (Mike Alfreds, Lyttelton); Fernandino in *Countrymania* (Alfreds, Olivier); James in Nick Ward's *The Strangeness of Others* (Cottesloe); Troll King in *Peer Gynt* (Declan Donnellan, Olivier); and Scherbuk in Trevor Griffiths's *The Piano* (Howard Davies, Cottesloe). In 1989 he played the title role in *King Lear* for the Oxford Stage Company (John Retallack, Tour).

Returning to the RSC after thirty years of relative obscurity, he was at last able to reveal his mastery of Shakespeare's characterisation and verse. He has been cast in roles that have suited his rather pedantic manner and his fruitily precise delivery of the verse, particularly the Lord Chief Justice in the two parts of *Henry IV* (Adrian Noble, RST, 1991); Sir Epicure Mammon in *The Alchemist* (Sam Mendes, Swan, 1991); Theseus in *The Thebans* (Noble, Swan, 1991); Piccolomini in Schiller's *Wallenstein* (Tim Albery, Pit, 1993); Lord Sheffield in Michael Hastings's *Unfin-*

ished Business (Steven Pimlott, Pit, 1993); Menenius in the Toby Stephens *Coriolanus* (David Thacker, Swan, 1994); a fussy Peter Quince, played absolutely 'straight' and all the funnier for that, in *A Midsummer Night's Dream* (Noble, RST, 1994); Bassanes in John Ford's *The Broken Heart* (Michael Boyd, Swan, 1994); a callous Ulysses in *Troilus and Cressida* (Ian Judge, RST, 1996); Malvolio in *Twelfth Night* (Noble, RST, 1997); Shylock in *The Merchant of Venice* (Gregory Doran, RST, 1997); and Prospero in *The Tempest* (James Macdonald, Small-scale Tour, 2001). In 2003 he was an unusually bitter Jacques in Peter Hall's *As You Like It* at the Theatre Royal, Bath.

W

Justine Waddell (b. Johannesburg, 1976) went up to Emmanuel College, Cambridge, in 1994 to read Social and Political Science and quickly became known as one of the best student actresses: she played Juliet in *Romeo and Juliet* and, at the end of her first year, Joan of Arc in Jean Anouilh's *The Lark*—the production visited the 1995 Edinburgh Festival where agents and producers took note.

She took time off from her studies to play a small role in *Anna Karenina* (Bernard Rose, 1997), and to join the Almeida company to appear opposite Ralph Fiennes in *Ivanov* (Jonathan Kent, 1997). Major television work followed. Her sabbatical from Cambridge lasted for over a year (she returned to complete the degree in 1998) as she cornered the market in literary heroines—Laura in *The Woman in White* (Tim Fywell, BBC, 1997), *The Moth* (ITV, 1997), Tess in *Tess of the D'Urbervilles* (Ian Sharp, ITV, 1998), Estella in Tony Marchant's adaptation of *Great Expectations* (Julian Jarrold, BBC, 1999), and Molly Gibson in *Wives and Daughters* (BBC, 1999). During the same period she was seen in supporting roles in the films *The Misadventures of*

Margaret (1998), *Mansfield Park* (Patricia Rozema, 1999), and *The Duchess of Malfi* (1999).

During the winter of 1999/2000, at the RSC, she played a proud, cruelly beautiful Nina in Adrian Noble's production of *The Seagull* (Swan and Barbican). The costume—red cardigan, denim-blue skirt—placed her both in and out of period.

She has since worked in Hollywood: *Dracula 2000* (2001); the title role in *The Mystery of Natalie Wood* (Peter Bogdanovich, 2004); *Chaos* (2005); and *The Fall* (2006).

Zoë Waites (b. Devon, 1975) came to prominence playing Ophelia opposite Michael Maloney in *Hamlet* (Philip Franks, Greenwich Theatre, 1996-97) and Juliet in Michael Attenborough's RSC production of *Romeo and Juliet* (Pit and Small-scale Tour, 1997-98). In the latter she found a new Juliet through simplicity (barelegged, she wore plain dresses of lilac and blue), sensuality and original touches (she washed clothes, prepared a meal and danced intimately with Paris in front of Ray Fearon's Romeo). A natural verse-speaker, she spoke the words with feeling ('love, lord, ay, husband, [*pause*] friend').

After the *Romeo* tour she joined the Almeida Company to play Girl—a role requiring the expression of lust, love and anxiety, as well as nudity—in the premiere of Edward Albee's *The Play About the Baby* (Howard Davies, Almeida, 1998). From 1999 to 2002 she was back at Stratford, the first RSC actress of her generation to create a body of work in Shakespeare: a poignant Desdemona, again partnered by Ray Fearon, in *Othello* (Attenborough, RST, 1999); Mary in *The Family Reunion* (Adrian Noble, Swan, 1999); Viola in *Twelfth Night* (Lindsay Posner, RST, 2001); Kelima in David Edgar's *The Prisoner's Dilemma* (Attenborough, TOP, 2001); and Joanna in David Farr's *Night of the Soul* (Farr, Pit, 2002). Between RSC seasons she appeared at the Lyric Hammersmith as Vittoria in Webster's *The White Devil* (Franks, 2000), and she has since played the title role in *Antigone* (Eugenia Arsenis, Royal Albert Hall, 2003, Prom concert staging with Mendelssohn's 1841 score); Pat Green opposite Philip Frank's Alan Turing in Hugh Whitemore's *Breaking the Code* (Philip Wilson, Theatre Royal, Northampton, 2003); and, at Chichester, Regan in the David Warner *King Lear* (Steven Pimlott, Minerva, 2005), Mistress Hibbins in Phyllis Nagy's *The Scarlet Letter* (Minerva, 2005), Rebecca in David Hare and Howard Brenton's *Pravda* (Jonathan Church, 2006), and Fanny Squeers/Miss Snevellicci/Madeline Bray in David Edgar's *Nicholas Nickleby* (Church, 2007).

She was brought up in Totnes, Devon, by parents she has described as 'hippies' (*The Times*, 19 November 1997). She appeared with the National Youth Theatre (roles included Titania in *A Midsummer Night's Dream*), and graduated from RADA in 1996. As well as Ophelia, during her first year of professional work she played Laura in *Goblin Market* (Battersea Arts Centre).

Catherine Walker (b. Dublin). On graduating from the Gaiety School in Dublin, Catherine Walker played Kate in *Blood* (Project Arts Centre), and co-devised *Diary of a New York Lady* (Beckett Centre). She made a striking London debut in John B. Keane's *Sive* at the Tricycle (Ben Barnes, 1997-98), and joined the RSC the following year, cast as Cassandra in *Troilus and Cressida* (Michael Boyd) and Vera in Brian Friel's *A Month in the Country* (Michael Attenborough, Small-scale Tour, 1998-99). Two roles in the 'This England' history cycle (2000-01) followed—Queen Isabelle in *Richard II* (Steven Pimlott, TOP) and Katherine in *Henry V* (Edmund Hall, RST). She has since played the lovesick secretary in Tennessee Williams's *Stairs to the Roof* (Lucy Bailey, Minerva, Chichester, 2001); the shop girl in *Wild Orchids*, Timberlake Wertenbaker's translation of Jean Anouilh's *Leocadia* (Edward Kemp, Chichester, 2002); Nora in Shaw's *John Bull's Other Island* (Dominic Dromgoole, Tricycle, 2003); Olivia in *Twelfth Night* (Stephen Unwin, English Touring Theatre, 2004); the title role in Tom McIntyre's *What Happened Bridgie Cleary*

(Alan Gilsenan, Peacock Theatre, Dublin, 2005); and the title role in Strindberg's *Miss Julie* (Project Arts Centre, Dublin, 2008).

David Waller (1920-1997, b. Street, Somerset) trained at the Embassy School of Acting and worked his way up from provincial weekly repertory to the Old Vic during the 1950s. He joined the RSC in 1962 and remained a member for twenty-four of the next twenty-nine years. It is impossible to consider the RSC of this period without reference to him. He was Bottom in Peter Brook's *A Midsummer Night's Dream* (RST, 1970); Duff opposite Peggy Ashcroft in Harold Pinter's *Landscape* (Peter Hall, Aldwych, 1969); Pandarus to the Cressidas of Helen Mirren (John Barton, RST, 1968) and Francesca Annis (Barton, RST, 1976); Kent and Gloucester to the Lears of Eric Porter (Trevor Nunn, RST, 1968) and Michael Gambon (Adrian Noble, RST, 1982); and Claudius to the Hamlet of Alan Howard (Nunn, RST, 1970). He was in *The Wars of the Roses* (Hall, RST, 1964) and *The Plantagenets* (Noble, RST, 1988). For such a commanding actor, Waller was a natural clown. If that famous Bottom is the best example, he was also the First Gravedigger in the David Warner *Hamlet* (Hall, RST, 1965); Dull in *Love's Labour's Lost* (Barton, RST, 1965); and Dogberry in *Much Ado About Nothing* (Nunn, RST, 1968).

On television he played Stanley Baldwin in *Edward and Mrs Simpson* (Waris Hussein, 1980) and *The Woman He Loved* (Charles Jarrott, 1988). His films included Peter Hall's *Work is a Four Letter Word* (1967) and *Perfect Friday* (1970), and Trevor Nunn's *Lady Jane* (1986).

Harriet Walter (b. London, 1950) trained at the London Academy of Music and Dramatic Art and initially worked on the fringe as a member of 7:84, Paines Plough and Joint Stock. She first made an impression in two productions by William Gaskill, *The Ragged Trousered Philanthropists* (Joint Stock, Tour, 1978) and *A Fair Quarrel* (NT Olivier, 1979). Her talent was confirmed at the Royal Court, where she played Ophelia in the Jonathan

Pryce *Hamlet* (Richard Eyre, 1980), Victoria/Edward in Caryl Churchill's *Cloud Nine* (Max Stafford-Clark, 1980), and Lily (Nina) in *The Seagull* (Stafford-Clark, 1981).

Between *Cloud Nine* and *The Seagull* she joined the RSC to play Madeleine Bray in *Nicholas Nickleby* (Trevor Nunn, Aldwych, 1980). In her first full season, 1981-82, she was a beguiling Helena in Trevor Nunn's production of *All's Well That Ends Well* (RST); Helena in *A Midsummer Night's Dream* (Ron Daniels, RST); Constance in *The Twin Rivals* (John Caird, TOP); Winnifrede in *The Witch of Edmonton* (Barry Kyle, TOP); and Lady Percy in *Henry IV* (Nunn, Barbican). She added to her range with the ferocious witch Skinner in Howard Barker's *The Castle* (Nick Hamm, Pit, 1985), and in 1987-88 excelled as Viola in *Twelfth Night* (Bill Alexander, RST), Imogen in *Cymbeline* (Alexander, TOP), Dacha in John Berger's *A Question of Geography* (Caird, TOP), and Masha in *Three Sisters* (John Barton, Barbican), work which brought her the Olivier for Best Actress. She ended the decade at the RSC with the title role in *The Duchess of Malfi* (Alexander, Swan, 1989). Elsewhere during the 1980s, she joined Alan Rickman for the inaugural production of the Women's Playhouse Trust, Aphra Behn's *The Lucky Chance* (Jules Wright, Royal Court, 1984), and played Portia in *The Merchant of Venice* (Braham Murray, Manchester Royal Exchange, 1987).

Her theatre appearances since 1990 have been mostly in modern plays: Timberlake Wertenbaker's *Three Birds Alighting on a Field* (Royal Court, 1991); Lady Croom in Tom Stoppard's *Arcadia* (Nunn, NT Lyttelton, 1993); the accused teacher opposite Clare Higgins in Lillian Hellman's *The Children's Hour* (Howard Davies, NT Lyttelton, 1994); Pinter's *Old Times* (Wyndham's, 1995); the child psychologist in Stephen Poliakoff's *Sweet Panic* (Hampstead Theatre, 1996); the betrayed wife opposite Ralph Fiennes in Chekhov's *Ivanov* (Jonathan Kent, Almeida, 1997); Sonia in Yasmina Reza's *Life x 3* (Matthew Warchus, NT Lyttelton, 2000-01); Julie in *The Royal Family* (Peter Hall, Theatre Royal Haymarket, 2001-02); Paige in Moira Buffini's *Dinner* (NT Loft, 2002); and Hester in Rattigan's *The*

Deep Blue Sea (Thea Sharrock, Tour, 2003). Back at the RSC, she was Lady Macbeth in *Macbeth* (Gregory Doran, Swan, 1999); Beatrice in *Much Ado About Nothing* (Doran, RST, 2002); and Cleopatra in *Antony and Cleopatra* (Doran, Swan, 2006).

On television, Harriet Walter starred as the young Wren in Ian McEwan's *The Intimation Game* (BBC, 1980)—a performance to place beside her classical work. Also of note: *Lord Peter Wimsey* (BBC, 1987), Michael Frayn's *Benefactors* (BBC, 1989), Simon Gray's *They Never Slept* (BBC, 1990), *The Men's Room* (Antonia Bird, 1991), and Peter Barnes's adaptation of *Hard Times* (BBC, 1994); and the films *Turtle Diary* (John Irvin 1985), *The Good Father* (Mike Newell, 1986), *Milou en mai* (Louis Malle, 1990), *Sense and Sensibility* (Ang Lee, 1995), *Onegin* (Martha Fiennes, 1999), and *Atonement* (Joe Wright, 2007).

Zoë Wanamaker (b. New York, 1949). The daughter of Sam Wanamaker, Zoë Wanamaker was three when her father, about to be called to appear before Senator McCarthy's House Un-American Activities Committee, moved his family from New York to London. She trained at the Central School of Speech and Drama and began her career with the 69 Theatre Company (*A Midsummer Night's Dream*, 1970). She then appeared in repertory at the Royal Lyceum, Edinburgh (1971-72), the Oxford Playhouse (1974-75), and the Nottingham Playhouse (1975-76).

She was with the RSC for much of the next twelve years. One of the Company's most naturally gifted, subtly expressive, performers, her work ranged from the playful to the profound: Essie in *The Devil's Disciple* (Jack Gold, Aldwych, 1976); Babakina in *Ivanov* (David Jones, Aldwych, 1976); Jane in *Wild Oats* (Clifford Williams, Aldwych, 1976); a bitchy Bianca in *The Taming of the Shrew* (Michael Bogdanov, RST, 1978); Gemma in Peter Whelan's *Captain Swing* (Bill Alexander, TOP, 1978); Toine in *Piaf* (Howard Davies, TOP, 1978); May Daniels in *Once in a Lifetime* (Trevor Nunn, Aldwych, 1979); Kitty in *The Time of Your Life* (Davies, TOP, 1983); Adriana in *The Comedy of Errors*

(Adrian Noble, RST, 1983); Viola in *Twelfth Night* (John Caird, RST, 1983); the mute Kattrin in *Mother Courage* (Davies, Barbican, 1984); and Emilia in *Othello* (Nunn, TOP, 1989).

She has also played leading roles at the National, the Donmar Warehouse and elsewhere: Gwendolen in *The Importance of Being Earnest* (Peter Hall, NT Lyttelton, 1982); Sophia in *The Bay at Nice* and Grace in *Wrecked Eggs* (David Hare, NT Cottesloe, 1986); Paula in *Mrs Klein* (Peter Gill, NT Cottesloe, 1988); Elizabeth in Arthur Miller's *The Crucible* (Howard Davies, NT Olivier, 1990); Patricia in Miller's *The Last Yankee* (David Thacker, Young Vic, 1993); Eleanor in Terry Johnson's *Dead Funny* (Johnson, Hampstead Theatre, 1994); Amanda in *The Glass Menagerie* (Sam Mendes, Donmar Warehouse, 1995); the title role in A.R. Gurney's *Sylvia* (Michael Blakemore, Apollo, 1996); the title role in *Electra* (David Leveaux, Minerva, Chichester, 1997); Jolly in David Mamet's *The Old Neighborhood* (Patrick Marber, Royal Court at the Duke of York's, 1998); David Mamet's *Boston Marriage* (Phyllida Lloyd, Donmar Warehouse, 2001); Hildy opposite Alex Jennings in *His Girl Friday* (Jack O'Brien, NT Olivier, 2003); and Beatrice opposite Simon Russell Beale in *Much Ado About Nothing* (Nicholas Hytner, NT Olivier, 2007-08).

Matthew Warchus (b. 1966) was educated at Bristol University. He was an assistant director at the RSC during the first two years of Adrian Noble's directorship (he worked on *The Thebans* among other productions). He made his reputation as an associate at the West Yorkshire Playhouse and as the director of an admired West End *Much Ado About Nothing* starring Mark Rylance and Janet McTeer (Queen's Theatre, 1993). Returning to the RSC in 1994 he directed a first-rate main house *Henry V* with Iain Glen, followed by a vigorous version of Ben Jonson's *The Devil is an Ass* (Swan, 1995). Neither prepared audiences for Warchus's controversial *Hamlet* (RST, 1997). Although this was one of the most assured main house stagings of the late 1990s, the decision to present *Hamlet* as a domestic chamber-piece (the political dimension was cut) reduced the play's mystery and power.

Before staging *Hamlet*, Warchus engineered a huge commercial success (on both sides of the Atlantic) from Yasmina Reza's *Art*, a phenomenon that, during the course of its long life, employed many of the best-known middle-aged thespians of London and New York (Wyndham's, from 1996). Warchus and translator Christopher Hampton went on to mount the British premieres of Reza's *The Unexpected Man* (RSC Pit, 1998), *Life x 3* (NT Lyttelton, 2000-01) and *God of Carnage* (Gielgud, 2008).

Other productions: *The Life of Stuff* (Donmar Warehouse, 1993); Sam Shepard's *True West* (Donmar Warehouse, 1994); a scathing account of *Volpone* (Olivier, 1995) with Michael Gambon and Simon Russell Beale on top form; *Peter Pan* (West Yorkshire Playhouse, 1996); Stravinsky's opera *The Rake's Progress* (Welsh National Opera, 1996); Verdi's *Falstaff* (Opera North, 1997); *Follies* (Roundabout Theater Company, Belasco Theater, New York, 2001); the Madness musical *Our House* (Cambridge Theatre, 2002); Beckett's *Endgame* (Albery, 2004) with Gambon; Marc Camoletti's farce *Boeing-Boeing* (Comedy, 2007) with Rylance; *The Lord of the Rings* (Theatre Royal, Drury Lane, 2007); David Mamet's *Speed-the-Plow* (Old Vic, 2008); and Alan Ayckbourn's *The Norman Conquests* (Old Vic, 2008).

Anthony Ward (b. 1957). The most important designer to emerge in the 1980s and 90s, Anthony Ward came to notice working with Phyllida Lloyd at the Bristol Old Vic. He now designs for Adrian Noble, Sam Mendes, Richard Eyre and Trevor Nunn. An often haunting application of both form and colour imbues his work.

He grew up in Shropshire and studied at the Wimbledon School of Art. At the RSC he was involved in some of the best work of the 1990s: Adrian Noble's *The Winter's Tale* (1992), *King Lear* (1993), *A Midsummer Night's Dream* (1994), *Cymbeline* (1997),

Twelfth Night (1997), *The Tempest* (1998), *The Lion, the Witch and the Wardrobe* (1998) and *The Secret Garden* (2000); Sam Mendes's *Troilus and Cressida* (Swan, 1990), *The Alchemist* (Swan, 1991) and *The Tempest* (RST, 1993); and Phyllida Lloyd's *The Virtuoso* (Swan, 1991).

Ward's other productions have included: *The Rehearsal* (Ian McDiarmid, Almeida, 1990); *Napoli Millionaria* (Richard Eyre, NT Lyttelton, 1991); *Assassins* (Mendes, Donmar Warehouse, 1992); *Sweet Bird of Youth* (Eyre, NT Lyttelton, 1994); *Oliver!* (Mendes, Palladium, 1994); *La Grande Magia* (Eyre, NT Lyttelton, 1995); Britten's *Gloriana* (Lloyd, Opera North, 1995); *The Way of the World* (Lloyd, NT Lyttelton, 1996); *The Nutcracker* (Adventures in Motion Pictures, 1996); *John Gabriel Borkman* (Eyre, NT Lyttelton, 1996); Tom Stoppard's *The Invention of Love* (Eyre, NT Cottesloe, 1997); *Othello* (Mendes, NT Cottesloe, 1997); the musical *Nine* (David Leveaux, Donmar Warehouse, 1997); *Oklahoma!* (Trevor Nunn, NT Olivier, 1998); *The Novice* (Eyre, Almeida, 2000); Monteverdi's *Le retour d'Ulysse en sa patrie* (Noble, Aix-en-Provence, 2000); *My Fair Lady* (Nunn, NT Olivier, 2001); *Chitty Chitty Bang Bang* (Noble, Palladium, 2002); *Uncle Vanya/Twelfth Night* (Mendes, Donmar Warehouse, 2002); *Gypsy* (Mendes, New York, 2003); Matthew Bourne's *Nutcracker* (Sadler's Wells, 2003-04); and *Die Zauberflöte* (Noble, Glyndebourne, 2004).

David Warner (b. Manchester, 1941) left school at fifteen and worked as a shop assistant, selling books, in Leamington Spa before successfully applying to RADA (in the years before, shunted between his separated parents, he had passed through an unsettling succession of towns and schools but had picked up an interest in drama along the way—school plays led to amateur dramatics in Leamington).

After RADA he was signed up by the Royal Court to play Snout in Tony Richardson's *A Midsummer Night's Dream* (1962). This led to his first film role, Blifil in Richardson's *Tom Jones* (1963). He worked briefly in Coventry at the Belgrade (Conrade in *Much Ado About Nothing*), then joined the RSC to play Jim in David Rudkin's *Afore Night Come* (Clifford Williams, Arts, 1962). Warner was very tall, had a mop of fair hair and wore glasses. He was far from being a stereotypical leading actor, but Peter Hall, impressed by his verse-speaking and ability to command a stage, cast him as Henry VI in *The Wars of the Roses* (RST, 1963). Warner's performance (noted for its gravitas) brought him to sudden prominence. Also in the season he showed real versatility by playing the clown Trinculo in *The Tempest* (Williams/Peter Brook). He repeated Henry VI and added Richard II for the complete history cycle of 1964 (RST), and then created the role of Valentine in Henry Livings's *Eh?* at the Aldwych (Hall, 1964).

Hall's choice of the unconventional Warner to star in his revival of *Hamlet* was a masterstroke (RST, 1965). The production became an event, with queues for returns and crowds of young people at the stage door. Warner's Hamlet was an undergraduate in a long red scarf—lanky and awkward with an acute sense of irony (when he put on a crown it dropped over his eyes). Disaffected, classless and anti-establishment, he spoke directly to young theatregoers and achieved pop star status during the two-year run.

His originality was also apparent in his other major success of this period, *Morgan: a Suitable Case for Treatment* (Karel Reisz, 1966). He stayed with the RSC for another year, playing Postmaster in *The Government Inspector* (Hall, Aldwych, 1966), Aguecheek in *Twelfth Night* (Williams, RST, 1966) and Lysander in Hall's film of *A Midsummer Night's Dream* (1968), and he returned in 1970 to play Julian in Edward Albee's *Tiny Alice* (Robin Phillips, Aldwych).

Following two engagements in 1972—Hammett in David Hare's *The Great Exhibition* (Hampstead) and Claudius in John Mortimer's *I, Claudius* (Queen's)—Warner retired from the theatre. His career became a gobbledegook of B-movies, horror films and Hollywood pulp. For years it looked like he was writing the longest and most perplexing suicide note in contemporary acting. But on returning to the stage to star in a New York production of Shaw's *Major Barbara* in 2001 Warner revealed that his long exile had been caused by severe stage-fright. His performance as Andrew Undershaft was acclaimed, but he made a bizarre choice for his London comeback, an old-fashioned star-vehicle called *The Feast of Snails* (Ron Daniels, Lyric, 2002). Happily, he was a fine Lear for Steven Pimlott at Chichester (Minerva, 2005), and in 2007 he returned to the RSC and Shakespeare's histories to play Falstaff in the two parts of *Henry IV* (Michael Boyd). Few performances in 2007 had comparable meaning or emotional resonance.

After *Morgan*, Warner's best films are Sam Peckinpah's *The Ballad of Cable Hogue* (1970), *Straw Dogs* (1971, he played the village idiot, mysteriously uncredited) and *Cross of Iron* (1977); Alain Resnais's *Providence* (1977); and *Time After Time* (1979, he played Jack the Ripper).

Deborah Warner (b. Oxford, 1959) trained to be a stage manager at the Central School. She worked for a while as Steven Berkoff's administrator, but wanted to direct, and at the age of twenty-one made it happen by forming, without backing or funding, her own company, Kick Theatre. Imaginative, pared-down, well-acted small-scale productions of the classics will always have an impact, and at a time when the RSC and the National were not staging Shakespeare in the studios, Warner's company found a niche and built a reputation. Between 1980 and 1986 they presented one production a year at the Edinburgh Festival: *The Good Person of Sichuan* (1980); *Woyzeck* (1981, 1982); *The Tempest* (1983); *Measure for Measure* (1984); *King Lear* (1985); and *Coriolanus* (1986).

King Lear, with Robert Demeger, and *Coriolanus*, with Douglas Hodge, played for a season at the Almeida in 1986. The following year Terry Hands asked Warner to direct a production at the RSC. Back to basics simplicity suited the chosen play, *Titus Andronicus*. Warner's scientific approach (she kept the house lights up for most of the performance) made the moments of gruesome horror seem utterly mundane; the result was both disturbing and moving. She stayed with the RSC until 1990, directing productions of *King John* (TOP, 1988) and *Electra* (Pit, 1989). If *King John* suggested that there are a limited number of times a director can approach Shakespeare in exactly the same way, *Electra* was a departure: she worked with a world-class designer, Hildegard Bechtler, who provided minimalist décor, and began her partnership with the actress Fiona Shaw. She reworked the 'poor theatre' aesthetic of Kick one last time (1990): her NT *King Lear* with Brian Cox was too small for the Lyttelton stage.

Warner is more interested in stretching the forms of theatre than most of her contemporaries, creating haunting installation works and fascinating accounts of operatic masterpieces, but her work is in danger of becoming self-consciously arty: *Hedda Gabler* (Abbey Theatre, Dublin, 1991); *Coriolan* (Salzburg Festival, 1993); *Footfalls* (Garrick, 1994); *Don Giovanni* (Glyndebourne, 1994); *The St Pancras Project* (LIFT Festival, 1995); Fiona Shaw reciting *The Waste Land* in locations of crumbling grandeur (1995); *Richard II* (NT Cottesloe, 1995-96); *Wozzeck* (Opera North, 1996); Honegger's *Joan of Arc at the Stake* (Prom, Royal Albert Hall, 1997); Ibsen's *Une maison de poupée* (Odéon, Paris, 1997); *The Turn of the Screw* (Royal Opera, Barbican Theatre, 1997); *The Tower Project* (LIFT Festival, Euston Tower, 1999); Ian Bostridge singing Janácek's song cycle *The Diary of One Who Vanished* before video images (1999); the ENO chorus, in modern dress, placing flowers on the stage at the end of Bach's *St John Passion* (2000); *Medea* (Abbey Theatre, Dublin, 2000); *Fidelio* (Glyndebourne, 2001); *The Power Book* (NT, 2002); and *Julius Caesar* (Barbican, 2005).

Emily Watson (b. London, 1967) came to sudden prominence with the release of Lars von Trier's *Breaking the Silence* in 1996. Her fearless performance was universally admired (best actress at Cannes; Oscar nomination). Previously, she had been an obscure theatre actress, but one prepared to take chances. In the RSC's production of *A Jovial Crew* (Swan, 1992) she took part in a dance that ended with a man spraying her bare breasts with a mouthful of drink.

She studied English literature at Bristol University and trained at the Drama Studio, London. That 1992 Stratford season was her first professional work. As well as her small part (as a mort, or beggar woman) in *A Jovial Crew* (Max Stafford-Clark), she played Violenta in Peter Hall's *All's Well That Ends Well* (Swan) and a non-speaking part in *The Taming of the Shrew* (Bill Alexander, RST). It was enough to get her noticed: after the RSC she played the schoolgirl who denounces two female teachers in Lilian Hellman's *The Children's Hour* (Howard Davies, NT Lyttelton, 1994).

There is something reminiscent of Sarah Miles about Emily Watson. She followed *Breaking the Silence* with diverse roles: a middle-class wife in *Metroland* (Philip Saville, 1997); Maggie in *The Mill on the Floss* (Graham Theakston, BBC, 1997); Daniel Day-Lewis's love interest in *The Boxer* (Jim Sheridan, 1997); Jacqueline du Pré in *Hilary and Jackie* (Anand Tucker, 1998); Angela in *Angela's Ashes* (Alan Parker, 1999); the head housemaid in *Gosford Park* (Robert Altman, 2001); Lena in *Punch-Drunk Love* (Paul Thomas Anderson, 2002); Reba in *Red Dragon* (Brett Ratner, 2002); Anne Sellers in *The Life and Death of Peter Sellers* (Stephen Hopkins, 2004); Anne in *Separate Lives* (Julian Fellowes, 2005). In 2002 she joined Sam Mendes's final ensemble at the Donmar Warehouse to play Sonya in *Uncle Vanya* and Viola in *Twelfth Night*.

Ruby Wax (b. Chicago, 1953). If Ruby Wax's past life as a member of the RSC now seems hard to believe, it is because her television persona has wiped everything else out. Those with detailed theatrical memories will recall the Ruby Wax of the 1970s, the actress who worked at the Sheffield Crucible before joining the RSC in 1978.

Her roles were Betty in *The Way of the World* (John Barton, Aldwych, 1978); Spirit in *The Tempest* (Clifford Williams, RST, 1978); both whore and nun with Juliet Stevenson in *Measure for Measure* (Barry Kyle, RST, 1978); Jaquenetta in *Love's Labour's Lost* (Barton, RST, 1978); Jane in *Wild Oats* (Williams, Aldwych, 1979); Suzie in Tom McGrath's *The Innocent* (Howard Davies, Warehouse, 1979); and the highly-sexed Sally in Howard Brenton's controversial *Sore Throats* (Kyle, Warehouse, 1979).

Ruby Wax trained at the Royal Scottish Academy of Music and Drama. She was a member of the RSC at the same time as the friend who would have a major influence on her progress from actress to personality, Alan Rickman. They met at the Sheffield Crucible in 1976 and for the next few years moved around together as an improbable double-act, with Alan Rickman playing the straight man: they worked at the Bristol Old Vic (1976), then returned to Sheffield (1977) to play Jaques and Audrey in a production of *As You Like It* (Peter James) before landing at the RSC in 1978. For Ruby Wax membership of the RSC was useful because it provided a platform for her own writing. With the help of friends in the Company she developed and produced two shows during the Stratford and London seasons, *The Johnson Wax Floorshow*, co-written with Darlene Johnson and performed by Rickman, Jane Lapotaire, Ian Charleson, Zoë Wanamaker, Jonathan Pryce and David Suchet, and *Desperately Yours*, performed with Juliet Stevenson under Rickman's direction. Rickman also directed her subsequent shows, *Live Wax* (Edinburgh Festival, 1986) and *Wax Acts* (West End, 1992), and must partly take the blame for the Ruby phenomenon of the 1990s.

Paul Webster. From 1967 to 1974 Paul Webster was based at the Library Theatre, Manchester, as actor and co-director—his productions included *Old Times*, *Dracula* and *The Imaginary Invalid*.

From 1978 to 2000 he was an indispensable supporting player at the RSC, a veteran of over forty parts: Gremio in *The Taming of the Shrew* (Michael Bogdanov, RST, 1978); Alonso in *The Tempest* (Clifford Williams, RST, 1978); Robert Whatley in *Captain Swing* (Bill Alexander, TOP, 1978); Colonel Ball in *The Churchill Play* (Barry Kyle, TOP, 1978); Agrippa in *Antony and Cleopatra* (Peter Brook, RST, 1978); Smooth in *Wild Oats* (Williams, Aldwych, 1979); Yakov Troshin in *The Children of the Sun* (Terry Hands, Aldwych, 1979); Grigson in *Shadow of a Gunman* (Bogdanov, TOP, 1980); Sir Henry Bushy in *Richard II* (Hands, RST, 1980); Robert Brakenbury in *Richard III* (Hands, RST, 1980); Vosmibratov in *The Forest* (Adrian Noble, TOP, 1981); Ross in Howard Brenton's *Thirteenth Night* (Kyle, Warehouse, 1981); Escalus in *Romeo and Juliet* (Ron Daniels, Aldwych, 1981); Clarke in *Arden of Faversham* (Hands, TOP, 1982); Warrington in *Lear* (Kyle, TOP, 1982); Alonso in *The Tempest* (Daniels, RST, 1982); Lepidus/Proculeius in *Antony and Cleopatra* (Noble, TOP, 1982); Sir Davy Dapper in *The Roaring Girl* (Kyle, Barbican, 1983); Dr Brink in *The Custom of the Country* (David Jones, Pit, 1983); Antigonus in *The Winter's Tale* (Noble) and Reverend Parris in *The Crucible* (Nick Hamm, Small-scale Tour, 1984); Master Page in *The Merry Wives of Windsor* (Bill Alexander, RST, 1985); Black George in *The Dillen* (Kyle, TOP, 1985); Gratiano in *Othello* (Hands, RST, 1985); Josthinkel in *Mephisto* (Noble, Barbican, 1986); Leonato in *Much Ado About Nothing* (Daniels) and Antonio in *The Merchant of Venice* (Roger Michell, Small-scale Tour, 1986); Bonavent in *Hyde Park* (Kyle, Swan, 1987); the Director in *Temptation* (Michell, TOP, 1987); Antonio in *Twelfth Night* (Alexander, RST, 1987); Belarius in *Cymbeline* (Alexander, TOP, 1987); Quince in *A Midsummer Night's Dream* (John Caird, RST, 1989); Belarius in *Cymbeline* (Alexander, RST, 1989); Leonato in *Much Ado About Nothing* (Alexander, RST, 1990); Albany in *King Lear* (Nicholas Hytner, RST, 1990); Sir Nathaniel in *Love's Labour's Lost* (Hands, RST, 1990); Hector in Peter Whelan's *The Bright and Bold Design* (Alexander, Pit, 1991); Questenberg in *Wallenstein*

(Tim Albery, Pit, 1993); and Ross in *Macbeth* (Gregory Doran, Swan, 1999).

Samuel West (b. London, 1966) was a leading student actor at Oxford, appearing in ambitious shows (including David Mamet's *American Buffalo*) and performing at the Edinburgh Festival (he read English at Lady Margaret Hall, 1985-88). Already a scholarly actor, he was President of the Oxford University Experimental Theatre Club and Archivist of the Oxford University Dramatic Society.

He had made his television debut at the age of seven in *Edward VII*, a series that starred his father, Timothy West (1973). On leaving Oxford he rapidly achieved some notable successes on the stage—Timothy in Somerset Maugham's *The Bread-Winner* (Kevin Billington, Theatre Royal, Windsor, 1989); John in David Mamet's *A Life in the Theatre* (Bill Bryden, Theatre Royal Haymarket, 1989); the son in Simon Gray's *Hidden Laughter* (Gray, Vaudeville, 1990); Edward Bond's *The Sea* (Sam Mendes, NT Lyttelton, 1992); the title role in Byron's *Cain* (Edward Hall, Minerva, Chichester, 1992); and the title role in Vivian Ellis's musical *Mr Cinders* (Martin Connor, King's Head, 1993). On screen he played the pivotal role of Leonard in *Howards End* (James Ivory, 1992).

As the young upper-class mathematician in Tom Stoppard's *Arcadia* he conveyed the excitement of ideas while making the egghead likeable (Trevor Nunn, NT Lyttelton, 1993). He next played Algernon in *The Importance of Being Earnest* (James Maxwell, Manchester Royal Exchange, 1993-94); Hal to his father's Falstaff in *Henry IV* (Steven Unwin, English Touring Theatre, 1996-97); Stanhope in *Journey's End* (David Evans Rees, King's Head, 1998); and Octavius in *Antony and Cleopatra* (Sean Mathias, NT Olivier, 1998).

In 2000 he joined the RSC to play the title role in *Richard II* ('This England: the Histories', TOP, 2000). Instead of the usual poetry reading, West presented a petulant, ironic, isolated young man. The title role in *Hamlet* followed (RST, 2001). The two productions, both directed by Steven Pimlott in the same style (clean abstract settings; modern dress), overlapped, meaning that West was playing Richard in London and Hamlet in Stratford during the same week. Wearing a black T-shirt and hooded fleece jacket, he played the prince as a bright but difficult postgraduate student, self-obsessed, cruel to the vulnerable (particularly Kerry Condon's Ophelia), but with enough charm to engage the audience. It was an interpretation that allowed him to play to his strength, for the sound of his voice means that he always comes across as an arrogant public schoolboy. True to this impression, as a leading actor in Adrian Noble's last true ensemble, he criticised his boss at an award ceremony and made himself available to the BBC's *Newsnight* on the day of Noble's resignation. He was particularly well cast as Anthony Blunt in *Cambridge Spies* (Tim Fywell, BBC, 2003).

Janet Whiteside (b. Birmingham) trained at the theatre school of the Birmingham Rep and began her career as a member of the Rep's company (1950s). She was at the RSC from 1969 to 1976, and again from 1994. She walked-on in *The Winter's Tale* (Trevor Nunn) and *Women Beware Women* (Terry Hands), and then succeeded Brenda Bruce as Mistress Page in *The Merry Wives of Windsor* (Hands, Japanese Tour, 1970). Significant character roles followed: Pert in Dion Boucicault's *London Assurance* (Ronald Eyre, Aldwych, 1970); Duchess of York in *Richard II* (John Barton, RST, 1971); Cariola in *The Duchess of Malfi* (Clifford Williams, RST, 1971); Lady Montague in the Timothy Dalton/Estelle Kohler *Romeo and Juliet* (Hands, RST, 1973); Duchess of Gloucester in *Richard II* (Barton, RST, 1973); Hisperia in *As You Like It* (Buzz Goodbody, RST, 1973); Lady Faulconbridge in *King John* (Barton/Barry Kyle, RST, 1974); Olga in Gorky's *Summerfolk* (David Jones, Aldwych, 1974); Mrs Starck in Strindberg's *Comrades* (Kyle, The Place, 1974); Mrs Opie in Harley Granville-

Barker's *The Marrying of Ann Leete* (Jones, Aldwych, 1975); and Anna in Gorky's *The Zykovs* (Jones, Aldwych, 1976).

On her return, she played Mrs Dilber in *A Christmas Carol* (Ian Judge, Barbican, 1994-95); Matron/Nun in *The White Devil* (Gale Edwards, Swan, 1996); First Witch in *Macbeth* (Tim Albery, RST, 1996); Hecuba in *Troilus and Cressida* (Michael Boyd) and Anna in *A Month in the Country* (Michael Attenborough, Small-scale Tour, 1998-99); Duchess of Gloucester and Duchess of York in *Richard II* (Steven Pimlott, TOP, 2000); Aunt Filomena in Giovanni Verga's *La Lupa* (Simona Gonella, TOP, 2000); and Serpent/Oracle/She Ancient in George Bernard Shaw's *Back to Methuselah* (David Fielding, TOP, 2000).

Janet Whiteside has also given distinguished performances at the National: *The Caucasian Chalk Circle* (Michael Bogdanov, Cottesloe, 1982); Isabella in *The Spanish Tragedy* (Bogdanov, Cottesloe, 1982); *Lorenzaccio* (Bogdanov, Olivier, 1983); *Macbeth* (Bogdanov, Cottesloe, 1983); *Saint Joan* (Ronald Eyre, Olivier, 1984); Euridice in *Antigone* (John Burgess/Peter Gill, Cottesloe, 1984); Feydeau's *A Little Hotel on the Side* (Jonathan Lynn, Olivier, 1984); Annie in Alan Ayckbourn's *A Chorus of Disapproval* (Ayckbourn, Olivier, 1985); *Yonadab* (Peter Hall, Olivier, 1985); Beatrice in Sarah Daniels's *Neaptide* (John Burgess, Cottesloe, 1986); Lady in *King Lear* (David Hare, Olivier, 1986); Mrs Moule in David Edgar's *Entertaining Strangers* (Hall, Cottesloe, 1987); Shakespeare's late romances—Emilia in *The Winter's Tale*, Mother to Posthumus in *Cymbeline* and Masque in *The Tempest* (Hall, Cottesloe, 1988); and Berte in *Hedda Gabler* (Howard Davies, Olivier, 1989).

Benjamin Whitrow (b. Oxford, 1937). The likeably urbane Benjamin Whitrow served in the King's Dragoon Guards (1956-58), trained at RADA, and made his debut at the Liverpool Playhouse in 1959. Repertory seasons at Birmingham, Bristol and Harrogate followed. His formative years were spent in the supporting ranks of the National Theatre (1967-74), and he returned as a master craftsman in the 1980s and 90s: John Mortimer's Feydeau adaptation *A Little Hotel on the Side* (Jonathan Lynn, Olivier, 1984); *Racing Demon* (Richard Eyre, 1991); Ephraim Smooth in John O'Keeffe's *Wild Oats* (Jeremy Sams, Lyttelton, 1995); and Ruskin in Tom Stoppard's *The Invention of Love* (Eyre, Cottesloe, 1997).

At the RSC he created the role of James in Peter Nichols's *Passion Play* (Mike Ockrent, Aldwych, 1981), and was a leading Shakespearean player in 1992 and 2000: Camillo in *The Winter's Tale* (Adrian Noble, RST, 1992); Falstaff in *The Merry Wives of Windsor* (David Thacker, RST, 1992); Fiodor in Richard Nelson and Alexander Gelman's *Misha's Party* (David Jones, Pit, 1993); Sir Anthony Absolute in *The Rivals* (Lindsay Posner, Swan, 2000); Shallow in *Henry IV Part 2* (Michael Attenborough, Swan, 2000); and the Gravedigger in *Hamlet* (fringe festival production, Samuel West, TOP, 2000).

Whitrow's stylish brand of Englishness is best indicated by his work for major contemporary writers: Wood in Simon Gray's *Otherwise Engaged* (Harold Pinter, Queen's, 1975); McTeazle in Tom Stoppard's *Dirty Linen* (Arts, 1976); Donald in Alan Ayckbourn's *Ten Times Table* (Ayckbourn, Globe, 1978); the director in Michael Frayn's *Noises Off* (Michael Blakemore, Savoy, 1983); and Dr Rance in Joe Orton's *What the Butler Saw* (Jeremy Sams, Theatre Royal, Bath, 2001). He was a fine Serebryakov in the Michael Gambon/Jonathan Pryce *Uncle Vanya* at the Vaudeville (Blakemore, 1988). On the screen, he has delivered memorable supporting performances in Alan Bennett's *One Fine Day* and *Afternoon Off* (Stephen Frears, ITV, 1979); Michael Frayn's *Clockwise* (Christopher Morahan, 1986); *Ffizz* (ITV, 1987); *Pride and Prejudice* (Simon Langton, BBC, 1995), as Mr Bennet; and *Island at War* (Thaddeus O'Sullivan, ITV, 2004).

Lucy Whybrow (b. London, 1972). Soon after leaving the Central School of Speech and Drama, Lucy Whybrow succeeded Emma Fielding as Thomasina in Tom Stoppard's *Arcadia*

(Trevor Nunn, NT West End, 1994). She then joined the RSC to play the disturbed and saintly Eleanora in Strindberg's *Easter* (Katie Mitchell, Pit, 1995), an exceptional performance that brought her the Ian Charleson Award, and set up huge expectations for her Juliet (Adrian Noble, RST, 1995). A pale blonde in a sky-blue dress, this movingly young Juliet looked like Lewis Carroll's Alice, but Lucy Whybrow also conveyed wilfulness and near-hysteria.

In the same season she was outstanding as Anya—stretching with fatigue after the homecoming and making something evocative out of the accompanying line 'I went up in a balloon in Paris!'—in Adrian Noble's production of *The Cherry Orchard* (Swan), and Antigone in *The Phoenician Women* (Katie Mitchell, TOP). At the end of the season she played Lucy in a BBC film of *The Mill on the Floss* (Graham Theakston, 1997).

At the National she has played Petra in *An Enemy of the People* (Nunn, Olivier, 1997); Tatiana in Tom Stoppard's *The Coast of Utopia* (Nunn, Olivier, 2002); Natasha in *Three Sisters* (Mitchell, Lyttelton, 2003); and Agnes in Strindberg's *A Dream Play* (Mitchell, Cottesloe, 2005). Elsewhere: Constanze to Michael Sheen's Mozart in *Amadeus* (Peter Hall, Old Vic, 1998); Kevin Elyot's *Mouth to Mouth* (Ian Rickson, Royal Court, 2001); and Sabine in Roland Schimmelpfennig's *Push Up* (Theatre Upstairs, Royal Court, 2002).

Peter Wight (b. 1950) read English at St Edmund Hall, Oxford, and gained his early experience at Hornchurch, Leicester and Liverpool. His career advanced slowly until the turn of the 1970s into the 80s, when directors like Peter Gill (at the Riverside Studios) and the young Michael Boyd (at the Belgrade, Coventry) started to recognise the quality of his acting.

His theatre roles of the 1980s and 90s included Lysander in *A Midsummer Night's Dream* and John Axt in Howard Barker's *A Passion in Six Days* for Boyd at the Sheffield Crucible (1983); Medvyedenko in the Vanessa Redgrave *The Seagull* (Charles

Sturridge) and Ollie in Doug Lucie's *Progress* at the Lyric Hammersmith (1985-86); Edmund in *Edward II* at the Manchester Royal Exchange (Nicholas Hytner, 1986); Andrei in *Three Sisters* at the Birmingham Rep (Peter Farago, 1987); Lucky in *Waiting for Godot* (Michael Rudman, Lyttelton), Mephistopheles in Kevin Dewhurst's *Black Snow* (William Gaskill, Cottesloe), Giri in *The Resistible Rise of Arturo Ui* (Di Trevis, Olivier) and the Home Secretary in David Hare's *Murmuring Judges* (Richard Eyre, Olivier) at the National (1987, 1991-92); Gavin in Lucie's *Grace* (Mike Bradwell) and Alaric in Philip Osment's *The Dearly Beloved* (Mike Alfreds) at the Hampstead Theatre (1992-93); and Oscar in Simon Block's *Not a Game for the Boys* at the Royal Court (1995).

He has made his mark at the RSC in only a handful of roles: a pragmatic but formidable Claudius, interrogating Mark Rylance's prince by thrusting his head in a bucket of water, in *Hamlet* (Ron Daniels, RST, 1989); Prison Clergyman in *A Clockwork Orange* (Ron Daniels, Barbican, 1990); the desolate Makarov in Gorky's *Barbarians* (David Jones, Barbican, 1990); Don Pedro in *Much Ado About Nothing* (Boyd, RST, 1996); and Hieronimo in Kyd's *The Spanish Tragedy* (Boyd, Swan, 1997). The latter showed his talent for quietly-spoken interpretations of potentially histrionic roles.

Subsequent stage work: Hanif Kureshi's *Sleep With Me* (Anthony Page, NT Cottesloe, 1999); Dennis in Kevin Elyot's *Mouth to Mouth* (Ian Rickson, Royal Court, 2001); Martin Crimp's *Face to the Wall* (Katie Mitchell, Royal Court, 2002); Lebedev in *Ivanov* (Mitchell, NT Cottesloe, 2002); and Rothko in *Red on Black* (Katie Read, Hen and Chickens, 2003).

On television Wight has often played world-weary, dependable characters on the periphery of the action—*Anna Lee* (1993-94), *Devil's Advocate* (Adrian Shergold, BBC, 1995) and *Out of the Blue* (BBC, 1995-96) are good examples. He created characters in Mike Leigh's *Meantime* (1983), *Naked* (1993), *Secrets and Lies* (1996) and *Vera Drake* (2004).

Tom Wilkinson (b. Leeds, 1948). The son of a farmer, brought up in Yorkshire, Canada and Cornwall, Tom Wilkinson studied English at Kent University before winning a place at RADA. For twenty-five years he steadily built an impressive career as a character actor, highly respected but largely unknown to the public until the success of *The Full Monty* in 1997.

His early theatre work included Howard Brenton's *The Churchill Play* and Trevor Griffiths's *Comedians* at Richard Eyre's Nottingham Playhouse (1974-75); Eric Bentley's *Are You Now or Have You Ever Been?* at the Birmingham Rep (1976); and Marullus/Titinius in *Julius Caesar* (John Schlesinger, Olivier) and the Soldier in *The Passion* (Bill Bryden, Cottesloe) at the National (1977).

He was a member of the RSC for one two-year cycle: Corin in *As You Like It* (Terry Hands, RST, 1980); Melantius—played powerfully as a callous homosexual—in *The Maid's Tragedy* (Barry Kyle, TOP, 1980); Horatio—short hair and round spectacles—in the Michael Pennington *Hamlet* (John Barton, RST, 1980); Sir William Catesby in the Alan Howard *Richard III* (Hands, RST, 1980); Antonio to David Suchet's Shylock in *The Merchant of Venice* (Barton, RST, 1981); and Pavel Gai in *The Love-Girl and the Innocent* (Clifford Williams, Aldwych, 1981).

His status was confirmed by two fine performances during the 1980s—T.S. Eliot in *Tom and Viv* at the Royal Court (1984) and Pastor Manders to Vanessa Redgrave's Mrs Alving in *Ghosts* at the Young Vic (David Thacker, 1986). However, he has increasingly given precedence to the cinema. Highlights have included *Priest* (Antonia Bird, 1994); Mr Dashwood in *Sense and Sensibility* (Ang Lee, 1995); the Marquess of Queensberry in *Wilde* (1997); Hugh Stratton in *Oscar and Lucinda* (Gillian Armstrong, 1997); *Shakespeare in Love* (John Madden, 1998); *Ride With the Devil* (Ang Lee, 1999); *In the Bedroom* (Todd Field, 2001)—arguably his finest achievement; *Eternal Sunshine of the Spotless Mind* (Michel Gondry, 2004); *Batman Begins* (Christopher Nolan, 2005); and *Michael Clayton* (2007).

Michael Williams (1935-2001, b. Salford). A Liverpudlian, Michael Williams worked in insurance before winning a scholarship to RADA at the age of twenty-one. His career began at the Nottingham Playhouse, where he played Auguste in J.B. Priestley's *Take the Fool Away* and Bernard in Hall and Waterhouse's *Celebration*. The latter went into the West End (Duchess Theatre, 1961).

He joined the RSC in 1963 and stayed for fifteen years. He was a naturally-gifted performer who, instantaneously, made a connection with spectators based on either melancholy or joy. His Shakespearean work combined feeling, wit and personality. Alongside Puck in *A Midsummer Night's Dream* (Peter Hall, Aldwych, 1963), Oswald in the Paul Scofield *King Lear* (Peter Brook, Aldwych, 1964), Rosencrantz in the David Warner *Hamlet* (Hall, RST, 1965), a loveable Dromio in two productions of *The Comedy of Errors* (Clifford Williams, RST, 1965; Trevor Nunn, RST, 1976), Petruchio opposite Janet Suzman in *The Taming of the Shrew* (Nunn, RST, 1967), Troilus opposite Helen Mirren in *Troilus and Cressida* (John Barton, RST, 1968), a tender Fool to the Lears of Eric Porter and Donald Sinden (Nunn, RST, 1968, 1976) and the title role in *Henry V* (Barton, RST, 1971), he played Adolf Eichmann in Rolf Hochhüth's *The Representative* (Williams, Aldwych, 1963), Vladimir in Samuel Beckett's *Waiting for Godot* (Gareth Morgan, Theatregoround, 1968), the title role in Bertolt Brecht's *Schweyk in the Second World War* (Howard Davies, TOP, 1976) and appeared in the RSC's most controversial productions, Peter Brook's *Marat/Sade* (Aldwych, 1964) and *US* (Aldwych, 1966) — it was Williams who set fire to the 'butterfly'.

He married Judi Dench, his RSC contemporary, in 1971. They worked together in subsequent Stratford and London seasons, and later played a couple in the popular situation comedy *A Fine Romance* (ITV, 1981-84). During the 1980s and 90s he was an occasional live performer, his appearances restricted to *Quar-*

termaine's Terms (UK Tour, 1982); *Pack of Lies* (Lyric, 1983); *Two Into One* (Shaftesbury, 1984); *Mr and Mrs Nobody* (Garrick, 1986); *Out of Order* (Shaftesbury, 1990); and *The Forest* (Anthony Page, NT Lyttelton, 1999). Among the screen work of the last phase of his career there were some notable achievements—Goronwy Rees in Alan Bennett's *Blunt* (BBC, 1985), Williams in Kenneth Branagh's *Henry V* (1989), and the popular dramas *September Song* (ITV, 1993-95) and *Conjugal Rites* (ITV, 1993-94).

Olivia Williams (b. London, 1968). The daughter of barristers, brought up in Camden Town, Olivia Williams read English at Newham College, Cambridge, before training for the stage. She left the Bristol Old Vic Theatre School in 1991 and appeared in episodes of two popular television series, *Van der Valk* and *Ruth Rendell Mysteries*. She joined the RSC in 1993 to play Lydia in Richard Nelson and Alexander Gelman's *Misha's Party* (David Jones, Pit) and Princess Thekla in Schiller's *Wallenstein* (Tim Albery, Pit). Then in 1994/95 she was a member of the chorus in John Barton's Swan production of *Peer Gynt* and played a serene Mrs Friendal in the Restoration rarity *The Wives' Excuse* (Max Stafford-Clark, Swan) and a grave, deceptively icy Calantha in John Ford's *The Broken Heart* (Michael Boyd, Swan).

On television she played a battered wife in the series *Beck* (BBC, 1996), and Jane Fairfax in Andrew Davies's adaptation of *Emma* (ITV, 1996). After a period of unemployment she won the female lead in Kevin Costner's *The Postman* (1998). She has since starred in *Rushmore* (1999); *The Sixth Sense* (M. Night Shyamalan, 1999), as Bruce Willis's grieving wife; *Dead Babies* (2000); *Born Romantic* (David Kane, 2000); *The Body* (2001); *Lucky Break* (Peter Cattaneo, 2001); *To Kill a King* (2003); *Peter Pan* (P.J. Hogan, 2003), as Mrs Darling; *Agatha Christie* (BBC, 2004); *Miss Austen Regrets* (BBC, 2008); *Flashbacks of a Fool* (2008).

Between film shoots Olivia Williams has returned to the London stage: the Princess of France in Trevor Nunn's *Love's Labour's Lost* at the National (Olivier, 2003); Annie in John Osborne's *The Hotel in Amsterdam* at the Donmar Warehouse (Robin Lefevre, 2003); and Beatrice Joanna in Middleton and Rowley's *The Changeling* at the Barbican (Declan Donnellan, Cheek by Jowl, 2006).

Nicol Williamson (b. Hamilton, Scotland, 1938). When Nicol Williamson arrived in London from the Dundee Rep in 1961 he was already an intimidatingly intense performer, a 'delinquent cherub' in John Osborne's phrase. He appeared at the Royal Court in Henry Chapman's *That's Us* (William Gaskill, 1961), *A Midsummer Night's Dream* (Tony Richardson, 1962) and *Twelfth Night* (George Devine, 1962), then joined the RSC to play leading roles during the season at the Arts (1962): Albert Meakin in Henry Livings's *Nil Carborundum* (Anthony Page); Satin in Gorky's *The Lower Depths* (Toby Robertson); and Leantio in *Women Beware Women* (Anthony Page). Returning to the Court in 1963, he continued to build his reputation in Wedekind's *Spring Awakening* (Desmond O'Donovan), Livings's *Kelly's Eye* (David Scase), and J.P. Donleavy's *The Ginger Man*.

His next role, Bill Maitland in *Inadmissible Evidence* (Page, 1964), made him a star, so convincingly did he inhabit the paranoia, petulance and self-disgust of Osborne's play. The production went into the West End and then to New York (1965). He starred in the film, released in 1967, and stayed in movies for *The Bofors Gun* (Jack Gold, 1968), *Laughter in the Dark* (Tony Richardson, 1968) and *The Reckoning* (Jack Gold, 1969). As Hamlet, which he played at the Roundhouse and in New York in 1969, he famously made no aesthetic concessions to the verse, preferring to constantly surprise audiences with his abrasiveness, volatility and sneering intellect. Even after more than thirty years he remains the most anti-heroic of Hamlets.

Now specialising in self-destructive characters, he returned to the RSC to play Coriolanus (Trevor Nunn, Aldwych, 1973), Macbeth opposite Helen Mirren (Nunn, RST, 1974), and Uncle Vanya, in his own production (TOP, 1974). Untelegraphed mood-swings—rage giving way to vulnerability and despair—connected all three. He made the characters outsiders, loners, difficult people, and the image stuck to him in real life. There was an almost puritanical need to get the character right, to get to the truth, despite the loss of sympathy.

In 1975 he played a cocaine-addicted Sherlock Holmes in the film *The Seven Per Cent Solution* (Herbert Ross), and Henry VIII in the musical *Rex* on Broadway. In 1978 he returned to the Royal Court and *Inadmissible Evidence*, this time directed by the author. By the beginning of the 1980s his marriage to the actress Jill Townsend had ended and he was living in New York. In exile from the English stage, he appeared regularly on Broadway—*Inadmissible Evidence* (1981), *Macbeth* (1983), *The Entertainer* (1983), *The Lark* (1983), and *The Real Thing* (1985). He played the title role in Macbeth for the BBC (1982) and continued to work in films—*The Cheap Detective* (1977); *The Goodbye Girl* (Herbert Ross, 1977); *Robin and Marion* (Richard Lester, 1977), as Little John; Graham Greene's *The Human Factor* (Otto Preminger, 1979); *Excalibur* (John Boorman, 1980), as Merlin; *Venom* (1980); *I'm Dancing as Fast as I Can* (1981); *Return to Oz* (1984); *Black Widow* (Bob Rafelson, 1986); and *The Hour of the Pig* (Leslie Megahey, 1994)—but from the mid-1980s his career went into a slow decline.

He allegedly stopped a performance of the 1969 *Hamlet* mid-scene because he was too tired to give of his best (Tony Richardson was filming the production during the day), and re-started a performance of the 1978 *Inadmissible Evidence* because the audience had yet to settle. In 1994 he returned to the London stage as John Barrymore in his own one-man show *Jack: a Night on the Town with John Barrymore* (Leslie Megahey, Criterion). It was a *tour de force* of acting, singing and impersonation, but the reviews were poor, advanced sales disappointing, and Williamson walked off during the second night. Seven years later, in the relative obscurity of Wales, he played King Lear (Terry Hands, Theatr Clwyd).

Penelope Wilton (b. Scarborough, 1946) followed her mother, aunt and uncle (Bill Travers) into the acting profession. She trained at the Drama Centre, London, and played Masha in *The Seagull* for Jonathan Miller at Chichester (1968). She came to notice in the early 1970s at the Royal Court (Christopher Hampton's *The Philanthropist*), the Nottingham Playhouse (*King Lear*), the Bristol Old Vic (*Uncle Vanya*), and the Greenwich Theatre (*Measure for Measure*, *All's Well That Ends Well*, and Alan Ayckbourn's *The Norman Conquests*, as Ruth). She played Annie in the television production of Ayckbourn's trilogy (Herbert Wise, ITV, 1977), the beginning of a screen career that has seen her bring gravitas to comedy roles—she is able to suggest an inner-life through expression alone. Most prominently, she played opposite Richard Briers in *Ever Decreasing Circles* (BBC, 1984-87), and Ian Holm, her husband, in *The Borrowers* (BBC, 1992-93).

As a stage actress she is particularly distinguished in Pinter, Chekhov, Ayckbourn and Shaw. She created the roles of the adulteress Emma, caught between Michael Gambon and Daniel Massey (her first husband), in Pinter's *Betrayal* (Peter Hall, Lyttelton, 1978), and the Tory politician Marion in David Hare's *The Secret Rapture* (Howard Davies, Lyttelton, 1988). Also at the National she was seen to great effect in Shaw's *The Philanderer* (Christopher Morahan, Lyttelton, 1978); as Bianca in the Paul Scofield *Othello* (Peter Hall, Olivier, 1980); Dorcas in Ayckbourn's *Sisterly Feelings* (Morahan, Olivier, 1980); Ann to Daniel Massey's Tanner in *Man and Superman* (Morahan, Olivier, 1981); Beatrice to Michael Gambon's Benedick in *Much Ado About Nothing* (Peter Gill, Olivier, 1981); the title role in *Major Barbara* (Gill, Lyttelton, 1982); in Trevor Griffiths's *The Piano* (Howard Davies, Cottesloe, 1990); and alongside Ian Holm in Pinter's *Landscape* (Pinter, Cottesloe, 1994). At the Almeida she was heartbreaking in Rattigan's *The Deep Blue Sea* (Karel Reisz, 1992).

At the RSC, working with Adrian Noble, she gave extraordinary, multifaceted performances as Madame Ranyevskaya in *The Cherry Orchard* (Swan, 1995) and Arkadina in *The Seagull* (Swan, 2000). She has since played Regina in *The Little Foxes* (Marianne Elliott, Donmar Warehouse, 2001); Sonya opposite John Hurt in Brian Friel's *Afterplay* (Gate Theatre, Dublin, 2002); Bernarda Alba in García Lorca's *The House of Bernarda Alba* (Davies, NT Lyttelton, 2005); and, back with the RSC, Livia in *Women Beware Women* (Laurence Boswell, Swan, 2006).

In the cinema: *Joseph Andrews* (Tony Richardson, 1976); *The French Lieutenant's Woman* (Karel Reisz, 1981); driving John Cleese into the mud in *Clockwise* (Christopher Morahan, 1986); Kevin Kline's wife in Richard Attenborough's *Cry Freedom* (1987); *The Secret Rapture* (Howard Davies, 1994); *Carrington* (Christopher Hampton, 1995); *Iris* (Richard Eyre, 2001); *Calendar Girls* (Nigel Cole, 2003); *Shaun of the Dead* (2004); and Woody Allen's *Match Point* (2005).

Clive Wood (b. Croydon, 1954) has returned to the RSC at intervals throughout his career. In his first two years with the Company, 1982-83, he played Lennox in *Macbeth* (Howard Davies, RST), Edmund in the Michael Gambon *King Lear* (Adrian Noble, RST), Thomas in Edward Bond's *Lear* (Barry Kyle, TOP), Dolabella/Sextus Pompeius in *Antony and Cleopatra* (Noble, TOP) and Kenneth Gross in Nick Darke's *The Body* (Nick Hamm, Pit); in 1985/86, John Browdie and Sir Mulberry Hawk in *Nicholas Nickleby* (RST); in 1993, Valmont in *Les liaisons dangereuses* (UK Tour); in 1994-95, Pistol in *Henry V* (Matthew Warchus, RST), Orsino in *Twelfth Night* (Ian Judge, RST), Mr Wilding in Thomas Southerne's *The Wives' Excuse* (Max Stafford-Clark, Swan) and Oblensky in John Osborne's *A Patriot For Me* (Peter Gill, Barbican); in 2000-01, York in *Henry VI 1-3* (Michael Boyd, 'This England: the Histories', Swan); in 2002, Enobarbus in *Antony and Cleopatra* (Michael Attenborough) and Don Pedro in *Much Ado About Nothing* (Gregory Doran, RST); in

2004-05, Macduff in *Macbeth* (Dominic Cooke, RST), Claudius in *Hamlet* (Boyd, RST) and Pontius Pilate in *The Pilate Project* (Boyd, TOP); in 2005, Sir Toby Belch, succeeding Nicky Henson, in *Twelfth Night* (Boyd, RST); and, in 2006-08, reprising York in *Henry VI* and adding Bolingbroke in *Richard II* and the title role in *Henry IV* (Boyd, Courtyard).

Wood trained at the London Academy of Music and Dramatic Art and came to notice at the Bristol Old Vic at the end of the 1970s—*The Beaux' Stratagem*, the title role in *Henry V*, *Guys and Dolls*, and Gaveston in *Edward II* (Richard Cottrell, 1980). Also in 1980 he played Malcolm in the Peter O'Toole Old Vic *Macbeth*.

John Wood (b. Derbyshire, 1930). Two periods of work at the RSC are the highpoints of John Wood's remarkable, if sporadic, stage career.

At Oxford (Jesus College) he was President of OUDS, and played Osric in *Hamlet* (Nevill Coghill, 1951), Malvolio in *Twelfth Night* (1952) and the title role in his own production of *Richard III* (1953). His first professional appearance was as Bernardo in the Richard Burton *Hamlet* at the Old Vic (Michael Benthall, 1953). For years his career fell short of expectations. Both the Old Vic and the Royal Court—where in 1957 he played small roles in *The Making of Moo* (Tony Richardson), *Nekrassov* (George Devine) and *A Resounding Tinkle* (William Gaskill)—let him go abruptly. In the West End he played Don Quixote in Tennessee Williams's *Camino Real* (Phoenix, 1957) and The Wali in *Brouhaha* (Aldwych, 1958). In the early 1960s he went into television, and became a well-known face in quality drama. His career changed when he was cast in Tom Stoppard's short television plays *Teeth* and *Another Moon Called Earth* (BBC, 1967). The two became friends and Wood played Guildenstern in *Rosencrantz and Guildenstern are Dead* on Broadway (1967), the first major recognition of his talent.

From 1971 to 76 he was one of the RSC's most exciting players, a tall, lean, edgy ironist whose precise articulation of, and relish for, words found its perfect outlet in a disparate choice of wordy roles: Yakov Bardin in Gorky's *Enemies* (David Jones, Aldwych, 1971); Sir Fopling Flutter in *The Man of Mode* (Terry Hands, Aldwych, 1971); Richard Rowan in James Joyce's *Exiles* (Harold Pinter, Aldwych, 1971); Brutus in *Julius Caesar* (Trevor Nunn/Buzz Goodbody, RST, 1972); Antipholus of Syracuse in *The Comedy of Errors* (Clifford Williams, RST, 1972); Saturninus in *Titus Andronicus* (Nunn/Goodbody, RST, 1972); Monsieur Luc in *A Lesson in Blood and Roses* (Williams, The Place, 1973); the title role in *Sherlock Holmes* (Frank Dunlop, Aldwych, 1974); Henry Carr, a part written for him, in Stoppard's *Travesties* (Peter Wood, Aldwych, 1974); General Burgoyne in Shaw's *The Devil's Disciple* (Jack Gold, Aldwych, 1976); and the title role in *Ivanov* (Jones, Aldwych, 1976).

The New York runs of *Sherlock Holmes* and *Travesties* made Wood's name in America, and he returned to New York in 1978 for *Death Trap*, and in the early 1980s for *Amadeus* (Peter Hall). *Amadeus* followed three roles at the National—Friedrich Horleiter in Stoppard's Schnitzler adaptation *Undiscovered Country* (Wood, Olivier, 1979), the title role in *Richard III* (Christopher Morahan, Olivier, 1979), and Sir John Brute in *The Provok'd Wife* (Wood, Lyttelton, 1980).

Wood returned to the RSC in 1988 and stayed for four years: Prospero in *The Tempest* (Nicholas Hytner, RST, 1988); Sheridan Whiteside in *The Man Who Came to Dinner* (Gene Saks, Barbican, 1989); Solness in *The Master Builder* (Adrian Noble, Barbican, 1989); the title role in *King Lear* (Hytner, RST, 1990); and Don Armado in *Love's Labour's Lost* (Hands, RST, 1990). In 1997 he was reunited with Stoppard at the National, portraying Housman in *The Invention of Love* (Richard Eyre, Cottesloe). He subsequently played Spooner to Corin Redgrave's Hirst in Harold Pinter's *No Man's Land* (Pinter, Lyttelton, 2001-02), and Shallow in *Henry IV Part 2* (Hytner, Olivier, 2005).

The later years of his career have been dominated by the British and American cinema—*War Games* (John Badham, 1983); *Ladyhawke* (Richard Donner, 1985); *The Purple Rose of Cairo* (Woody Allen, 1985); John Dudley in *Lady Jane* (Nunn, 1986); *Orlando* (Sally Potter, 1992); *Shadowlands* (Richard Attenborough, 1993); Thurlow in *The Madness of King George* (Hytner, 1994); King Edward in *Richard III* (Richard Loncraine, 1995); *Sabrina* (Sydney Pollack, 1995); Mr Brocklehurst in *Jane Eyre* (Franco Zeffirelli, 1996); *Metroland* (Philip Saville, 1997); *An Ideal Husband* (Oliver Parker, 1999); *Chocolat* (Lasse Hallström, 2000); and *The White Countess* (James Ivory, 2005).

Nicholas Woodeson spent his early childhood in the Middle East. He was educated at boarding schools and at Sussex University. A member of the drama society (competing at the National Student Drama Festival), he went on to train at RADA. He began his career in Crewe, as an assistant stage manager and an occasional actor (first significant role: Benvolio in *Romeo and Juliet*).

As a stage actor he has followed an impressively versatile career: Fielding in Nick Dear's *The Art of Success* (Adrian Noble, Manhattan Theater Club, New York, 1989-90); Lenny in Pinter's *The Homecoming* (Peter Hall, Comedy, 1991); Richard in Daniel Mornin's *At Our Table* (Jenny Killick, NT Cottesloe, 1991); the title role in Howard Brenton's *Berlin Bertie* (Danny Boyle, Royal Court, 1992); Meredith Oakes's *The Editing Process* (Stephen Daldry, Royal Court, 1994); Goole in *An Inspector Calls* (Stephen Daldry, Garrick, 1995); Don in David Mamet's *American Buffalo* (Lindsay Posner, Young Vic, 1997); Lawrence in Simon Block's *Chimps* (Hampstead Theatre, 1997); Mr Brownlow in Simon Gray's *The Late Middle Classes* (Harold Pinter, Palace Theatre, Watford, 1999); *Art* (Matthew Warchus, 1999); Choke in Jim Cartwright's *Hard Fruit* (James Macdonald, Royal Court, 2000); and Bones in Stoppard's *Jumpers* (David Leveaux, NT Lyttelton, 2003).

At the RSC, from 1981 to 1990, he was the Dauphin to Kenneth Branagh's Henry V (Adrian Noble, RST, 1984), a surprisingly traditional Puck (Bill Alexander, RST, 1986), Malcolm to Jonathan Pryce's Macbeth (Noble, RST, 1986), and, most memorably, an Ian Holm-like King John (Deborah Warner, TOP, 1988). The rest of his RSC work consisted of new writing: Adolf Eichmann/Bouller in C.P. Taylor's *Good* (Howard Davies, Warehouse, 1981); Wadlow in Edward Bond's *The Fool* (Davies, Warehouse, 1981); Hayes/Joe Shawcross in Trevor Griffiths's *The Party* (Davies, TOP, 1984); Captain Woolf in Nicholas Wright's *The Desert Air* (Noble, TOP, 1984); Shakespeare in David Rudkin's *Will's Way* (Alison Sutcliffe, RSC fringe festival, TOP, 1984); Largewit in Kenneth Branagh's *Tell Me Honestly* (RSC fringe festival, Almeida, 1985); Frapper in Peter Barnes's *Red Noses* (Terry Hands, Barbican, 1985); Porcelain in Howard Barker's *Crimes in Hot Countries* (Bill Alexander, Pit, 1985); Mike Levine in David Lan's *Flight* (Davies, TOP, 1986); Bessmertny in Vladimir Gubaryev's *Sarcophagus* (Jude Kelly, Pit, 1987); and Queen Victoria/A Magical Priest in Frank McGuinness's *Mary and Lizzie* (Sarah Pia Anderson, Pit, 1989). He returned to the RSC in 2001 to play Garrick in Peter Barnes's *Jubilee* (Gregory Doran, Swan).

In Hollywood's *The Pelican Brief* (Alan J. Pakula, 1993) Woodeson played, with Pinteresque menace, one of the suits pursuing Julia Roberts. Other notable screen roles have included Seymour in Mike Leigh's *Topsy-Turvy* (1999) and Posca in *Rome* (BBC, 2005-07).

John Woodvine (b. Durham, 1929). In his first seasons with the RSC John Woodvine gave commanding performances as Capulet in the Ian McKellen/Francesca Annis *Romeo and Juliet* (Trevor Nunn, RST, 1976); Dogberry in *Much Ado About Nothing* (John Barton, RST, 1976); Polixenes in *The Winter's Tale* (Barton/Nunn, RST, 1976); Cornwall in *King Lear* (Nunn, RST, 1976); Dr Pinch, succeeding Robin Ellis, in *The Comedy of Errors* (Nunn,

RST, 1977); Subtle in *The Alchemist* (Nunn, TOP, 1977); Banquo in *Macbeth* (Nunn, TOP, 1976); Fainall in *The Way of the World* (Barton, Aldwych, 1978); Hersch in *A Miserable and Lonely Death* (Walter Donohue, Aldwych, 1978); a restrained Falstaff in *The Merry Wives of Windsor* (Nunn/John Caird, RST, 1979); Malvolio in *Twelfth Night* (Terry Hands, RST, 1979); the title role in *Julius Caesar* (Kyle, RST, 1979); the severe Ralph Nickleby in *Nicholas Nickleby* (Nunn/Caird, Aldwych, 1980); and Charles Merrythought in *The Knight of the Burning Pestle* (Michael Bogdanov, Aldwych, 1981).

He returned to Falstaff for Bogdanov's English Shakespeare Company production of *Henry IV*, presenting a cold egotist in a garish green suit. In *Henry V* he played the Chorus in modern dress, dominating the stage with his trademark vocal authority (Tour, 1986-87). Also on tour with the ESC he was Shylock in *The Merchant of Venice*, Volpone (Tim Luscombe) and Prospero in *The Tempest* (1992). His other theatre appearances have included: Claudius to McKellen's *Hamlet* (Robert Chetwyn, Prospect, 1971); *Joe Lives* (Greenwich, 1971); Orlovsky in *The Wood Demon* (David Giles, Actors' Company, 1973); Kent in *King Lear* (David William, Actors' Company, 1974); Jacob Gens in *Ghetto* (Nicholas Hytner, NT Olivier, 1989); Dr Gortler in J.B. Priestley's *I Have Been Here Before* (Matthew Francis, Palace Theatre, Watford, 1990); Christopherson to Natasha Richardson's Anna in *Anna Christie* (David Thacker, Young Vic, 1990); the husband in *Machinal* (Stephen Daldry, NT Lyttelton, 1993); *Venice Preserv'd* (Ian McDiarmid, Almeida, 1995); David Williamson's *Dead White Males* (Patrick Sandford, Nuffield Theatre, Southampton, 1996); Aslaken in *An Enemy of the People* (Nunn, NT Olivier, 1997); Brian Friel's *Give Me Your Answer, Do!* (Robin Lefevre, 1998); Edgar in *Life After Life* (NT Loft, 2002); Polonius in *Hamlet* (Sandford, Nuffield Theatre, Southampton, 2003); and Patrick in Alan Plater's musical *Blonde Bombshells of 1943* (Roxana Silbert, West Yorkshire Playhouse, 2004).

Woodvine returned to the RSC in the 1990s, and again in 2008: Monsewer in *The Hostage* (Bogdanov, Barbican, 1994);

Jaques in *As You Like It* (Steven Pimlott, RST, 1996); Clinton in *The General from America* (Howard Davies, Swan, 1996); King Philip in *Don Carlos* (Gale Edwards, TOP, 1999); Flavius in *Timon of Athens* (Gregory Doran, RST, 1999); and the Player King in *Hamlet* (Doran, Courtyard, 2008).

Sarah Woodward (b. London, 1963). The youngest of Edward Woodward's three actor children, Sarah Woodward trained at RADA and was given her first job by the RSC. She played minor roles until her second year: English Soldier in *Henry V* (Adrian Noble, RST, 1984); Yvette in Pam Gems's *Camille* (Ron Daniels, TOP, 1984); Lady of the Court in *Richard III* (Bill Alexander, RST, 1984); Lady in *Hamlet* (Daniels, RST, 1984); Kenneth Branagh's *Tell Me Honestly* (RSC fringe festival, Donmar Warehouse, 1985); Boy, succeeding Dexter Fletcher, in *Henry V* (Noble, Barbican, 1985); Evaline in Peter Barnes's *Red Noses* (Terry Hands, Barbican, 1985); and Katharine, succeeding Kate Buffery, in *Love's Labour's Lost* (Barry Kyle, Barbican, 1985).

She established her reputation over the next few years. She played Juliet to Ralph Fiennes's Romeo at the Open Air Theatre, Regent's Park (Declan Donnellan, 1985); Susie in Daniel Mornin's *Built on Sand* at the Royal Court (1987); Grace in Boucicault's *London Assurance* at Chichester (Sam Mendes, 1989); Anne in *Kean* (Mendes, Old Vic, 1990); and Rose in Edward Bond's *The Sea* (Mendes, NT Lyttelton, 1991).

She returned to the RSC as a leading actress: Chorus in T.S. Eliot's *Murder in the Cathedral* (Steven Pimlott, Swan, 1993); Rosaura in Goldoni's *The Venetian Twins* (Michael Bogdanov, Swan, 1993); Miranda to Alec McCowen's Prospero in *The Tempest* (Mendes, RST, 1993); and Rosaline in *Love's Labour's Lost* (Ian Judge, Barbican, 1995). Her subsequent appearances have included Alan Bennett's *Habeas Corpus*, her fifth production for Sam Mendes (Donmar Warehouse, 1996); Kitty alongside Michael Gambon and Alec McCowen in *Tom and Clem* (Richard Wilson, Aldwych, 1997); the wife in Tom Stoppard's *The Real*

Thing (David Leveaux, Donmar Warehouse, 1999); David Harrower's Beatles play *Presence* (Theatre Upstairs, Royal Court, 2001); Madame de Volanges in *Les liaisons dangereuses* (Tim Fywell, Playhouse, 2003-04); Dogberry in *Much Ado About Nothing* (Globe, 2004); Monica in Noël Coward's *Present Laughter* (Howard Davies, NT Lyttelton, 2007-08); and Peter Handke's *The Hour We Knew Nothing of Each Other* (James Macdonald, NT Lyttelton, 2008).

Angus Wright was born in Washington and raised in Cairo, Bahrain and Syria (his British father worked for the Foreign Office). This background may have inspired his decision to portray Warwick in Shaw's *Saint Joan* (Marianne Elliott, NT Olivier, 2007) as a John le Carré mandarin, urbane but deadly. It was a fine achievement.

Wright read art history at Edinburgh University and trained for the stage at Central. His career began at the RSC. As a member of Adrian Noble's first ensemble (1991-93), he played Second Officer in *Twelfth Night* (Griff Rhys Jones, RST); Douglas/Bullcalf in *Henry IV* (Noble, RST); Chorus in *The Thebans* (Noble, Swan); Balton in *The Dybbuk* (Katie Mitchell, Pit); and Guildenstern in the Kenneth Branagh *Hamlet* (Noble, Barbican).

At the National, leading up to *Saint Joan*, his roles included Pilot Officer in Arnold Wesker's *Chips With Everything* (Howard Davies, Lyttelton, 1997), Kulygin in *Three Sisters* (Mitchell, NT Cottesloe, 2003), the Provost in *Measure for Measure* (Simon McBurney, NT Olivier, 2004), and Alfred in Strindberg's *A Dream Play* (Mitchell, NT Cottesloe, 2005).

His RSC career continued with Clive in Stephen Poliakoff's *Talk of the City* (Poliakoff, Swan, 1998) and Shylock in *The Merchant of Venice* (Tim Carroll, Courtyard, 2008).

Tim Wylton (b. Bangor, Wales, 1940). A fine character actor, Tim Wylton was a mainstay of the RSC in the 1960s and 70s. On graduating from RADA, his early work included the international tour of Franco Zeffirelli's Old Vic *Romeo and Juliet* (1961). His Stratford career began with minor roles, but he quickly progressed to better things, including the part he was to make his own, Bardolph in *Henry IV* and *Henry V*. Wylton played Bardolph during the history cycle of 1966 (John Barton/Trevor Nunn/Clifford Williams, RST), and again in Terry Hands productions of the *Henries* and *The Merry Wives of Windsor* in 1975-76.

Before and after Bardolph: Claudius in *Julius Caesar* (John Blatchley, RST, 1963); Michael in *The Wars of the Roses* (Peter Hall, RST, 1963); Costard in *Love's Labour's Lost* (John Barton, RST, 1965); Friar Jacomo in *The Jew of Malta* (Clifford Williams, RST, 1965); Balthasar in *The Merchant of Venice* (Williams, RST, 1965); Servilius in *Timon of Athens* (John Schlesinger, RST, 1965); Reynaldo in the David Warner *Hamlet* (Hall, RST, 1965); Bobchinsky in *The Government Inspector* (Hall, Aldwych, 1966); Fabian in *Twelfth Night* (Williams, RST, 1966); Hortensio in *The Taming of the Shrew* (Nunn, RST, 1967); William/Le Beau in *As You Like It* (David Jones, RST, 1967); Lory in *The Relapse* (Nunn, Aldwych, 1967); Henry Jadd in Paddy Chayefsky's *The Latent Heterosexual* (Terry Hands, Aldwych, 1968); Sim in *Wild Oats* (Williams, Aldwych, 1976); Charles Bishop in *Privates on Parade* (Michael Blakemore, Aldwych, 1977); Bergetto in *'Tis Pity She's a Whore* (Ron Daniels, TOP, 1977); and Sicinius Velutus in *Coriolanus* (Hands, RST, 1977). He made a long overdue return to the Company in 1998 to play Sir Oliver Surface in *The School for Scandal* (Declan Donnellan, RST).

Wylton is a veteran of television drama, an obvious highlight of his work being David Nobbs's *A Bit of a Do* (ITV, 1989).

Y

Susannah York (b. London, 1941) trained at RADA and appeared briefly in provincial repertory before starting in films, a disarmingly pretty pale blonde, not yet twenty. *There Was a Crooked Man* (Stuart Burge, 1960), *Tunes of Glory* (Ronald Neame, 1960), *The Greengage Summer* (1961) and *Tom Jones* (Tony Richardson, 1963) made her a popular young star. She worked primarily in films for the next decade and a half, not only the vivacious or vulnerable love interest in comedies and thrillers, but also a skilled dramatic actress in darker pieces such as *Freud* (John Huston, 1962), *The Killing of Sister George* (1968), *They Shoot Horses, Don't They?* (1969), perhaps her finest achievement, and Robert Altman's *Images* (1972). *Images* was based on her own story.

Since the mid-1970s she has worked, with increasing regularity, on the stage, not in the manner of a movie star returning to the theatre but with adventurousness: Jean Genet's *The Maids* (Greenwich Theatre, 1974); *Peter Pan* (1977); the title role in *Hedda Gabler* (Donald McWhinnie, Cambridge Theatre, 1982); *The Apple Cart* (Theatre Royal Haymarket, 1986); *The Women* (Old Vic, 1986); Amanda in *The Glass Menagerie* (David Thacker, Young Vic, 1989); Blanche in *A Streetcar Named Desire* (Octagon, Bolton, 1990); her own translation of Jean Cocteau's one-woman play *The Human Voice* (New End Theatre, Hampstead, 1990); Yse in her own translation of Paul Claudel's *Partage de Midi* (Noon Break, French Institute, 1991); Daphne du Maurier's *September Tide* (1993); the country singer in Mark Davies Markham's one-woman show *Independent State* (Robert Chetwyn, The Grace, Battersea, 1995); the survivor of a Japanese camp in John Misto's *The Shoe-Horn Sonata* (Dan Crawford, King's Head Theatre, 1996); Leona, the white trash beautician, in *Small Craft Warnings* (Rufus Norris, Pleasance Theatre, 1999); Jacqueline Roque in Brian McAvera's *Picasso's Women* (Assembly Rooms, Edinburgh Festival, 2000); Esme in *Amy's View* (Robin Lefevre, UK Tour, 2001); her own one-woman show *The Loves of Shakespeare's Women* (Edinburgh Festival, 2001); the narrator in *Peter Pan, a Musical Adventure* (Ian Talbot, Royal Festival Hall, 2002); and the title role in D.M.W. Greer's *Alice Virginia* (Cathrine Meister-Petersen, New End, 2004).

She turned down an offer to join the RSC in the mid-1980s (Titania in *A Midsummer Night's Dream*, directed by Bill Alexander). A decade later she accepted Adrian Noble's invitation. As Mistress Ford in *The Merry Wives of Windsor* (Ian Judge, RST, 1996), Marguerite in Tennessee Williams's *Camino Real* (Steven Pimlott, Swan, 1997) and Gertrude in *Hamlet* (Matthew Warchus, RST, 1997) she gave exemplary performances. Lightness of touch, energy, and warmth in the comedy; elegance under strain in the tragedy; and faded glamour in *Camino Real*. During the rehearsals for *Hamlet* she fell and broke a bone in her heel (Diana Quick opened as Gertrude). In 2003 she performed, with Donald Sinden and Richard Johnson, John Barton's anthology *The Hollow Crown* (Tour).

Coda: the RSC in the 2000s

Adrian Noble's announcement, in May 2001, of a radical change of direction for the RSC secured an initially favourable response. In planning to build a new main house in Stratford, the RSC was, after all, responding to the commonly held view that the RST was a poorly designed auditorium, with too great a distance between the balcony and the stage. In proposing change the RSC was moving forward carefully — the idea of a new Stratford theatre was first mooted in July 1997, and the RSC was perhaps the last major arts organisation to apply for lottery funding. The theatre critics expressed little affection for the Royal Shakespeare Theatre. At the time of the announcement, Michael Billington, who would later become an influential opponent of the innovations, could not have been more encouraging (see *The Guardian*, 9 May 2001).

The theatregoing public were equally optimistic. An opinion poll carried out by a theatre website in July 2001 revealed that 69% of respondents favoured the re-development of the RST, and 51% agreed with the decision to leave the Barbican. Almost a year later, another survey showed a complete reversal. Since it is reasonable to surmise that many people voted on both occasions it is clear that public opinion was transformed during that year. At some point the journalistic agenda changed from an acceptance that the reforms were necessary to a determination to prevent them.

There was a case to be made against the reforms, but the oft-repeated accusation that the RSC was in a state of artistic crisis seemed unjust. During the years 2000-03 the RSC staged, to considerable acclaim, a Shakespeare history cycle, the first to include an unabridged sequence of all eight plays; a season of new plays at The Other Place, including Peter Whelan's elegiac

A Russian in the Woods and Martin McDonagh's controversial *The Lieutenant of Inishmore* (in all, the RSC performed twelve new works during this period); three of Shakespeare's late romances at the Roundhouse (the disappointing ticket sales at the Roundhouse were blamed on poor marketing, but a more likely cause was the bad publicity that coincided with the season); and a sell-out season of Jacobean rarities in the Swan, performed by a crack company of young actors.

However, a short documentary made by BBC 4 called *Trouble at the RSC* (broadcast on 3 September 2002) talked repeatedly of artistic crisis. The director Jude Kelly was just one of the experts who accused the RSC of delivering too many productions and of failing to generate excitement. A look at the number of productions mounted in the immediate years before Adrian Noble took over shows just how prolific the RSC used to be: twenty-seven (1986); twenty-five (1987); twenty-two (1988); and twenty-three (1989). In 2002 Noble programmed only eleven plays. There was a sense that some of Noble's detractors were against change while, paradoxically, criticising the RSC for not changing despite the fact that it had changed. This conundrum revealed just how confused thinking had become.

An important goal of the changes was to meet the requirements of actors, particularly the Company's alumni; but those who chose to speak out argued for the status quo with a self-contradictory innocence that was endearing if not very helpful (during the 2000 Stratford open day the associate actors taking part praised the Swan but dismissed the RST as 'the Odeon next door', and Judi Dench, a very prominent opponent of change, hadn't worked in the Stratford main house since 1979). An equally important tenet was to make the Stratford main house more inclusive; but the plan was savaged by critics who never watched shows from the balcony. One conclusion to be drawn from all these ironies and inconsistencies is that a positive response to radical change is unlikely until after the retirement of the current generation of senior actors and critics.

So what was the real case to be made against the innovations? One, the RSC tried to do too much too quickly. There was never any question that the RSC would leave the Barbican at the end of the lease in 2005, but it should surely have kept its London home until an alternative had been found. Two, in selling the Stratford re-development (most of the finance was being chased in America) a false impression was given about its nature and aims—the press started to talk about a Shakespeare theme park. The RSC failed to counter this accusation of 'dumbing down'. As a result, a long held plan to create a great new main house at Stratford (dating at least from the time of Peter Hall), a new flexible TOP and a base for a training academy was never seriously debated in the public forum of the press. Creating an education facility and giving interested people a means of learning about the backstage craft of theatre (educational and other events go on all the time) does not amount to a theme park. Three, the staffing issues were mismanaged. An insensitive approach to the impact of the reforms on individual employees created a division between those managers in favour of the changes and everyone else. Four, the abandonment of a long Stratford repertory season could, over time, threaten the very uniqueness and importance of the RSC.

Michael Boyd, Adrian Noble's successor, shelved the new RST, Other Place and the RSC Academy. His prudent approach represented either a loss of nerve or the rediscovery of good sense, depending on one's view. Prudence became the order of the day, with Boyd programming only the most popular plays in the main house and forming partnerships with the commercial sector to transfer them into the West End (a deal with Cameron Mackintosh, beginning in 2005/06 at the Novello Theatre, will tie the RSC to the commercial sector for five risk-free years). When Boyd and his team finally released details of the re-development of the RST, it became clear that they wanted a second, if bigger, Swan Theatre. The scheme, entrusted to Bennetts

Associates, follows the current fashion for Jacobean-style theatres.

As I write, builders are constructing the new theatre. Up the road, the RST's temporary replacement, the Courtyard Theatre, has been running for more than a year. One has to admire the RSC's handling of the transitional period. The Courtyard was built in time for the Complete Works Festival (2006). It allows the RSC to continue to deliver a full programme during the closure and acts as a testing ground for the new RST. If Michael Boyd meant it when he said the Courtyard was a prototype, I wonder whether the design of the new theatre has been revised in light of the experiences of the last year. For in my view the Courtyard has revealed that large indoor Jacobean-style theatres don't work.

Small galleried playhouses like the Swan encourage an intimate, conversational style of acting. But a main house theatre demands something more—images, atmosphere, and stagecraft. The playing area should be transformable. Courtyard-style theatres with their redundant high spaces and ranks of distracting spectators in every direction are clearly limiting in this respect. How many more times can Michael Boyd bring the actors down from above on ropes and trapezes? Perhaps most worrying of all, directors know that if they use any part of the stage other than a narrow section about a third of the way down from the rear wall, a large percentage of the audience will be watching the backs of the actors' heads.

It's true that proscenium theatres like the old RST are unforgiving to all but the most talented directors and actors, and I wonder whether the RSC's artistic director isn't simply admitting defeat. I'm not aware of any major theatre in France or Germany bringing down the curtain on the proscenium, but in the era of New Labour our theatre culture is always looking for the new trend, the new buzz word and the easiest option. During the last public event in the RST, Trevor Nunn, Terry Hands and Adrian Noble spoke eloquently of the theatre's importance, with Nunn explaining how Peter Hall and John Bury's decision to extend a raked stage through and beyond the proscenium created a unique RSC style. Michael Boyd, for his part, was unapologetic, dismissing the doubters by suggesting that if they want to sit in the dark they should go to the cinema. Well, it's true, there is a world elsewhere... and the current development looks too much like a compromise to be regarded by future generations as the end of the story.

Michael Boyd has continued to split the Stratford year between summer and winter seasons and to divide the Company by theatre or project. He has spoken constantly about the importance of the ensemble, by which he means ensembles, self-contained groups of actors working on their own productions, and not, unfortunately, a single troupe performing, in repertory across all three spaces, an entire season's work. The 2008 season at the Courtyard was shared by two ensembles. One group performed *The Merchant of Venice* and *The Taming of the Shrew*; the other *Hamlet* and *Love's Labour's Lost*. Since nearly all of the well-known actors were in the latter company, directed by Gregory Doran, there was a very definite sense of a first and second eleven. This kind of fragmentation is not only unnecessary; it runs counter to the sense of collective endeavour that must underpin a theatre troupe, if only as an aspiration.

Many of the changes of the last six years were ill-considered. The shorter contracts and less demanding schedules of work did not strengthen the Company; in fact, ironically, they had the opposite affect. If too many of the best actors were no longer choosing to join the RSC, it was because the Company had lost its distinctiveness and influence. The re-structuring made the RSC seem like any other theatre, and so compounded the problem. It is not too late to return to the ideas of Peter Hall, Peter Brook, Trevor Nunn and Terry Hands. The Comédie-Française is still governed by its founding principles after more than four centuries. While not wishing the RSC to be so rigidly doctrinal, the point is well made: some cultural institutions are important enough to operate above fashion and shifting circumstances.

Printed in the United Kingdom by
Lightning Source UK Ltd., Milton Keynes
137780UK00001B/173/P